Autism Spectrum Disorders: Assessment and Treatment

Autism Spectrum Disorders: Assessment and Treatment

Edited by Harold Herrera

hayle medical
New York

Hayle Medical,
750 Third Avenue, 9th Floor,
New York, NY 10017, USA

Visit us on the World Wide Web at:
www.haylemedical.com

ISBN: 978-1-63241-737-4

The publisher's policy is to use permanent paper from mills that operate a sustainable forestry policy. Furthermore, the publisher ensures that the text paper and cover boards used have met acceptable environmental accreditation standards.

Printed in China.

Cataloging-in-Publication Data

Autism spectrum disorders : assessment and treatment / edited by Harold Herrera.
p. cm.
Includes bibliographical references and index.
ISBN 978-1-63241-737-4
1. Autism spectrum disorders. 2. Autism spectrum disorders--Diagnosis.
3. Autism spectrum disorders--Treatment. 4. Autism. I. Herrera, Harold.
RC553.A88 A88 2019
616.858 82--dc23

Table of Contents

Preface

The main aim of this book is to educate learners and enhance their research focus by presenting diverse topics covering this vast field. This is an advanced book which compiles significant studies by distinguished experts in the area of analysis. This book addresses successive solutions to the challenges arising in the area of application, along with it; the book provides scope for future developments.

All neurodevelopmental disorders which include autism and related conditions fall under the category of autism spectrum disorder. Problems in social interaction and repetitive patterns of behavior are the two main symptoms of autism spectrum disorder. There is no specific cause associated with these disorders, but risk factors include neuroanatomical abnormalities, genetic conditions like fragile X syndrome, prenatal and perinatal risk factors like maternal gestational diabetes and a family history of similar condition. The assessment of behavior is the primary way to diagnose autism spectrum disorders. Autism Diagnostic Interview-Revised (ADI-R), Childhood Autism Rating Scale (CARS), and Autism Diagnostic Observation Schedule (ADOS) are some of the commonly used diagnostic measurements. Medications include atypical antipsychotic drugs and anticonvulsants. Some alternative therapies and interventions, including CEASE therapy and vaccine detoxing are also used to treat autism spectrum disorders. This book unravels the recent studies in the field of autism spectrum disorders. Some of the diverse topics covered herein address the varied aspects of assessment and treatment of such disorders. This book is a complete source of knowledge on the present status of these disorders.

It was a great honour to edit this book, though there were challenges, as it involved a lot of communication and networking between me and the editorial team. However, the end result was this all-inclusive book covering diverse themes in the field.

Finally, it is important to acknowledge the efforts of the contributors for their excellent chapters, through which a wide variety of issues have been addressed. I would also like to thank my colleagues for their valuable feedback during the making of this book.

Editor

1

Theory of Mind Deficit versus Faulty Procedural Memory in Autism Spectrum Disorders

Miguel Ángel Romero-Munguía

Outpatient Service, "Dr. Samuel Ramírez Moreno" Psychiatric Hospital, Health Secretariat, Autopista México-Puebla Km 5.5 Santa Catarina, Tláhuac, 13100 Mexico, DF, Mexico

Correspondence should be addressed to Miguel Ángel Romero-Munguía; romero_munguia@hotmail.com

Academic Editor: Manuel F. Casanova

Individuals with autism spectrum disorders (ASD) have impairments in social interaction, communicative capacity, and behavioral flexibility (core triad). Three major cognitive theories (theory of mind deficit, weak central coherence, and executive dysfunction) seem to explain many of these impairments. Currently, however, the empathizing-systemizing (a newer version of the theory of mind deficit account) and mnesic imbalance theories are the only ones that attempt to explain all these core triadic symptoms of ASD On the other hand, theory of mind deficit in empathizing-systemizing theory is the most influential account for ASD, but its counterpart in the mnesic imbalance theory, faulty procedural memory, seems to occur earlier in development; consequently, this might be a better solution to the problem of the etiology of ASD, if it truly meets the precedence criterion. Hence, in the present paper I review the reasoning in favor of the theory of mind deficit but with a new interpretation based on the mnesic imbalance theory, which posits that faulty procedural memory causes deficits in several cognitive skills, resulting in poor performance in theory of mind tasks.

1. Introduction

Autistic disorder is characterized by impairments in reciprocal social interaction, communicative capacity, and repetitive patterns of behavior (core triad) [1]. The term autism spectrum disorders (ASD), which has been used by some mental health professionals as a synonym of pervasive developmental disorder (PDD) [2], implies that these impairments are shared among autistic disorder, Asperger's syndrome, and pervasive developmental disorder not otherwise specified (PDD-NOS) [3]. However, considering that the diagnosis of PDD-NOS does not require the presence of the three diagnostic domains of the autistic triad (social interaction, communicative capacity and behavioral flexibility), the inclusion of PDD-NOS as an ASD has been questioned [4]. This observation is important because it is hard, if not impossible, to make a cognitive theory on disorders that do not share clinical and etiological features [5]. Consequently, I use the term ASD throughout this work to refer to the group comprised only by autistic disorder and Asperger's syndrome, whereas both disorders are mentioned separately when they are not forming a group in some mentioned study in this text.

On the other hand, when Kanner provided the first clinical description of autistic disorder, he also wrote "Their excellent rote memory... It is difficult to know for certain whether the stuffing as such has contributed essentially to the course of the psychopathologic condition" [6]; thus, a cognitive hypothesis was the first one proposed to explain the etiology of autistic disorder. Moreover, a second cognitive hypothesis was established early by Asperger, who surmised that autistic intelligence was an extreme variant of male intelligence. He based his hypothesis on the belief that men were innately more capable of abstract thought than women, whereas women were innately more focused on emotions than men [7]. Nevertheless, neither Kanner's nor Asperger's theory had any influence on the initial development of the three major cognitive theories that have guided research in ASD: theory of mind deficit, weak central coherence, and executive dysfunction [8–10]. Surprisingly, two more recent theories (empathizing-systemizing and mnesic imbalance) make reference to those old hypotheses [11, 12].

The theory of mind deficit account has attempted to explain impairments in social interaction and communicative capacity; the weak central coherence theory seems to explain remarkable abilities of some autistic individuals, and the executive dysfunction theory has been proposed to explain impairments in their behavioral flexibility [13, 14]. In contrast, two theories have attempted to account for the whole autistic triad. Thus, the empathizing-systemizing theory proposes that ASD may be explained by hyperdeveloped systemizing with hypodeveloped empathizing, defining systemizing as drive to analyze or construct systems while empathizing has been defined as drive to infer mental states (theory of mind) and to have an appropriate emotional reaction to them [11, 15]. On the other hand, the mnesic imbalance theory posits that ASD may be explained by faulty procedural memory with relatively preserved declarative memory: defining procedural memory as behavioral algorithms that operate at the unconscious level, while declarative memory is defined as information that is subject to verbal reflection [12, 16].

In the present review article only faulty procedural memory and theory of mind deficit are discussed, whereas relatively preserved declarative memory and hyperdeveloped systemizing will be reviewed next in another work.

2. Tests of False Belief

2.1. First Study in Autistic Disorder. As mentioned above, the ability to recognize mental states (thoughts and emotions) is one of the two major elements of empathizing. This ability is called theory of mind (mentalizing or mind-reading) [8, 11, 15]; its deficit in autistic disorder was initially tested using the unexpected transfer test of false belief, in which children watch a story about two dolls: one of them (Sally) has a marble, which she puts in a basket and leaves the scene; when she is away, the marble is transferred by the other doll (Anne) from the basket to a box. Then, the experimenter asks the children to infer where Sally will look for the marble. The children pass the test if they point to the basket by taking into account the knowledge (false belief) from Sally. That study found that 85% of typically developing control children passed this test, whereas 80% of children with autistic disorder failed. Thus, its authors surmised that theory of mind deficit is independent from intellectual ability, since the children with autistic disorder had a mean verbal mental age (VMA) as measured by the British Picture Vocabulary Test (BPVT), of 5 years 5 months, while the typically developing control children had a mean chronological age (CA) of 4 years 5 months [8].

2.2. Language as an Index of Mental Age. If only vocabulary tests were considered as index of the overall linguistic ability of individuals with ASD in some studies on tests of false belief, such ability could be overestimated, since the picture vocabulary tests adequately estimate verbal mental age in typically developing persons but not in people with ASD because the performance in vocabulary tests is a peak of ability in these individuals [17]. Moreover, some studies have observed impaired grammatical abilities in comparison to the level of lexical abilities in ASD [18, 19]; a study reported lack of significant correlation between grammar and vocabulary in ASD [20]; another study showed slower reaction times to grammatical errors than to lexical errors [21]. These findings are noteworthy because a stronger association has been reported between grammar and test of false belief in children with ASD and mean VMA by the British Picture Vocabulary Scale 2nd edition (BPVS-II) of 7.28 years than in those in control group of children with moderate learning difficulties (MLD) and VMA of 7.58 years by BPVS-II, who in addition had a significantly better performance in tests of theory of mind [22]; also other deficits in communicative function such as pragmatics, reception of gestural language and verbal commands, prosody and discourse comprehension have been found in people with ASD matched for receptive vocabulary with controls, but it is not easy to know whether such deficits are the cause or consequence of theory of mind deficit (mindblindness) or if both traits are caused by a third variable [23–26].

2.2.1. Vocabulary: Lexical Mental Age. Furthermore, the declarative/procedural model assumes that grammar is stored in procedural memory, whereas vocabulary is stored in declarative memory [27]. So, the mnesic imbalance theory may explain grammatical abnormalities in ASD, as well as why some individuals with autistic disorder can repeat many words, phrases, and sentences from their memory, without being able to create expressions appropriate to the context (echolalia) [25, 28], since declarative memory involves consciously recollected information, whereas procedural memory involves unconscious behavioral algorithms [12, 16]. Other deficits in communicative functions (e.g., prosody) in people with ASD also might be due to the lack of simultaneous application of procedural knowledge (simultaneousness) and not just by faulty procedural memory [24, 25], while the relationship between mnesic imbalance and other features of the language (e.g., neologisms) of individuals with ASD has been recently pointed out [29]. So, if there are difficulties in language from individuals with ASD despite their relatively preserved vocabulary, then the poor performance in some theory of mind tasks might be due to those difficulties of language. For this reason, the term "lexical mental age" (LMA) will be used, following other authors [24, 26], throughout this paper instead of VMA when some vocabulary test has been used as an index of mental age.

However, a greater amount of empirical studies is required in individuals with ASD that compare aspects of language that are based on declarative versus procedural memory in order to have conclusive evidence for the mnesic imbalance theory.

2.3. Typical Development versus Development in ASD. It should be noted that the majority of typically developing 3-year-old children gives incorrect responses in tests of false belief, such as the unexpected content test of false belief, in which they are shown a tube of Smarties (or M&Ms) and the experimenter asks them what it contains. After they give their answer (candy), they are shown that the tube only contains a pencil. Then, subjects are asked to infer what another child, who has not seen the tube, will think it contains. They pass the test if they respond candy (the false belief). Thus, it has been assumed that 3 year olds have an inability to assign conflicting truth values to propositions despite having the ability to make theory of mind [30]. In contrast, this same deficit in subjects with autistic disorder (CA 13.6; LMA: 6.2) has been interpreted as profound difficulty in making theory of mind [31]. The latter assumption is debatable, since many individuals with autistic disorder who fail in unexpected transfer test of false belief pass nonstandard false belief tasks such as the explicit false belief task in which, for instance, they watch a story about a protagonist (Mary) who wants to find her kitten. It is explicitly mentioned that the pet is in the bedroom and that she thinks her kitten is in the kitchen. Then, they should answer the question: where will Mary look for her kitten [32]? Furthermore, both typically developing 3 year olds and children with autistic disorder significantly improve on tests of false belief when they use thought bubbles to represent mental states [33, 34]. These findings suggest that the difficulty with tests of false belief might be secondary to a poor ability to make inferences. Indeed, a study found that children and adolescents with autistic disorder were impaired relative to LMA-matched controls (7.9 versus 7.46 years) at physical-state counterfactual conditional reasoning, which requires answering questions such as "If there had been no fire, where would Peter be?" but do not understand mental states; the authors of that study suggested that difficulty with standard false belief tasks in autistic disorder might be due to deficits in counterfactual conditional and inferential reasoning, rather than by inadequate theory of mind [32]. On the other hand, it has been reported that the ability to extract the content of a proposition embedded in another proposition (knowledge of complement syntax) significantly predicts the performance on standard false belief tasks [26]. This relationship has been tested in a study in children with ASD utilizing a complement syntax task in which the participants hear stories such as "She said there was a spider in her cereal, but it was really a raisin"; then they respond to the question "What did she say?" The results showed a significantly stronger correlation between complement syntax scores and unexpected transfer (Sally-Anne) test of false belief performance in the ASD group (LMA: 6.87 years) compared with the control group (LMA: 6.37 years), but neither the ASD group (LMA: 6.34 years) nor the control group (LMA: 6.20 years) showed a significant correlation between the unexpected content (Smarties) test of false belief and the complement syntax [35]. In addition, another study mentioned above showed that children with MLD performed significantly better on the Smarties test than on the Sally-Anne test. More specifically, 61% of those children with MLD and inconsistent performance between both tests of false belief failed only the Sally-Anne test whilst passing Smarties test, whereas only 19% of those children with ASD who performed inconsistently the tests showed the same pattern of performance [22]. These different patterns of results deserve to be explained to justify the utilization of both tests in any study. A possible explanation for these results might be found in the way that performance on standard false belief tasks can be improved in typically developing children. For instance, most 3 year olds give correct answers in the unexpected content test of false belief when using a "syntactic method". That is, the experimenter asks them the same question (what will [name of the other child] think is in the tube?) but with a clause tagged at the end that makes it temporally more specific: What will [name of the other child] think is in the tube before I [experimenter] take the top off [36]? On the other hand, to my knowledge, there is no syntactic method to improve unexpected transfer test of false belief performance, although there is a nonsyntactic method to do that (thought bubbles) [33, 34]. So, any unconscious algorithm (procedural knowledge) similar to the syntactic method might normally be used to resolve unexpected content test of false belief, whereas another unconscious algorithm (procedural knowledge) similar to the thought bubbles would normally be used during unexpected transfer test of false belief, which might explain why the passers and failures in the ASD group obtained equal complement syntax scores than those in the control group to solve unexpected content test of false belief; in contrast, the largest difference in complement syntax scores has been observed between passers and failures, only among the ASD group, to solve unexpected transfer test of false belief [35]. Indeed, this same difference has been observed with the Test for Reception of Grammar (TROG) scores [22]. This greater variation in complement syntax and reception of grammar suggests that these language skills have little true impact on tests of false belief performance; hence, the significant correlation between these language skills and performance in tests of false belief might be an artifact since the ASD groups showed a significantly worse performance relative to comparison groups on tests of false belief, despite the fact that mean performance on complement syntax and reception of grammar were similar in both types of groups, but with a greater variation of these two variables [22, 35].

Finally, counterfactual conditional and inferential reasoning might be considered as a single type of reasoning, called analogical inference, which is linked to procedural memory because it may be done without awareness of the processes that one performs; moreover, the unconscious algorithms that are perhaps normally involved in the solution of tests of false belief might also be analogical inference; consequently, it would be interesting to conduct correlation studies between analogical inference tasks and tests of false belief in people with ASD [37–40].

3. Executive Dysfunction

Notwithstanding, overall language skills appear to be associated with overall performance in false belief tasks, as was demonstrated in one of the first studies on executive dysfunction in ASD, in which the Verbal Intellectual Quotient (VIQ) was derived from performance in only three subtests (information, similarities, and vocabulary) of intelligence scales developed by Wechsler. Individuals with ASD were divided into two groups: ASD individuals with or without current autistic language abnormalities, with CA of 11.79 versus 12.38 years. The former group achieved lower VIQ (mean = 75.69) scores than the latter (mean = 92.30). In addition, participants were asked to solve first- (including unexpected content test of false belief) and second-order theory of mind theory tasks [41]. The latter test involves the ability to infer the person's beliefs about another person's beliefs; one example is the story about two children (John and Mary) who see an ice-cream man in the park. John wants ice-cream but does not have money, and the ice-cream man tells John that he will stay the rest of the afternoon in the park, but after John goes home to get money the ice-cream man decides to go and sell ice-cream in the school. Mary knows this entire situation, but after the ice-cream man passes John's house and tells John that he will stay in the school to sell ice-cream. Mary did not know that they had met, because she at that time was still in the park. Then she looks for John in his house and his mother tells her that John has gone to buy an ice-cream. The participants are asked to infer where Mary thinks that John has gone to buy the ice-cream. They pass the test if they respond "the park" (the false belief) and correctly explain why Mary thinks that [42]. On the other hand, in the above mentioned study on executive dysfunction, significant deficits on first- and second-order theory of mind tasks were found only within the ASD group with the lowest VIQ, in comparison to the control group matched for VIQ, whereas the ASD group with the highest VIQ did not show these deficits. However, both groups with ASD had significantly more deficits in executive function tests (Tower of Hanoi; Wisconsin Card Sorting Test) than did control groups. Therefore, the authors concluded that neither executive dysfunction nor theory of mind deficit causes the other, but both might have a common causal factor [10, 41]. Indeed, I have argued that the alterations described by the three major cognitive theories may be caused by imbalance between a faulty procedural memory and a relatively preserved declarative memory [12]. For instance, as previously mentioned, the Tower of Hanoi and the Wisconsin Card Sorting Test have been used to evaluate executive function, but these tests have also been linked to procedural learning [43, 44].

4. Theory of Mind Tasks beyond False Belief

Since several individuals with ASD pass tests of false belief, including the second-order false belief task, the majority of adults with Asperger's syndrome (people with ASD and average or above average Intellectual Quotient (IQ), as well as no history of language delay) passes this latter task; researchers have developed more difficult tests such as the strange stories test, the test of faux pas detection, the eyes task, and the Cambridge mindreading face-voice battery in order to show theory of mind deficit in all subjects with ASD [13, 14, 28].

4.1. Strange Stories Test. In a study utilizing the strange stories test, which consists of stories where the characters say utterances that are not literally true for various justifications, the participants responded to the questions "Was it true, what X said? Why did X say that?" Justifications given by participants to the "Why" question were scored as either correct or incorrect. Then, correct mental justifications were taken as evidence of theory of mind. The results showed that the ASD group that passed second order false belief tasks (CA 17.7 years; VIQ 95.8) had significantly lower correct mental justifications than control groups. For instance, in a sarcasm story, the mother of Ann cooks the favorite food of Ann, but when the mother brings it to Ann, she is watching TV and does not say thank you. Then the mother of Ann says "That's what I call politeness!" An individual with ASD explained this utterance with the justification that she said it to avoid disturbing her daughter. On the other hand, it is interesting to note the significantly lower number of incorrect mental state justifications on the contrary emotion story from an ASD group (who passed, at least, first-order false belief tasks: CA 20.6 years; VIQ 87.3) relative to children with typical development (CA 8.6 years), while the opposite pattern occurred for most of the other strange stories [45]. A possible explanation is that strange stories as sarcasm and white lie might require the activation of chains of emotional behaviors similar to the chains of motor acts (mirror neurons), but other stories such as the contrary emotion do not. Indeed, it has been observed that in typically developing children, the muscles of the mouth are activated as soon as they move their arm to reach food, as well as during the observation of this same action performed by another individual, whereas, in children with ASD, none of these activations are observed [46]. Therefore, it has been suggested that children with ASD cannot understand the intentions of others because these mirror neurons are not activated [47, 48]. However, when one hears strange stories on persuasion or sarcasm, chains of emotional behaviors (beyond the mirror neurons: chains of motor acts) might be activated to understand the emotions of the protagonists, whereas the strange stories on contrary emotion or lie do not require such activations because the emotions are explicitly mentioned in them [49]. In previous paper I argued that the mirror neurons might be part of the procedural memory since they operate at the unconscious level [12]; such reasoning might be applied to chains of emotional behaviors.

Nevertheless, a study of adults with high functioning autism (HFA), that is, autistic disorder with average or above average IQ, and a history of language delay (CA 30.71 years; VIQ 107.59), as well as adults with Asperger's syndrome (CA 27.77 years; VIQ 110.82), reported the highest number of errors on the stories of double bluff rather than on the other types of stories; it was surmised that the reason for this is that the double bluff story is a third-order theory of mind task [50]. However, the ability to understand double bluff stories does not seem to be associated with the level of performance on theory of mind tasks, since individuals who failed to pass all of the false belief tests obtained the same number of correct mental justifications on the double bluff story than those who passed first order false belief tests [45]. Also it was suggested that the metarepresentation "he *knows* they *think* he will *lie*" indicates second order false belief in double bluff story, but this is similar to metarepresentation "she *knows* they will be *sad* if she does not *want*" in white lie story. However, the latter was easier to understand for group with ASD than the former [45, 50]. This result is in agreement with a study that showed that the ability to respond to new situations (such as the double bluff story) appears to be diminished in individuals with ASD when they have been exposed to the local context (such as false belief tests) [51]; that is, the individuals with ASD had learnt in tests of false belief that the protagonists cannot know a location if they have not seen or heard that [8, 42], which might be a restrictive procedural knowledge that makes difficult to understand double bluff stories, whereas in pretend and figure of speech stories do not [45, 49, 50]. So, correlation studies are necessary among tests of false belief, each item of the strange stories test, and analogical inference tasks to verify these hypotheses.

4.2. Test of Faux Pas Detection. Another test of theory of mind is the test of faux pas detection, which evaluates the ability of individuals to recognize when a speaker says something that the listener might not want to know. The results of a study demonstrated that children with ASD (CA 144.0 months; LMA 159.0 months) perform poorly on this test; in addition, although some of them could recognize the faux pas, still they could not inhibit them [52]. This latter finding could be due to any failure in chains of emotional behaviors.

In sum, strange stories test and test of faux pas detection show hypothetical scenarios to individuals who should infer the appropriate mental states. However, another measurable variable in this type of tests may be the reaction time, which significantly decreased with age between adolescence and adulthood in typically developing people [53, 54]. Moreover, the reduction of reaction time during repeated sequences utilizing tests such as the Serial Response Time Task (SRTT) is an index of procedural learning; the SRTT has indicated significant impairments in procedural learning from people with ASD [16, 55]. Thus, studies comparing reaction times between theory of mind and procedural learning tasks would be useful to test the mnesic imbalance theory.

4.3. Eyes Task. The eyes task (reading the mind in the eyes task) consists of showing the participants photographs of the eye region, through which they should infer the mental state of people just from the information in those photographs. A study demonstrated that adults with ASD (CA 28.6 years; IQ 105.31) are impaired in their ability to infer mental states from photographs of persons' eyes compared with two control groups, one of adults with Tourette's syndrome (CA 27.77 years; IQ 103.5) and another group of typically developing adults (CA 30.0 years) [56]. The deficits already mentioned, such as lack of simultaneousness, analogical inference, or chains of emotional behaviors, do not appear to be appropriate to explain the results from the eyes task, but procedural learning has been linked to another skill; this is, so-called perceptual categorization, which can be achieved through two types of category-learning tasks: rulebased and information-integration. In rulebased tasks, the categories can be acquired through declarative learning, whereas in information-integration tasks, the categories can be acquired via procedural learning [57]. Afterward, if participants can assign every photograph of the eye region to any category of mental state, then the ability to solve this task must have been acquired through procedural learning, since it is difficult (if not impossible) to verbally explain (i.e., by declarative memory) what characteristics of each photograph can justify its assignment to certain category of mental state; consequently, impaired performance in the eyes task in the group with ASD might be the result of lack of unconscious algorithms [12]. So, even some typically developing adults performed the eyes task worse than some individuals with ASD [56]. Then, a revised version of the eyes test was developed which increased the number of photographs from 25 to 36, as well as from two to four answer choices for each photograph: thereby, these changes improved the reliability of the test [58]. Still, the original version of the eyes test showed theory of mid deficit, whereas a basic emotion recognition task did not [56]. This result could be because the basic emotions can be easily explained by declarative knowledge; for example, the emoticons of happiness {:-)}, sadness {:-(}, and surprise {:-O} only require a simple change in the shape of the mouth, whereas the photographs of the eye region on complex emotion such as worry, insistence, or uneasy cannot be distinguished from each other by any explicit feature. Thus, the mnesic imbalance theory also might explain the results of other studies, for instance, one measured the visual fixation time in adolescents and young adults with autistic disorder (CA 15.4 years; VIQ 101.3) on eye, mouth, body, and object regions when they watched movies, finding a significant positive correlation between the percentage of fixation time on the mouth region and level of social competence in this group, whereas the fixation time on the eye region did not correlate with their social skills. In addition, the study showed that they focused twice as much on the mouth region and two times less on the eye region, in comparison with the control group (CA 17.9 years; VIQ 102.5) [59].

These data are in agreement with another study which reported that children with autistic disorder (CA 83.7 months; IQ 82.2) who were asked to identify four basic emotions on photographs of faces had a performance above chance when they viewed the lower face, whereas their performance was within chance levels when they viewed the upper face alone. In addition, the author of that study proposed the hypothesis that an automatic system (procedural) orients us to the upper face to understand the emotional states of others, whereas an intentional system (declarative) is linked to the lower face [60].

4.4. Cambridge Mindreading Face-Voice. The Cambridge mindreading face-voice is a battery that uses several emotion concepts via video and audio in order for the participants to show their ability to recognize complex emotions in the face and in the voice. In a study utilizing this battery, the results demonstrated that a group of adults with Asperger's syndrome (CA 30.2 years; VIQ 114.4) was significantly impaired relative to control adults (CA 27.1 years; VIQ 118.47) [61]. According to the mnesic imbalance theory, this result might be explained by lower development of perceptual categorization and chains of emotional behaviors [12].

In several studies have been observed significant differences in brain activity in theory of mind tasks between adolescence and adulthood; for instance, typically developing adolescents (aged 9–17 years) showed activation of the anterior cingulate cortex during viewing of fearful faces relative to neutral faces, whereas typically developing adults (age 25–36 years) did not [62]. Similarly, a study showed higher activity in anterior cingulate cortex of men with HFA (ages 20–33 years) in comparison with the control group [63]. In addition, using the antisaccade task (a test of inhibition) in individuals with typical development (ages 12 to 23 years) showed that inhibition (as index of executive function) has the most important correlation with affective theory of mind (emotion inferences) than updating and shifting (others two executive functions) [64]. These data are in accordance with my hypothesis of higher activity in anterior cingulate cortex by overload for declarative memory in people with HFA [16], while such overload can cause very significant inhibitory errors [65].

Several tests using film scenes, such as the awkward moments test [66], the movie for assessment of social cognition [67], and the "reading the mind in film" task [68, 69], have been developed in order to assess theory of mind skills of children and adults with ASD during tasks more similar to genuine social settings than in previous tests. As expected, in all experiments, the ASD groups scored significantly lower on these film tasks, compared to control groups.

During another experiment, a group with ASD (CA 30.29; VIQ 116.29) and a control group (CA 30.21; VIQ 116.93) watched film clips of a test named the Moral Dilemmas Film Task and were asked to write about what happened in each clip. Then, the narratives given by participants were scored for total number of references to objects and mental states, as well as of protagonists to whom mental states were attributed. The results showed that the ASD group had a slightly lower number of references to objects and a significantly lower number of references to mental states relative to the control group. However, there was no statistically significant difference between the two groups in the number of individuals who spontaneously applied second order theory of mind to at least one protagonist ($P = 0.085$); besides, only the ASD group had a significant correlation between the number of references to mental states and the VIQ but not the Empathy Quotient (EQ), a questionnaire used to assess empathizing (theory of mind; appropriate emotional reaction) [70]. These data suggest that the ASD group generated complex inferences of mental states despite not believing that they had good theory of mind on others.

This discrepancy between ability and intention to make theory of mind might be explained by an interesting model which suggests that theory of mind can be divided into affective (emotion inferences) and cognitive theory of mind (belief inferences); the latter has to integrate with empathy (the drive to establish theory of mind) and emotional contagion for making affective theory of mind [71]. In particular, the empathy might be the drive to infer mental states in the Moral Dilemmas Film Task, which does not require participants to correctly make theory of mind on film characters [70]. Furthermore, the affective theory of mind may be based on perceptual categorization and chains of emotional behaviors, while cognitive theory of mind may be based on analogical inference. Also in the mnesic imbalance theory, the empathy might be the drive to show procedural knowledge; the simultaneousness would facilitate a better demonstration of the procedural knowledge.

5. Conclusions

This paper argues that a faulty procedural memory causes deficits in several cognitive skills such as simultaneousness, analogical inference, chains of emotional behaviors, and perceptual categorization and that all these deficits may explain the theory of mind deficit measured by the tests of false belief (analogical inference), the strange stories test and the test of faux pas detection (analogical inference; chains of emotional behaviors), the eyes task, and the Cambridge mindreading face-voice (perceptual categorization). In other words, although several studies are necessary in order to verify the hypotheses on the faulty procedural memory, they seem to explain impairments in social interaction from people with ASD, but these cannot explain the other features of individuals with ASD: insistence on sameness, idiosyncratic behaviors, fixated interests, abnormal reactions to sensory stimuli, and special isolated skills. Consequently, the mnesic imbalance theory requires a second factor named "relatively preserved declarative memory" [12], which will be discussed next in another review article, although I have already published preliminary works on that topic [29, 72].

Acknowledgment

The author would like to thank Edith Monroy for reviewing the language of the paper.

References

[1] American Psychiatric Association, *Diagnostic and Statistical Manual of Mental Disorders*, American Psychiatric Publishing, Washington, DC, USA, 4th edition, 2000.

[2] M. Tateno, S. Kikuchi, K. Uehara et al., "Pervasive developmental disorders and autism spectrum disorders: are these disorders one and the same?" *Psychiatry Investigation*, vol. 8, no. 1, pp. 67–70, 2011.

[3] L. Gabis, H. Wei, A. Azizian et al., "1H-magnetic resonance spectroscopy markers of cognitive and language ability in clinical subtypes of autism spectrum disorders," *Journal of Child Neurology*, vol. 23, no. 7, pp. 766–774, 2008.

[4] M. T. Mercadante, R. J. van der Gaag, and J. S. Schwartzman, "Non-autistic pervasive developmental disorders: rett's syndrome, childhood disintegrative disorder and pervasive developmental disorder not otherwise specified," *Revista Brasileira de Psiquiatria*, vol. 28, supplement 1, pp. S12–S20, 2006.

[5] L. Waterhouse, "Autism overflows: increasing prevalence and proliferating theories," *Neuropsychology Review*, vol. 18, no. 4, pp. 273–286, 2008.

[6] L. Kanner, "Autistic disturbances of affective contact," *The Nervous Child*, vol. 2, pp. 217–250, 1943.

[7] H. Asperger, "Die "autistischen psychopathen" im kindesalter," *Archiv für Psychiatrie und Nervenkrankheiten*, vol. 117, no. 1, pp. 76–136, 1944.

[8] S. Baron-Cohen, A. M. Leslie, and U. Frith, "Does the autistic child have a 'theory of mind'?" *Cognition*, vol. 21, no. 1, pp. 37–46, 1985.

[9] U. Frith, *Autism: Explaining the Enigma*, Blackwell, Malden, Mass, USA, 1989.

[10] S. Ozonoff, B. F. Pennington, and S. J. Rogers, "Executive function deficits in high-functioning autistic individuals: relationship to theory of mind," *Journal of Child Psychology and Psychiatry and Allied Disciplines*, vol. 32, no. 7, pp. 1081–1105, 1991.

[11] S. Baron-Cohen, "The extreme male brain theory of autism," *Trends in Cognitive Sciences*, vol. 6, no. 6, pp. 248–254, 2002.

[12] M. Á. Romero-Munguía, "Mnesic imbalance: a cognitive theory about autism spectrum disorders," *Annals of General Psychiatry*, vol. 7, no. 1, article 20, 2008.

[13] E. Pisula, "The autistic mind in the light of neuropsychological studies," *Acta Neurobiologiae Experimentalis*, vol. 70, no. 2, pp. 119–130, 2010.

[14] G. Rajendran and P. Mitchell, "Cognitive theories of autism," *Developmental Review*, vol. 27, no. 2, pp. 224–260, 2007.

[15] S. Baron-Cohen, "Autism: the empathizing-systemizing (E-S) theory," *Annals of the New York Academy of Sciences*, vol. 1156, pp. 68–80, 2009.

[16] M. A. Romero-Munguía, "Mnesic imbalance and the neuroanatomy of autism spectrum disorders," in *Autism—A Neurodevelopmental Journey from Genes to Behaviour*, V. Eapen, Ed., pp. 425–444, InTech, Rijeka, Croatia, 2011.

[17] L. Mottron, "Matching strategies in cognitive research with individuals with high-functioning autism: current practices, instrument biases, and recommendations," *Journal of Autism and Developmental Disorders*, vol. 34, no. 1, pp. 19–27, 2004.

[18] I. M. Eigsti, L. Bennetto, and M. B. Dadlani, "Beyond pragmatics: morphosyntactic development in autism," *Journal of Autism and Developmental Disorders*, vol. 37, no. 6, pp. 1007–1023, 2007.

[19] M. Walenski, H. Tager-Flusberg, and M. T. Ullman, "Language in autism," in *Understanding Autism: From Basic Neuroscience to Treatment*, S. O. Moldin and J. L. R. Rubenstein, Eds., pp. 175–203, Taylor & Francis, Boca Raton, Fla, USA, 2006.

[20] S. Ellis Weismer, M. A. Gernsbacher, S. Stronach et al., "Lexical and grammatical skills in toddlers on the autism spectrum compared to late talking toddlers," *Journal of Autism and Developmental Disorders*, vol. 41, no. 8, pp. 1065–1075, 2011.

[21] S. Koolen, C. T. W. M. Vissers, A. W. C. J. Hendriks, J. I. M. Egger, and L. Verhoeven, "The interplay between attentional strategies and language processing in high-functioning adults with autism spectrum disorder," *Journal of Autism and Developmental Disorders*, vol. 42, no. 5, pp. 805–814, 2012.

[22] N. Fisher, F. Happé, and J. Dunn, "The relationship between vocabulary, grammar, and false belief task performance in children with autistic spectrum disorders and children with moderate learning difficulties," *Journal of Child Psychology and Psychiatry and Allied Disciplines*, vol. 46, no. 4, pp. 409–419, 2005.

[23] J. Åsberg, "Patterns of language and discourse comprehension skills in school-aged children with autism spectrum disorders," *Scandinavian Journal of Psychology*, vol. 51, no. 6, pp. 534–539, 2010.

[24] S. Peppe, J. Cleland, F. Gibbon, A. O'Hare, and P. M. Castilla, "Expressive prosody in children with autism spectrum conditions," *Journal of Neurolinguistics*, vol. 24, no. 1, pp. 41–53, 2011.

[25] M. A. Romero-Munguía, "Memoria procesal deficiente y alteraciones de la comunicación en la patogenia del autismo infantil," *Neurología, Neurocirugía y Psiquiatría*, vol. 35, no. 4, pp. 203–208, 2002.

[26] H. Tager-Flusberg, "Language and understanding minds: connections in autism," in *Understanding Other Minds: Perspectives From Autism and Developmental Cognitive Neuroscience*, S. Baron-Cohen, H. Tager-Flusberg, and D. J. Cohen, Eds., pp. 124–149, Oxford University Press, Oxford, UK, 2nd edition, 2000.

[27] M. T. Ullman, "The declarative/procedural model of lexicon and grammar," *Journal of Psycholinguistic Research*, vol. 30, no. 1, pp. 37–69, 2001.

[28] F. Happé, *Autism: An Introduction to Psychological Theory*, Taylor & Francis, London, UK, 1994.

[29] M. A. Romero-Munguía, "Mnesic imbalance or hyperthymestic syndrome as cause of autism symptoms in Shereshevskii," in *Recent Advances in Autism Spectrum Disorders—Volume I*, M. Fitzgerald, Ed., pp. 165–187, InTech, Rijeka, Croatia, 2013.

[30] J. Perner, S. R. Leekam, and H. Wimmer, "Three-year-olds' difficulty with false belief: the case for a conceptual deficit," *British Journal of Developmental Psychology*, vol. 5, no. 2, pp. 125–137, 1987.

[31] J. Perner, U. Frith, A. M. Leslie, and S. R. Leekam, "Exploration of the autistic child's theory of mind: knowledge, belief, and communication," *Child Development*, vol. 60, no. 3, pp. 688–700, 1989.

[32] C. M. Grant, K. J. Riggs, and J. Boucher, "Counterfactual and mental state reasoning in children with autism," *Journal of Autism and Developmental Disorders*, vol. 34, no. 2, pp. 177–188, 2004.

[33] S. Kerr and K. Durkin, "Understanding of thought bubbles as mental representations in children with autism: implications for theory of mind," *Journal of Autism and Developmental Disorders*, vol. 34, no. 6, pp. 637–648, 2004.

[34] H. M. Wellman, S. Baron-Cohen, R. Caswell et al., "Thought-bubbles help children with autism acquire an alternative to a theory of mind," *Autism*, vol. 6, no. 4, pp. 343–363, 2002.

[35] S. E. Lind and D. M. Bowler, "Language and theory of mind in autism spectrum disorder: the relationship between complement syntax and false belief task performance," *Journal of Autism and Developmental Disorders*, vol. 39, no. 6, pp. 929–937, 2009.

[36] C. Lewis and A. Osborne, "Three-year-olds' problems with false belief: conceptual deficit or linguistic artifact?" *Child Development*, vol. 61, no. 5, pp. 1514–1519, 1990.

[37] S. B. Day and D. Gentner, "Nonintentional analogical inference in text comprehension," *Memory and Cognition*, vol. 35, no. 1, pp. 39–49, 2007.

[38] E. de Gortari, *Introducción a la lógica dialéctica*, Fondo de Cultura Económica, México, Mexico, 1956.

[39] L. Girelli, C. Semenza, and M. Delazer, "Inductive reasoning and implicit memory: evidence from intact and impaired memory systems," *Neuropsychologia*, vol. 42, no. 7, pp. 926–938, 2004.

[40] W. L. Gross and A. J. Greene, "Analogical inference: the role of awareness in abstract learning," *Memory*, vol. 15, no. 8, pp. 838–844, 2007.

[41] S. Ozonoff, S. J. Rogers, and B. F. Pennington, "Asperger's syndrome: evidence of an empirical distinction from high-functioning autism," *Journal of Child Psychology and Psychiatry and Allied Disciplines*, vol. 32, no. 7, pp. 1107–1122, 1991.

[42] S. Baron-Cohen, "The autistic child's theory of mind: a case of specific developmental delay," *Journal of Child Psychology and Psychiatry and Allied Disciplines*, vol. 30, no. 2, pp. 285–297, 1989.

[43] R. de Oliveira-Souza, J. Moll, F. T. Moll, and D. L. Gusmão De Oliveira, "Executive amnesia in a patient with pre-frontal damage due to a gunshot wound," *Neurocase*, vol. 7, no. 5, pp. 383–389, 2001.

[44] W. E. Winter, M. Broman, A. L. Rose, and A. S. Reber, "The assessment of cognitive procedural learning in amnesia: why the tower of Hanoi has fallen down," *Brain and Cognition*, vol. 45, no. 1, pp. 79–96, 2001.

[45] F. G. E. Happé, "An advanced test of theory of mind: understanding of story characters' thoughts and feelings by able autistic, mentally handicapped, and normal children and adults," *Journal of Autism and Developmental Disorders*, vol. 24, no. 2, pp. 129–154, 1994.

[46] L. Cattaneo, M. Fabbri-Destro, S. Boria et al., "Impairment of actions chains in autism and its possible role in intention understanding," *Proceedings of the National Academy of Sciences of the United States of America*, vol. 104, no. 45, pp. 17825–17830, 2007.

[47] L. Fogassi, P. F. Ferrari, B. Gesierich, S. Rozzi, F. Chersi, and G. Rizzolotti, "Neuroscience: parietal lobe: from action organization to intention understanding," *Science*, vol. 308, no. 5722, pp. 662–667, 2005.

[48] G. Rizzolatti and M. Fabbri-Destro, "Mirror neurons: from discovery to autism," *Experimental Brain Research*, vol. 200, no. 3-4, pp. 223–237, 2010.

[49] A. E. O'Hare, L. Bremner, M. Nash, F. Happé, and L. M. Pettigrew, "A clinical assessment tool for advanced theory of mind performance in 5 to 12 year olds," *Journal of Autism and Developmental Disorders*, vol. 39, no. 6, pp. 916–928, 2009.

[50] T. Jolliffe and S. Baron-Cohen, "The strange stories test: a replication with high-functioning adults with autism or Asperger syndrome," *Journal of Autism and Developmental Disorders*, vol. 29, no. 5, pp. 395–406, 1999.

[51] K. Anastasia, S. R. Leekam, and J. M. Findlay, "Implicit learning of local context in autism spectrum disorder," *Journal of Autism and Developmental Disorders*, vol. 42, no. 2, pp. 244–256, 2012.

[52] S. Baron-Cohen, M. O'Riordan, V. Stone, R. Jones, and K. Plaisted, "Recognition of faux pas by normally developing children and children with asperger syndrome or high-functioning autism," *Journal of Autism and Developmental Disorders*, vol. 29, no. 5, pp. 407–418, 1999.

[53] S. Choudhury, S. J. Blakemore, and T. Charman, "Social cognitive development during adolescence," *Social Cognitive and Affective Neuroscience*, vol. 1, no. 3, pp. 165–174, 2006.

[54] E. H. H. Keulers, E. A. T. Evers, P. Stiers, and J. Jolles, "Age, sex, and pubertal phase influence mentalizing about emotions and actions in adolescents," *Developmental Neuropsychology*, vol. 35, no. 5, pp. 555–569, 2010.

[55] S. H. Mostofsky, M. C. Goldberg, R. J. Landa, and M. B. Denckla, "Evidence for a deficit in procedural learning in children and adolescents with autism: implications for cerebellar contribution," *Journal of the International Neuropsychological Society*, vol. 6, no. 7, pp. 752–759, 2000.

[56] S. Baron-Cohen, T. Jolliffe, C. Mortimore, and M. Robertson, "Another advanced test of theory of mind: evidence from very high functioning adults with autism or Asperger syndrome," *Journal of Child Psychology and Psychiatry and Allied Disciplines*, vol. 38, no. 7, pp. 813–822, 1997.

[57] F. Gregory Ashby and M. J. Crossley, "Interactions between declarative and procedural-learning categorization systems," *Neurobiology of Learning and Memory*, vol. 94, no. 1, pp. 1–12, 2010.

[58] S. Baron-Cohen, S. Wheelwright, J. Hill, Y. Raste, and I. Plumb, "The "reading the mind in the eyes" test revised version: a study with normal adults, and adults with Asperger syndrome or high-functioning autism," *Journal of Child Psychology and Psychiatry and Allied Disciplines*, vol. 42, no. 2, pp. 241–251, 2001.

[59] A. Klin, W. Jones, R. Schultz, F. Volkmar, and D. Cohen, "Visual fixation patterns during viewing of naturalistic social situations as predictors of social competence in individuals with autism," *Archives of General Psychiatry*, vol. 59, no. 9, pp. 809–816, 2002.

[60] T. F. Gross, "The perception of four basic emotions in human and nonhuman faces by children with autism and other developmental disabilities," *Journal of Abnormal Child Psychology*, vol. 32, no. 5, pp. 469–480, 2004.

[61] O. Golan, S. Baron-Cohen, and J. Hill, "The Cambridge Mindreading (CAM) face-voice battery: testing complex emotion recognition in adults with and without Asperger Syndrome," *Journal of Autism and Developmental Disorders*, vol. 36, no. 2, pp. 169–183, 2006.

[62] S. Blakemore, "The social brain in adolescence," *Nature Reviews Neuroscience*, vol. 9, no. 4, pp. 267–277, 2008.

[63] G. B. C. Hall, H. Szechtman, and C. Nahmias, "Enhanced salience and emotion recognition in autism: a PET study," *American Journal of Psychiatry*, vol. 160, no. 8, pp. 1439–1441, 2003.

[64] N. C. Vetter, M. Altgassen, L. Phillips, C. E. Mahy, and M. Kliegel, "Development of affective theory of mind across adolescence: disentangling the role of executive functions," *Developmental Neuropsychology*, vol. 38, no. 2, pp. 114–125, 2013.

[65] R. J. Roberts, L. D. Hager, and C. Heron, "Prefrontal cognitive processes: working memory and inhibition in the antisaccade task," *Journal of Experimental Psychology*, vol. 123, no. 4, pp. 374–393, 1994.

[66] L. Heavey, W. Phillips, S. Baron-Cohen, and M. Rutter, "The awkward moments test: a naturalistic measure of social understanding in autism," *Journal of Autism and Developmental Disorders*, vol. 30, no. 3, pp. 225–236, 2000.

[67] I. Dziobek, S. Fleck, E. Kalbe et al., "Introducing MASC: a movie for the assessment of social cognition," *Journal of Autism and Developmental Disorders*, vol. 36, no. 5, pp. 623–636, 2006.

[68] O. Golan, S. Baron-Cohen, J. J. Hill, and Y. Golan, "The "reading the mind in films" task: complex emotion recognition in adults with and without autism spectrum conditions," *Social neuroscience*, vol. 1, no. 2, pp. 111–123, 2006.

[69] O. Golan, S. Baron-Cohen, and Y. Golan, "The "reading the mind in films" task [child version]: complex emotion and mental state recognition in children with and without autism spectrum conditions," *Journal of Autism and Developmental Disorders*, vol. 38, no. 8, pp. 1534–1541, 2008.

[70] J. L. Barnes, M. V. Lombardo, S. Wheelwright, and S. Baron-Cohen, "Moral dilemmas film task: a study of spontaneous

2

Neural Mechanisms Involved in Hypersensitive Hearing: Helping Children with ASD who are Overly Sensitive to Sounds

Jay R. Lucker[1] and Alex Doman[2]

[1]*Howard University, Washington, DC, USA*
[2]*Advanced Brain Technologies, Ogden, UT, USA*

Correspondence should be addressed to Jay R. Lucker; apddrj@gmail.com

Academic Editor: Roberto Canitano

Professionals working with children diagnosed with autism spectrum disorder (ASD) may find that these children are overly sensitive to sounds. These professionals are often concerned as to why children may have auditory hypersensitivities. This review article discusses the neural mechanisms identified underlying hypersensitive hearing in people. The authors focus on brain research to support the idea of the nonclassical auditory pathways being involved in connecting the auditory system with the emotional system of the brain. The authors also discuss brain mechanisms felt to be involved in auditory hypersensitivity. The authors conclude with a discussion of some treatments for hypersensitive hearing. These treatments include desensitization training and the use of listening therapies such as The Listening Program.

1. Introduction

Professionals working with children who overly react to sounds want to know why the children have hypersensitive hearing. Additionally, parents of these children want to have a better understanding of their children's problems. Often these children are described as being afraid of such sounds, losing control of their behaviors when hearing such sounds, and even fearing that the sounds may be heard when there are no such sounds in the listening environment. Typically these behaviors are seen in children diagnosed with autism spectrum disorder (ASD).

For many people, the method applied to deal with children who have hypersensitive hearing is to avoid the listening situations or deal with the child at the time that the sounds are occurring. Sometimes, people try to prepare children by saying that such annoying sounds will occur; yet, even with this preparation, many of these children still lose control of their behaviors when the actual sounds are heard. Many professionals relate these hypersensitivities in hearing to problems with the children's auditory systems.

Lucker and Doman [1] and Lucker [2] discussed the fact that auditory hypersensitivity in children with ASD is more of an emotional based problem than a specific auditory system problem. In these publications, the authors state that underlying auditory hypersensitivity (or oversensitivity to sounds) involves what are called the nonclassical auditory pathways and limbic system connections. However, the authors do not go very far in describing the brain (or neural) mechanisms involved other than identifying that there is a connection between the auditory system and the limbic system deep in the temporal lobe of the brain. The present paper is a follow-up to these 2012 and 2013 publications. The present paper reviews that what our present research has indicated might be underlying neural mechanisms involved in hypersensitive hearing. Understanding these neural mechanisms will provide the reader with two important factors. First, understanding what is going on with a child who has auditory hypersensitivities is a normal neural reaction and, second, identifying what treatments may be appropriate to help children who are overly sensitive deal more successfully with sound so that they do not have over reactions during listening tasks and, possibly, "shut down" so as to avoid listening and responding to any sounds.

Before beginning the discussion of these various neural pathways, the reader should have a clearer understanding of some of the terms used in this paper. One term is auditory hypersensitivity. This problem is often identified as a person being overly sensitive to sounds. Some professionals have referred to the oversensitivity to sounds as misophonia. Others [3, 4] have called this phonophobia or fear of sound. Thus, in the present paper, the use of hypersensitivity will include oversensitivity to sounds that includes misophonia and phonophobia. It is hypothesized that the same neural mechanisms are involved in all these oversensitivities to sound; however, for some children the sensitivity is only to sounds of an intensity above typical tolerance by people (e.g., greater than 90 dBHL, as 90 dBHL is often identified as a level of maximum tolerance in people). For other children, their oversensitivity may be for a variety of sounds, while for some children it is for specific sounds.

2. The Classical Auditory Pathway

Two other important terms used in this paper are classical and nonclassical auditory pathways. Professionals studying hearing typically learn about the standard or classical auditory pathways. These pathways (see Figure 1) start at the cochlea of the inner ear where the cells of hearing, called hair cells, release neurochemicals which are picked up by the auditory nerve also known as the eighth cranial nerve. This nerve can be found in both ears (right and left sides). The auditory nerve travels transmitting the auditory stimulation to a region on the right and left sides of the brainstem called the pons. Specifically, the nerve innervates areas of the cochlear nucleus. Some of the nerve pathways come from the cochlear nucleus project to the same (ipsilateral) side of the brainstem while others cross to the opposite (contralateral) side.

The next level in the system involves a complex of neuronal sites called the superior olivary complex. This is still in the lower brainstem within the pons. From the superior olivary region the nerves travel to the next level called the lateral lemniscus. (This is an important region when we look at the nonclassical pathways.) From the lateral lemniscus, the nerves travel to the inferior colliculus in the classical pathways. The inferior colliculus is at the upper brainstem level, and projections from this level go to the thalamus at the cortical level. The nerves projecting from the medial geniculate bodies project to the auditory cortex which is in the temporal lobe of the brain. Then, via a "bridge" connection between the two auditory cortices of the right and left hemispheres of the brain, the corpus callosum connects these hemispheres so that we can integrate auditory information from each hemisphere.

3. The Nonclassical Auditory Pathway

The previous description was of the classical auditory pathways. However, by eight years of age, Moller and Rollins [5]

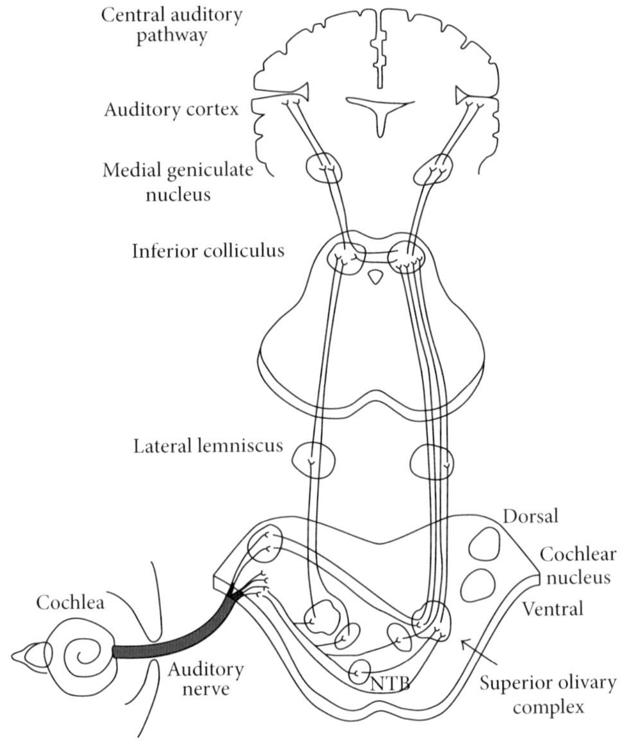

FIGURE 1: Diagram of the classical auditory pathways from the ear to the auditory cortex (diagram retrieved from https://dnbhelp.wordpress.com/otology/).

identified that this classical pathway becomes the dominant pathway by which sound travels so that we can process and comprehend what we hear. Moller and his associates [5, 6] identified another pathway which was first investigated in the 1970s which is also an auditory pathway and is mostly active in young children. This pathway has been referred to as the nonclassical auditory pathway (see Figure 2). In typically developing children, by the age of 8 years this pathway becomes suppressed under most listening conditions.

One of the first neural mechanisms identified as being involved in auditory hypersensitivity is this nonclassical pathway. The nonclassical pathway branches off from the classical pathway at the level of the lateral lemniscus. Nerves traveling from the external nucleus of the lateral lemniscus project and receive stimulation from the reticular formation in the upper brainstem. The reticular formation is involved in awareness, detection, and attention to sensory stimulation including sound. The reticular formation then sends neural information back to this region of the lateral lemniscus involved with auditory sensory processing. These neural inputs travel from the external nucleus of the lateral lemniscus to regions of the thalamus but not the medial geniculate bodies which are involved with the classical auditory pathway. From these regions of thalamus, not involved with auditory sensory processing, the nerves project to what is called the auditory association cortex, not the primary auditory cortex which is involved with the major processing of what we hear. These association areas include projections to the limbic system deep within the temporal lobe of the brain. The limbic system

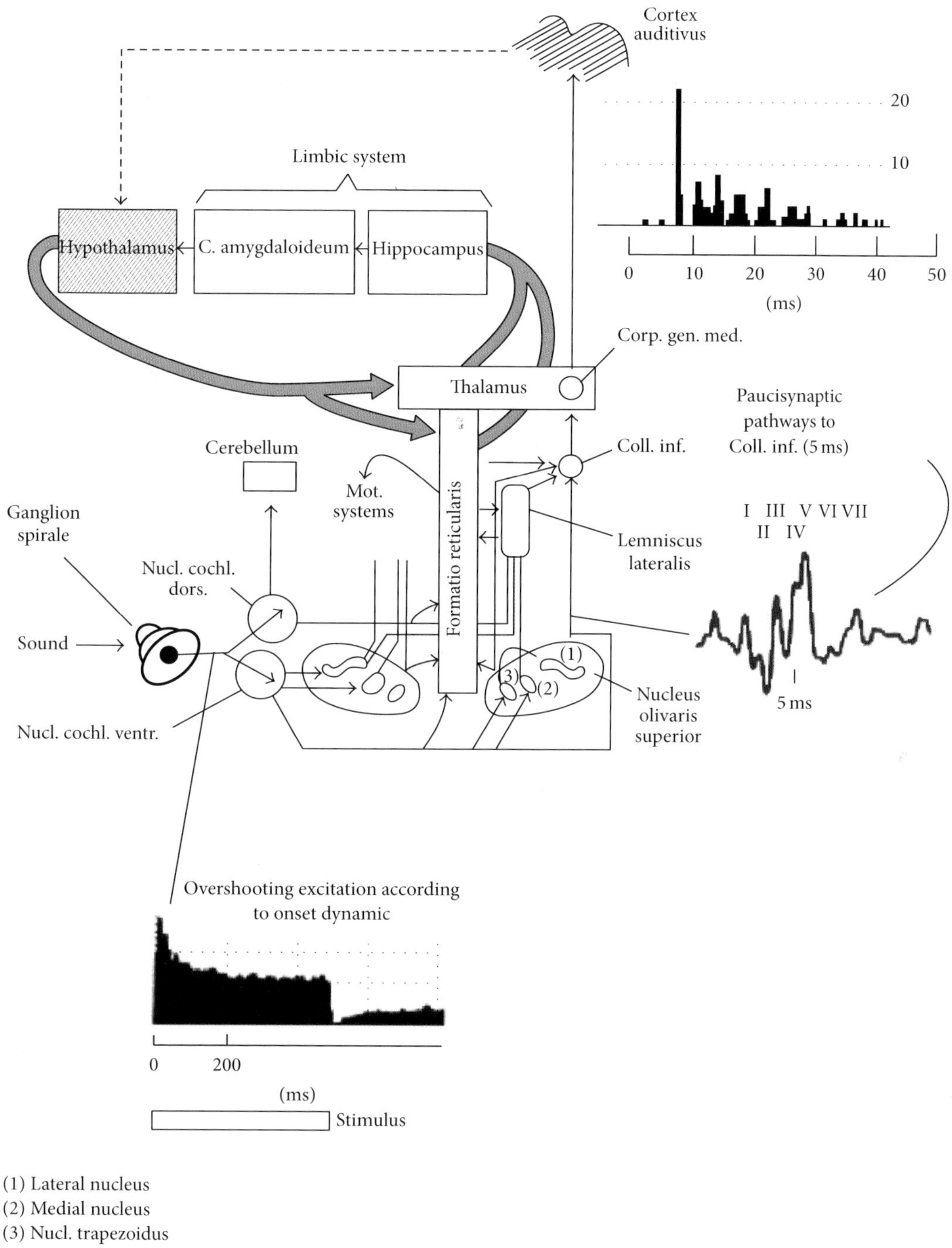

FIGURE 2: Diagram of the nonclassical auditory pathways showing the relationship between the pathways from the auditory system to the limbic system and to the auditory cortex (diagram retrieved from Noise and Health, 2000, http://www.noiseandhealth.org/viewimage.asp?img=NoiseHealth_2000_2_7_49_31742_1.jpg).

is involved with a number of factors including emotional responsiveness. One major center is the amygdala which is involved with emotional memories. What is also interesting is that projections to the thalamic regions that receive input from the external nucleus of the lateral lemniscus go directly to the amygdala. Thus, this nonclassical auditory pathway connects auditory sensory input with the emotional centers of the brain and with brainstem levels of awareness and attention to sensory input.

An important finding from the work of Moller and Rollins [5] and Møller et al. [6] is that not only does the nonclassical pathway obtain auditory sensory information but also it receives stimulation from the somatosensory systems of the body. These systems are involved in processing touch and temperature and help process body position in space. In Moller and Rollins' research [5], they found that overstimulation of touch (sensory processing) in young, typically developing children led to these children becoming overly (hyper) sensitive to sound. This occurred for young children up to 8 years of age. After that age, overstimulation of touch did not lead to an increase in auditory hypersensitivity. However, these were typically developing children. In another study, Møller et al. [6] discussed that children with autism spectrum disorder (ASD) may continue to be overly sensitive to touch and, thus, to sound because their nonclassical auditory systems do not become inhibited to respond under normal listening conditions. In an article published by Musiek et al. [7], they write, "Some children with developmental disorders may have emotional learning problems caused by the brain's inability to reduce the involvement of the non-classical pathway and the amygdala" (p. 6). These children may include those with ASD. These findings support the original discussions from Lucker and Doman's [1] and Lucker's [2] publications that auditory hypersensitivity is largely an emotional (limbic system) based response to sound and not an auditory system response to sound. Thus, the treatment for auditory hypersensitivity, based on this factor, would focus upon calming the emotional system during listening tasks.

4. From the Limbic System to Behavioral Reactions to Sound

4.1. Involvement of the Vagus Nerve. Once sound has been processed by the brain, the brain reacts to the sound. As noted from the previous discussions, one of the systems that is involved in hypersensitive hearing is the limbic system. Additionally, observing children who show negative behavioral reactions to sounds we see that they tend to react in manners one can call negative emotional behavioral reactions. These negative emotional behavioral reactions can include what we call avoidance or "flight" responses (running away, avoiding, or hiding) or striking out against the "world" or a "fight" response. This "flight and fight" responding is automatic behavior controlled largely by limbic system reactions to stimuli. However, a question arises as to what mechanisms may be involved in this negative behavioral reactivity. One of these mechanisms is through the innervation of an efferent nerve called the vagus nerve or the tenth cranial nerve which receives stimulation from the limbic system.

Porges [8] and Porges and Lewis [9] discuss the functioning of the vagus nerve in setting up automatic bodily responses to sound as part of what Porges calls the "Polyvagal Theory." This theory relates automatic or autonomic functions in response to incoming stimuli, such as sound. These autonomic functions are regulated through what is called the autonomic nervous system or ANS. Essentially, this theory describes how the vagus nerve is innervated through limbic system connections. The information transmitted via the vagus nerve innervates bodily responses to various emotional states including stress and fear. For example, the vagus nerve innervates the heart and, under stress and fearful conditions, a person's heart rate increases. The vagus nerve also innervates the larynx or vocal folds which allow people to vocalize and speak. Under stress and fearful conditions, one may notice how a person's voice "cracks," raises in pitch, or becomes weak. When sound causes people to have negative emotional reactions (i.e., hypersensitivity), the vagus nerve may become innervated by the limbic system leading to ANS reactions of "flight and fight" which are often seen in children who overly react to sounds, such as children with ASD. Also, these children may "shut down" in listening and start babbling incoherently. These changes may be affected by vagal nerve innervation.

4.2. Other Reactions Based on Limbic System Innervation. Mazurek et al. [10, 11] discussed their research looking at the effects of stress (increased negative emotionality) in rats. They found that under stress, these rats were highly oversensitive to sound (i.e., auditory hypersensitivity). They identified that there were negative reactions after hearing these sounds in these "stressed" rats. The reactions were measured in their hypothalamus (a brain mechanism part of the limbic system), their pituitary glands, and their adrenal glands (the latter two being part of the ANS). This research suggests that children who are hypersensitive to sound may have problems because of similar reactions in their hypothalamus, as well as their amygdala; both areas are identified earlier in this paper as part of the limbic system. Furthermore, the reactions to these nontolerated sounds can set off ANS responses as well as the vagal nerve reactions previously discussed.

In the initial study by Mazurek et al. [10] discussed above, the stress in their lab rats was produced by exposure to annoying sounds that were not very intense. This could be related to child's normal, ANS reactions to sounds which are not tolerated which lead to infants and very young children being frightened by these sounds. For children with ASD, their limbic systems may develop negative memories of these sounds (through the amygdala) and react negatively because of ANS innervation as seen with the animal experiments discussed.

5. Other Neural Mechanisms Involved with Hypersensitive Hearing

The nonclassical auditory pathways and the limbic system are important neural mechanisms involved in hypersensitive hearing in children, especially those with ASD. However, there has been recent research indicating that some other factors may be involved. One of these other factors involves problems with neural innervation due to abnormal production of neurochemicals such as GABA or gamma-aminobutyric acid as well as 5-hydroxytryptamine (5-HT). This problem with neurochemical production may further increase the auditory hypersensitivities in children. What the research indicates is that this abnormal production is found in children with ASD.

5.1. Abnormal Neurochemical Production and Inhibition

5.1.1. GABA. Rubenstein and Merzenich [12] identified that one of the neural mechanisms found in people with auditory hypersensitivity is a problem with the neurochemical GABA. They discuss how abnormal GABA production has been found in children with autism. Furthermore, they explain how GABA helps in the inhibitory control of sensory processing including auditory sensory processing.

Inhibition relates to functioning in the following manner. When we receive incoming sensory stimuli, we can allow the stimulation to be transmitted from the sensory receptive organ (such as the inner ear) to the brain for further processing. In the brain, there are cells that transmit neurochemicals that "block" the transmission of the incoming sensory stimulation. This blocking is called inhibition which leads to a reduction in responding. Thus, in the case of nontolerated, annoying sounds, the brain can "block" or reduce the transmission of the incoming auditory sensory stimuli from getting to the receptor centers in the brain. One neurochemical that does this blocking is GABA. Rubenstein and Merzenich [12], as well as investigations by others cited by these authors, have identified that release of GABA in the brain inhibits overreaction to sensory stimulation such as sound. Furthermore, they discuss that children with ASD have a reduction in their GABA production. Abnormal GABA production and transmission leads to a hyperreactivity in the neurons of the brain because of this lack of inhibitory responding. Thus, the person's brain is not appropriately processing sounds, and the body's reaction to this may be referred to as overreactivity. This overreactivity can lead to negative emotional reactions that lead the child with ASD to fear and dislike sounds they hear. Research is needed to investigate GABA in children with autism and identify whether hypersensitive hearing may be due to abnormal production of GABA, inappropriate transmission of this neurochemical, or a combination of both factors.

5.1.2. 5-Hydroxytryptamine (5-HT), Serotonin. Marriage and Barnes [13] identified that another neurochemical involved in sensory modulation and, thus, sensory processing, is 5-HT, also known as serotonin. Based on animal studies, these researchers describe that abnormal functioning of 5-HT caused a heightened startle response to auditory stimuli in animals. This suggested that auditory hypersensitivity in people might be due to abnormal functioning of 5-HT (serotonin). Baguley [14] stated that people with William syndrome, who are typically found to have auditory hypersensitivities, also have serotonin abnormalities in their brains. As such, it is possible that children with ASD may also have abnormal production of 5-HT. Further research is needed to look at 5-HT/serotonin functioning in these children and relate this to listening and auditory hypersensitivities.

5.2. Sensory Gating. When we consider the neurochemical factors contributing to inhibition, we can see that these factors may relate to what some people call sensory gating. Some of the behavioral reactions we see in children who are hypersensitive to sound may involve how the brain "gates" or deals with sensory information such as sound and, due to this gating, how the brain sets up behavioral reactions to sound. Gating relates to the regulation of how the brain handles incoming sensory information. This "gating" deals with two factors related to sound processing. One is the acceptance and "passing on" of sound information to higher cortical centers such as when we listen in conversations, our neural sensory gating system allows what the speaker is saying to be passed through the auditory system to higher levels of auditory processing into the language centers for language processing and on to the cognitive centers where we think about what the speaker is saying. At the same time, there may be background noises which our sensory gating systems inhibit so they are not processed beyond a certain low neural level. This is often referred to as auditory filtering.

Some children with auditory filtering problems are described as having abnormalities in something called executive functioning or self-regulation. Executive functions involve those regulatory mechanisms in the prefrontal cortex that send neural messages to other parts of the brain to manage the processing of information, including what we hear. These abnormalities are deficits in the frontal lobe of the brain which suggest that children with ASD having auditory hypersensitivities may have abnormalities in this part of their brains.

Orekhova et al. [15] and Mayer et al. [16] discuss this sensory monitoring or gating and state that our reactions to how we respond to sensory input are strongly related by prefrontal cortical activity. Abnormal prefrontal cortical functioning can contribute to poor sensory gating and overreacting to sensory stimuli. Thus, one factor in the frontal lobe contributing to why children may react so strongly to sound (which we call auditory hypersensitivity) is poor executive functioning which does not allow their brains to inhibit these negative emotional reactions from occurring.

5.3. Abnormal Functioning in the Frontal Lobe of the Brain. Another group of researchers have investigated what may be involved with frontal lobe malfunctioning. Gomot et al. [17] looked at the electrophysiological measure called the mismatched negativity or the MMN response which is related to functioning in the frontal lobe of the brain and is a response that occurs just prior to neural activity related to listening attention. The MMN response is a discriminatory response to changes in auditory stimuli. For example, if two tones of the same frequency or two monosyllabic words are heard, there is a relatively low neural response measured by the MMN. Then, if one of the tones or words is changed, the MMN becomes larger indicating that the brain has discriminated and identifying the difference.

Gomot et al. [17] found that in children with auditory hypersensitivities, the MMN from the left frontal lobe was abnormal compared with children who had normal reactions to high intensity sounds. Thus, one can conclude that children with auditory hypersensitivities may not be able to appropriately discriminate changes in loudness in sound so that unexpected changes may lead to negative emotional reactions. Thus, one other factor that may lead to abnormalities in brain (neural) functioning in children with ASD is this abnormal functioning in discriminating sound. Further research is needed looking at the MMN in children with ASD.

6. What May Occur in Children with Auditory Hypersensitivity

Children's reactions to certain, intolerant sounds may be a natural, negative response which, over time, becomes filtered by the brain mechanisms discussed above. When we think about how parents (and others) react to young children's responses to sounds the child cannot tolerate, the reactions are usually hugging the child, comforting the child through touch, and similar physical reactions. As discussed earlier, somatosensory information is integrated with sound in the nonclassical auditory system. In the typically developing child, these manual touches may be processed as comforting leading to a reduction in stress which then becomes processed through the nonclassical auditory system to interpret sounds that are annoying and intolerant as not being fearful. Thus, the child learns not to fear such sounds and not to be stressed out when hearing or expecting these annoying sounds. In contrast, it is hypothesized that the child with ASD and auditory hypersensitivities may overreact not only to the sounds that cause the negative behavioral reactions but also to somatosensory stimulation, so that when people try to comfort them as young children, their nonclassical auditory systems react with further negative responses, and they learn to associate negative emotional reactions to the sounds. Thus, a focus of the treatment for auditory hypersensitivity has to be to reduce this negative emotional reactivity, reduce the stress, and reduce the "fight or flight" reactions in people with hypersensitive hearing.

7. Treatment for Hypersensitive Hearing

In view of the above discussions, the underlying theme is that hypersensitive hearing involves neural mechanisms that are related to emotional processing, emotional memory, and emotional reactivity which is considered negative. This negative reactivity can lead to fight/flight responses affecting the autonomic nervous system and secretion by glands throughout the body as well as neural motor responses that can lead to a deterioration or loss of vocalizing (vagus nerve reactions) as well as behavioral responses of fighting and running away. As such, the underlying factor for treating these problems is to focus on the negative emotional reactions.

In order to better understand how one focuses on the emotional responses, one needs to have a basic understanding of behavioral therapies. There are two general approaches to behavioral therapy. One is called operant conditioning and the other is called classical conditioning. Operant conditioning is typically associated with the work of BF Skinner while classical conditioning is associated with the work of Ivan Pavlov. Operant conditioning follows the basic concept that when we are presented with a stimulus (e.g., a sound of high intensity) and there is a response (e.g., the child running away), there is a reaction which occurs that reinforces or punishes the response increasing (reinforcement) or decreasing (punishment) the likelihood that the response will occur again when the same stimulus is presented. The therapist, educator, or parent providing the reinforcement presents a reaction to the child's behavior in order to reduce the running away behavior (punishment) or to reinforce the child listening to the sound (reinforcement). Classical conditioning works slightly differently. We present a stimulus (e.g., the same intense sound) but we teach the child a behavior that is different from what is called the unconditioned response (in this example, the child running away is the unconditioned response). We may teach the child to count how long the sound is present and reinforce this conditioned response. Over time, the expectation is that the child hearing the sound will just count how long it lasts, but not run away. When we consider retraining or reprogramming children who have auditory hypersensitivity, we need to think more in line with classical conditioning for children who are responsive and can handle such behavioral training. For some children, such as those with ASD, we may need to consider operant conditioning treatments similar in many respects to what is often used with these children called ABA or applied behavioral analysis.

Therapy or training, which can also be called retraining, is to associate the negative sounds with some behavior that will lead to a more calming response and, thus, reduce the negative emotional reactions to the sound. There are two proposed methods for doing this. One is through a straight behavioral training program. The other is through the use of a listening therapy. The following is a discussion of each of these approaches.

7.1. Behavioral Training for Sound Desensitization. The underlying concept of a behavioral approach is to recondition the person's system so that the emotional memory is changed from negative to more neutral and, if possible, positive. Then, if the person is faced with those stimuli which originally "set off" the negative emotional responses, the person would have a more neutral response. The goal of behavioral training is to desensitize the person to the previously feared sounds. An example of a behavioral approach would be as follows. Consider a person being annoyed by sounds and having strong negative emotional reactions to people eating because of the sound of crunching food. The person might be taught how to relax his/her body and feel more calm which would lead to a more positive emotional feeling. Then, the person would engage in the relaxation exercise while hearing food crunching first presented at a low volume level for short periods of time then having the volume and length of time increased. Eventually, the person would start associating this relaxed, more positive feeling with the crunching sound and feel that he/she can control his/her reactions to the sound.

As one can see, this desensitization using a behavioral approach takes time and a level of involvement on the part of the person that may not be available for many children with ASD. For them, another approach might be more successful. This approach may be called "in vivo exposure." In this approach, the person who presents with hypersensitive hearing is slowly introduced to the sounds and situations involving the sounds that led to the negative emotional reactions. This is done in a controlled manner in real life (in vivo) situations. For the same example as used above, the person may be exposed to someone softly crunching food once. The volume of crunching and the number of crunches as well as the length of time having to listen would then be systematically increased until the person is able to sit through a meal with people. The child going through this systematic desensitization training would be rewarded for success in sitting still while the person is hearing the food crunching sound (an operant conditioning approach).

An example of in vivo exposure is seen in the research of Koegel et al. [18]. In their research, they used this approach with a small group of children identified as being on the autism spectrum and found that even one year after training, the children were desensitized to the sounds which they originally feared. Furthermore, generalization of the training occurred so that the children became desensitized to many sounds that were not part of the original training program.

7.2. Use of Listening Therapies. Along with desensitization training (whether a classical conditioning approach or in vivo exposure is used) one can use a sound intervention or listening therapy. A listening therapy is the use of specially recorded music and environmental sounds having nothing necessarily to do with the sounds to which the person has negative emotional reactions. The music and recorded sounds are carefully chosen and systematically produced to enhance positive emotional and calming reactions when listening. This type of training involves a more passive method to desensitize the limbic system and reprogram the emotional memory system with the aim of making sounds something to which one desires to listen rather than avoid. The listening method described here uses specially recorded instrumental music. The music is acoustically modified to lead the child to react less negatively to sounds and, thus, reduce the child's hypersensitivity.

Although a number of listening methods have been developed, one specific method found beneficial for children with ASD is The Listening Program (TLP). In TLP, a trained provider, usually a professional such as an occupational therapist or speech-language pathologist, oversees the training. The provider typically establishes the actual protocol based on the individual child's needs and may carry out the training in the child's home or at the child's school. When using TLP, especially through specially designed air and bone conduction headphones, the sound signal is believed to travel along both classical and nonclassical auditory pathways. One of the first outcomes that parents, educators, and professionals often see in children undergoing TLP training is that the children are calmer. This is a good indicator that the listening has tapped into the emotional areas of the limbic system via the nonclassical auditory pathways. Over the course of training, children often are reported to be more attentive to sounds, better able to detect (discriminate) sounds they hear, and are more verbally communicative likely because they are more open to listening. As the training proceeds, the child continues to relax and become calmer when listening. It is hypothesized that this is because a reprogramming of emotional memory in the amygdala is occurring. The training also helps improve stress regulation so the child no longer has fight/flight responses to nonthreatening sounds. When the child then finds him- or herself in real-world situations and hears sounds that may have been frightening or annoying in the past, the training allows the child to process the sounds in a more neutral manner.

For many children, the use of a program such as TLP is sufficient to reprogram their systems so that sound is no longer frightening. The child may still react verbally saying that he or she does not like such sounds or the situations in which the sounds occur, but after TLP training, the child should no longer lose control of his or her behavior when hearing such sounds. Additionally, the child may be more willing to listen to parents or teachers who can model desensitization by saying, "The sound is annoying, so let's move over here," or "If we walk more quickly toward [our goal], we can get away from having to hear that sound."

Research using TLP has largely been anecdotal, but the evidence base is growing as studies continue to be conducted. For example, Gee et al. [19] present a case study of a child with ASD who was overly sensitive to sound and completed TLP training. They report that the child showed a decrease in negative behavioral reactions to previously "annoying" and feared sounds after completing this training. A review of other studies and descriptions of individual cases can also be found at the Advanced Brain Technologies website (http://www.advancedbrain.com/). The research has demonstrated that after going through this listening program, children, adolescents, and adults find their abilities to tolerate sounds are improved. Many find listening to be more pleasurable and positive so that negative emotional reactions rarely occur. Thus, professionals working with children who have ASD and auditory hypersensitivities as well as parents of these children might wish to try TLP training on an investigative basis focusing on seeing changes in the children's reactions to sounds in their environment. It is the expectation of these authors that completing TLP training should lead to reduced negative emotional reactions when listening increasing the child's listening and communication skills. Since listening is an important part of learning, it is hoped that the improvements in listening will improve learning for these children as well. Further research is needed carefully investigating these educational and communicative factors.

8. Conclusions

The underlying theme throughout this paper is that the primary neural mechanisms in hypersensitive hearing involve negative emotional reactions to sound via connections between the auditory system and the limbic system as well as the limbic system and other parts of the body. Research has demonstrated issues involving the auditory system connecting with the limbic system as well as frontal lobe involvement that can contribute to negative emotional reactions. Research has also identified some problems based on poor neurochemical functioning, specifically GABA and serotonin, which eventually lead to negative emotional reactions when listening.

Children with ASD may have negative emotional reactions to some sounds (i.e., auditory hypersensitivity) that can involve some degree of a fight or flight responses. The treatment for these hypersensitive hearing problems is felt to focus on changing the negative emotional reactions to more neutral and, hopefully, positive responses. This can be done through desensitization training which can be in an active form of behavioral reconditioning or a holistic form called in vivo exposure. Additionally, the use of a listening therapy, such as The Listening Program, can lead to more neutral or positive reactions when listening to these annoying sounds.

The focus of this paper was to help the reader understand the underlying mechanisms involved in hypersensitive hearing and the treatments that can help reprogram the person's mechanisms to be more open to listening. In the end, the focus is to help the child with ASD be more involved in communicating with the world around him/her. It is hoped that professionals and parents will consider these factors and the treatment recommendations discussed. Future research should focus on these factors and their direct relationship to hypersensitive hearing in children with ASD so that we can obtain a greater understanding of specific mechanisms involved with hypersensitive hearing and the evidence base for the use of treatments such as desensitization training and listening therapy.

References

[1] J. R. Lucker and A. Doman, "Auditory hypersensitivities and autism spectrum disorders: an emotional response," *Autism Science Digest*, vol. 4, pp. 103–108, 2012.

[2] J. R. Lucker, "Auditory hypersensitivity in children with autism spectrum disorders," *Focus on Autism and Other Developmental Disabilities*, vol. 28, no. 3, pp. 184–191, 2013.

[3] P. J. Jastreboff and M. M. Jastreboff, "Tinnitus retraining therapy (TRT) as a method for treatment of tinnitus and hyperacusis patients," *Journal of the American Academy of Audiology*, vol. 11, no. 3, pp. 162–177, 2000.

[4] P. J. Jastreboff and M. M. Jastreboff, "Tinnitus retraining treatment for patients with tinnitus and decreased sound tolerance," *Otolaryngological Clinics of North America*, vol. 36, pp. 321–336, 2003.

[5] A. R. Moller and P. R. Rollins, "The non-classical auditory pathways are involved in hearing in children but not in adults," *Neuroscience Letters*, vol. 319, no. 1, pp. 41–44, 2002.

[6] A. R. Møller, J. K. Kern, and B. Grannemann, "Are the non-classical auditory pathways involved in autism and PDD?" *Neurological Research*, vol. 27, no. 6, pp. 625–629, 2005.

[7] F. Musiek, A. Mohanani, E. Wierzbinski, G. Kilgore, J. Hunter, and J. Marotto, "The non-classical pathway: too great to be ignored," *Hearing Journal*, vol. 64, no. 10, pp. 6–7, 2011.

[8] S. W. Porges, "The polyvagal perspective," *Biological Psychology*, vol. 74, no. 2, pp. 116–143, 2007.

[9] S. W. Porges and G. F. Lewis, "The polyvagal hypothesis: common mechanisms mediating autonomic regulation, vocalizations and listening," in *Handbook of Behavioral Neuroscience*, vol. 19, pp. 255–264, 2010.

[10] B. Mazurek, H. Haupt, R. Joachim, B. F. Klapp, T. Stöver, and A. J. Szczepek, "Stress induces transient auditory hypersensitivity in rats," *Hearing Research*, vol. 259, no. 1-2, pp. 55–63, 2010.

[11] B. Mazurek, H. Haupt, B. F. Klapp, A. J. Szczepek, and H. Olze, "Exposure of Wistar rats to 24-h psycho-social stress alters gene expression in the inferior colliculus," *Neuroscience Letters*, vol. 527, no. 1, pp. 40–45, 2012.

[12] J. L. R. Rubenstein and M. M. Merzenich, "Model of autism: increased ratio of excitation/inhibition in key neural systems," *Genes, Brain and Behavior*, vol. 2, no. 5, pp. 255–267, 2003.

[13] J. Marriage and N. M. Barnes, "Is central hyperacusis a symptom of 5-hydroxytryptamine (5-HT) dysfunction?," *The Journal of Laryngology and Otology*, vol. 109, no. 10, pp. 915–921, 1995.

[14] D. M. Baguley, "Hyperacusis," *Journal of the Royal Society of Medicine*, vol. 96, no. 12, pp. 582–585, 2003.

[15] E. V. Orekhova, T. A. Stroganova, A. O. Prokofyev, G. Nygren, C. Gillberg, and M. Elam, "Sensory gating in young children with autism: relation to age, IQ, and EEG gamma oscillations," *Neuroscience Letters*, vol. 434, no. 2, pp. 218–223, 2008.

[16] A. R. Mayer, F. M. Hanlon, A. R. Franco et al., "The neural networks underlying auditory sensory gating," *NeuroImage*, vol. 44, no. 1, pp. 182–189, 2009.

[17] M. Gomot, M.-H. Giard, J.-L. Adrien, C. Barthelemy, and N. Bruneau, "Hypersensitivity to acoustic change in children with autism: electrophysiological evidence of left frontal cortex dysfunctioning," *Psychophysiology*, vol. 39, no. 5, pp. 577–584, 2002.

[18] R. L. Koegel, D. Openden, and L. K. Koegel, "A systematic desensitization paradigm to treat hypersensitivity to auditory stimuli in children with autism in family contexts," *Research and Practice for Persons with Severe Disabilities*, vol. 29, no. 2, pp. 122–134, 2004.

[19] B. M. Gee, K. Thompson, and H. St John, "Efficacy of a sound-based intervention with a child with an autism spectrum disorder and auditory sensory over-responsivity," *Occupational Therapy International*, vol. 21, no. 1, pp. 12–20, 2014.

3

No Differences in Emotion Recognition Strategies in Children with Autism Spectrum Disorder: Evidence from Hybrid Faces

Kris Evers,[1,2,3] Inneke Kerkhof,[4] Jean Steyaert,[2,3,5] Ilse Noens,[3,6,7] and Johan Wagemans[1,3]

[1] Laboratory of Experimental Psychology, KU Leuven, Tiensestraat 102 (Box 3711), 3000 Leuven, Belgium
[2] Department of Child Psychiatry, UPC-KU Leuven, 3000 Leuven, Belgium
[3] Leuven Autism Research (LAuRes), KU Leuven, 3000 Leuven, Belgium
[4] Quantitative Psychology and Individual Differences, KU Leuven, 3000 Leuven, Belgium
[5] Department of Clinical Genetics, University Hospital Maastricht, 6200 Maastricht, The Netherlands
[6] Parenting and Special Education Research Unit, KU Leuven, 3000 Leuven, Belgium
[7] Psychiatric and Neurodevelopmental Genetics Unit, Massachusetts General Hospital, MA, Boston, USA

Correspondence should be addressed to Kris Evers; kris.evers@ppw.kuleuven.be

Academic Editor: Connie Kasari

Emotion recognition problems are frequently reported in individuals with an autism spectrum disorder (ASD). However, this research area is characterized by inconsistent findings, with atypical emotion processing strategies possibly contributing to existing contradictions. In addition, an attenuated saliency of the eyes region is often demonstrated in ASD during face identity processing. We wanted to compare reliance on mouth versus eyes information in children with and without ASD, using hybrid facial expressions. A group of six-to-eight-year-old boys with ASD and an age- and intelligence-matched typically developing (TD) group without intellectual disability performed an emotion labelling task with hybrid facial expressions. Five static expressions were used: one neutral expression and four emotional expressions, namely, anger, fear, happiness, and sadness. Hybrid faces were created, consisting of an emotional face half (upper or lower face region) with the other face half showing a neutral expression. Results showed no emotion recognition problem in ASD. Moreover, we provided evidence for the existence of top- and bottom-emotions in children: correct identification of expressions mainly depends on information in the eyes (so-called top-emotions: happiness) or in the mouth region (so-called bottom-emotions: sadness, anger, and fear). No stronger reliance on mouth information was found in children with ASD.

1. Introduction

Facial expressions inform us about the feelings and state of mind of others and enable us to adjust our behavior and to react appropriately. Therefore, the ability to interpret facial expressions accurately and to derive socially relevant information from them is considered a fundamental requirement for typical reciprocal social interactions and communication [1].

Autism spectrum disorders (ASD) are pervasive developmental disorders characterized by quantitative and qualitative deficits in reciprocal social interactions and communication and by the presence of restricted and repetitive behavior patterns, interests, and activities [2]. Difficulties in recognizing, identifying, and understanding the meaning of emotions are often considered as one of the trademarks of their social problems. Different procedures have been used to examine emotion processing abilities in children and adults with ASD, with or without intellectual disability: sorting, (cross-modal) matching, and labeling tasks (for a literature review and a meta-analysis on this topic, see [3, 4], resp.). Each of these procedures has revealed problems with affect processing in individuals with ASD (e.g., [5–8]). Other studies, however, failed to find atypical emotion recognition skills in individuals with ASD (e.g., [9–13]). Inconsistencies (for an overview, see [3]) may be due to differences in sample and participants' characteristics, task demands [14], and stimuli. Performances of individuals with ASD seem to be especially impaired for negative, more subtle, or more complex emotions (e.g., [7, 15, 16]) or expressions embedded in a social context [17, 18]. Besides, it is important to note that an intact performance does not exclude the use of atypical—more cognition- or language-mediated—or more feature-based emotion processing strategies leading to impairments in some emotion recognition tasks, but camouflaging these deficits in other tasks (and therefore often referred to as compensation mechanisms; [3, 11, 19]).

Interestingly, face identity research has provided evidence for atypical face processing strategies in individuals with ASD (for a review, see [20]). People with ASD show an attenuated reliance on the eyes region: they are less attentive towards the upper face part in comparison to neurotypicals, but instead the lower face seems to be more salient. This was found using face identification tasks with familiar [21] and unfamiliar faces (e.g., [22, 23]) and with eye-movement studies using neutral faces or faces embedded in a social context (e.g., [24, 25]). This atypical attention pattern with an increased "mouth bias" in ASD was sometimes interpreted as a specific expertise for mouth regions [26], or as a (language-and-cognition mediated) compensation strategy [27], or even as an active aversion for the quickly and unpredictably moving eyes [28]. However, not all studies found differences in gaze patterns between children with and without ASD (e.g., [29, 30]). Here also, inconsistencies are supposed to be caused by differences in samples, tasks, and stimuli [3].

The above-mentioned studies concern facial identity processing. It is sometimes suggested that face identity recognition (which is based on invariant face properties) and face expression recognition (which is based on changeable aspects of a face) can be dissociated at a neural and theoretical level [31, 32]. According to this view, findings about face identity processing will not necessarily generalize to the domain of emotion perception (see also findings on patients with amygdalectomy [33] or acquired prosopagnosia [34]). The aim of the present study is to examine whether the atypical saliency of upper versus lower face area also holds for emotion perception in children with ASD.

Attendance to a narrow range of specific features in the face (e.g., the mouth region) when judging facial affect could partly explain the difficulties that children with ASD experience in reading emotional expressions. Some evidence for increased reliance on mouth information and less sensitivity for the eyes was already found ([16, 27, 35, 36], but also see, e.g., [37]). A disturbed attention pattern might affect emotion recognition performance most strongly in emotions where information of the eyes is more crucial. Research in typical individuals provided evidence for a distinction between top-emotions (most salient information in the eyes region) and bottom-emotions (most salient information in the mouth region). Behavioral research in adults demonstrated that the recognition of sadness, anger, and fear mostly relies on information in the eyes region, and the recognition of happiness and disgust relies on information in the mouth region ([38], Experiment 1). More recently, eye-movement studies also demonstrated that the most characteristic face regions (top or bottom) depend on nature of the emotional expression [39–41].

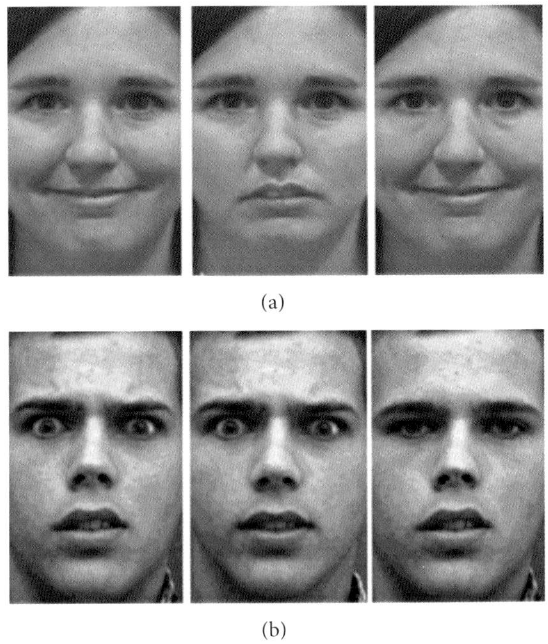

Figure 1: Representative sample stimulus of bottom-emotion happiness (a) and top-emotion fear (b), from left to right: original expression, hybrid expression with neutral mouth, and hybrid expression with neutral eyes (the pictures used in our paper are part of the California Facial Expression database, which is freely available online for research purpose. For more information regarding this database, we refer you to their website: http://cseweb.ucsd.edu/users/gary/CAFE/readme.txt).

Using an emotion labeling task with hybrid stimuli, we wanted to compare the reliance on eyes versus mouth information in children with and without ASD when recognizing emotional expressions. Hence the original expressions of anger, fear, happiness, and sadness and neutral expressions were shown together with their hybrid counterparts. The hybrid facial expressions used here are computer-morphed emotional expressions with the upper (or lower) face half being replaced by a neutral expression, such that emotional information is only available in the mouth (or eyes, resp.) region (see Figure 1 for an example). The generation of hybrid facial stimuli is a rather novel technique with some significant benefits in comparison to eye-movement studies. Whereas both methods aim at evaluating automatic and implicit emotion recognition strategies, the most salient advantage of hybrid stimuli is a practical one. An expensive eye-tracking setup is obviously not required, making the experimental design easier to implement, and also significantly reduces the burden on participants. The data obtained within the context of an eye-movement experiment are clearly richer, yet much more difficult and less clear-cut to process. In addition to these more pragmatic advantages of using hybrid stimuli, an important methodological difference is the active manipulation of available information in hybrid expressions. Showing full facial expressions allows participants to (freely) scan the whole picture. However, this is impossible when using hybrid expressions, simply because no all emotional information is

Table 1: Demographic characteristics of both participant groups: means (M) and standard deviations (SD) for age (expressed in months), full-scale IQ, and ADI-R scores. Group differences in age or IQ were evaluated with independent samples t-tests (homoscedasticity assumption checked with F-test).

	ASD group (n = 22)		Comparison group (n = 22)		Group comparison	
	M (SD)	Range	M (SD)	Range	2-sided t-test	P value
Age	92.14 (10.54)	75–106	95.36 (8.16)	79–107	1.11	.2483
Full-scale IQ	94.36 (11.93)	78–119	98.50 (7.78)	84–108	1.39	.1816
ADI-R scores	44.50 (12.59)	15–65	N/A	N/A		N/A
Communication	15.68 (5.27)	3–24				
Social	20.45 (5.63)	8–28				
Repetitive behaviors	5.41 (2.65)	1–9				

available. Clearly, both paradigms offer a slightly different perspective on the evaluation of saliency of upper versus lower facial areas. Eye-movement studies indeed provide a stronger indication of spontaneous viewing strategies, but the drawback is that participants can adapt their viewing style, with both strategies being impossible to disentangle. Hybrid facial expressions, on the other hand, offer the opportunity to evaluate the reliance on a specific face half when recognizing emotions, by comparing performances on full expressions and their hybrid counterparts. Studies using face parts, such as, for instance, the part-whole paradigm or composite face illusions, also actively intervene in the available information. However, the lack of naturalness is a major disadvantage of using face parts. The processing of these nonfacial and artificial stimuli might be unnatural anyway, not telling us much about (full) face perception.

This study had two goals. We firstly wanted to evaluate whether children with ASD would experience difficulties when labeling four basic emotional expressions and a neutral expression. Secondly, we aimed at comparing eyes versus mouth reliance between children with and without ASD. If typically developing children mostly relied on information in the eyes region, they were expected to experience more difficulties recognizing a hybrid expression with neutral eyes, and especially for those emotions with more characteristic features in the eyes region (top-emotions), such as fear, anger, and sadness. An attenuated bias for the eyes region in the ASD group, or in increased reliance on the mouth area, would result in the reverse pattern. The ASD sample would then be mostly impaired when recognizing hybrid expressions with neutral mouths, and especially for bottom-emotions which have more salient features in the mouth area, such as happiness.

2. Methods

2.1. Participants. Two groups of six-to-eight-year-old boys without an intellectual disability (IQ $\geq$ 70) participated in this study: an experimental group and a matched comparison group. The experimental group consisted of 22 boys with ASD, recruited through the child psychiatry unit at the university hospital (n = 16) and through a special needs school for children with ASD (n = 6). They all received a formal clinical diagnosis of ASD based on a comprehensive assessment by a multidisciplinary team (first subgroup) or by a medical specialist (second subgroup), and according to DSM-IV-TR criteria [2]. Clinical diagnoses were confirmed within the research protocol using the Autism Diagnostic Interview-Revised (ADI-R; [42]) and by file review by a child psychiatrist experienced in ASD. Whereas all diagnoses were confirmed based on file review, all but two participants scored above cut-off on the reciprocal social interactions and the language/communication ADI-R domains. Four additional patients did not meet the restrictive and repetitive behaviors ADI-R domain. In the ASD group, full-scale IQ was measured within the recent clinical diagnostic protocol using the Wechsler Scales of Intelligence (WISC-III-R; [43]) or the Snijders-Oomen Non-Verbal Intelligence Test (SON-R; [44]).

The comparison group comprised 22 typically developing boys (TD group), representative for the general population, and recruited through two mainstream schools. Within the experimental protocol, full-scale IQ was estimated based on an abbreviated version of the WISC-III-R [45], comprising four subtests (vocabulary, similarities, picture arrangement, and block design). The ASD and TD groups were groupwise matched based on age and full-scale IQ (for detailed participant characteristics and group comparisons, see Table 1).

2.2. Materials. Black-and-white photographs of twelve adult faces (seven males and five females) were selected from the California Facial Expressions database [46]. These stimuli were posed according to the Facial Action Coding System (FACS; [47]) and were normalized for the location of eyes and mouth. Hybrid facial expressions were created with Adobe Photoshop. In a hybrid expression, the upper (or lower) face part is replaced by a neutral upper (or lower) face of the same actor. For every emotion-identity combination, two types of hybrid expressions were made: one in which the upper part was replaced by a neutral expression ("hybrid with neutral eyes") and one in which the lower part was replaced by a neutral expression ("hybrid with neutral mouth"). The clone sample tool was used as smoothing tool to mask the lines between both face halves (see Figure 1 for an example).

Five different facial expressions were used: one neutral expression and four emotional faces, expressing happiness, sadness, anger, and fear. Based upon a pilot study (with six TD children and eight TD adults), the three (out of four) best recognizable emotions were selected for every actor, in such a way that, in total, all emotional expressions were presented the same number of times (i.e., all four emotions were presented nine times).

2.3. Procedure and Design. Approval by the Medical Ethical Committee of the University Hospital was obtained and the participants' parents gave their written informed consent before start. All participants were tested individually in a quiet room. Stimuli were presented on a portable computer with a 38 cm screen, at a viewing distance of approximately 76 cm. Stimuli were presented within the E-prime environment. The experimental procedure followed a step-by-step protocol, including a phase wherein participants were made familiar with the different response alternatives and their understanding of the (emotion) labels was checked. This was done by asking for an example situation for the different emotions. If participants could not provide a correct example situation, the experimenter presented a standard example, as outlined in the protocol. Children were instructed to label the facial expressions. All participants understood the task and the emotion labels. Trials consisted of a face stimulus (presented at the left side) and the response alternatives (presented at the right side). Participants responded verbally or by pointing to the label at the screen. Experimenters always entered the participant's response. In between two trials a blank screen with fixation cross was presented for one second. The face stimuli were presented with an unlimited presentation time.

In total, this experiment consisted of 120 trials, so that each expression was presented 10 times per identity: 12 neutral facial expressions (1 per identity) + 36 original emotional expressions (3 emotions × 12 identities) + 72 hybrid emotional expressions (3 emotions × 12 identities × 2 hybrid types, namely, neutral mouth and neutral eyes). Trial order was randomized.

2.4. Data and Data Analysis. All analyses were performed with SAS. Split-plot ANOVAs were conducted on accuracy scores. Accuracy data for the original expressions were analyzed separately, with group (ASD-TD group) as between-subjects factor and expression (neutral-happiness-sadness-anger-fear) as within-subjects factor. In a second analysis, all versions, the hybrid and the original expressions, were analyzed, with the neutral expressions being omitted from these analyses because they had no hybrid counterpart. Again, a split-plot ANOVA with group (ASD-TD group) as between-subjects factor and emotional expression (happiness-sadness-anger-fear) and hybrid type (hybrid neutral mouth-hybrid neutral eyes-original emotional expression) as within-subjects factors was conducted for accuracy data. A significance level of $P < .05$ (two-sided) was adopted, and effects with a P value between .05 and .10 were indicated as marginally significant.

All analyses performed on the whole ASD group ($n = 22$) yielded similar results as analyses with the subgroup of ASD participants who scored above the cut-off on the social and communication domain of the ADI-R ($n = 20$), or on those participants who scored above cut-off on all ADI-R domains ($n = 16$). Therefore, we will report the results of the analyses on the whole group.

TABLE 2: Accurate labeling of the expressions for both participant groups: mean accuracy and standard deviation (between brackets).

	ASD	TD
Anger	.71 (.22)	.67 (.26)
Fear	.76 (.21)	.75 (.21)
Happiness	.92 (.11)	.98 (.04)
Neutral	.60 (.31)	.76 (.13)
Sadness	.52 (.23)	.56 (.26)

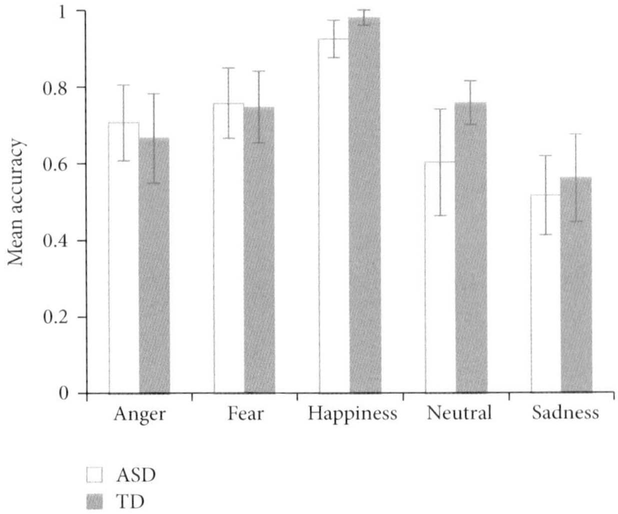

FIGURE 2: Mean performances for both participant groups on the different original expressions (error bars represent 95% confidence intervals of the means).

3. Results

3.1. Recognition of the Original Expressions and Relationship with Age, Full-Scale IQ, or ASD Severity. Results (see Table 2) indicated a main effect of expression ($F(4,168) = 27.28$, $P < .0001$, see Figure 2). Post hoc Tukey-Kramer tests ($\alpha = .05$) revealed that sadness ($M = .54$) was overall recognized less accurately than all other emotions, and happiness ($M = .95$) was overall recognized more accurately than all other emotions. We did not find evidence for a main effect of participant group ($F(1,42) = 1.14$, $P = .29$) and the participant group-by-expression-interaction was not significant either ($F(4,168) = 1.69$, $P = .15$).

No evidence for a correlation between emotion recognition and age, intelligence, or ASD traits (measured with the ADI-R) was found (all correlations with P values > .10).

3.2. Which Face Region Is Used to Recognize Emotional Expressions: Mouth or Eyes? Again, sadness was recognized less accurately (across group and hybrid type) than the other expressions, and happiness was the best recognized emotion ($F(3,126) = 34.35$, $P < .0001$; post-hoc Tukey-Kramer tests). Evidence for a main effect of hybrid type was also found ($F(2,84) = 78.14$, $P < .0001$), such that original stimuli were recognized the most accurate, and hybrid expressions with neutral eyes were recognized the least accurate. Interestingly,

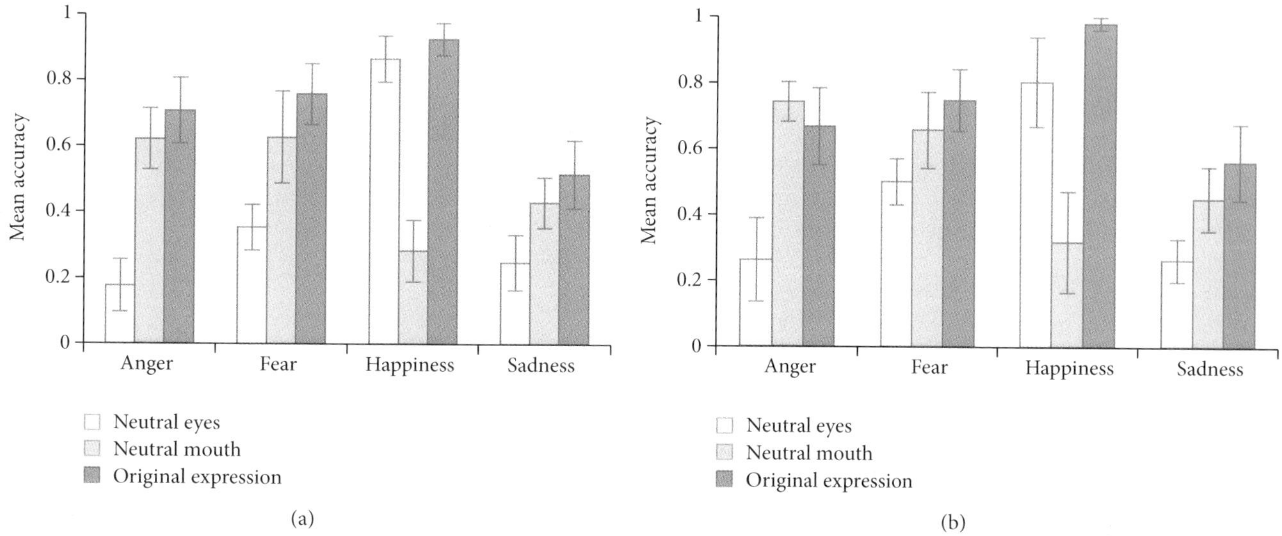

FIGURE 3: The effect of stimulus presentation (hybrid expression with neutral eyes, hybrid expression with neutral mouth, and original expression) on emotion recognition performance was similar in both the ASD group (a) and in the TD group (b). Happiness is a bottom-emotion; sadness, anger, and fear are top-emotions. Error bars represent 95% confidence intervals of the means.

the interaction between emotion and hybrid type was highly significant ($F(6,252) = 57.28$, $P < .0001$), indicating that the most characteristic region (eyes or mouth) is emotion-dependent. Post hoc Bonferroni adjusted tests supported the distinction between top-emotions (anger, fear, and sadness) and bottom-emotions (happiness). Moreover, these tests indicated that adding the other, less characteristic face half did not significantly improve the performance (i.e., no statistically significant difference between the recognition of original expressions and the most salient hybrid ones).

The main effect of participant group was not significant ($F(1,42) = 2.31$, $P = .14$), nor were the interactions between participant group and emotion, or between participant group and hybrid type (all $F < 1$). Contrary to our expectations, the 3-way interaction among participant group, emotion, and hybrid type was not significant ($F(6,252) = 1.59$, $P = .15$, depicted in Figure 3 and Table 3). This suggests that both children with and without ASD show a similar distinction between expressions for which the mouth region contains the most salient information (bottom-emotions) and expressions for which the eyes region is the most informative (top-emotions).

TABLE 3: Accurate labeling of the hybrid expressions for both participant groups: mean accuracy and standard deviation (between brackets).

Emotion	Hybrid type	ASD	TD
Anger	Neutral eyes	.18 (.18)	.26 (.29)
	Neutral mouth	.62 (.21)	.74 (.13)
	Original	.71 (.22)	.67 (.26)
Fear	Neutral eyes	.35 (.16)	.50 (.16)
	Neutral mouth	.63 (.32)	.66 (.26)
	Original	.76 (.21)	.75 (.21)
Happiness	Neutral eyes	.86 (.16)	.80 (.31)
	Neutral mouth	.28 (.21)	.32 (.35)
	Original	.92 (.11)	.98 (.04)
Sadness	Neutral eyes	.25 (.19)	.26 (.15)
	Neutral mouth	.43 (.17)	.45 (.22)
	Original	.52 (.23)	.56 (.26)

4. Discussion

The goal of this research was to investigate (1) whether children with ASD were impaired in recognizing facial expressions of four basic emotions and a neutral one and (2) whether children with ASD tend to rely more on features in the lower part of the face (mouth region) when recognizing emotions. We evaluated this with a novel stimulus generation technique, namely, hybrid expressions, hereby actively manipulating the amount of emotional information available in the face stimulus. A computer-morphed facial expression was generated, with the upper (or lower) face half being replaced by a neutral expression, such that emotional information is only present in the other face half (lower or upper region, resp.).

No impairment in the recognition of angry, happy, sad, and fearful and neutral original expressions was found in children with ASD, compared to an age- and IQ-matched group of TD children. Both participant groups performed well above chance on these original expressions, which indicated that our stimulus selection was successful. Indeed, it was necessary for this study to use expressions with a high recognition rate, so that correct identification was still feasible based on a reduced amount of information (when recognizing the hybrid emotions). Although some studies found children with ASD to be outperformed by TD children in basic emotion recognition tasks, nowadays it has been generally accepted that children with ASD (without intellectual disability) mostly succeed in structured emotion processing tasks, using basic and easily recognizable stimuli [3]. In line with this, a challenge for future applied research is to develop experimental procedures that can tap into the more profound understanding of the meaning of emotions. Besides, one should evaluate whether existing emotion training programs for children with ASD teach them more than mere labelling the basic affects correctly.

Interestingly, we found an interaction between emotion and hybrid type, providing evidence for the existence of top- and bottom-emotions in children. Mouth information holds crucial information to correctly identify the emotion happiness. For the emotions anger, fear, and sadness, the most salient information is located in the region of the eyes. Hereby we nicely replicate and extend the previously demonstrated distinction between top- and bottom-emotions to a group of children with and without a developmental disorder (studies in adults: [38–40]). At the same time, this effect demonstrates that the experiment had sufficient statistical power to pick up subtle performance differences. Moreover, it proves that this method—using hybrid stimuli—is valuable for a coarse evaluation of attentional bias, without the need for eye-movement registration.

In general, original expressions were recognized more accurately than hybrid faces with neutral eyes and hybrid faces with neutral mouth. However, this effect can be mainly attributed to the apparent overrepresentation of top-emotions in the stimulus selection. In addition, providing the most salient or relevant emotional information (mouth or eyes region, for bottom- and top-emotions, resp.) is not only sufficient for a successful identification of the expression, but moreover, adding more emotional cues (namely, the other face half), does not cause a significant increase in performance level. Although it must be noted that a trend in that direction is visible in both groups. These findings could suggest that both groups of children did not integrate emotional information across both face parts, depending mostly on a more local analysis of the salient regions. Since our participant group consisted of young children—all the participants were younger than 10 years—it could indeed be that they tend to use a more feature-based recognition strategy in daily life too. However, it should be noted that the age at which children shift from using a primarily feature-based representation for faces to more holistic encoding processes is not uncontroversial [48, 49]. Although there are inconsistencies, some studies suggest that children with ASD use a more feature-based face processing strategy (for a recent overview, see [20]), which is in line with the neurocognitive theories attributing an atypical, more locally biased perceptual style to individuals with ASD (for two different views on this topic, see [50, 51]). Further research is necessary to explore the role of holistic processing in the emotion recognition in individuals with ASD and the developmental trajectory of this evolution.

This study did not provide evidence for the use of an atypical emotion recognition strategy in children with ASD: children with ASD were not found to rely more on information in the lower part of the face in comparison to TD children. These findings contrast with those of previous work which argued for the higher reliance on the mouth region in children with ASD ([16, 27, 35, 36], and also see, e.g., [37]). Apparent inconsistencies could be explained by several factors. Stimulus-specific aspects probably play an important role. Previous studies attributed a crucial influence to stimulus complexity, and most importantly, the embedding of the facial stimulus in a social context [3, 18]. It was sometimes suggested that the increased fixation on mouths can be linked to speech perception: children with ASD, and especially the group of children without language disorder, focused on the mouth region as a compensatory mechanism for their difficulties in processing eye information [52]. The use of dynamic and auditory material is consistent with the proposal that more naturalistic and ecologically valid paradigms should be developed in ASD research [27]. In addition, most previous work did not make a distinction between viewing patterns for different expressions, hereby disregarding that the significance of information in the eyes or mouth region could be strongly emotion dependent, as suggested by the difference between top- and bottom-emotions. In addition, compensatory mechanisms could also cause inconsistencies. Although one of the advantages of using hybrid stimuli is the fact that you get an insight into the implicit processing strategies, more cognition- or language-mediated compensatory mechanisms cannot be fully excluded. The unlimited presentation time (which maybe gave the children the time to use compensation strategies), the fact that the experimental group consisted of children without intellectual disability (deficits are more often found in younger children and in children with intellectual disability), the multiple choice response format, the types of stimuli, and the use of basic emotions, could make children to use these compensation strategies. One child, for example, commented while viewing an angry expression that "the eyebrows are turned downwards so this must be angry." Please note that it is nearly impossible to exclude the possibility that the ASD sample used a more time-consuming, less efficient processing strategy. One could argue that designs with a limited presentation time partially exclude this. However, a confusion is created in these instances: it becomes very hard to distinguish between task difficulty and the use of time-consuming compensatory mechanisms. Whenever participants fail at a task using shorter presentation times, it becomes unclear whether this is due to the increased difficulty as such or because of an atypical default processing manner (i.e., a compensation strategy).

Employing an emotion labeling task with static emotional expressions, we found no evidence for an emotion recognition impairment in six-to-eight-year-olds with ASD. Furthermore, using hybrid stimuli, we demonstrated that the face region providing the most salient information is strongly emotion dependent. We hereby extended research findings on top- and bottom-emotions to children with and without a developmental disorder. This factor should be taken into account in future research, and the distinction between top- and bottom-emotions and the impact hereof on scanning patterns should be evaluated. In addition, we showed that coarse attention patterns can be evaluated with this innovative stimulus manipulation technique, which does not require eye-movement registration. Lastly, no evidence for a stronger mouth reliance in ASD was found in our task. Future research needs to investigate whether the same holds for more complex emotions and for emotions where information of both the upper and lower parts is required to achieve good recognition.

Acknowledgments

The authors are grateful to all participating children and their parents, as well as to the participating special needs schools. they would like to acknowledge the assistance in participant recruitment and testing by Eline Verbeke and want to thank Patricia Bijttebier, Wilfried Peeters, and Eline Verbeke for their careful reading and feedback on a previous version of this paper. This research was funded by a Grant of the Flemish government, awarded to Johan Wagemans (METH/02/08), and an Interdisciplinary Grant of KU Leuven, awarded to Jean Steyaert, Johan Wagemans, and Ilse Noens (IDO 08/013). Kris Evers and Inneke Kerkhof are joint first authors.

References

[1] I. Nachson, "On the modularity of face recognition: the riddle of domain specificity," *Journal of Clinical and Experimental Neuropsychology*, vol. 17, no. 2, pp. 256–275, 1995.

[2] American Psychiatric Association, *Diagnostic and Statistical Manual of Mental Disorders*, Washington, DC, USA, 4th edition, 2000.

[3] M. B. Harms, A. Martin, and G. L. Wallace, "Facial emotion recognition in autism spectrum disorders: a review of behavioral and neuroimaging studies," *Neuropsychology Review*, vol. 20, no. 3, pp. 290–322, 2010.

[4] M. Uljarevic and A. Hamilton, "Recognition of emotions in autism: a formal meta-analysis," *Journal of Autism and Developmental Disorders*, vol. 43, no. 7, pp. 1517–1526, 2013.

[5] D. Tantam, L. Monaghan, H. Nicholson, and J. Stirling, "Autistic children's ability to interpret faces: a research note," *Journal of Child Psychology and Psychiatry and Allied Disciplines*, vol. 30, no. 4, pp. 623–630, 1989.

[6] G. Celani, M. W. Battacchi, and L. Arcidiacono, "The understanding of the emotional meaning of facial expressions in people with autism," *Journal of Autism and Developmental Disorders*, vol. 29, no. 1, pp. 57–66, 1999.

[7] M. J. Law Smith, B. Montagne, D. I. Perrett, M. Gill, and L. Gallagher, "Detecting subtle facial emotion recognition deficits in high-functioning Autism using dynamic stimuli of varying intensities," *Neuropsychologia*, vol. 48, no. 9, pp. 2777–2781, 2010.

[8] R. P. Hobson, "The autistic child's appraisal of expressions of emotion: a further study," *Journal of Child Psychology and Psychiatry and Allied Disciplines*, vol. 27, no. 5, pp. 671–680, 1986.

[9] S. Kuusikko, H. Haapsamo, E. Jansson-Verkasalo et al., "Emotion recognition in children and adolescents with autism spectrum disorders," *Journal of Autism and Developmental Disorders*, vol. 39, no. 6, pp. 938–945, 2009.

[10] M. Prior, B. Dahlstrom, and T.-L. Squires, "Autistic children's knowledge of thinking and feeling states in other people," *Journal of Child Psychology and Psychiatry and Allied Disciplines*, vol. 31, no. 4, pp. 587–601, 1990.

[11] J.-P. Teunisse and B. De Gelder, "Face processing in adolescents with autistic disorder: the inversion and composite effects," *Brain and Cognition*, vol. 52, no. 3, pp. 285–294, 2003.

[12] J. L. Tracy, R. W. Robins, R. A. Schriber, and M. Solomon, "Is emotion recognition impaired in individuals with autism spectrum disorders?" *Journal of Autism and Developmental Disorders*, vol. 41, no. 1, pp. 102–109, 2011.

[13] B. Wright, N. Clarke, J. Jordan et al., "Emotion recognition in faces and the use of visual context Vo in young people with high-functioning autism spectrum disorders," *Autism*, vol. 12, no. 6, pp. 607–626, 2008.

[14] K. Evers, I. Noens, J. Steyaert, and J. Wagemans, "Combining strengths and weaknesses in visual perception of children with an autism spectrum disorder: perceptual matching of facial expressions," *Research in Autism Spectrum Disorders*, vol. 5, no. 4, pp. 1327–1342, 2011.

[15] G. L. Wallace, L. K. Case, M. B. Harms, J. A. Silvers, L. Kenworthy, and A. Martin, "Diminished sensitivity to sad facial expressions in high functioning autism spectrum disorders is associated with symptomatology and adaptive functioning," *Journal of Autism and Developmental Disorders*, vol. 41, no. 11, pp. 1475–1486, 2011.

[16] S. Baron-Cohen, S. Wheelwright, and T. Jolliffe, "Is there a "language of the eyes"? Evidence from normal adults, and adults with autism or Asperger Syndrome," *Visual Cognition*, vol. 4, no. 3, pp. 311–331, 1997.

[17] D. Da Fonseca, A. Santos, D. Bastard-Rosset, C. Rondan, F. Poinso, and C. Deruelle, "Can children with autistic spectrum disorders extract emotions out of contextual cues?" *Research in Autism Spectrum Disorders*, vol. 3, no. 1, pp. 50–56, 2009.

[18] L. Speer, A. Cook, W. McMahon, and E. Clark, "Face processing in children with autism: effects of stimulus contents and type," *Autism*, vol. 11, no. 3, pp. 265–277, 2007.

[19] M. Behrmann, G. Avidan, G. L. Leonard et al., "Configural processing in autism and its relationship to face processing," *Neuropsychologia*, vol. 44, no. 1, pp. 110–129, 2006.

[20] S. Weigelt, K. Koldewyn, and N. Kanwisher, "Face identity recognition in autism spectrum disorders: a review of behavioral studies," *Neuroscience and Biobehavioral Reviews*, vol. 36, no. 3, pp. 1060–1084, 2012.

[21] T. Langdell, "Recognition of faces: an approach to the study of autism," *Journal of Child Psychology and Psychiatry and Allied Disciplines*, vol. 19, no. 3, pp. 255–268, 1978.

[22] D. M. Riby, G. Doherty-Sneddon, and V. Bruce, "The eyes or the mouth? Feature salience and unfamiliar face processing in Williams syndrome and autism," *Quarterly Journal of Experimental Psychology*, vol. 62, no. 1, pp. 189–203, 2009.

[23] R. M. Joseph, K. Ehrman, R. McNally, and B. Keehn, "Affective response to eye contact and face recognition ability in children with ASD," *Journal of the International Neuropsychological Society*, vol. 14, no. 6, pp. 947–955, 2008.

[24] K. Chawarska and F. Shic, "Looking but not seeing: atypical visual scanning and recognition of faces in 2 and 4-Year-old children with Autism spectrum disorder," *Journal of Autism and Developmental Disorders*, vol. 39, no. 12, pp. 1663–1672, 2009.

[25] W. Jones, K. Carr, and A. Klin, "Absence of preferential looking to the eyes of approaching adults predicts level of social disability in 2-year-old toddlers with autism spectrum disorder," *Archives of General Psychiatry*, vol. 65, no. 8, pp. 946–954, 2008.

[26] R. M. Joseph and J. Tanaka, "Holistic and part-based face recognition in children with autism," *Journal of Child Psychology and*

Psychiatry and Allied Disciplines, vol. 44, no. 4, pp. 529–542, 2003.

[27] A. Klin, W. Jones, R. Schultz, F. Volkmar, and D. Cohen, "Visual fixation patterns during viewing of naturalistic social situations as predictors of social competence in individuals with autism," *Archives of General Psychiatry*, vol. 59, no. 9, pp. 809–816, 2002.

[28] B. Gepner and F. Féron, "Autism: a world changing too fast for a mis-wired brain?" *Neuroscience and Biobehavioral Reviews*, vol. 33, no. 8, pp. 1227–1242, 2009.

[29] K. Pelphrey, J. Goldstein, S. Reznick, J. Piven, T. Allison, and G. McCarthy, "The influence of observed gaze shift context and timing upon activity within the superior temporal sulcus," *Journal of Cognitive Neuroscience*, p. 69, 2002.

[30] J. N. Van Der Geest, C. Kemner, G. Camfferman, M. N. Verbaten, and H. van Engeland, "Looking at images with human figures: comparison between autistic and normal children," *Journal of Autism and Developmental Disorders*, vol. 32, no. 2, pp. 69–75, 2002.

[31] V. Bruce and A. Young, "Understanding face recognition," *The British journal of psychology*, vol. 77, pp. 305–327, 1986.

[32] J. V. Haxby, E. A. Hoffman, and M. I. Gobbini, "The distributed human neural system for face perception," *Trends in Cognitive Sciences*, vol. 4, no. 6, pp. 223–233, 2000.

[33] R. Adolphs, D. Tranel, H. Damasio, and A. Damasio, "Impared recognition of emotion in facial expressions following bilateral damage to the human amygdala," *Nature*, vol. 372, no. 6507, pp. 669–672, 1994.

[34] R. Bruyer, C. Laterre, X. Seron et al., "A case of prosopagnosia with some preserved covert remembrance of familiar faces," *Brain and Cognition*, vol. 2, no. 3, pp. 257–284, 1983.

[35] T. F. Gross, "The perception of four basic emotions in human and nonhuman faces by children with autism and other developmental disabilities," *Journal of Abnormal Child Psychology*, vol. 32, no. 5, pp. 469–480, 2004.

[36] K. Rice, J. M. Moriuchi, W. Jones, and A. Klin, "Parsing heterogeneity in autism spectrum disorders: visual scanning of dynamic social scenes in school-aged children," *Journal of the American Academy of Child and Adolescent Psychiatry*, vol. 51, no. 3, pp. 238–248, 2012.

[37] M. D. Rutherford and A. M. Towns, "Scan path differences and similarities during emotion perception in those with and without autism spectrum disorders," *Journal of Autism and Developmental Disorders*, vol. 38, no. 7, pp. 1371–1381, 2008.

[38] A. J. Calder, A. M. Burton, P. Miller, A. W. Young, and S. Akamatsu, "A principal component analysis of facial expressions," *Vision Research*, vol. 41, no. 9, pp. 1179–1208, 2001.

[39] H. Eisenbarth and G. W. Alpers, "Happy mouth and sad eyes: scanning emotional facial expressions," *Emotion*, vol. 11, no. 4, pp. 860–865, 2011.

[40] M. L. Smith, G. W. Cottrell, F. Gosselin, and P. G. Schyns, "Transmitting and decoding facial expressions," *Psychological Science*, vol. 16, no. 3, pp. 184–189, 2005.

[41] E. Scheller, C. Büchel, and M. Gamer, "Diagnostic features of emotional expressions are processed preferentially," *PLoS ONE*, vol. 7, no. 7, Article ID e41792, 2012.

[42] C. Lord, S. Risi, L. Lambrecht et al., "The Autism Diagnostic Observation Schedule-Generic: a standard measure of social and communication deficits associated with the spectrum of autism," *Journal of Autism and Developmental Disorders*, vol. 30, no. 3, pp. 205–223, 2000.

[43] D. Wechsler, *Wechsler Intelligence Scale for Children*, The Psychological Corporation, London, UK, 3rd edition, 1992.

[44] P. J. Tellegen, J. A. Laros, and M. Winkel, *SON-R 2 1/2-7 Niet-Verbale Intelligentietest*, Hogrefe, Amsterdam, The Netherlands, 2003.

[45] J. Grégoire, *L'Evaluation clinique de l'intelligence de l'enfant: Théorie et pratique du WISC-III*, Mardaga, Sprimont, Belgium, 2000.

[46] M. N. Dailey, G. W. Cottrell, and J. Reilly, "California Facial Expressions (CAFE)," Computer Science and Engineering Departement, UCSD, La Jolla, Calif, USA, 2001, http://www.cs.ucsd.edu/users/gary/CAFE/.

[47] P. Ekman and W. V. Friesen, *The Facial Action Coding System (FACS): A Technique for the Measurement of Facial Action*, Consulting Psychologists Press, Palo Alto, Calif, USA, 1978.

[48] E. Pellicano and G. Rhodes, "Holistic processing of faces in preschool children and adults," *Psychological Science*, vol. 14, no. 6, pp. 618–622, 2003.

[49] S. Carey and R. Diamond, "Are faces perceived as configurations? More by adults than by children?" *Visual Cognition*, vol. 1, no. 2/3, pp. 253–274, 1994.

[50] F. Happé and U. Frith, "The weak coherence account: detail-focused cognitive style in autism spectrum disorders," *Journal of Autism and Developmental Disorders*, vol. 36, no. 1, pp. 5–25, 2006.

[51] L. Mottron, M. Dawson, I. Soulières, B. Hubert, and J. Burack, "Enhanced perceptual functioning in autism: an update, and eight principles of autistic perception," *Journal of Autism and Developmental Disorders*, vol. 36, no. 1, pp. 27–43, 2006.

[52] C. F. Norbury, J. Brock, L. Cragg, S. Einav, H. Griffiths, and K. Nation, "Eye-movement patterns are associated with communicative competence in autistic spectrum disorders," *Journal of Child Psychology and Psychiatry and Allied Disciplines*, vol. 50, no. 7, pp. 834–842, 2009.

4

Preliminary Efficacy of Adapted Responsive Teaching for Infants at Risk of Autism Spectrum Disorder in a Community Sample

Grace T. Baranek, Linda R. Watson, Lauren Turner-Brown, Samuel H. Field, Elizabeth R. Crais, Linn Wakeford, Lauren M. Little, and J. Steven Reznick

University of North Carolina at Chapel Hill, Chapel Hill, NC 27599-7122, USA

Correspondence should be addressed to Grace T. Baranek; gbaranek@med.unc.edu

Academic Editor: Herbert Roeyers

This study examined the (a) feasibility of enrolling 12-month-olds at risk of ASD from a community sample into a randomized controlled trial, (b) subsequent utilization of community services, and (c) potential of a novel parent-mediated intervention to improve outcomes. The First Year Inventory was used to screen and recruit 12-month-old infants at risk of ASD to compare the effects of 6–9 months of Adapted Responsive Teaching (ART) versus referral to early intervention and monitoring (REIM). Eighteen families were followed for ~20 months. Assessments were conducted before randomization, after treatment, and at 6-month follow-up. Utilization of community services was highest for the REIM group. ART significantly outperformed REIM on parent-reported and observed measures of child receptive language with good linear model fit. Multiphase growth models had better fit for more variables, showing the greatest effects in the active treatment phase, where ART outperformed REIM on parental interactive style (less directive), child sensory responsiveness (less hyporesponsive), and adaptive behavior (increased communication and socialization). This study demonstrates the promise of a parent-mediated intervention for improving developmental outcomes for infants at risk of ASD in a community sample and highlights the utility of earlier identification for access to community services earlier than standard practice.

1. Introduction

The rising prevalence of autism spectrum disorder (ASD) [1] and relatively late age of diagnosis for a neurodevelopmental disorder of early onset [2, 3] highlight the need for more efficacious methods of identifying and intervening with infants at risk of a later diagnosis of ASD. Early identification and intervention can serve to optimize developmental outcomes, decrease disability, and ultimately reduce associated burdens on families and society. In the United States, federal law mandates state agencies to administer early intervention (EI) services under Part C of the Individuals with Disabilities Education Act [4]; however, state eligibility criteria vary tremendously and, in most cases, infants at risk for ASD are not eligible for these services unless they have an established condition (e.g., clinical diagnosis) and/or a significant level (e.g., >25%) of developmental delay on standardized assessments [5].

Moreover, physicians typically do not screen for ASD prior to 18–24 months of age and are reluctant to make referrals to EI without evidence of available and efficacious treatments for such young children [6–8]. Although some studies with toddlers (ages 15–36 months) fail to show significant effects of tested interventions on child language, cognition, or ASD symptoms [9–11], growing evidence shows that early behavioral interventions are beneficial for some toddlers with clear ASD symptoms [12–16]. However, intervention studies differ vastly in terms of design, content, format, intensity, time course, age at enrollment, and their outcome measures and moderating variables, which obfuscates the key ingredients responsible for positive outcomes. More research utilizing strong comparison groups would help to determine benefits of specific treatments [17], and integrating the perspectives of families and other stakeholders is needed to help translate promising interventions into community settings [18].

Five published randomized controlled trials (RCTs) specifically included toddlers with ASD < 24 months of age and thus are described further. These studies utilized clinical samples of children with ASD referred from EI programs or clinics and/or high-risk infant siblings. Although the specific approach and context of the interventions (clinic versus in-home) varied, all five studies demonstrated positive effects of early behavioral intervention [12–16]. Specifically, Dawson et al. [13] found evidence that the Early Start Denver Model (ESDM; [19]) was more effective than usual services for improving cognitive and adaptive functioning for 48 children, ages 18–30 months ($M = 23$). ESDM, a relatively high intensity intervention based on principles of applied behavior analysis and developmental strategies, was administered by trained clinicians in the families' homes ~15 hours per week and supplemented by parents over the course of two years.

Landa et al. [15] compared an intervention called interpersonal synchrony against a noninterpersonal synchrony intervention with 50 toddlers ages 20 to 33 months ($M = 28$). Both interventions were provided in a classroom 10 hours per week for 6 months and were supplemented by 38 hours of parent education and 1.5 hours per month of home-based parent training. Children in both groups showed significant gains in social, language, and cognitive outcomes across time, with children in the interpersonal synchrony intervention showing significantly larger gains in socially engaged imitation.

Carter et al. [12] compared a relatively lower intensity behavioral intervention, Hanen's More than Words (HMTW) [20], to services as usual with 62 toddlers ages 15–25 months ($M = 20$). The HMTW program comprised eight group parent training sessions and three individual in-home parent-child sessions provided by speech-language pathologists over ~5 months to teach parents practical communication strategies. Child communication outcomes were moderated by baseline levels of "object interest," such that children with lower levels of object interest fared better with HMTW, whereas those with higher levels of object interest did better in the control condition. These findings suggest that subgroups of children may respond differentially to various types of behavioral interventions.

Kasari et al. [14] applied a wait-list control design with 38 children with ASD ages 21–36 months ($M = 31$) and demonstrated that an 8-week caregiver-mediated intervention was effective for improving some skills (i.e., joint engagement, response to joint attention, and functional play acts) but not others (i.e., initiations to joint attention and diversity in play acts). The immediate treatment group maintained skills one year after treatment. Interestingly, utilization of community EI services was not predictive of outcomes in this relatively short timeframe. Finally, an RCT by Schertz et al. [16] similarly studied the effects of a focused, developmentally sequenced intervention model called Joint Attention Mediated Learning (JAML) on the acquisition of social-communication competencies. They randomized 23 toddlers with ASD all under 30 months of age ($M = 26$ months) and found that the intervention group outperformed the usual services group on observed measures of responding to joint attention and focusing on faces. Intervention x time effects also favored the JAML group on standardized measures of receptive language and functional communication. Although both of the latter joint attention studies used a parent-mediated approach, the Kasari study was conducted in a clinical setting, whereas the JAML was conducted in the families' homes. Overall, despite differences in approach and intensity, all five of these RCTs show positive effects of early behavioral interventions relative to comparison conditions (services as usual in four cases, and an active treatment in Landa et al. [15]) for toddlers with clear symptoms of ASD from clinical populations, particularly for social-communication outcomes. However, no studies have been published that test the effects of a parent-mediated intervention for infants at risk of ASD (before diagnosis) from a nonclinical community population, which is the prime aim of the current study.

Neurodevelopmental theories stress the importance of timing and transactions between genetic susceptibilities to ASD and environmental factors that shape neural connections through experience [2, 3, 22, 23]. These theories, along with evidence that neural shaping processes become highly prevalent at the end of the first year of life [24], lend support to the hypothesis that behavioral interventions beginning as soon as risk for ASD can be detected will be efficacious [25]. Dawson [26] further theorized that prevention of ASD is plausible through new advances in detecting at-risk infants (before the full presentation of the syndrome) and implementing interventions that can alter the course of early behavioral and brain development for at risk infants.

Thus, development of novel and efficacious interventions for infants at risk of a later diagnosis of ASD is needed to test scientific hypotheses and address growing public health issues. Models that are socioculturally and ecologically congruent with the needs of families with very young infants and toddlers, particularly parent-mediated models, need to be considered. Parental responsiveness is a key variable associated with developmental gains in typically developing children as well as for those who are at risk of or who have been diagnosed with developmental disabilities including ASD [27–32]. Furthermore, approaches that are consistent with the guidelines set forth in Part C of the Individuals with Disabilities Education Act [4] (e.g., individualized, conducted in natural environments, and integrated into daily activities) are particularly important for utility in community EI settings. No RCTs have been published that demonstrate the efficacy of such parent-mediated interventions for very young infants and toddlers (<18 months) specifically at risk of a later diagnosis of ASD in a nonclinical sample.

This study aimed at (a) establishing the feasibility of enrolling 12-month-olds at risk of ASD in a community sample into an intervention study, (b) describing families' subsequent utilization of community EI services, and (c) evaluating the potential of a novel parent-mediated intervention, called "Adapted Responsive Teaching" (ART), to improve parental responsiveness as well as children's developmental outcomes. Empirical evidence clearly links early pivotal behaviors (e.g., social play, joint attention, arousal and attention, engagement, adaptability, and coping), similar to those used in ART, to later outcomes in children with and/or without ASD [33–37]. Thus, we hypothesized that

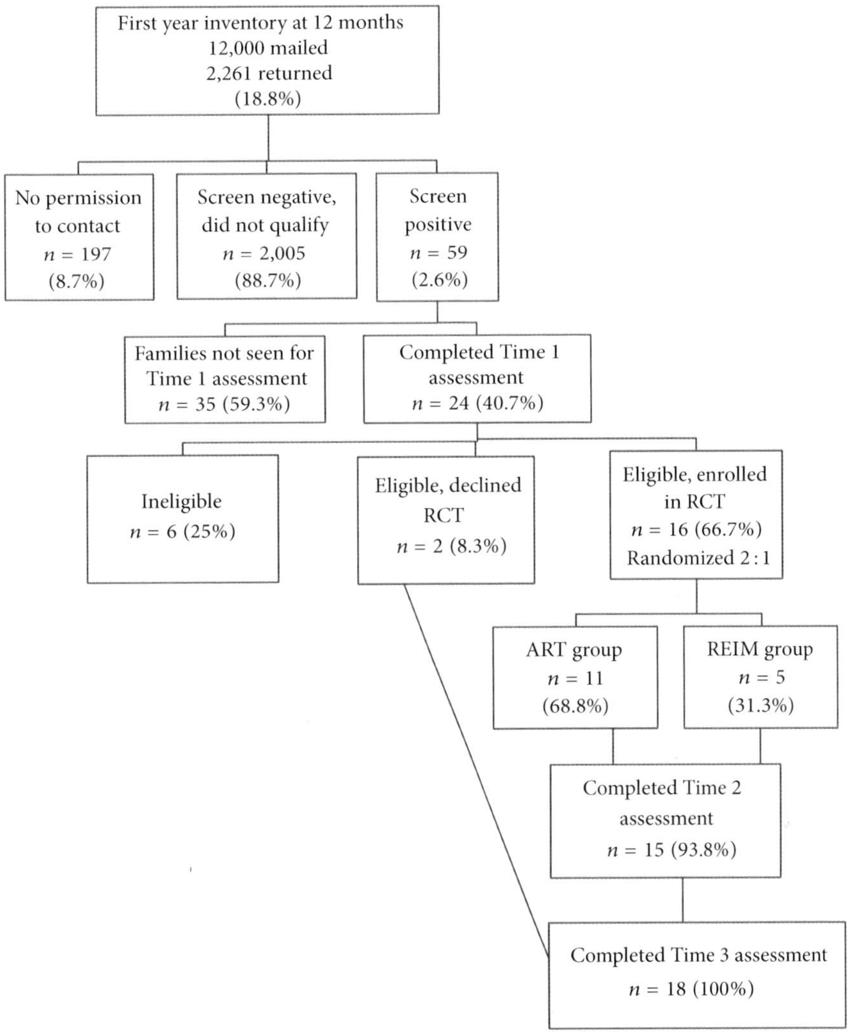

FIGURE 1: Study flow chart with participation rates for each phase.

parents in the ART group, as compared to a "referral to early intervention and monitoring" (REIM) group, would be more responsive and less directive during parent-child free-play interactions. We also hypothesized that ART would improve the infants' pivotal behaviors in two domains—social-communication and sensory-regulatory functions—and that these effects would be evident at both outcome assessments (immediately after treatment and at later follow-up). We also explored ASD diagnostic outcomes to generate hypotheses for future studies.

2. Method

This prospective behavioral intervention study employed a two-part procedure across ~20 months: (1) screening and ascertainment of 12-month-old infants at risk of a later diagnosis of ASD from a community sample using the First Year Inventory, version 2.0 (FYI) [38], with subsequent referral to the community EI system, and (2) enrollment of eligible parent-infant dyads into a randomized controlled trial (RCT) to investigate the preliminary efficacy of ART versus REIM and track utilization of community EI services through the duration of the study for all participants. Both ART and REIM groups received a battery of standardized assessments at each of three time points: before randomization (Time 1, around 14 months), postintervention phase (Time 2, around 22 months), and diagnostic follow-up (Time 3, around 32 months). Eligible families who declined randomization were assessed only at Time 1 and Time 3. Figure 1 presents a flow chart detailing the study phases and participation rates at each phase. Linear and multiphase growth models were used to compare the two groups in the RCT phase on outcome variables of interest. The quantity and types of community EI services and diagnostic outcomes were analyzed descriptively for all participants.

2.1. Ascertainment and Recruitment of Infants at Risk of a Later Diagnosis of ASD Using FYI. Approximately 12,000 FYI screening packets were mailed to families in the catchment area on the basis of birth registry records ~2 weeks prior to the child's first birthday across a 15-month time span. The catchment area included 5 counties in central North Carolina

(NC) representing both rural and urban areas. Hispanic surnames were excluded from the mailing due to the lack of availability of Spanish language FYI and ART protocols. A letter in the packet informed parents of the purpose of our study (i.e., screening for risk for autism and related developmental disorders; potential eligibility for an RCT). This recruitment strategy ensured a broader at-risk sample than one relying solely on genetically high risk younger infant siblings of children with ASD. A total of 2,261 FYIs were completed and returned by families, representing a 19% response rate. The purpose of this screening was to identify a cohort of infants from a community sample that had sufficient risk markers deemed eligible to participate in the RCT. This was not intended as an epidemiological study of screening procedures or a psychometric study of tool development; see Turner-Brown et al. [39] for details of FYI validation in a community sample, which indicated the 12-month-olds receiving at risk scores on the FYI that had a 31% chance of obtaining an ASD diagnosis by three years of age.

Families of infants who met one of the following risk criteria were invited to participate in a comprehensive developmental assessment (Time 1, before randomization) to confirm risk status: (1) infants with an FYI risk score at or above the 95th percentile, (2) infants with an FYI risk score at or above the 90th percentile with documented parent concerns in the core ASD symptom areas, and (3) any infant whose parent indicated a family history of autism spectrum disorder (ASD). Children were excluded from further study if their parents reported significant vision or hearing impairments, Down syndrome, cerebral palsy, and/or significant prematurity (<2500 grams at birth), regardless of whether or not they met FYI algorithm cut-points. A total of 59 children met preliminary inclusion criteria. Twenty-eight families agreed to participate in the Time 1 assessment, but four subsequently cancelled, yielding 24 (40.1%). Thirty-one families were either unreachable or declined the opportunity to participate further.

2.2. Time 1 Baseline Prerandomization Assessment. Following parental written consent, 24 infants completed a baseline developmental assessment in a family friendly assessment suite in a community adjacent to the university campus. Measures used in the assessment are explicated below. An eligibility algorithm was developed to ensure that only children with clear delays or concerns related to ASD (based on a combination of parent report and observational measures) were invited to enroll in the intervention phase of the study. This algorithm took into account all Time 1 measures (see below) and deemed eligible any infant who (1) met ASD cutoffs on diagnostic measures (i.e., AOSI $\geq$ 7, and/or ADOS-T $\geq$ 12), and/or (2) showed delays in 2/3 domains of social-communication [i.e., expressive, receptive, and social/play as measured by the MSEL ($T < 40$), CSBS (SS < 7), MCDI (<15%), and ITSEA (rated "of concern")], and/or (3) showed disruptions in 2/3 domains of sensory-regulatory functions [i.e., sensory processing, regulatory processing, and repetitive/atypical behaviors, as measured by the SPA (>1.5 s.d. above norm for age), SEQ (>1.5 s.d. above norm for age), and ITSEA (rated "of concern")]. Families received the results via an interpretive conference and a written report.

2.3. Enrollment and Randomization of Eligible Participants into the RCT Intervention Phase. Infant-parent dyads were recruited into the RCT by the project coordinator following the Time 1 assessment if they met eligibility criteria above. Of the 24 infants who completed a Time 1 assessment, six (25%) did not meet full eligibility criteria; thus, their families were not offered enrollment in this phase. The remaining 18 infants met eligibility criteria and sixteen of these families (88.9%) subsequently signed consent and were enrolled into the RCT intervention phase. All 18 also were referred to local community EI services.

Randomization of parent-infant dyads was conducted using a random number generator in Excel by an investigator blind to the assessment results. Given the small sample size and our primary aim to test the promise of a novel intervention, a 2 : 1 randomization procedure was used [40]. Thus, a total of 11 dyads were randomized into ART and 5 were randomized into the REIM condition. The project coordinator notified the families of their assignment following randomization and answered any questions. The two eligible families that declined participation in the RCT (intervention phase) agreed to complete the final diagnostic follow-up assessment (Time 3) and thus were included in the descriptive data on diagnostic outcomes. Demographics for these 18 families are provided in Table 1.

2.4. Assessments/Measures (All Participants)

The First Year Inventory (FYI) [38]. It is a 63-item parent-report screener used to identify infants at risk of ASD at 12 months. Item/scoring details are available elsewhere [41]. It has a positive predictive value of .31 [39]. The FYI was the primary screening measure for recruiting infants into the study.

The Mullen Scales of Early Learning (MSEL) [42]. It is a standardized developmental assessment for birth of 58 months. It has 4 scales (Fine Motor, Visual Reception, Receptive, and Expressive Language). Two outcomes of interest (Receptive and Expressive T scores) were analyzed at Times 1, 2, and 3.

The Vineland Adaptive Behavior Scales, Second Edition (VABS-II) [43]. It is a parent interview that assesses adaptive behaviors. The Parent/Caregiver Rating Form was used. Standard scores were computed for the three outcomes of interest: communication (breaking out receptive and expressive), and socialization at Times 1, 2, and 3.

The Communication and Symbolic Behavior Scale (CSBS) Developmental Profile [44]. It is a standardized, norm-referenced instrument used to assess children with functional communication ages between 6 and 24 months. The Caregiver Questionnaire and Behavior Sample were both computed at Times 1 and 2 to examine communication and symbolic outcomes.

TABLE 1: Participant demographics of RCT eligible families (n = 18).

	ART intervention group (n = 11)	REIM control group (n = 5)	Eligible/Declined group (n = 2)
Chronological age in months			
Range at Time 1	13–17	13–17	17
Mean (SD)	15.22 (1.2)	15.6 (1.3)	17.7 (0.19)
Gender (boys)	9/11	5/5	2/2
Ethnicity (white)	9/11	4/5	1/2
Mother's education			
High school/vocational	1/11	—	—
College	9/11	5/5	1/2
Missing	1/11	—	1/2
MSEL early learning composite mean (SD)	86.6 (18.7)	85.8 (14.1)	81.0 (2.8)
MSEL expressive language age mean (SD)	11.9 (3.7)	10.8 (2.4)	13.5 (2.1)
MSEL receptive language age mean (SD)	13.0 (5.0)	12.8 (4.2)	14.5 (0.7)
MSEL visual reception age mean (SD)	14.9 (3.3)	16.2 (1.9)	17.5 (0.7)

Note: MSEL: Mullen Scales of Early Learning.

The MacArthur-Bates Communicative Development Inventory (MCDI) [45]. It is a standardized, norm-referenced parent report of children's communication skills. The Words and Gestures form for infants aged 8–18 months was used at Time 1 for eligibility assessment.

The Sensory Processing Assessment (SPA) for Young Children [46]. It is a play-based assessment that was used to measure hyperresponsiveness (i.e., approach-avoidance to sensory toys) and hyporesponsiveness (i.e., orienting responses across 3 sensory modalities). It has good interrater reliability (ICC = .91–.99), discriminates between children with ASD and those with other developmental disabilities, and shows sensitivity to maturational change [47, 48]. Summary scores for hyporesponsiveness and hyperresponsiveness were analyzed at Times 1, 2, and 3.

The Sensory Experiences Questionnaire (SEQ), Version 2.1 [49]. It is a 43-item parent questionnaire for children 6 months to 6 years that measures responses to various sensory stimuli in the context of daily activities. The internal consistency is α = .80 [50] and it has good discriminative validity [51]. Summary scores for hyporesponsiveness and hyperresponsiveness were analyzed at Times 1, 2, and 3.

The Infant-Toddler Social Emotional Assessment (ITSEA) [52]. It is a 166-item measure of social-emotional competencies/problems at 12–36 months. It was used for eligibility determinations at Time 1.

The Autism Observation Scale for Infants (AOSI) [53]. It uses 18 markers to identify infants at risk of autism during semistructured play. A total score >7 was used as cut-off at Time 1 for eligibility criteria.

The Autism Diagnostic Observation Schedule (ADOS) [54]. It is a standardized, semistructured assessment used to evaluate social-communication symptoms in children suspected of having ASD. We used either Module 1 or 2 at Time 3 to describe clinical outcomes in this study.

A Parent Diagnostic Interview. It was conducted by the Clinical Psychologist (LTB) with all participants at Time 3. Based upon DSM-IV-TR criteria for autistic disorder, this interview covered early developmental history and diagnostic symptoms in core autism domains. This interview was used to provide parent input to support the clinical diagnosis (if any) assigned by the psychologist.

The Maternal Behavior Rating Scale (MBRS) [55]. It is a 12-item (5 point) rating assessing parent interactive style across 4 factors (or dimensions): responsive/child oriented (sensitivity, responsivity, and effectiveness; 3–15 points), affect/animation (acceptance, enjoyment, expressiveness, inventiveness, warmth; 5–25 points), achievement oriented (achievement, verbal praise; 2–10 points), and directive (directiveness, pace; 2–10 pts). It is sensitive to treatment change [30]. A 10-minute parent-child free-play session with standard toys was videotaped at Times 1, 2, and 3. Ratings were scored from video by a trained coder, blind to group assignment. A second coder scored independently; consensus scores were computed for final analyses for two outcomes—responsive and directive.

A Demographic Form. It was used to document information about the infant/family (e.g., race, ethnicity, gender, education, number/ages of people in the home, and child care arrangements).

A Monthly Status Check and Community Early Intervention Services Interview (MSC). It was conducted each month by the project coordinator with all families. This 15–20 minute session aimed to (a) obtain updates on the infant's general health and developmental status (e.g., doctor visits, medications, and behavior changes), (b) track referrals to and utilization of community EI services (e.g., type, dosage, provider, location, parent trainings, and provider referrals/recommendations and changes in services since previous interview), (c) answer any questions, and (d) provide general support to facilitate community referrals.

2.5. Additional Measures Used with ART Group Only

The Family Routines Exploration and Description Revised (FRED) [56]. It was developed to facilitate intervention planning. This semistructured parent interview examined the child's current level of participation in daily family routines, strategies parents use to support their child in those routines, and parents' satisfaction with their child's participation in those routines.

The ART Interventionist Implementation Fidelity Checklist (IFC). It is adapted from Mahoney and MacDonald [57] and is a 24-item checklist used to measure the extent to which interventionists appropriately engaged parents in ART. Monthly videos with each parent-infant dyad were scored for consensus by two raters. Fidelity was monitored by reviewing videos of sessions once per month for each child; fidelity scores ranged from 80 to 90% across sessions.

The Parent Adherence Rating Form (PARF). It was developed as a 10-item rating of the interventionist's perceptions of parent adherence. It was completed following each intervention session. A percent score was computed and tracked weekly. Strategies and/or pivotal behaviors were reviewed if adherence dropped below 80%. Parent adherence scores were 73–97% across sessions.

The Parent Weekly Log (PWL). It was used to track parent's self-reported ratings of understanding, ease, and success of strategy use on a weekly basis, and when to review specific strategies.

2.6. Intervention Phase Protocols

2.6.1. General Early Intervention Referral Protocol. Following the Time 1 assessment, all infants with established risk factors were referred to the EI program in their county. Following consent and randomization, all services received by families participating in the study were systematically documented (MSC) by the project coordinator who answered general developmental questions and helped families attain access to community resources. This design did not require parents in either group to seek community EI services and did not guarantee that the family would be able to access community EI services under Part C of IDEA.

2.6.2. Referral to Early Intervention and Monitoring (REIM) Group. The REIM group received EI services normally available in the local communities, depending on parent choices, resources, and infant eligibility for publicly funded EI services. They also received monthly phone calls from our project coordinator to answer questions and track their community services as noted above. They received identical assessments on the same schedule (Times 1, 2, and 3) matched to the ART group.

2.6.3. Adapted Responsive Teaching Group. ART is a 6-month relationship-focused, home based intervention aimed at improving parental responsiveness and child developmental outcomes [58] that is based on the responsive teaching curriculum [30, 57]. Research indicates that parents can be taught responsive strategies (e.g., follow child's lead; imitate child, or take one turn and wait) [27] and that relationship-focused programs, particularly ≥6 months, have been associated with positive child outcomes [29, 30, 59–61]. ART employed modeling and coaching to encourage parents to use responsive strategies during daily routines with their children, which were designed to target "pivotal" behaviors (e.g., social play, joint attention, arousal and attention, engagement, adaptability, and coping) shown to benefit later development (e.g., [33–37, 62]).

ART was administered in this preliminary study with the 4 main intervention components depicted in Figure 2. *Pivotal Behavior Intervention Objectives* targeted key child developmental behaviors within the two key domains (i.e., social-communication and sensory-regulatory Functions). *Discussion points* consisted of 135 scripted miniconversations used by interventionists to discuss the rationale of ART with parents (1 or 2 selected per session). *Responsive Teaching Strategies* were taught to parents to use during daily routines to interact with their infants across 5 dimensions (i.e., *reciprocity*, *contingency*, *control*, *affect*, and *match*.). *Family Action Plans* were "follow-through" plans for parents to reflect on, discuss with others, and/or integrate newly learned strategies into interactions with their infants between sessions. ART was adapted from responsive teaching [57] by our team to enhance its appropriateness for one-year-olds at risk of ASD. Specifically, the ART model was redesigned with two domains to match the FYI structure. Pivotal behaviors were streamlined to address a smaller subset of behaviors often observed in infants at risk of ASD. Both content and process were enhanced by adding parent education sessions using adult learning strategies. Also, supporting materials were developed (e.g., FRED; intervention notebook; weekly documentation forms).

Interventionists were three staff members with experience in child development/EI (e.g., therapists, teachers). Session plans were printed for parents weekly. Interventionists documented children's progress and parents' adherence ratings. An intervention coordinator led biweekly meetings with the intervention team and monitored progress.

The target intervention dosage was 36 contacts: 2 in-home sessions per week for the first 6 weeks = 12; 1 home session plus 1 phone call/email contact per week for second 6 weeks = 12; 1 in-home session per week for the last 12 weeks = 12. Thus, intensity was highest in the beginning and was slowly reduced as parents mastered the skills. Interventionists could flexibly increase the number of in-home sessions up to 36 (or 8 mos. maximum) to support higher implementation fidelity. Families in the ART group received an average of 33.5 (range 20–39) total contacts (in-home + phone/email) across a 6- to 8-month period. The average number of in-home

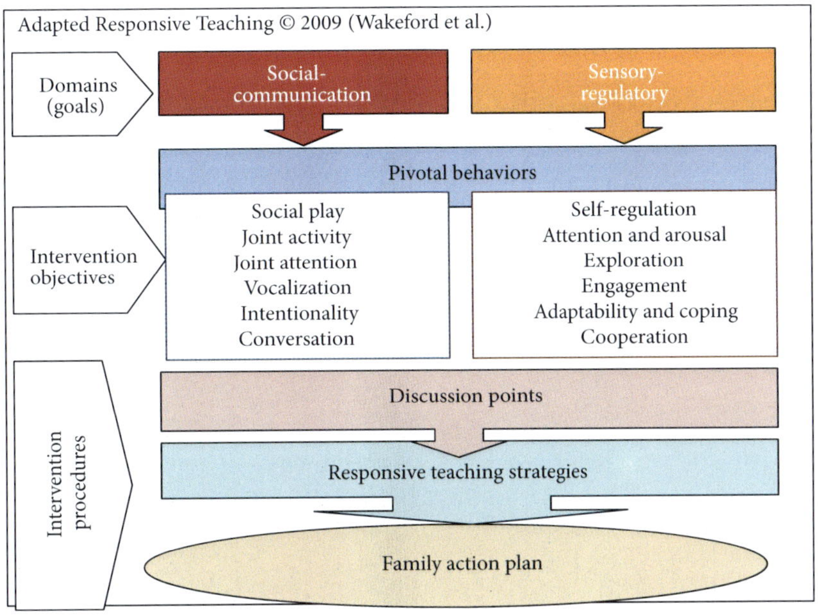

FIGURE 2: Adapted Responsive Teaching (ART) conceptual model.

sessions was 27.6 (range 18–33), and the average number of phone/email contacts was 5.8 (range 2–10).

2.7. Time 2 after Intervention (ART/REIM) and Time 3 Diagnostic Follow-Up Assessments. After concluding the intervention phase (ART or REIM), the toddlers (ages 22–26 months; $M = 23.6$) were scheduled for Time 2 assessments with a multidisciplinary team to measure developmental outcomes (i.e., MSEL, VABS, SEQ, SPA, CSBS, and MBRS). The diagnostic follow-up (Time 3) assessments were conducted ~6 months later (ages 30–35 months; $M = 32.3$) for all toddlers in the RCT as well as the two from the Eligible/Declined group. Time 3 included developmental outcomes but also added the blinded diagnostic evaluation by a clinical psychologist (ADOS + diagnostic interview). The assessment team was blinded to group assignment; parents were instructed to not share information regarding EI services or group assignment. An interpretive conference and a written report were provided to all families. Parents received a $20 gas card per assessment for travel costs. No families dropped out of the RCT; however, one family in the REIM group missed the Time 2 assessment. All 16 families who were enrolled in the RCT completed their Time 3 assessments as did the 2 families from the Eligible/Declined group.

2.8. Statistical Analyses of Treatment Effects. Initial estimates for the unknown parameters from both the linear and multiphase growth models were obtained using maximum likelihood estimation (MLE). The linear model specified that Y_{it} equals an outcome for child i at time t, and T_{it} equals the observed time (in months) from the date of the first assessment. We fit the following hierarchical linear growth model: $Y_{it} = \beta_{0i} + \beta_{1i}T_{it} + \varepsilon_{it}$, where $\varepsilon_{it} \sim N(0, \delta^2)$. The level two (subject) equations were $\beta_{0i} = \gamma_{00} + \mu_{0i}$ for the intercept and $\beta_{1i} = \gamma_{10} + \gamma_{11}D_i + \mu_{1i}$ for the slope; μ_{0i} and μ_{1i} were assumed to follow a multivariate normal distribution. Thus,

$$[\mu_{0i}, \mu_{1i}] \sim MVN\left([0,0], \begin{bmatrix} \tau_{00}^2 & \tau_{01} \\ \tau_{10} & \tau_{11}^2 \end{bmatrix}\right). \quad (1)$$

For each outcome examined, we also estimated a set of models that relaxed the assumption of strictly linear growth over the period observed. Multiphase mixed effects models for repeated measure data assume that growth over time exhibits distinctively different rates of change from one time period to another [63] and requires dividing time into discrete segments or phases. In the current study, growth after the initial assessment until the cessation of intervention (Times 1 to 2) constituted the first phase, that is, active treatment, while the subsequent, postintervention follow-up period (Time 2 to 3) constituted the second phase. Similar to the linear model, the multiphase growth model specified that Y_{it} equals an outcome for child i at time t; however, the time variable only took on discreet values, $\varphi_{it} \in \{1, 2, 3\}$, representing the baseline, posttreatment, and follow-up periods, respectively. We defined two within subject-level regressors:

$$\theta_{1it} = \begin{cases} 0 & \text{if } \varphi_{it} \le 1 \\ 1 & \text{if } \varphi_{it} > 1, \end{cases} \qquad \theta_{2it} = \begin{cases} 0 & \text{if } \varphi_{it} \le 2 \\ 1 & \text{if } \varphi_{it} > 2. \end{cases} \quad (2)$$

The outcome was assumed to be sampled from the following model: $Y_{it} = \beta_{0i} + \beta_{1i}\theta_{1it} + \beta_{2i}\theta_{2it} + \varepsilon_{it}$, where $\varepsilon_{it} \sim N(0, \delta^2)$. The level two (subject) equations were modified slightly from the linear growth model. Because growth was now captured in two parameters, random subject level variation in growth was not fully identified. We therefore only estimated fixed variation in two growth parameters as a function of treatment assignment, $\beta_{1i} = \gamma_{10} + \gamma_{11}D_i$, and $\beta_{2i} = \gamma_{20} + \gamma_{21}D_i$. The

TABLE 2: Dosage of community EI services utilized by groups across study phases.

	ART group	REIM control group	Eligible/Declined group
Number of children receiving community EI services prior to Time 3 (NC state or private), including service coordination	N = 4/11 (36%)	N = 4/5 (80%)	N = 0/2 (0%)
Mean number of hours (range) of community EI services (OT, SLP, PT, feeding, or play therapy/group) between Times 1 and 2	8.78 (0–65)	29.8 (0–62)	0
Mean number of hours (range) of community EI services (OT, SLP, PT, feeding, play therapy/group, and developmental preschool) between Times 2 and 3	13.80 (0–76.3)	154.47 (0–525)	0
Mean number of hours (range) of community EI services total across study from Times 1 through 3.	22.6 (0–93.5)	184.3 (0–546)	0

intercept equation still contained a random component, but in order to detect potential heteroscedasticity in the residuals induced by random, subject level differences in linear growth *within segments*, we included another random effect in an interaction with time as it was originally coded; $\beta_{0i} = \gamma_{00} + \mu_{0i} + \mu_{1i}T_{it}$. Again, μ_{0i} and μ_{1i} were assumed to follow a multivariate normal distribution:

$$[\mu_{0i}, \mu_{1i}] \sim MVN\,[0,0], \begin{bmatrix} \tau_{00}^2 & \tau_{01} \\ \tau_{10} & \tau_{11}^2 \end{bmatrix}. \quad (3)$$

3. Results

3.1. Screening and Feasibility-to-Enroll Phase. The first aim was to examine feasibility of enrolling one-year-olds at risk of ASD into an intervention study on the basis of using the FYI screening tool in a community sample. Initial response rate to the FYI mailing for this intervention study was 19%. We successfully recruited 24 families (41%) of 12-month-old infants who met the FYI risk cutoffs to participate in further developmental assessments. Only 2 of these families had made contacts with community EI providers prior to receiving the FYI mailing. Recruitment of eligible participants into the RCT was 89%.

3.2. Utilization of Community EI Services. The second aim was to describe participating families' subsequent utilization of community EI services. All 18 infants confirmed to be at risk of developmental concerns (regardless of willingness to enroll in the RCT) at the Time 1 assessment were referred to community EI services at 13–17 months of age. Of the 16 families who enrolled in the RCT, only 2 had been previously referred to community EI services by their pediatricians. Descriptive data compiled from the monthly community EI services interviews revealed that half (8/16) of the RCT families received community EI services at some point during their participation between Time 1 and Time 3, but rates varied substantially by group. Only 4 of the 11 (36%) families in the ART treatment group received community EI services, and two of these began only after the ART intervention phase ended. Four of the 5 (80%) families in the REIM control group received community EI services, all beginning during the time of the intervention phase. The descriptive patterns were similar between groups for those children actually receiving EI services defined as (a) the average age of entry to the EI system (ART = 19.7, range = 18–22 months; REIM = 19.0, range = 16–22 months); (b) when the first EI service was provided (ART mean age = 22.0, range = 18–26, median = 21; REIM mean age = 20.5, range = 16–27, median = 21); and (c) the average number of EI services received, excluding service coordination (ART = 3.0, range 1–5; REIM = 2.5, range 1–5). The ART and REIM groups both received the same types of community services overall, which typically comprised service coordination (~1 contact per month) and 1-2 therapeutic services (i.e., speech-language therapy, occupational therapy, feeding therapy, and/or developmental/play therapy or a TEACCH play group, usually for 1 hour per week). Neither of the families in the Eligible/Declined group sought or received community EI services prior to the Time 3 diagnostic follow-up assessment. Table 2 shows the dosage of community EI received by each group of families.

3.3. Findings from RCT Intervention Phase. The next aim focused on the potential of ART to improve child developmental outcomes and parental responsiveness as compared to the REIM group. Descriptive statistics for all outcome variables are in Table 3.

For each of the outcomes examined, Table 4 reports the estimates for the primary parameters of interest from the linear and multiphase growth models, as well as the AIC statistics, with lower values indicating better fit of the model to the data. Because the multiphase and linear growth models are not nested due to differences in time coding, we did not rely on likelihood ratio tests to decide which model is preferred. For the strictly linear regression model, the difference in the slope between treated and untreated subjects, γ, can be interpreted as the expected difference between treated and control subjects at Time 3 (or ~20 months after the first assessment). This interpretation of the parameter was obtained by dividing the time variable, T_{it}, which was originally coded in months, by 20. The multiphase growth models, in contrast, contain two parameters of interest: the differential rate of growth between treatment and control (γ_1) between Time 1 and Time 2 assessments (the active treatment period) and the same quantity (γ_2) for the period between Time 2 and Time 3 assessments (the follow-up period).

In the linear model, significant associations between treatment assignment and posttreatment growth were observed for three outcomes: CSBS Caregiver Questionnaire

TABLE 3: Means and standard deviations (SD) for all variables: ART and REIM groups.

	Time 1 assessment		Time 2 assessment		Time 3 assessment	
	Mean	SD	Mean	SD	Mean	SD
MSEL Expressive Language *T* Score						
ART	38.00	10.53	41.64	9.00	50.55	13.91
REIM	34.00	4.12	34.75	15.22	46.80	15.17
MSEL Receptive Language *T* Score						
ART	39.73	15.50	44.00	12.71	52.27	8.19
REIM	38.40	13.69	33.75	16.13	42.40	10.64
MSEL Visual Reception *T* Score*						
ART	46.09	12.72	51.0	9.09	54.55	10.75
REIM	50.80	12.28	48.25	10.78	47.80	18.44
MSEL Early Learning Composite						
ART	86.55	18.69	90.70	16.60	101.09	19.42
REIM	85.80	14.15	82.50	23.95	90.40	25.14
Vineland Expressive Comm. *V* Scale Score						
ART	13.91	1.70	14.82	1.99	15.55	1.968
REIM	11.80	2.04	11.25	2.36	13.20	2.58
Vineland Receptive Comm. *V* Scale Score						
ART	14.55	1.86	15.64	1.80	15.82	1.99
REIM	14.40	2.07	13.00	2.44	14.40	2.88
Vineland Communication Standard Score						
ART	94.45	8.15	99.91	8.08	102.73	9.43
REIM	86.80	12.68	82.25	14.57	92.60	10.83
Vineland Daily Living Skills Domain						
ART	91.55	9.83	101.09	13.45	99.91	12.98
REIM	86.00	5.66	82.00	13.54	95.00	7.84
Vineland Socialization Domain						
ART	93.45	7.22	101.27	13.91	104.82	14.72
REIM	89.60	8.41	84.00	6.73	91.20	10.78
Vineland Adaptive Behavior Composite						
ART	94.45	6.71	99.73	11.51	101.45	12.65
REIM	88.00	7.58	81.50	9.04	90.00	9.80
SEQ Hyperresponsiveness Scale Mean						
ART	2.01	0.34	2.10	0.43	2.31	0.40
REIM	1.93	0.47	1.91	0.19	1.80	0.24
SEQ Hyporesponsiveness Scale Mean						
ART	1.88	0.51	1.64	0.48	1.65	0.54
REIM	1.60	0.42	2.17	0.79	1.93	0.72
SPA Hyperresponsiveness Scale Mean						
ART	1.55	0.29	1.60	0.52	1.37	0.34
REIM	1.59	0.45	1.38	0.32	1.26	0.23
SPA Hyporesponsiveness Scale Mean						
ART	2.80	0.89	2.35	1.07	2.30	0.44
REIM	3.35	0.89	3.08	0.64	2.43	0.95
MBRS Directive Scale						
ART	2.90	0.61	2.95	0.52	3.18	0.34
REIM	3.20	0.27	3.88	0.25	3.40	0.65

Table 3: Continued.

	Time 1 assessment		Time 2 assessment		Time 3 assessment	
	Mean	SD	Mean	SD	Mean	SD
MBRS Responsive Scale						
ART	3.08	0.75	3.70	0.77	3.97	0.57
REIM	3.38	0.35	3.30	0.24	3.46	1.12
CSBS Caregiver Questionnaire Total Standard Score						
ART	83.18	9.32	102.72	12.24	—	—
REIM	81.60	8.17	81.5	14.46	—	—
CSBS Behavior Sample Total Standard Score						
ART	87.54	15.77	97.45	15.86	—	—
REIM	81.00	11.09	83.25	21.94	—	—

*The Mullen Visual Reception T Score was not used as an outcome measure but is provided in this table to describe the sample more fully.

Table 4: Estimated difference in growth between treatment and control from two difference model specifications.

Outcome	Linear growth model[1]	Multiphase growth model[1]		Model fit comparison: AIC[3]	
	γ	γ_1	γ_2	Linear	Multiphase
MBRS Directive Scale Score	−0.701 (0.54)	**−1.419 (0.45)***	**1.053 (0.561)⁺**	130.1	**123.2**
MBRS Responsive Scale Score	0.925 (0.536)	0.647 (0.541)	0.13 (0.677)	**125.5**	126.9
CSBS-Behavior Sample Total Standard Score[2]	0.896 (0.623)	NA	NA	**83.7**	NA
CSBS-Caregiver Question. Total Standard Score[2]	**1.228 (0.447)***	NA	NA	**69.7**	NA
MSEL Expressive Language T score	0.187 (0.716)	0.211 (0.404)	−0.252 (0.454)	116.2	**115.1**
MSEL Receptive Language T score	**0.928 (0.403)***	0.76 (0.485)	−0.029 (0.589)	123.4	**123.2**
SEQ: Hyperresponsive Scale Mean Score	**1.38 (0.533)***	0.452 (0.373)	0.696 (0.419)	**114.3**	117.3
SEQ: Hyporesponsive Scale Mean Score	−1.023 (0.628)	**−1.541 (0.478)***	0.738 (0.534)	131.6	**127.6**
SPA: Hyperresponsive Scale Mean Score	0.525 (0.58)	0.794 (0.519)	−0.447 (0.598)	129.0	**127.4**
SPA: Hyporesponsive Scale Mean Score	−0.31 (0.517)	−0.701 (0.53)	0.555 (0.679)	131.0	**130.6**
Vineland Expressive Communication V-scale score	0.614 (0.575)	**0.79 (0.328)***	−0.474 (0.356)	108.8	**106.9**
Vineland Receptive Communication V-scale score	0.874 (0.594)	**1.34 (0.356)***	**−0.765 (0.393)⁺**	120.4	**113.0**
Vineland Socialization Standard Score	**1.299 (0.734)⁺**	**1.178 (0.431)***	−0.092 (0.51)	117.1	**115.3**

[1]Standard errors in parentheses; [2]outcome was only measured on two occasions; [3]**lower** AIC statistics indicate better fit between linear and multiphase models (indicated in bold font between last two columns).
⁺**P < 0.10**; ***P < 0.05**.

Total standard score, MSEL Receptive Language T score, and SEQ Hyperresponsiveness mean score (see Table 4). The associations observed for the first two outcome variables were in the expected direction, with exposure to the ART intervention associated with *improved* child communication outcomes. However, parents participating in the ART intervention reported *higher* levels of SEQ Hyperresponsiveness in their children than did parents in the control condition.

In the case of the multiphase model, statistically significant associations between treatment status and growth were concentrated in the active treatment phase (Time 1 to Time 2). Because randomization insures that parents from both experimental groups were drawn from the same baseline distributions on the outcome variables (at least in expectation), the γ_1 parameter can be interpreted as the expected difference between treatment and control at the second, posttreatment measurement occasion. After the Time 1 and Time 2 assessments, 5 outcome variables were statistically significant. As expected, parents in the ART intervention group showed lower levels of MBRS Directiveness and had children who displayed better outcomes, specifically lower symptoms for SEQ Hyporesponsiveness and higher Vineland expressive and receptive communication as well as socialization. In contrast, statistically significant differential growth x treatment status in the follow-up period (Time 2 to Time 3) was largely absent. The AIC statistic indicated that the multiphase model for these 5 outcome variables provided a better fit than the linear model (Table 4); this is exemplified in the plots shown in Figures 3(a), 3(b), and 3(c).

The effect sizes for the outcome variables in Table 5 gauge the magnitude of the statistically significant effects previously revealed in Table 4. The denominator for the effect size is the estimated residual variance at the first measurement occasion. The majority of the outcomes were measured on 3 occasions, so this quantity is simply the square root of the intercept variance plus the residual variance, or $\sqrt{(\tau_{00}^2 + \delta^2)}$. This particular formulation of the effect size is a regression-based analog of the familiar Cohen's D [21], which is itself a ratio of the difference in the group means and the within group standard deviations (pooled). In the current context,

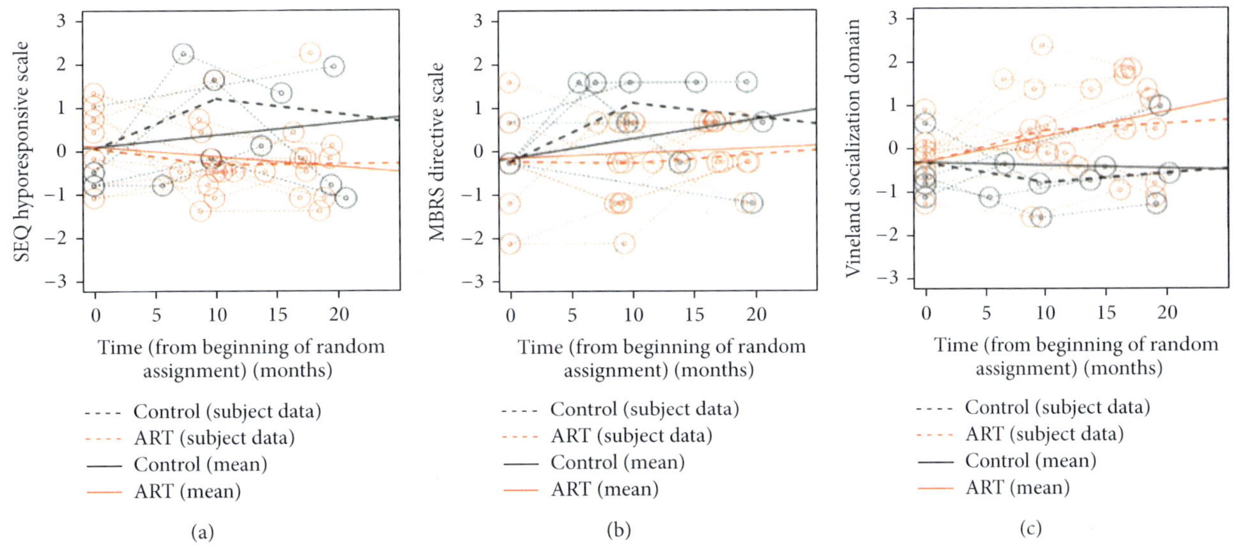

FIGURE 3: Three examples of nonlinear growth trajectories for outcomes with significant differences between ART and REIM groups: (a) SEQ hyporesponsive scale; (b) MBRS directive scale, and (c) Vineland socialization domain.

TABLE 5: Effect sizes from linear and multiphase growth models with statistically significant outcomes.

	Effect size[2]		
	Linear	Multiphase	
	Difference at Time 3	Difference at Time 2	Difference at Time 3
MBRS Directive Scale Score	−0.642	**−1.379**	**−0.356**
CSBS Caregiver Questionnaire Total Standard Score[1]	**2.022**	NA	NA
MSEL Receptive Language *T* Score[1]	0.876	**0.704**	0.678
SEQ Hyperresponsiveness Scale Mean Score[1]	1.441	**0.470**	1.194
SEQ Hyporesponsiveness Scale Mean Score	−1.187	**−1.684**	−0.877
Vineland Expressive Communication *V*-scale Score	0.701	**0.940**	0.376
Vineland Receptive Communication *V*-scale Score	0.972	**1.514**	**0.650**
Vineland Socialization Standard Score	1.968	**1.852**	1.708

[1]Linear model provided better fit than multi-phase.
[2]Effect sizes: low (<0.30), medium (0.30–0.60), and high >0.60 (Cohen, 1988 [21]).
Bold font indicates effects that were statistically significant.

the reporting of effect sizes facilitates comparison of intervention impacts across outcome variables that lack a common metric.

3.4. Clinical Outcomes. Exploratory descriptive analyses indicated that 8 of the 18 children (44%) followed in the study obtained a diagnosis of ASD by a clinical psychologist (blind to group assignment) at Time 3. Specifically, 4/11 (36%) in the ART group (2 autistic disorder; 2 PDDNOS), 2/5 (40%) in the REIM group (both autistic disorder), and 2/2 (100%) in the Eligible/Declined group (one autistic disorder; one PDDNOS) were identified. The average scores on the MSEL across groups were within the average range, though there was considerable variability among the sample; some of the children with ASD diagnoses scored in the average to above average range on the MSEL. All of the children without an ASD diagnosis were noted by the clinical team to have other concerns (i.e., sensory processing, anxiety, articulation, fine motor, or behavior problems) at Time 3.

4. Discussion

This study addressed the feasibility of enrolling 12-month-old infants at risk of a later diagnosis of ASD into an RCT and tested the preliminary efficacy of ART, a parent-mediated intervention, and relative to REIM (i.e., referral to early intervention and monitoring). Utilization of community EI services and clinical diagnostic outcomes were also measured for the 18 families who met eligibility criteria for the RCT. To our knowledge, this is the first study to describe effects of a behavioral parent-mediated intervention with a community-based sample of infants at risk of ASD identified at the young age of 12 months. Overall, the findings indicated improved child receptive language, socialization, and sensory hyporesponsiveness, as well as a less directive parental interactive style for the ART group relative to the REIM group, particularly during the 6–8 month active phase of intervention.

4.1. Feasibility. Although response rates to the FYI screening based on mailings to families identified through the state birth registry were relatively low, they were consistent with our previous research (e.g., [41]). Some families were not reachable, but others gave reasons for declining that included lack of time or lack of concern regarding their child's development. Only 41% of families whose infants met the FYI risk score cutoffs came in for further assessment, but when the in-person assessments were concluded, 89% of those who were eligible agreed to enroll in the RCT and were subsequently randomized. This study thus demonstrated feasibility for enrolling families from a community sample into an RCT "before diagnosis," but also stressed the challenges of ascertaining a community-based sample of infants whose parents may have limited awareness and/or acceptance of ASD-related concerns. Utilizing a two-tiered ascertainment approach (a parent report screener followed by in-person assessments) provided more opportunities for parents to witness and reflect upon their infant's behaviors in a novel context. While less than half of parents invited to participate based upon FYI results agreed to participate further, most of the eligible families enrolled in the RCT after the in-person assessment, suggesting stronger feasibility at this latter point of the process. However, not all parents who enrolled in the RCT voiced concerns about their child's development even after the assessments were completed, and, moreover, not all of those who acknowledged concerns chose to enroll. Motivations (e.g., altruism, potential health benefits) and barriers (e.g., inconvenience, mistrust) to family participation in RCTs are described in qualitative research [64–66] and cover a wide range of child, family, trial design, and provider factors. Although studies enrolling diagnosed clinical samples may have somewhat fewer challenges, the average age of enrollment tends to be higher [14, 15] and, thus, may have potential implications for prognosis and outcomes. The retention rates for families who enrolled in the present study were very high, with 100% of families completing the final assessment ~20 months after their infant was first screened. This was true of the families in the ART condition who had weekly home visits and often formed close relationships with project therapists, as well as those in the REIM (and Eligible/Declined) groups who did not have an opportunity to form those relationships, but who were contacted monthly by the project coordinator. Although other behavioral intervention studies using parent-mediated methods have shown similarly high retention rates, the majority of those studies was shorter in duration and was aimed at toddlers showing symptoms fully consistent with ASD diagnoses [11, 12, 16]. Thus, the present study expands the literature to demonstrate the feasibility for retaining a community sample of infants who are at risk of ASD "before diagnosis" in an early intervention study.

4.2. Subsequent Utilization of Services. Only 2 of 16 families enrolled in the RCT were referred to community EI services by their pediatricians *prior* to enrolling in the RCT; thus, 6 families (37.5%) entered the EI system sooner than would have occurred through usual primary care practices. Through participation in our early screening phase, infants deemed to be at risk of developmental concerns were referred to community EI services at 13–17 months of age. Given that the average age of diagnosis of autistic disorder in NC is 37 months [1] and that only 2 of the 18 children who we identified as at risk had been referred to EI for any type of developmental concerns prior to the FYI screening, our findings suggest that children in both the REIM and the ART groups were identified and referred earlier than standard practice for ASD screening and referral in the state of NC [1].

It is important to note that half of the families randomized to either ART or REIM were receiving community EI services by their Time 3 assessment (~30 months of age) whereas neither child in the Eligible/Declined group was receiving services by this same time point, probably because their families did not pursue the clinical team's Time 1 recommendations. Both of these children were diagnosed with ASD at their Time 3 assessments, so further research is definitely needed to determine factors influencing earlier access to services, including the extent to which monthly monitoring and support for at-risk infants (as we provided to both ART and REIM families) can facilitate such access.

An important contrast between our model and current practice is that we intervened with one-year-olds based on indicators of being *at risk* of an eventual diagnosis of ASD. In NC and many other states, documented risk of a developmental delay or disorder is not included in the eligibility criteria for publicly mandated EI services. Rather, children must either have significant current delays in one or more areas of development or must be diagnosed with an established condition. See http://www.beearly.nc.gov/index.php/providers/eligibility-referral, retrieved 8/4/2014, for a description of this policy. Thus, the findings in the present study have implications for clinical practice and government policy.

4.3. Promise of ART. The children who received the ART intervention outperformed the REIM group on several child developmental outcomes in the key domains of social-communication and sensory-regulatory functions. Our study was not powered to detect anything less than large effects at the .05 confidence level; thus, our significant findings are associated with large effect sizes (>.60). Such large effects were more apparent on the parent-report measures (e.g., Vineland, SEQ), but also emerged in observed measures (e.g., MSEL, MBRS). Our results add to growing empirical evidence that clearly links early pivotal behaviors (e.g., social play, joint attention, arousal and attention, engagement, adaptability, and coping, etc.) to later developmental outcomes in children with and/or without ASD [13, 33–37] and extends these findings to one-year-olds at risk of a later diagnosis of ASD who were identified via community-based screening.

Interestingly, one variable showed a pattern of change in a direction opposite to what was predicted—SEQ Hyperresponsiveness increased rather than decreased over time for the ART group. One interpretation is that as children's language and social skills increased and parents became more responsive to their child's behaviors, they may have also become more aware of their child's sensitivities and aversions and thus were more likely to report them. Future studies will be needed to explore this unexpected finding.

Although both the ART and REIM groups made gains over time, their rates and patterns of developmental change varied across variables, with some demonstrating linear growth (e.g., MSEL Receptive Language, CSBS Caregiver Questionnaire Total Score, and SEQ Hyperresponsiveness) and some demonstrating nonlinear change (i.e., SEQ Hyporesponsiveness, Vineland Receptive and Expressive Communication and Socialization, and MBRS Directive). The ART group showed the most benefit during the active treatment phase (i.e., first 6–8 months), with some attenuation in improvement in the follow-up phase. Concomitant patterns were seen with parental behaviors, such that directiveness in the ART group showed large significant improvement between Time 1 and Time 2 and then decreased in the follow-up phase. These findings underscore the importance of using multiple assessment time points (3 or more) to optimize sensitivity to potentially nonlinear treatment changes during both active and maintenance phases. Future studies with larger samples should address whether treatment fidelity and improvements in parental behaviors (e.g., responsiveness) mediate child developmental outcomes.

The present findings also suggest that studies with larger scaled trials should explore the need for booster sessions in the follow-up phase of intervention or the need to better prepared families for transitions from RCTs to conventional community EI services. Although maturational changes (i.e., "catch up" of the REIM group) could be hypothesized, these effects could not be disentangled from treatment effects in the present study. However, given that the REIM group likely benefitted from earlier identification and referral to community EI services than usual and that their boost in performance between Times 2 and 3 coincided with increases in the intensity of the EI services, we believe that maturational changes are an insufficient explanation.

4.4. Limitations, Future Directions, and Clinical Implications. This study adds to the growing literature indicating that earlier identification of infants at risk of ASD can lead to earlier access to EI services and can facilitate improved developmental outcomes. Although the ART group outperformed the REIM group in both child and parent outcomes, the present study has too few participants to make definitive conclusions about the efficacy of ART. However, the present study does suggest that larger scaled trials should be conducted to extend exploration of this promising intervention. Limitations of the intent-to-treat design that is commonly used in RCT such as the present study include the assumption that the treatment condition is the same as treatment exposure. Clearly, not all family decisions and variables can be controlled by randomization: families often behave differently despite being in the same condition, resulting in heterogeneity in the intent-to-treat effects.

The present study does not reveal whether a diagnosis of ASD may have been prevented through earlier behavioral intervention as theorized by some experts in the field (e.g., [26]). Approximately half of the children in the ART and REIM groups, as well as both children in the Eligible/Declined group, received an eventual diagnosis of ASD. Dawson and colleagues [13] reported that two years of intensive treatment with the Early Start Denver Model led to children having less problematic variants of ASD at around 4 years of age. This suggests that a larger-scaled study could reveal more subtle effects of ART in ameliorating ASD symptom severity or reversing early symptoms. The diagnosis of children in our sample at an average of 32 months is considerably earlier than reported in the literature for community samples (61 months) [67] and, thus, promotes earlier access to ASD specific services in the community.

Future studies should investigate the extent to which enrollment in an RCT of a behavioral intervention may postpone community EI services for some families, and whether or not this decision affects outcomes. In our study, engagement in community services differed by group. The families receiving our novel intervention were less likely to initiate community EI services, particularly during the active phase of ART. This effect may have reflected parental perceptions that their child's needs were being sufficiently addressed by our intervention. It is important to note that for both the ART and REIM groups, some infants referred for community EI services that met the state's eligibility criteria for Part C services and some did not. Moreover, some families did not seek community EI services for their infants, or they waited until an older age to do so. The community EI services received by a subset of families varied widely in goals, strategies, and intensity. Specific goals and services for children eligible for Part C services are determined through the process of developing the Individualized Family Service Plan. Some families also pursued services privately. Although researchers hope to validate beneficial effects of novel behavioral interventions, the potential costs (e.g., time, anxiety, and delay of community EI services) of entering into an RCT of an intervention that is potentially non-efficacious should not be neglected and requires further research.

Future research may also want to explore alternate strategies to identify and enroll children from community samples showing early risk signs for ASD. Working with pediatric or family medicine practices where developmental and ASD screening takes place could potentially increase family enrollment at an earlier stage. This strategy might also yield more diverse samples through targeted recruitment. Although the present study was not intended as a large-scale epidemiological study, we recognize the need to replicate findings with large, diverse samples.

To summarize, the present study confirmed the feasibility of using the FYI with a community sample to enroll 12-month-olds at risk of a later diagnosis of ASD into a behavioral RCT. The families enrolled in this study were from a narrower demographic (e.g., white/college educated) than the community at large; thus, the possibility of nonresponse bias requires further study. Although both groups made significant gains and received community services earlier than they would have through conventional surveillance and pediatric referrals, ART showed more beneficial effects relative to REIM for both child and parent outcomes, particularly in the active phase of treatment. Our study supports the promise of using a parent-mediated early intervention with very young infants at risk of ASD in authentic home contexts using an intensity of professional effort compatible with the intensity of business-as-usual EI services in our state. Future large scaled studies are needed to replicate these findings and to further assess potential mediators and moderators of comparable early behavioral interventions. Mixed methods research would be ideal to better understand quantitative outcomes as well as qualitative explanations for variability in such outcomes. Finally, scale-up and implementation efforts will need to better address the potential reasons motivating some families to seek early behavioral interventions.

Acknowledgments

The authors thank Autism Speaks and The Ireland Family Foundation for their generous funding of this study. The authors also acknowledge NC Vital Records and the families and staff of the Early Development Project and PEARLS for their support.

References

[1] Centers for Disease Control, "Prevalence of autism spectrum disorder among children aged 8 years—autism and developmental disabilities monitoring network, 11 sites, United States, 2010," *Surveillance Summaries*, vol. 63, no. 2, pp. 1–21, 2014.

[2] E. Courchesne, C. M. Karns, H. R. Davis et al., "Unusual brain growth patterns in early life in patients with autistic disorder: an MRI study," *Neurology*, vol. 57, no. 2, pp. 245–254, 2001.

[3] J. J. Wolff, H. Gu, G. Gerig et al., "Differences in white matter fiber tract development present from 6 to 24 months in infants with autism," *The American Journal of Psychiatry*, vol. 169, no. 6, pp. 589–600, 2012.

[4] Office of Special Education Programs, *Summary Table of States' and Territories' Definitions of/Criteria for IDEA Part C Eligibility*, 2004.

[5] S. Ringwalt, *Summary Table of States' and Territories' Definitions of/Criteria for IDEA Part C Eligibility*, 2012, http://ectacenter.org/~pdfs/topics/earlyid/partc_elig_table.pdf.

[6] E. R. Crais, C. S. McComish, B. P. Humphreys et al., "Pediatric healthcare professionals' views on autism spectrum disorder screening at 12–18 months," *Journal of Autism and Developmental Disorders*, vol. 44, no. 9, pp. 2311–2328, 2014.

[7] J. S. Miller, T. Gabrielsen, M. Villalobos et al., "The each child study: systematic screening for autism spectrum disorders in a pediatric setting," *Pediatrics*, vol. 127, no. 5, pp. 866–871, 2011.

[8] K. Pierce, C. Carter, M. Weinfeld et al., "Detecting, studying, and treating autism early: the one-year well-baby check-up approach," *The Journal of Pediatrics*, vol. 159, no. 3, pp. 458.e6–465.e6, 2011.

[9] A. Drew, G. Baird, S. Baron-Cohen et al., "A pilot randomised control trial of a parent training intervention for pre-school children with autism: preliminary findings and methodological challenges," *European Child & Adolescent Psychiatry*, vol. 11, no. 6, pp. 266–272, 2002.

[10] I. Oosterling, J. Visser, S. Swinkels et al., "Randomized controlled trial of the focus parent training for toddlers with autism: 1-year outcome," *Journal of Autism and Developmental Disorders*, vol. 40, no. 12, pp. 1447–1458, 2010.

[11] S. J. Rogers, A. Estes, C. Lord et al., "Effects of a brief early start Denver model (ESDM)-based parent intervention on toddlers at risk for autism spectrum disorders: a randomized controlled trial," *Journal of the American Academy of Child and Adolescent Psychiatry*, vol. 51, no. 10, pp. 1052–1065, 2012.

[12] A. S. Carter, D. S. Messinger, W. L. Stone, S. Celimli, A. S. Nahmias, and P. Yoder, "A randomized controlled trial of Hanen's "more than words" in toddlers with early autism symptoms," *Journal of Child Psychology and Psychiatry*, vol. 52, no. 7, pp. 741–752, 2011.

[13] G. Dawson, S. Rogers, J. Munson et al., "Randomized, controlled trial of an intervention for toddlers with autism: the early start Denver model," *Pediatrics*, vol. 125, no. 1, pp. e17–e23, 2010.

[14] C. Kasari, A. C. Gulsrud, C. Wong, S. Kwon, and J. Locke, "Randomized controlled caregiver mediated joint engagement intervention for toddlers with autism," *Journal of Autism and Developmental Disorders*, vol. 40, no. 9, pp. 1045–1056, 2010.

[15] R. J. Landa, K. C. Holman, A. H. O'Neill, and E. A. Stuart, "Intervention targeting development of socially synchronous engagement in toddlers with autism spectrum disorder: a randomized controlled trial," *Journal of Child Psychology and Psychiatry and Allied Disciplines*, vol. 52, no. 1, pp. 13–21, 2011.

[16] H. H. Schertz, S. L. Odom, K. M. Baggett, and J. H. Sideris, "Effects of joint attention mediated learning for toddlers with autism spectrum disorders: an initial randomized controlled study," *Early Childhood Research Quarterly*, vol. 28, no. 2, pp. 249–258, 2013.

[17] K. S. Wallace and S. J. Rogers, "Intervening in infancy: implications for autism spectrum disorders," *Journal of Child Psychology and Psychiatry and Allied Disciplines*, vol. 51, no. 12, pp. 1300–1320, 2010.

[18] A. C. Stahmer, L. Brookman-Frazee, E. Lee, K. Searcy, and S. Reed, "Parent and multidisciplinary provider perspectives on earliest intervention for children at risk for autism spectrum disorders," *Infants and Young Children*, vol. 24, no. 4, pp. 344–363, 2011.

[19] S. Rogers and G. Dawson, *Play and Engagement in Early Autism: The Early Start Denver Model*, Guilford Press, New York, NY, USA, 2009.

[20] F. Sussman, *More than Words: A Paren't Guide to Building Interaction and Language Skills for Children with Autism Spectrum Disorder or Social Communication Difficulties*, The Hanen Centre, Toronto, Canada, 2012.

[21] J. Cohen, *Statistical Power Analysis for the Behavioral Sciences (2nd ed.)*, Erlbaum Associates, Hillsdale, NJ, USA, 1988.

[22] T. P. Beauchaine, E. Neuhaus, S. L. Brenner, and L. Gatzke-Kopp, "Ten good reasons to consider biological processes in prevention and intervention research," *Development and Psychopathology*, vol. 20, no. 3, pp. 745–774, 2008.

[23] T. C. Bethea and L. Sikich, "Early pharmacological treatment of autism: a rationale for developmental treatment," *Biological Psychiatry*, vol. 61, no. 4, pp. 521–537, 2007.

[24] S. J. Webb, C. S. Monk, and C. A. Nelson, "Mechanisms of postnatal neurobiological development: implications for human development," *Developmental Neuropsychology*, vol. 19, no. 2, pp. 147–171, 2001.

[25] J. Green, M. W. Wan, J. Guiraud et al., "Intervention for infants at risk of developing autism: a case series," *Journal of Autism and Developmental Disorders*, vol. 43, no. 11, pp. 2502–2514, 2013.

[26] G. Dawson, "Early behavioral intervention, brain plasticity, and the prevention of autism spectrum disorder," *Development and Psychopathology*, vol. 20, no. 3, pp. 775–803, 2008.

[27] M. J. Bakermans-Kranenburg, M. H. van IJzendoorn, and F. Juffer, "Less is more: meta-analyses of sensitivity and attachment interventions in early childhood," *Psychological Bulletin*, vol. 129, no. 2, pp. 195–215, 2003.

[28] C. J. Dunst, C. M. Trivette, M. Raab, and T. L. Masiello, "Early childhood contingency learning and detection: research evidence and implications for practice," *Exceptionality*, vol. 16, no. 1, pp. 4–17, 2008.

[29] G. Mahoney, G. Boyce, R. R. Fewell, D. Spiker, and C. A. Wheeden, "The relationship of parent-child interaction to the effectiveness of early intervention services for at-risk children and children with disabilities," *Topics in Early Childhood Special Education*, vol. 18, no. 1, pp. 5–17, 1998.

[30] G. Mahoney and F. Perales, "Relationship-focused early intervention with children with pervasive developmental disorders and other disabilities: a comparative study," *Journal of Developmental and Behavioral Pediatrics*, vol. 26, no. 2, pp. 77–85, 2005.

[31] J. P. Shonkoff and D. A. Phillips, *From Neurons to Neighborhoods: The Science of Early Childhood Development*, National Academy Press, Washington, DC, USA, 2000.

[32] M. Siller and M. Sigman, "The behaviors of parents of children with autism predict the subsequent development of their children's communication," *Journal of Autism and Developmental Disorders*, vol. 32, no. 2, pp. 77–89, 2002.

[33] S. M. Clifford and C. Dissanayake, "The early development of joint attention in infants with autistic disorder using home video observations and parental interview," *Journal of Autism and Developmental Disorders*, vol. 38, no. 5, pp. 791–805, 2008.

[34] W. E. Dixon Jr. and P. H. Smith, "Links between early temperament and language acquisition," *Merrill-Palmer Quarterly*, vol. 46, no. 3, pp. 417–440, 2000.

[35] R. Feldman, S. Masalha, and D. Alony, "Microregulatory patterns of family interactions: cultural pathways to toddlers' self-regulation," *Journal of Family Psychology*, vol. 20, no. 4, pp. 614–623, 2006.

[36] J. Poehlmann and B. H. Fiese, "The interaction of maternal and infant vulnerabilities on developing attachment relationships," *Development and Psychopathology*, vol. 13, no. 1, pp. 1–11, 2001.

[37] K. Toth, J. Munson, A. N. Meltzoff, and G. Dawson, "Early predictors of communication development in young children with autism spectrum disorder: joint attention, imitation, and toy play," *Journal of Autism and Developmental Disorders*, vol. 36, no. 8, pp. 993–1005, 2006.

[38] G. T. Baranek, L. R. Watson, E. Crais, and S. Reznick, *First-Year Inventory (FYI) 2.0.*, University of North Carolina, Chapel Hill, NC, USA, 2003.

[39] L. M. Turner-Brown, G. T. Baranek, J. S. Reznick, L. R. Watson, and E. R. Crais, "The first year inventory: a longitudinal follow-up of 12-month-old to 3-year-old children," *Autism*, vol. 17, no. 5, pp. 527–540, 2013.

[40] J. C. Dumville, S. Hahn, J. N. V. Miles, and D. J. Torgerson, "The use of unequal randomisation ratios in clinical trials: a review," *Contemporary Clinical Trials*, vol. 27, no. 1, pp. 1–12, 2006.

[41] J. S. Reznick, G. T. Baranek, S. Reavis, L. R. Watson, and E. R. Crais, "A parent-report instrument for identifying one-year-olds at risk for an eventual diagnosis of autism: the first year inventory," *Journal of Autism and Developmental Disorders*, vol. 37, no. 9, pp. 1691–1710, 2007.

[42] E. M. Mullen, *Mullen Scales of Early Learning: AGS Edition*, American Guidance Service, Circle Pines, MN, USA, 1995.

[43] S. S. Sparrow, D. V. Cicchetti, and D. A. Balla, Eds., *Vielad Adaptive Behavior Scales*, AGS, 2nd edition, 2005.

[44] A. M. Wetherby and B. Prizant, *Communication and Symbolic Behavior Scales Developmental Profile–First Normed Edition*, Brookes, Baltimore, Md, USA, 2002.

[45] L. Fenson, P. S. Dale, J. S. Reznick et al., *MacArthur Communicative Development Inventories: User's Guide and Technical Manual*, Paul H. Brookes, Baltimore, Md, USA, 2003.

[46] G. T. Baranek, *Sensory Processing Assessment for Young Children (SPA)*, University of North Carolina, Chapel Hill, NC, USA, 1999.

[47] G. T. Baranek, B. A. Boyd, M. D. Poe, F. J. David, and L. R. Watson, "Hyperresponsive sensory patterns in young children with autism, developmental delay, and typical development," *The American Journal on Mental Retardation*, vol. 112, no. 4, pp. 233–245, 2007.

[48] G. T. Baranek, L. R. Watson, B. A. Boyd, M. D. Poe, F. J. David, and L. McGuire, "Hyporesponsiveness to social and nonsocial sensory stimuli in children with autism, children with developmental delays, and typically developing children," *Development and Psychopathology*, vol. 25, no. 2, pp. 307–320, 2013.

[49] G. T. Baranek, *Sensory Experiences Questionnaire (SEQ)*, University of North Carolina at Chapel Hill, Chapel Hill, NC, USA, 1999.

[50] L. M. Little, A. C. Freuler, M. B. Houser et al., "Psychometric validation of the sensory experiences questionnaire," *The American Journal of Occupational Therapy*, vol. 65, no. 2, pp. 207–210, 2011.

[51] G. T. Baranek, F. J. David, M. D. Poe, W. L. Stone, and L. R. Watson, "Sensory Experiences Questionnaire: discriminating sensory features in young children with autism, developmental delays, and typical development," *Journal of Child Psychology and Psychiatry and Allied Disciplines*, vol. 47, no. 6, pp. 591–601, 2006.

[52] A. Carter and M. Briggs-Gowan, *Manual for the Infant-Toddler Social & Emotional Assessment (ITSEA) and Brief-ITSEA (BITSEA)*, Psychological Corporation, Harcourt Press, San Antonio, Tex, USA, 2005.

[53] L. Zwaigenbaum, S. Bryson, T. Rogers, W. Roberts, J. Brian, and P. Szatmari, "Behavioral manifestations of autism in the first year of life," *International Journal of Developmental Neuroscience*, vol. 23, no. 2-3, pp. 143–152, 2005.

[54] C. Lord, S. Risi, L. Lambrecht et al., "The Autism Diagnostic Observation Schedule-Generic: a standard measure of social and communication deficits associated with the spectrum of autism," *Journal of Autism and Developmental Disorders*, vol. 30, no. 3, pp. 205–223, 2000.

[55] G. Mahoney, A. Powell, and I. Finger, "The maternal behavior rating scale," *Topics in Early Childhood Special Education*, vol. 6, no. 2, pp. 44–56, 1986.

[56] L. Wakeford, B. A. Boyd, L. M. Little et al., *The Family Routines Exploration & Description-Revised*, University of North Carolina, Chapel Hill, NC, USA, 2009.

[57] G. Mahoney and J. MacDonald, *Autism and Developmental Delays in Young Children: The Responsive Teaching Curriculum for Parents and Professionals Manual*, PRO-ED Inc., Austin, Tex, USA, 2007.

[58] L. Wakeford, G. T. Baranek, E. R. Crais, L. R. Watson, and L. Turner-Brown, "Adapted responsive teaching: a case example," Under review.

[59] R. R. Fewell and B. Deutscher, "Contributions of early language and maternal facilitation variables to later language and reading abilities," *Journal of Early Intervention*, vol. 26, no. 2, pp. 132–145, 2004.

[60] M. L. Hemmeter and A. P. Kaiser, "Enhanced milieu teaching: effects of parent-implemented language intervention," *Journal of Early Intervention*, vol. 18, no. 3, pp. 269–289, 1994.

[61] S. I. Greenspan and S. Weider, "Developmental patterns and outcomes in infants and children with disorders relating and communicating: a chart review of 200 cases of children with autistic spectrum diagnoses," *Journal of Developmental and Learning Disorders*, vol. 1, pp. 87–142, 1997.

[62] A. S. Nadig, S. Ozonoff, G. S. Young, A. Rozga, M. Sigman, and S. J. Rogers, "A prospective study of response to name in infants at risk for autism," *Archives of Pediatrics and Adolescent Medicine*, vol. 161, no. 4, pp. 378–383, 2007.

[63] R. Cudeck and K. J. Klebe, "Multiphase mixed-effects models for repeated measures data," *Psychological Methods*, vol. 7, no. 1, pp. 41–63, 2002.

[64] A. C. Freuler, G. T. Baranek, C. Tashjian, L. R. Watson, E. R. Crais, and L. M. Turner-Brown, "Parent reflections of experiences of participating in a randomized controlled trial of a behavioral intervention for infants at risk of autism spectrum disorders," *Autism*, vol. 18, no. 5, pp. 519–528, 2014.

[65] M. Siller, L. Morgan, L. Turner-Brown et al., "Designing studies to evaluate parent-mediated interventions for toddlers with autism spectrum disorder," *Journal of Early Intervention*, 2014.

[66] P. H. Y. Caldwell, P. N. Butow, and J. C. Craig, "Parents' attitudes to children's participation in randomized controlled trials," *The Journal of Pediatrics*, vol. 142, no. 5, pp. 554–559, 2003.

[67] L. D. Wiggins, J. Baio, and C. Rice, "Examination of the time between first evaluation and first autism spectrum diagnosis in a population-based sample," *Journal of Developmental and Behavioral Pediatrics*, vol. 27, no. 2, supplement, pp. S79–S87, 2006.

5

Parent-Child Agreement using the Spence Children's Anxiety Scale and a Thermometer in Children with Autism Spectrum Disorder

T. May,[1] K. Cornish,[2] and N. J. Rinehart[3]

[1]*Deakin Child Study Centre, Deakin University, Melbourne Burwood Campus, 221 Burwood Highway, Burwood, VIC 3125, Australia*
[2]*School of Psychological Sciences and Monash Institute for Brain Development & Repair, Monash University, Clayton Campus, Building 17, Wellington Road, Clayton, VIC 3800, Australia*
[3]*Deakin Child Study Centre, School of Psychology, Deakin University, Melbourne Burwood Campus, 221 Burwood Highway, Burwood, VIC 3125, Australia*

Correspondence should be addressed to T. May; tamara.may@deakin.edu.au

Academic Editor: Michael G. Aman

Children with Autism Spectrum Disorder (ASD) experience high anxiety which often prompts clinical referral and requires intervention. This study aimed to compare parent and child reports on the Spence Children's Anxiety Scale (SCAS) and a child-reported "worry thermometer" in 88 children aged 8–13 years, 44 with ASD and 44 age, gender, and perceptual IQ matched typically developing children. There were no gender differences in child report on the SCAS and worry thermometers. Results indicated generally good correlations between parent and child self-reported SCAS symptoms for typically developing children but poor agreement in parent-child ASD dyads. The worry thermometer child-report did not reflect child or parent reports on the SCAS. Findings suggest 8–13-year-old children with ASD may have difficulties accurately reporting their anxiety levels. The clinical implications were discussed.

1. Introduction

Children with Autism Spectrum Disorder (ASD) consistently show high levels of anxiety. Around 40% of children and adolescents with ASD have clinically elevated anxiety levels or experience at least one anxiety disorder [1–4]. A recent meta-analysis of anxiety in ASD found that specific phobia was the most common subtype (30%), followed by Obsessive Compulsive Disorder (OCD; 17%), social anxiety disorder and agoraphobia (17%), generalized anxiety disorder (15%), separation anxiety disorder (9%), and panic disorder (2%) [3]. Anxiety related issues may prompt clinical referral and also require clinical intervention in this population. As children with ASD may quickly escalate their emotional states during "meltdowns," assessing anxiety symptoms in a timely and valid manner is important for management at home, at school, and in clinical setting [5, 6]. A rapid assessment measure of anxiety in ASD would be useful in these contexts. This would allow parents, teachers, and clinicians to easily determine the level of anxiety in a child with ASD and, if elevated, employ an appropriate intervention. However, whether self-reported anxiety symptoms in children with ASD are valid is somewhat unclear.

A number of researchers have questioned the ability of children with ASD to self-report internal emotional states [7–10]. In empirical studies of ASD, there are mixed findings. Many have used the parent and child version of the Spence Children's Anxiety Scale (SCAS) in children with ASD. Russell and Sofronoff [11] investigated 10–13-year-old children with Asperger's Disorder compared to a clinically anxious normed group and found that parents of children with ASD rated their children as having higher levels of overall anxiety, obsessive compulsive symptoms, and specific phobias than parents of clinically anxious children. Children with ASD rated themselves as having similar levels of anxiety to clinically anxious children. Parents rated their children as having higher levels of separation anxiety, social phobia, and generalized anxiety than did their child, with child ratings significantly higher than parent ratings for obsessive compulsive symptoms. Magiati and colleagues [12] examined a nonreferred sample of children with ASD aged over 8 years (mean age 12 y 10 m) and found moderately good parent-child agreement for only three subscales (Physical Injuries, Generalised Anxiety Disorder, and separation anxiety). Farrugia and Hudson [13] found generally good parent-child correlations (r = .697) in 12–16-year-olds with Asperger's Disorder. Ozsivadjian et al. [14] also found good parent-child agreement on the total SCAS score in 10–16-year-old males with ASD. Potentially, the older child age may account for the better consistency between parent-child reports compared with younger children examined by Russell and Sofronoff and Magiati et al.

Other measures of anxiety have also been used to examine parent-child agreement on anxiety symptoms. Lopata and colleagues [15] found parents reported higher levels of anxiety than their 7–13-year-old children with ASD using the Behavior Assessment System for Children Second Edition. However, children with ASD self-reported similar levels of anxiety to comparison children. Parent and child anxiety symptoms showed poor correlations in the ASD group. White and colleagues [16] used the Multidimensional Anxiety Scale for Children, child and parent version in 12–17-year-olds with ASD. They also found child and parent reports were not significantly correlated. The validity of self-report measures in adolescents with ASD was questioned given only 23% self-reported clinically elevated anxiety scores despite all being diagnosed with an anxiety disorder. They noted that adolescents with ASD may underreport their anxiety, perhaps due to a lack of insight, because they have a different perspective about their own anxiety, or an unwillingness to truthfully report their difficulties. Using the Screen for Child Anxiety Related Emotional Disorders [17] in 8–14-year-olds with ASD, Blakeley-Smith et al. [18] found moderate interclass correlations between parent-child reports with parents reporting higher levels of anxiety than their children, except for separation anxiety. van Steensel and colleagues [19] compared child and parent reports also using the SCARED in 7–17-year-old children with ASD and an anxiety disordered group. Parent-child agreement on this instrument was poorer in the ASD group than in the anxiety disordered group.

Overall, there are equivocal findings, with some studies showing parents generally report higher levels of anxiety in their child with ASD compared with the child's own report [11, 15, 19], whereas other studies have found relatively good parent-child agreement [12–14, 16, 18]. These discrepancies may relate to different methodologies employed given various ages, diagnoses, gender proportions, measurement instruments, and child IQ levels used across studies. For example, a meta-analytic review of anxiety in ASD found age was associated positively with levels of Generalised Anxiety Disorder and negatively with Obsessive Compulsive Disorder (OCD) and separation anxiety [3]. The meta-analysis also found a complex relationship between type of ASD (Asperger's Disorder, PDD-NOS, or Autistic Disorder) and type of anxiety, including higher rates of Generalised Anxiety Disorder in Asperger's Disorder, higher OCD, and specific phobia in Autistic Disorder and lower rates of OCD in PDD-NOS.

The studies reviewed so far have examined parent-child agreement using multiple item questionnaires (such as on the SCAS). Given the cognitive and verbal deficits in this population, high levels of alexithymia, and difficulties answering open ended questions, more simple ways of assessing internal states are indicated [20]. Visual cues such as Visual Analogue Scales, for example, "emotional thermometers," can be used to measure the strength of feelings [20]. Thermometer scales are frequently used in mood and anxiety interventions for individuals with ASD [21–23] and have the advantage of being a largely visual tool which is important in ASD where language delays and deviance are commonplace with relative strengths in visual skills.

Thermometer scales have long been used and validated in paediatric pain management to assess the level of pain [24–26] and emotional distress in hospital [27, 28] and nonhospital settings [29–31]. Generally, visual analogue pain scales show reasonably sound psychometrics [32]; however, there are some mixed findings. Some studies have shown poor agreement between parent and child ratings, with parents reporting generally lower levels of pain than their child [33]. Research suggests that children generally need to have normal IQ and be 7 years of age and older to use thermometer scales reliably [34].

The validity of these types of visual scales is largely unexamined in ASD. Lopata and colleagues [35] used a thermometer scale to examine stress in children aged 6–13 years with ASD. They found mild to moderate correlations between a stress thermometer scale and cortisol levels which was unexpected given the fact that child self-reports often do not correlate well with physiological measures [35, 36]. This indicated that children with ASD may have some capacity to rate their internal states accurately using a thermometer scale. No studies examining the validity of anxiety specific thermometers for ASD were found in the literature.

It is also noteworthy that studies in this area of ASD have generally failed to examine gender differences in parent-child agreement on anxiety symptoms. There are many more boys than girls diagnosed with ASD, yet how gender interacts with anxiety in ASD is not well explored. Girls from adolescence onwards are reported to experience higher levels of anxiety than boys [37], which may also be the case in ASD [38]. Younger girls with ASD may also show higher levels of social anxiety relative to boys with ASD, with this difference also reflected in typically developing children [39]. It is possible that girls and boys may also self-report different levels of anxiety, with this yet to be explored by gender in ASD.

The major aim of this study was to determine how well child and parent reports on the SCAS correlated in children with ASD. Secondly, the study aimed to determine if a "worry thermometer" correlated with the SCAS. We also sought to examine whether there were any gender differences in child reports on the SCAS and the "worry thermometer." We investigated the following research questions. (1) How well do typically developing (TYP) and ASD children's self-reports correlate with their parent report on the SCAS? (2) How well do anxiety thermometer child-report ratings correlate with parent and child report on the SCAS and does this differ if a child has ASD? (3) Do boys and girls with ASD self-report similar levels of anxiety symptoms on the SCAS and a worry thermometer?

2. Method

2.1. Participants. In total, 88 children participated in this study. Participants with ASD were 44 children, 21 male and 23 female, with Autistic Disorder or Asperger's Disorder and aged between 8 and 13 years. This sample was taken from our larger study of gender differences in children with ASD, and hence females were oversampled compared to the normal male prevalence found in ASD [39]. Participants were recruited prior to the release of DSM-5. All clinical children were diagnosed using DSM-IV-TR criteria by registered psychologists and pediatricians prior to taking part in the study. The DSM-IV-TR criteria for Autistic Disorder or Asperger's Disorder were confirmed for ASD participants using our standard process involving reviewing diagnostic reports completed by pediatricians/psychologists and interviewing parents using a symptom checklist to ensure DSM-IV-TR criteria were fulfilled. In addition, all ASD participants were screened and confirmed to be within the clinical range on the Social Responsiveness Scale (SRS) parent report [40] which has demonstrated validity with the Autism Diagnostic Interview Revised [41]. To increase the diagnostic validity and homogeneity of the ASD sample, children with PDD-NOS were excluded given the fact that this condition is diagnosed only when there are subclinical autism symptoms or atypical presentation [42]. All participants were recruited through the Monash University Centre for Developmental Psychology and Psychiatry, the Autism Victoria "Get Involved" volunteer register, and private clinics in the Melbourne metropolitan area. Only children with a full-scale IQ of 70 and above were included in the study.

Forty-four typically developing children, 25 male and 19 female, who were matched based on gender, age, and perceptual IQ, were recruited from a Melbourne metropolitan primary school. These children were also aged between 8 and 13 years. None of these children had any prior history of parent or teacher reported developmental disability or psychopathology. Further, possible ASD symptoms in this population were screened with these children scoring within the typical range on the SRS parent report [40]. Children across both groups were excluded if they had a history of brain injury or any genetic disorders (such as Fragile X syndrome).

2.2. Measures

2.2.1. Intellectual Functioning. For all children with ASD, intellectual ability was assessed using the Wechsler Intelligence Scale for Children IV (WISC-IV, [43]), Australian version. This yields a full-scale IQ, Verbal Comprehension Index, and a Perceptual Reasoning Index. The Wechsler Abbreviated Scale of Intelligence (WASI, [44]), which yields a full-scale IQ, a Verbal IQ, and a Performance IQ, was completed for all typically developing children. The typically developing children completed the WASI as it was a shorter assessment which reduced the time burden of their participation in the study. The WASI full-scale IQ is comparable to the WISC-IV full-scale IQ, the Verbal IQ comparable to the Verbal Comprehension Index of the WISC-IV, and the Performance IQ comparable to the Perceptual Reasoning Index from the WISC-IV [44].

2.2.2. Parent- and Child-Reported Anxiety. The Spence Children's Anxiety Scale [45] parent report is a 38-item questionnaire based on DSM-IV-TR criteria for anxiety disorders in children. The child-report is a 45-item questionnaire which includes six positive filler items (i.e., "I am happy") and one general item which are not scored in either the total or subscale scores. Hence, the child report has 38 items which are scored and correspond directly with the parent version. The scale assesses six domains of anxiety including generalized anxiety, panic/agoraphobia, social phobia, separation anxiety, Obsessive Compulsive Disorder, and Physical Injury Fears. Parents and children report how often each of the items happens to their child using a four-point scale: "never," "sometimes," "often," and "always." Validity and reliability have been established [45–47]. The SCAS has previously been employed and shown to be a valid measure of anxiety levels in individuals with ASD [11, 13]. This measure does not have a unitary cutoff point but employs age and gender based norms to place children in clinically significant or the normal range of anxiety.

This study also used a 100-point Visual Analogue Scale (VAS) for the assessment of self-reported anxiety (worry thermometer adapted from [48]). Higher scores on this scale reflected higher levels of anxiety. The thermometer was presented on an A4 sized page with the thermometer presented vertically in the middle of the page marked from 0 (bottom) to 100 (top) with marks at 1-point intervals. A score of 0 indicated "Not at all worried," 50 "worried," and 100 "very very worried," with these words placed next to their corresponding point on the scale. Three worry thermometers were utilised which referred to current worry, the worst worries in the last 2 weeks, and the worst worries in the child's lifetime. Children are asked for the two-week thermometer, "Including the last two weeks, what's the most worried/scared you've ever felt?"; for the ever thermometer, "What is the most worried/scared you've ever felt?"; and the now thermometer, "How worried/scared do you feel now?"

2.3. Procedure. The study was approved by Human Research Ethics Committees of Monash University and the Victorian Government Department of Education and Early Childhood. Parents received an explanatory statement and provided written informed consent. Children provided assent. Participation was voluntary and participants did not receive any monetary reward for participation other than reimbursement for travel costs.

Table 1: Demographic characteristics of the Autism Spectrum Disorder and typically developing groups.

Variable	ASD group (N = 44)	TYP group (N = 44)
Age in months M (SD)	124.7 (19.3)	122.9 (19.5)
Boys : girls	21 : 23	25 : 19
Verbal IQ M (SD)	100.7 (13.2)	107.1 (9.6)
Performance IQ M (SD)	100.7 (15.3)	105.2 (13.9)

ASD: Autism Spectrum Disorder; TYP: typically developing.

Parents of participants were invited to participate via email or letter and follow-up telephone call. Participants were tested at a home visit, at the Monash University campus, or at their primary school. The WASI and WISC-IV were administered according to standardized instructions.

Parents filled out the questionnaires as per their standard instructions. Age-based standardized scores were utilized for the WISC-IV and WASI. Raw scores were used in analyses unless otherwise stated. Children completed the SCAS and worry thermometers in the presence of the examiner (TM) who explained and clarified any questions about the measures and read the questions from the SCAS for all children. All data were entered into statistical package for the social sciences (SPSS) version 22.0 for statistical analyses.

3. Results

3.1. Preliminary Analyses. Analyses utilised included t-tests to compare demographic variables between groups and mixed model analysis of variance (ANOVA) to compare group differences in anxiety measures across raters and gender. Pearson correlations were used to determine the associations between variables. Bonferroni corrections were employed for post hoc tests.

Independent t-tests showed no difference in age $t(86) = -.440$, $P = .661$ and perceptual IQ $t(86) = 1.436$, $P = .155$, between the ASD and TYP groups, Table 1. Children with ASD had lower Verbal IQs than TYP children, $t(86) = 2.573$, $P = .012$. The group was matched on gender according to a Chi square test, $\chi^2(88) = .729$, $P = .393$.

3.2. Group and Gender Differences on the SCAS. The means of the SCAS total score and subscales by parent, child, and group are found in Figure 1, with group differences described in the following analyses. For the SCAS total score, a Repeated Measures ANOVA with group (ASD or TYP) and gender (male or female child) as the between-subject factors and SCAS rater (parent or child) as the repeated measure was conducted. This showed a significant main effect of group, $F(1, 84) = 11.978$, $P = .001$, $\eta_P^2 = .125$, and rater, $F(1, 84) = 19.132$, $P = .001$, $\eta_P^2 = .186$. There was a significant group by rater interaction, $F(1, 84) = 11.653$, $P = .001$, $\eta_P^2 = .122$. To explore the interaction, independent t-tests were used with Bonferroni corrections ($.05/4 = .0125$). These found no difference between TYP and ASD child self-reports, $t(86) = -.569$, $P = .517$, but parents of children with ASD reported

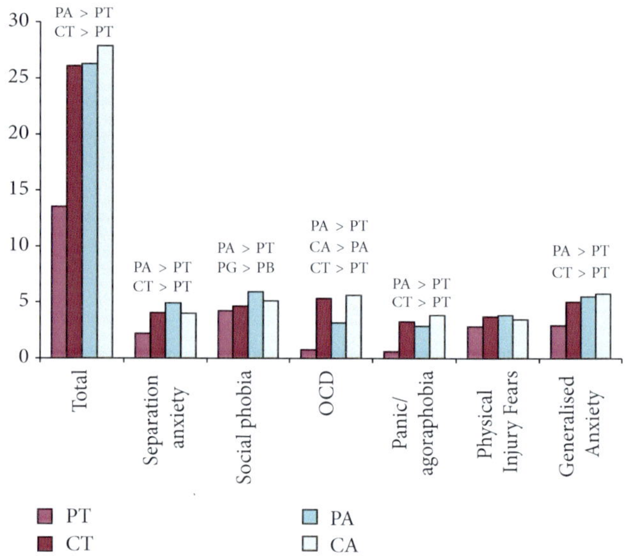

Figure 1: Means of the SCAS total and subscales for parents and children by group. Significant group differences are coded as follows: PA, parents of children with ASD; PT, parents of typically developing children; CA, children with ASD; CT, typically developing children; PG, parents of girls; PB, parents of boys.

higher levels of anxiety than parents of TYP children, $t(86) = -7.023$, $P < .001$. Paired samples t-test showed there was no difference between parent and child reporting total anxiety for children with ASD, $t(43) = -.654$, $P < .517$, but there was a difference for the TYP group with TYP children reporting higher levels of anxiety than their parents, $t(43) = -6.252$, $P < .001$.

The six subscales were then explored using a Repeated Measures ANOVA to compare rater (parent versus child), group (TYP versus ASD), and gender (male versus female child). There was a significant main effect of subscale, $F(1, 84) = 24.573$, $P < .001$, $\eta_P^2 = .226$, rater $F(1, 84) = 19.132$, $P < .001$, $\eta_P^2 = .186$, and group, $F(1, 84) = 11.978$, $P < .001$, $\eta_P^2 = .125$. There was a significant interaction between rater and group, $F(1, 84) = 11.653$, $P = .001$, $\eta_P^2 = .122$, and subscale and rater $F(1, 84) = 21.811$, $P < .001$, $\eta_P^2 = .206$. These were explored using post hoc ANOVAs with Bonferroni corrections for each subscale ($.05/4 = .0125$) and the differences are summarised in Figure 1. For Physical Injury Fears, there were no significant differences between parent-child reports.

For separation anxiety, there was a significant difference in parent reports ($P < .001$) for TYP and ASD children. TYP parents reported lower levels of separation anxiety than their children ($P < .001$) whereas in ASD parent-child dyads levels were similar.

For social phobia, parent-child dyads reported similar levels regardless of diagnosis. There was a significant difference between TYP and ASD parent reports ($P = .007$) with ASD parents reporting higher levels, but no difference between child reports.

Similarly, for Obsessive Compulsive Disorder, parents of children with ASD reported higher levels than parents of TYP

TABLE 2: Agreement between parent and child SCAS subscales and total score for the ASD and TYP groups.

	Child SA	Child SP	Child OCD	Child PA	Child PIF	Child GA	Child total
Typically developing							
Parent Separation Anxiety	.299*	.112	.262	.319*	.018	.084	.262
Parent Social Phobia	.067	.336*	−.031	−.036	.247	−.122	.100
Parent Obsessive Compulsive Disorder	.236	.117	.083	.068	.122	−.059	.130
Parent Panic/Agoraphobia	.295	.291	.155	.343*	.250	.166	.342*
Parent Physical Injury Fears	.020	.327*	−.142	−.042	.517**	.222	.171
Parent Generalised Anxiety	.238	.130	.195	.282	.354*	.213	.315*
Parent total	.268	.360*	.113	.206	.392**	.104	.320*
ASD							
Parent Separation Anxiety	.306*	.345*	.049	.219	.220	.223	.287
Parent Social Phobia	−.037	.180	−.167	−.033	.052	.001	−.005
Parent Obsessive Compulsive Disorder	−.016	.056	.106	.085	.105	.128	.100
Parent Panic/Agoraphobia	.223	.322*	.058	.145	.169	.232	.244
Parent Physical Injury Fears	.121	.053	−.026	.036	.290	.012	.089
Parent Generalised Anxiety	.248	.218	−.007	.168	.219	.196	.215
Parent total	.227	.324*	−.006	.163	.280	.209	.247

SA, separation anxiety; SP, social phobia; OCD, Obsessive Compulsive Disorder; PA, panic/agoraphobia; PIF, Physical Injury Fears; GA, Generalised Anxiety, SCAS, Spence Children's Anxiety Scale; $^{*}P < .05$, $^{**}P < .01$.

children ($P < .001$) but there was no difference in child report. Both parents of children with ASD ($P < .001$) and parents of TYP children ($P < .001$) reported lower levels of OCD than their children.

Parents of TYP children reported significantly lower levels of panic/agoraphobia than their children ($P < .001$), with no difference between ASD parent-child reports. Parents of children with ASD reported higher levels of panic/agoraphobia than parents of TYP children ($P < .001$), with children reporting similar levels.

For Generalised Anxiety, parents of TYP children reported lower levels than their children ($P < .001$), with no difference between ASD parent-child dyads. Parents of children with ASD reported higher levels than parents of TYP children, with no difference in self-reported Generalised Anxiety in children with or without ASD.

For gender there was only one subscale by gender interaction, $F(1, 84) = 2.391$, $P = .037$, $\eta_P^2 = .028$, with a significant difference for parent-reported social phobia ($P < .001$), with inspection of means revealing that girls were reported to experience higher levels ($M = 6.26$, SD = 3.22) than boys ($M = 4.02$, SD = 2.41). There were no other gender differences in any other analyses, including the thermometer scales.

3.3. Child Thermometer Scales. Pearson correlations between the now, ever, and two-week scales were calculated for the TYP and ASD groups. For the TYP group, the ever and two-week scales were correlated, $r = .459$, $P = .002$, but the now and ever ($r = .151$, $P = .328$) and now and two-week scales ($r = .280$, $P = .065$) were not. For the ASD group, the same pattern was present. The ever and two-week scales were correlated, $r = .304$, $P = .045$, but the now and ever ($r = .144$, $P = .352$) and now and two-week scales ($r = .199$, $P = .196$) were not.

An ANOVA showed no group differences in the child-reported anxiety thermometer scales (now, two weeks, ever) in regard to ASD (two weeks $M = 35$, SD = 33; now $M = 11$, SD = 21; ever $M = 79$, SD = 76) versus TYP children (two weeks $M = 29$, SD = 21; now $M = 5$, SD = 10; ever $M = 72$, SD = 26). Given the fact that Verbal IQ was correlated with the 2-week thermometer, an ANCOVA was conducted and similarly found no difference between TYP and ASD children.

3.4. SCAS Parent and Child Correlations. Correlations between the SCAS parent and child reports for both groups are shown in Table 2. In children with ASD, there was a significant correlation between parent- and child-reported separation anxiety. In TYP children, there were significant correlations between parent- and child-reported separation anxiety, social phobia, panic/agoraphobia, Physical Injury Fears, and the SCAS total score.

3.5. Child Thermometer Correlations with Parent and Child SCAS Scores. Pearson correlations between the child thermometers and parent and child SCAS scores were calculated. For child reports on the SCAS and thermometer, in the ASD group, separation anxiety ($r = .380$, $P < .05$), social phobia ($r = .441$, $P < .01$), and the SCAS total score ($r = .305$, $P < .05$) correlated with the ever thermometer; Physical Injury Fears ($r = .373$, $P < .05$) with the now thermometer; and social phobia ($r = .304$, $P < .05$), panic/agoraphobia ($r = .357$, $P < .05$), and Generalised Anxiety ($r = .319$, $P < .05$) with the two-week thermometer. In TYP children, there was only one correlation which was between separation anxiety and the now thermometer ($r = .350$, $P < .05$).

In regard to parent-child agreement, in the TYP group, the two-week thermometer was unexpectedly negatively correlated with parent-reported separation anxiety ($r = -.327$,

$P < .05$). For children with ASD, the now thermometer was correlated with parent-reported OCD ($r = .309$, $P < .05$) and Generalised Anxiety ($r = .352$, $P < .05$). The lack of associations indicated that the thermometer was not measuring the same anxiety construct as the SCAS.

4. Discussion

In the present study, we sought to compare parent and child reports of child anxiety using the SCAS in children with ASD and typically developing children aged 8–13 years. We found that typically developing parent-child reports on the SCAS showed good correlations, whereas ASD parent-child reports were generally poorly correlated. We also examined whether a "worry thermometer" was able to measure anxiety and found poor construct validity with the SCAS.

4.1. TYP versus ASD on the SCAS. Children with ASD rated themselves as having similar levels of anxiety to typically developing children across all subscales and for the total score, which was in contrast to some past studies [11] but consistent with others [15]. This was despite ASD parents reporting significantly higher levels of anxiety in regard to total anxiety, social phobia, separation anxiety, OCD, and Generalised Anxiety than did TYP parents, a finding consistent with some past studies [15, 18]. Hence, even though children with ASD have high levels of anxiety according to parent report, they self-report similar levels to typically developing children. This may relate to poorer emotion recognition in children with ASD who may have difficulty recognizing and expressing their anxiety, despite them being cognitively high-functioning in the present study. For example, although children with Asperger's Disorder generally have superficially normal language development, their comprehension may be particularly poor [49] which may impact on their ability to understand and express complex constructs such as their own anxiety. Research in adults with ASD suggests up to 50% have alexithymia which impacts on the ability to recognize and express emotional states [50, 51].

Parents of TYP children reported lower levels of anxiety than did their children with the exception of Physical Injury Fears and social phobia. These types of anxiety may be more readily observed by parents in child behavior, potentially resulting in better concordance on these two measures. ASD parents reported lower levels of OCD than their children, with otherwise similar mean scores for the other five subscales and total SCAS score. Russell and Sofronoff [11] similarly found that children with ASD rated themselves as having higher levels of OCD than their parents indicated. Overall, ASD parents and children actually reported more similar mean levels of anxiety, with TYP parents generally reporting lower mean levels of anxiety than their children. It may be that TYP children overreport their levels of anxiety and children with ASD underreport theirs, resulting in this pattern of similar child-reported anxiety levels.

4.2. Correlations between Parent and Child SCAS. Although at the group level there was general consistency between mean parent- and child-reported levels of anxiety, the parent-child *correlations* suggested poor agreement in ASD parent-child dyads compared with better agreement in TYP parent-child dyads. These findings are in contrast to some past studies [12–14], which found generally good child-parent correlations on the total SCAS score in youth with ASD, but consistent with White and colleagues [16] who found poor parent-child correlations (12–17 years). These differences may be due to the older children in these three aforementioned studies (10–16 years) compared to the current study (8–13 years). The SCAS may be better able to accurately capture self-reported anxiety in older children with ASD. Consistent with the current study, Lopata and colleagues [15] and van Steensel and colleagues [19] also found poor correlations between parent-child-reported anxieties in children with ASD using other anxiety measures. Their age ranges also included younger participants (7–17) further supporting the notion that age may be a factor in the accurate self-reporting of anxiety in ASD.

4.3. Thermometer Scale. This is the first study to our knowledge to compare a Visual Analogue Scale to the SCAS in children with ASD. The child-rated worry thermometer used in the study showed poor construct validity with parent and child reports on the SCAS for both TYP and ASD groups. There have been some studies which have not found Visual Analogue Scales to be well correlated with parent reports, at least in the paediatric pain literature [33]. Parent-child agreement is good for severe difficulties (such as severe injuries and things complained of daily), but less for more infrequent or less severe difficulties [52]. The thermometer scale used in the current study asked children to report on how "worried" or "scared" they were, which can be considered two separate constructs; hence, this could explain the lack of validity of the thermometer. Future work may benefit from separating these constructs into separate thermometers.

4.4. Gender. Finally, this was the first study to compare self-reported anxiety in girls and boys with ASD. There were no gender differences found in boys and girls ratings of their own anxiety in the ASD or TYP groups, on both the SCAS and worry thermometers. Potentially, as girls reach puberty, they may experience greater levels of anxiety than boys and show differences in anxiety self-report from this period onwards.

4.5. Clinical Implications. The present findings contribute to a growing body of research showing that children with ASD prior to puberty may have difficulties accurately reporting their anxiety. This is not the case for typically developing children which may relate to their better verbal and emotional understanding. Parent report, at least using the SCAS, is likely to be a more accurate measure of anxiety than children with ASD's self-report. Hence, clinicians and those who work with children with ASD within the 8–13-year age range may need to primarily rely on parent reports of anxiety. Additionally, the use of thermometer scales to measure internal states in children with ASD is commonplace in a number of ASD specific interventions [20, 22, 23]. Clinicians should interpret these child self-reported thermometer scales cautiously until validity is demonstrated.

4.6. Limitations. An important extension of this study will be for clinicians to rate anxiety in the children using structured parent and child interviews. In the present study, the child ratings were compared to their parents and not to a clinical assessment of anxiety symptoms. This will then allow clinician reports to be correlated with child and parent reports of anxiety to further examine the validity of a thermometer scale. The lack of a clinician report is a major limitation of the study. However, it is noteworthy that past studies that have compared parent, child, and clinician structured interviews in youth with ASD have found good to excellent correspondence between clinician consensus diagnosis and parent reports of anxiety [53]. Comparing a group of children with anxiety disorders without ASD to those with ASD on the thermometer scale may have also been informative to determine whether the poor correspondence between parent-child reports is associated with anxiety per se or ASD.

Only children with full-scale IQs greater than 70 were included, and hence these findings may not generalize to children with ASD and intellectual disability. Of note, none of the studies examining self-reported anxiety in ASD discussed have included children with intellectual disability as participants. Given the fact that most individuals with ASD have intellectual disability, examining whether similar self-report measures of anxiety are valid in this population is needed.

5. Conclusion

Overall, children with ASD aged between 8 and 13 years show difficulty in accurately reporting their anxiety relative to parent reports. In contrast, typically developing children of this age range self-report anxiety levels similar to their parent ratings. The use of a visual analogue "worry thermometer" to gauge anxiety levels in children with ASD was not supported by the present studies findings. Given the extensive use of these types of scales in interventions for children with ASD, further research into the validity of these measures is warranted.

References

[1] V. Hallett, L. Lecavalier, D. G. Sukhodolsky et al., "Exploring the manifestations of anxiety in children with autism spectrum disorders," *Journal of Autism and Developmental Disorders*, vol. 43, no. 10, pp. 2341–2352, 2013.

[2] E. Simonoff, A. Pickles, T. Charman, S. Chandler, T. Loucas, and G. Baird, "Psychiatric disorders in children with autism spectrum disorders: prevalence, comorbidity, and associated factors in a population-derived sample," *Journal of the American Academy of Child and Adolescent Psychiatry*, vol. 47, no. 8, pp. 921–929, 2008.

[3] F. J. van Steensel, S. M. Bögels, and S. Perrin, "Anxiety disorders in children and adolescents with autistic spectrum disorders: a meta-analysis," *Clinical Child and Family Psychology Review*, vol. 14, no. 3, pp. 302–317, 2011.

[4] S. W. White, D. P. Oswald, T. H. Ollendick, and L. Scahill, "Anxiety in children and adolescents with autism spectrum disorders," *Clinical Psychology Review*, vol. 29, no. 3, pp. 216–229, 2009.

[5] N. Humphrey and S. Lewis, "'Make me normal': tthe views and experiences of pupils on the autistic spectrum in mainstream secondary schools," *Autism*, vol. 12, no. 1, pp. 23–46, 2008.

[6] M. Sciutto, S. Richwine, J. Mentrikoski, and K. Niedzwiecki, "A qualitative analysis of the school experiences of students with Asperger syndrome," *Focus on Autism and Other Developmental Disabilities*, vol. 27, no. 3, pp. 177–188, 2012.

[7] M. G. Baron, *Stress and Coping in Autism*, Oxford University Press, 2006.

[8] M. Ghaziuddin, N. Ghaziuddin, and J. Greden, "Depression in persons with autism: implications for research and clinical care," *Journal of Autism and Developmental Disorders*, vol. 32, no. 4, pp. 299–306, 2002.

[9] J. Green, A. Gilchrist, D. Burton, and A. Cox, "Social and psychiatric functioning in adolescents with Asperger syndrome compared with conduct disorder," *Journal of Autism and Developmental Disorders*, vol. 30, no. 4, pp. 279–293, 2000.

[10] J. Groden, M. G. Baron, and G. Groden, "Assessment and coping strategies," in *Stress and Coping in Autism*, pp. 15–41, 2006.

[11] E. Russell and K. Sofronoff, "Anxiety and social worries in children with Asperger syndrome," *Australian and New Zealand Journal of Psychiatry*, vol. 39, no. 7, pp. 633–638, 2005.

[12] I. Magiati, J. Y. Chan, W.-L. J. Tan, and K. K. Poon, "Do non-referred young people with Autism Spectrum Disorders and their caregivers agree when reporting anxiety symptoms? A preliminary investigation using the Spence Children's Anxiety Scale," *Research in Autism Spectrum Disorders*, vol. 8, no. 5, pp. 546–558, 2014.

[13] S. Farrugia and J. Hudson, "Anxiety in adolescents with asperger syndrome: negative thoughts, behavioral problems, and life interference," *Focus on Autism and Other Developmental Disabilities*, vol. 21, no. 1, pp. 25–35, 2006.

[14] A. Ozsivadjian, C. Hibberd, and M. J. Hollocks, "Brief report: the use of self-report measures in young people with autism spectrum disorder to access symptoms of anxiety, depression and negative thoughts," *Journal of Autism and Developmental Disorders*, vol. 44, no. 4, pp. 969–974, 2014.

[15] C. Lopata, J. A. Toomey, J. D. Fox et al., "Anxiety and depression in children with hfasds: symptom levels and source differences," *Journal of Abnormal Child Psychology*, vol. 38, no. 6, pp. 765–776, 2010.

[16] S. W. White, A. R. Schry, and B. B. Maddox, "Brief report: the assessment of anxiety in high-functioning adolescents with autism spectrum disorder," *Journal of Autism and Developmental Disorders*, vol. 42, no. 6, pp. 1138–1145, 2012.

[17] B. Birmaher, D. A. Brent, L. Chiappetta, J. Bridge, S. Monga, and M. Baugher, "Psychometric properties of the screen for child anxiety related emotional disorders (SCARED): a replication study," *Journal of the American Academy of Child & Adolescent Psychiatry*, vol. 38, no. 10, pp. 1230–1236, 1999.

[18] A. Blakeley-Smith, J. Reaven, K. Ridge, and S. Hepburn, "Parent–child agreement of anxiety symptoms in youth with

autism spectrum disorders," *Research in Autism Spectrum Disorders*, vol. 6, no. 2, pp. 707–716, 2012.

[19] F. J. van Steensel, A. A. Deutschman, and S. M. Bögels, "Examining the Screen for Child Anxiety-Related Emotional Disorder-71 as an assessment tool for anxiety in children with high-functioning autism spectrum disorders," *Autism*, vol. 17, no. 6, pp. 681–692, 2013.

[20] T. Attwood, *The Complete Guide to Asperger's Syndrome*, Jessica Kingsley Publishers, Philadelphia, Pa, USA, 2006.

[21] T. Attwood, "Cognitive behaviour therapy for children and adults with Asperger's syndrome," *Behaviour Change*, vol. 21, no. 3, pp. 147–161, 2004.

[22] A. M. Chalfant, R. Rapee, and L. Carroll, "Treating anxiety disorders in children with high functioning autism spectrum disorders: a controlled trial," *Journal of Autism and Developmental Disorders*, vol. 37, no. 10, pp. 1842–1857, 2007.

[23] K. Sofronoff, T. Attwood, and S. Hinton, "A randomised controlled trial of a CBT intervention for anxiety in children with Asperger syndrome," *Journal of Child Psychology and Psychiatry*, vol. 46, no. 11, pp. 1152–1160, 2005.

[24] D. D. Price, P. A. McGrath, A. Rafii, and B. Buckingham, "The validation of visual analogue scales as ratio scale measures for chronic and experimental pain," *Pain*, vol. 17, no. 1, pp. 45–56, 1983.

[25] P. J. Scott, B. M. Ansell, and E. C. Huskisson, "Measurement of pain in juvenile chronic polyarthritis," *Annals of the Rheumatic Diseases*, vol. 36, no. 2, pp. 186–187, 1977.

[26] D. L. Wong and C. M. Baker, "Pain in children: comparison of assessment scales," *Pediatric Nursing*, vol. 14, no. 1, pp. 9–17, 1988.

[27] A. J. Mitchell, E. A. Baker-Glenn, B. Park, L. Granger, and P. Symonds, "Can the Distress Thermometer be improved by additional mood domains? Part II. What is the optimal combination of Emotion Thermometers?" *Psycho-Oncology*, vol. 19, no. 2, pp. 134–140, 2010.

[28] A. J. Mitchell, E. A. Baker-Glenn, L. Granger, and P. Symonds, "Can the distress thermometer be improved by additional mood domains? Part I. Initial validation of the emotion thermometers tool," *Psycho-Oncology*, vol. 19, no. 2, pp. 125–133, 2010.

[29] G. A. Bernstein and B. D. Garfinkel, "The visual analogue scale for anxiety—revised: psychometric properties," *Journal of Anxiety Disorders*, vol. 6, no. 3, pp. 223–239, 1992.

[30] R. Digiuseppe and M. E. Bernard, "REBT assessment and treatment with children," in *Rational Emotive Behavioral Approaches to Childhood Disorders*, pp. 85–114, Springer, New York, NY, USA, 2006.

[31] M. E. Wewers and N. K. Lowe, "A critical review of visual analogue scales in the measurement of clinical phenomena," *Research in Nursing & Health*, vol. 13, no. 4, pp. 227–236, 1990.

[32] J. N. Stinson, T. Kavanagh, J. Yamada, N. Gill, and B. Stevens, "Systematic review of the psychometric properties, interpretability and feasibility of self-report pain intensity measures for use in clinical trials in children and adolescents," *Pain*, vol. 125, no. 1-2, pp. 143–157, 2006.

[33] A.-M. Kelly, C. V. Powell, and A. Williams, "Parent visual analogue scale ratings of children's pain do not reliably reflect pain reported by child," *Pediatric Emergency Care*, vol. 18, no. 3, pp. 159–162, 2002.

[34] B. J. Shields, T. M. Palermo, J. D. Powers, S. D. Grewe, and G. A. Smith, "Predictors of a child's ability to use a visual analogue scale," *Child: Care, Health and Development*, vol. 29, no. 4, pp. 281–290, 2003.

[35] C. Lopata, M. A. Volker, S. K. Putnam, M. L. Thomeer, and R. E. Nida, "Effect of social familiarity on salivary cortisol and self-reports of social anxiety and stress in children with high functioning autism spectrum disorders," *Journal of Autism and Developmental Disorders*, vol. 38, no. 10, pp. 1866–1877, 2008.

[36] R. G. Romanczyk and J. M. Gillis, "Autism and the physiology of stress and anxiety," in *Stress and Coping in Autism*, pp. 183–204, Oxford University Press, New York, NY, USA, 2006.

[37] APA, *Diagnostic and Statistical Manual of Mental Disorders 5*, American Psychiatric Association, Washington, DC, USA, 2013.

[38] M. Solomon, M. Miller, S. L. Taylor, S. P. Hinshaw, and C. S. Carter, "Autism symptoms and internalizing psychopathology in girls and boys with autism spectrum disorders," *Journal of Autism and Developmental Disorders*, vol. 42, no. 1, pp. 48–59, 2012.

[39] T. May, K. Cornish, and N. Rinehart, "Does gender matter? A one year follow-up of autistic, attention and anxiety symptoms in high-functioning children with autism spectrum disorder," *Journal of Autism and Developmental Disorders*, vol. 44, no. 5, pp. 1077–1086, 2014.

[40] J. N. Constantino, *The Social Responsiveness Scale*, Western Psychological Services, West Los Angeles, Calif, USA, 2002.

[41] J. N. Constantino, S. A. Davis, R. D. Todd et al., "Validation of a brief quantitative measure of autistic traits: comparison of the social responsiveness scale with the autism diagnostic interview-revised," *Journal of Autism and Developmental Disorders*, vol. 33, no. 4, pp. 427–433, 2003.

[42] American Psychiatric Association, *Diagnostic and Statistical Manual of Mental Disorders, IV-TR*, American Psychiatric Association, Washington, DC, USA, 2000.

[43] D. Wechsler, *WISC-IV Australian Administration and Scoring Manual*, Harcourt Assessment, 2005.

[44] D. Wechsler, *Wechsler Abbreviated Scale of Intelligence (WASI)*, Harcourt Assessment, San Antonio, Tex, USA, 1999.

[45] S. H. Spence, "A measure of anxiety symptoms among children," *Behaviour Research and Therapy*, vol. 36, no. 5, pp. 545–566, 1998.

[46] M. H. Nauta, A. Scholing, R. M. Rapee, M. Abbott, S. H. Spence, and A. Waters, "A parent-report measure of children's anxiety: Psychometric properties and comparison with child-report in a clinic and normal sample," *Behaviour Research and Therapy*, vol. 42, no. 7, pp. 813–839, 2004.

[47] S. H. Spence, P. M. Barrett, and C. M. Turner, "Psychometric properties of the Spence Children's Anxiety Scale with young adolescents," *Journal of Anxiety Disorders*, vol. 17, no. 6, pp. 605–625, 2003.

[48] M. S. Gordon, B. Tonge, and G. A. Melvin, "Outcome of adolescent depression: 6 months after treatment," *Australian and New Zealand Journal of Psychiatry*, vol. 45, no. 3, pp. 232–239, 2011.

[49] S. Saalasti, T. Lepistö, E. Toppila et al., "Language abilities of children with Asperger syndrome," *Journal of Autism and Developmental Disorders*, vol. 38, no. 8, pp. 1574–1580, 2008.

[50] S. Berthoz and E. L. Hill, "The validity of using self-reports to assess emotion regulation abilities in adults with autism spectrum disorder," *European Psychiatry*, vol. 20, no. 3, pp. 291–298, 2005.

[51] M. V. Lombardo, J. L. Barnes, S. J. Wheelwright, and S. Baron-Cohen, "Self-referential cognition and empathy in autism," *PLoS ONE*, vol. 2, no. 9, article e883, 2007.

6

Parenting Behavior in Mothers of Preschool Children with ASD: Development of a Self-Report Questionnaire

Greet Lambrechts,[1,2] Jarymke Maljaars,[1,2] Hannah Boonen,[1,2] Lotte van Esch,[1,2] Karla Van Leeuwen,[1] and Ilse Noens[1,2]

[1] *Parenting and Special Education Research Unit, University of Leuven (KU Leuven), Leopold Vanderkelenstraat 32, P.O. Box 3765, 3000 Leuven, Belgium*
[2] *Leuven Autism Research (LAuRes), University of Leuven (KU Leuven), 3000 Leuven, Belgium*

Correspondence should be addressed to Greet Lambrechts; greet.lambrechts@ppw.kuleuven.be

Academic Editor: Hansen Wang

Parents of young children with autism spectrum disorder (ASD) encounter many daily challenges and often experience much stress. However, little research exists about parenting behavior among these parents. With this study, we aim to address this gap. We examined the structure and internal consistency of a questionnaire intended to measure parenting behavior among mothers of young children with ASD. Furthermore, we compared parenting behavior among mothers of young children with and without ASD between two and six years old. Factor analyses resulted in a factor solution with seven subscales of parenting behavior. Two additional subscales especially relevant for parenting preschoolers with ASD were also considered. Analyses of covariance, controlling for gender and age, showed significantly higher scores for *Discipline* and *Stimulating the Development* in the control group in comparison with the ASD group. These findings suggest that mothers of preschoolers with ASD are still trying to find strategies to guide and stimulate their child's behavior and development effectively.

1. Introduction

Parents of children with autism spectrum disorder (ASD) encounter many challenges on a daily basis. A great number of studies refer to higher levels of stress among parents of children with ASD when compared to parents of typically developing children or parents of children with other disabilities (e.g., [1–5]). Whether parents experience stress or not depends on their coping strategies, informal social support sources, beliefs about the efficacy of the interventions, and the level of autism symptomatology [3]. Apart from the daily stress of raising a child with ASD, parents of young children (between two and six years old) also have to cope with the emotions of a recent ASD diagnosis and the initiation of intervention services [6]. Furthermore, during this period, young children are likely to show many "early autism" deficits, such as a lack of social responsiveness, communication skills, joint attention, and interactive play skills. These deficits can cause considerable concern for parents who may question their own parenting abilities as a result [7]. Literature suggests that parents of young children with ASD who are emotionally unable to accept their family's situation may have more difficulties attuning to their children's needs [8].

Despite the evidence that parenting young children with ASD is rather challenging, little research exists about parenting behavior among parents of young children with ASD as such. Previous research has primarily investigated characteristics of the parent-child relationship, such as emotional availability and attachment in families with a young child with ASD [9]. van Ijzendoorn et al. [9], for example, studied sensitivity and attachment in parents of children with ASD using the strange situation procedure [10] and the Emotional Availability Scales (EAS Infancy/Early Childhood Version; [11]). However, in the present study, parenting behavior is rather considered as the observable behavior of parents which plays a role in the socialization of children or the way in which children acquire the social, emotional, and cognitive skills to function in the social community [12]. Literature about typically developing children generally distinguishes between two main dimensions: parental warmth (support or responsiveness) and parental control (behavioral and psychological control) [13]. Maccoby and Martin [13] identified four patterns of parenting based on these two dimensions: authoritarian, authoritative, permissive, and indifferent parenting. More recently, growing attention is being given to autonomy support in addition to these two dimensions [14]. Examples of autonomy support are showing empathy for the perspective of the child, giving choices, and encouraging the child to act on the basis of intrinsic satisfying motives [15].

Only a few studies have examined these dimensions of parenting or closely related variables in parents of young children with ASD. First, Kasari et al. [16] compared the caregiver's (mother or father) responsiveness in three groups of preschool children (a group with ASD, a group with a developmental disability, and a control group without a disability), but they did not observe any significant differences between the groups. Second, in a study by Watson [17], mothers of preschool children with ASD showed as much responsiveness as mothers of typically developing preschool children. And, finally, Baker et al. [18] did not find differences in sensitivity between mothers of toddlers with emergent ASD and mothers of toddlers without an eventual ASD diagnosis.

As regards the parental control dimension, Kasari et al. [16] showed that caregivers of children with ASD and children with a developmental disability used more control strategies than caregivers of the control group. Similar results were found in a study by Lemanek et al. [19] of preschoolers with ASD and in a study by Wan et al. [20] of infants at risk for ASD.

Some studies focused on specific aspects of parenting behavior. Meirsschaut et al. [21] concluded that mothers of preschoolers with ASD used more social and imperative initiatives, less declarative initiatives, and more denying responses towards their child in comparison to mothers of typically developing children. Furthermore, mothers of preschoolers with ASD used as many social initiatives and reacted as responsively with an unfamiliar child as with their own child. Blacher et al. [22] examined positive and negative parenting behaviors among parents of children with developmental delays (i.e., ASD, Down syndrome, and cerebral palsy) in comparison to parents of typically developing children at three, four, and five years of age. Parents of children with developmental delays showed more negative parenting behavior (i.e., negative affect, intrusiveness, and detachment) in comparison with the control group at the three time points. Parents of the clinical group showed less positive parenting behavior (i.e., positive affect, sensitivity, and stimulation of cognition) in comparison with the control group but only when the child was three years old.

Finally, Rutgers et al. [23] focused specifically on parenting styles instead of parenting dimensions and they compared parenting styles among parents of preschoolers with ASD with parenting styles among parents of children of the same age with an intellectual disability, with a language disorder, and without a diagnosis. Parents of typically developing children reported higher levels of authoritative parenting (a combination of high levels of demandingness and responsiveness) in comparison with all other clinical groups.

In summary, the majority of studies reported no differences between the clinical groups and the control group in terms of responsiveness. Conversely, regarding control strategies, differences were often observed, with higher scores in the clinical groups. However, results across studies are inconclusive, thus highlighting the need for more research. Furthermore, the clinical groups often consist of a combination of parents of children with ASD and parents of children with another developmental disorder. This makes it difficult to draw conclusions about parents of children with ASD specifically.

Except for the study by Rutgers et al. [23], all these studies used observations to study parenting behavior. Although observations have the advantage of presenting a more "objective" view on parenting, self-report measures on parenting can also provide useful information: they give insight into the parents' point of view about behavior in different daily situations. Moreover, an instrument that could prompt parents to have a conversation about their parenting behavior would be valuable, particularly in clinical applications. In the study by Rutgers et al. [23], parents completed a questionnaire assessing authoritative and authoritarian child-rearing styles. Osborne and Reed [5] presented the parents of children with ASD between 2 and 16 years old with a self-report instrument with four parenting subscales, involvement, communication, limit setting, and autonomy, in combination with a parental stress measure. In addition to these already available questionnaires, it would be interesting to have a self-report instrument to measure a broad range of general parenting behaviors combined with a focus on parenting behavior specifically relevant for young children with ASD. In the current study, we aimed at evaluating such a self-report questionnaire of parenting behavior and characterizing parenting behavior among mothers of young children with ASD.

In a preliminary questionnaire study about parenting behavior among parents of children with ASD between 8 and 18 years old [24], we found, apart from the general parenting behaviors, indications for parenting behaviors specifically relevant for children with ASD. We developed an instrument similar to this earlier questionnaire for children younger than 6 years old based on the Parental Behavior Scale for toddlers (PBS-T; [25]).

First, we examined the factor structure and internal consistency of this adjusted questionnaire to measure parenting behavior among mothers of young children with ASD. Second, we compared parenting behavior among mothers of young children with and without ASD. Based on earlier research, we did not expect to find any differences on the subscale Positive Parenting between the two groups but more behavioral control and behaviors specifically relevant for parenting children with ASD in the ASD group.

2. Materials and Methods

2.1. Participants and Procedure. A total of 1314 Dutch-speaking mothers (Flemish part of Belgium and Netherlands) participated in this study. The ASD group consisted of 57 biological mothers of a child with ASD (n = 37 from Netherlands and n = 20 from the Flemish part of Belgium). All children were between 31 months and 72 months old (M = 55.37; SD = 11.21) and 84.2% (n = 48) were boys. Ten children had an intellectual disability, 8 children had an IQ below average (between 70 and 84), 20 children had an average IQ (between 85 and 115), and 6 children had an IQ above average (higher than 115). For 13 children, there was no information available about their cognitive functioning. Mothers indicated on a questionnaire that their child had received a clinical ASD diagnosis. The control group consisted of 1257 biological mothers with a child without ASD (n = 138 from Netherlands and n = 1119 from the Flemish part of Belgium). All children were between 20 and 73 months old (M = 36.93; SD = 9.72) and 52.3% (n = 658) were boys. For the factor analyses, data of the entire control group were used, while the group comparisons were based on the data of a subgroup matched with the ASD group.

All mothers participated in the context of several research projects on parenting behavior and/or ASD in young children. After informed consent was given, they received the questionnaire by mail or during a home visit. The majority of the mothers of the control group (n = 882) filled out the Parental Behavior Scale for toddlers (PBS-T; [22]). All the other mothers filled out the adjusted version of the measure supplemented with additional items tapping parenting behaviors hypothesized to be specifically relevant in the context of ASD. The research design was approved by the university's ethical committee and mothers were not reimbursed for participating.

2.2. Measure. The Parental Behavior Scale for toddlers (PBS-T; [25]) is designed to measure general parenting behavior among parents of children younger than four years old. This questionnaire is based on the Parental Behavior Scale (PBS; [26]) for parents of school-aged children. For the purpose of studying parenting in families with school-aged children with ASD, this PBS version for parents of school-aged children has been extended with items tapping parenting behaviors specifically relevant in the context of ASD, such as adapting the child's environment and stimulating the child's development (PBS-A; [27]). In line with that extension, we also adjusted the Parental Behavior Scale for toddlers and added several items. First of all, we selected all the items of this scale about general parenting behavior that were applicable to children between two and six years old (n = 40): *Positive Parenting* (e.g., I play with my child), *Autonomy Support* (e.g., I give my child the opportunity to try new things), *Supervision and Safety* (e.g., I provide a safe environment for my child), *Discipline* (e.g., when my child does something I do not like, I raise my voice), *Rules and Structure* (e.g., I make sure my child's daily routine is the same day in, day out), and *Rewarding* (e.g., when my child masters doing something new, I applaud or say good boy/good girl). Furthermore, 21 items specifically relevant for parenting children with ASD were added about *Stimulating the Development* (e.g., when a person is crying, I explain to my child how this person is feeling and why) and *Adapting the Environment* (e.g., when my child is doing an activity (e.g., drawing or reading a book), I keep distraction to a minimum). This self-report measure is to be completed by parents of children up to six years old. By means of a 5-point Likert scale, parents rate the frequency of each behavior (1 = (almost) never, 2 = little, 3 = sometimes, 4 = often, and 5 = (almost) always).

2.3. Data Analysis. All statistical tests were performed using IBM SPSS Statistics 22. Because the ASD group is much smaller than the control group, we decided to carry out the factor analyses only on the data of the control group that consisted of 1257 biological mothers of a child without ASD. First, we checked the assumptions to execute a Principal Axis Factoring (PAF). The Kaiser-Meyer-Olkin (KMO) value was greater than .8 and Bartlett's test of sphericity was significant ($p < .001$) indicating that we could execute a PAF [28]. We chose to use a direct oblimin rotation, because we expected the factors to be correlated.

To conduct the comparative analyses, we created a matching control group by randomly selecting respondents from the control group, based on the criteria of child age (M = 55.6 months in the control group and M = 55.4 in the ASD group) and child sex (9 girls and 48 boys in both groups). We used a MANCOVA with group and sex as factors, age as a covariate, and mean scores for the parenting subscales as dependent variables. The error variance was equal across groups for most of the subscales (Levene's tests, $p > .05$), except for *Supervision and Safety* and for *Stimulating the Development*. To address the violation of homogeneity for the latter subscales, we checked the Brown-Forsythe F and Welch F statistics of the One-Way ANOVA analysis of these subscales. Eta squared values were used as indicators of effect size with values of .01–.06 pointing to a small effect, .06–.14 pointing to a medium effect, and >.14 pointing to a large effect [29].

3. Results

3.1. Factor Structure of the General Parenting Items. The Kaiser criterion (select all factors with eigenvalue > 1) suggested a ten-factor solution with many factors explaining only little variance and/or comprising just a few items. However, the drop in the scree plot suggested a seven-factor solution [30] and because this solution is also more acceptable from a conceptual point of view we decided to continue with seven factors. This solution accounted for 34.10% of the variance. We included items only if they loaded higher than $|.35|$ on one factor in the pattern matrix and lower than $|.30|$ on the other factors. This resulted in a *Positive Parenting* subscale of 6 items, an *Autonomy Support* subscale of 4 items, a *Rules and Structure* subscale of 3 items, a *Discipline* subscale of 5 items, a *Rewarding* subscale of 3 items, a *Supervision and Safety* subscale of 6 items, and an *Indulging* subscale of 2 items (e.g., when my child wants something, I give in so he or she will not get cross or start to cry). Eleven items were removed.

The internal consistency was good for five subscales ($.70 < \alpha < .81$; corrected item total correlations >.36). For the *Discipline* subscale, the internal consistency was rather poor, with Cronbach's alpha value of .57 (corrected item

Table 1: Number of items and α values for all the factors and their intercorrelations (Pearson's correlations).

Factors	Number of items	α	(2)	(3)	(4)	(5)	(6)	(7)
(1) Positive Parenting	6	.72	.43***	.17***	.01	.35***	−.01	.34***
(2) Autonomy Support	4	.79		.15***	.06*	.27***	−.12***	.24***
(3) Rules and Structure	3	.75			.00	.14***	−.14***	.22***
(4) Discipline	5	.57				.07*	.00	−.05
(5) Rewarding	3	.81					−.05	.36***
(6) Indulging	2	—						−.01
(7) Supervision and Safety	6	.71						

$^{*}p < .05$; $^{***}p < .001$.

Table 2: Group differences in parenting behavior between the ASD and control group.

	Control (n = 57) M (SD)	ASD (n = 57) M (SD)	MANCOVA: ASD versus control F	p	η^2
General parenting behavior					
Positive Parenting	4.02 (.40)	3.86 (.41)	3.55	.062	—
Autonomy Support	4.23 (.38)	4.00 (.40)	2.38	.126	—
Rules and Structure	4.41 (.49)	4.29 (.58)	0.03	.864	—
Discipline	**3.26 (.42)**	**2.93 (.51)**	**13.22**	**<.001**	**.101**[a]
Rewarding	4.61 (.41)	4.71 (.40)	1.29	.259	—
Indulging	2.19 (.56)	2.61 (.66)	2.31	.132	—
Supervision and Safety	4.22 (.38)	4.24 (.46)	0.16	.695	—
ASD-adapted parenting behavior					
Stimulating the Development	**3.96 (.38)**	**3.63 (.55)**	**5.11**	**.026**	**.044**[b]
Adapting the Environment	3.68 (.37)	3.73 (.49)	0.18	.672	—

[a]Medium effect size; [b]small effect size.

total correlations >.25). Pearson's correlation between the two items of the *Indulging* subscale was high (r = .48; $p < .001$). α values and the intercorrelations of the seven factors are presented in Table 1.

3.2. Items Specifically Relevant for Parenting Preschoolers with ASD. Although it is advisable to conduct a factor analysis on the ASD-related items as well, the ASD group was too small to obtain meaningful results. Therefore we decided to use the original 21 items belonging to the two subscales based on the solution in the study by Lambrechts et al. [24]: *Stimulating the Development* (n = 13 items) and *Adapting the Environment* (n = 8 items).

The calculation of the internal consistency was based on the data of all mothers who filled in the adjusted version of the measure (n = 432). The internal consistency was good for *Stimulating the Development* subscale (α = .81; corrected item total correlations >.22) and rather weak for *Adapting the Environment* subscale (α = .56; corrected item total correlations >.14).

3.3. Comparing Parenting Behavior between the Control and the ASD Group. Significant main effects of the factor "group" were present for the subscales *Discipline* ($F_{(1,109)}$ = 13.22; $p < .001$; η^2 = .10) and *Stimulating the Development* (Brown-Forsythe $F_{(1,99.495)}$ = 14.14, $p < .001$, and Welch $F_{(1,99.495)}$ = 14.14, $p < .001$), with higher mean scores for the control group in comparison with the ASD group. Table 2 shows the main results of these analyses. For *Supervision and Safety*, Brown-Forsythe F and Welch F statistics showed the same result as F-test.

Regarding the age of the children, MANCOVA showed a significant main effect for the *Discipline* subscale ($F_{(1,109)}$ = 7.75; $p < .01$; η^2 = .06). When checking Spearman's ρ correlations, a significant correlation was found between age and *Discipline* subscale in the control group only (ρ = −.27, $p < .05$ for the control group; ρ = −.23, p = .09 for the ASD group), with parents of older children reporting using less discipline.

4. Discussion

In this study we examined the factor structure and internal consistency of a new questionnaire to measure parenting behavior among mothers of young children with ASD. With regard to the general parenting items, all the theoretically expected scales were found, with one extra subscale referring to indulging behavior. All but one subscale yielded good internal consistency; *Discipline* subscale should be considered with caution. Regarding the items specifically relevant for parenting preschoolers with ASD, further analyses of a larger group of parents of a child with ASD are needed. For now, the original subscales, based on an instrument used in a previous study on parenting behavior among parents of older children with ASD [24], showed a good internal consistency score for *Stimulating the Development* subscale and a poorer internal consistency score for *Adapting the Environment* subscale.

With respect to the comparison between the control group and the ASD group, no differences were present for *Positive Parenting*. That was also the case for the other subscales that are related to Positive Parenting (*Autonomy Support*, *Rewarding*, and *Supervision and Safety*). These results are similar to the conclusions of other studies based on observational measurements [16–18].

For one aspect of *behavioral control* we found a significant difference between both groups with higher scores for *Discipline* in the control group. However, one should take the lower internal consistency score of this subscale into account. For other aspects of behavioral control (*Rules and Structure* and *Indulging*), there were no significant differences. Conversely, other studies revealed mostly higher scores for behavioral control in parents of children with or at risk for ASD [16, 19, 20]. A possible explanation for this contrast with previous research could be that in our study a distinction was made between several aspects of behavioral control and thus behavioral control was not treated as a general concept. Disciplining is a very specific act and only one aspect of behavioral control. It might be that mothers of young children with ASD interpret undesirable/unwanted behavior of their child differently. Often these behaviors cannot be labeled as unwillingness or deliberate misbehavior, and parents might be more inclined to search for preceding events that might provide insight into the behavior of their child [31].

Another finding regarding *Discipline* subscale revealed that disciplinary behaviors decreased with increasing age of the children in the control group. This effect was not present in the ASD group. Typically, young children's gains in representation, language, and self-concept support their emotional development. Consequently, intense emotional outbursts become less frequent over the preschool years [32] and this is possibly accompanied by less use of disciplining strategies when parenting older children. Young children with ASD, however, often have difficulties with representation, language, and self-concept [33, 34] and their emotional development may be slower and/or different, which can result in a different pattern of disciplining.

With respect to behaviors specifically relevant for parenting preschoolers with ASD, no group differences were found in *Adapting the Environment* subscale. Several items of this subscale are closely related to the general subscale *Rules and Structure* (e.g., "I make sure that everything has a definite place in our house" or "when my child is doing a certain activity, I limit possible distraction to a minimum"). Also for *Rules and Structure* subscale we did not find significant group differences. Given the age of the children involved in this study, this is perhaps not surprising. Almost all mothers of young children seem to provide structure. However, the mothers of the control group reported *Stimulating the Development* of their child more than the ASD group. One explanation could be that mothers of young children with ASD do not know exactly how to stimulate the development of their child and are still experimenting with ways to promote their children's psychosocial maturation. Additionally, some of the parenting behaviors included in *Stimulating the Development* subscale may not apply to young children with ASD (e.g., "when a person is crying, I explain to my child how this person is feeling and why" or "I stimulate pretend play"). However, the answers of parents to these items could be a good starting point for a conversation with parents about their needs in this context. Maybe they need more knowledge about parenting young children with ASD and/or maybe they need specific advice on how to stimulate their child's behavior in everyday situations.

Further research is needed to confirm these results. Concerning the subscales *Stimulating the Development* and *Adapting the Environment*, it may be interesting to look for items that are more specifically relevant for preschoolers with ASD.

The current results have to be interpreted with caution. First, for most children we obtained a confirmation of their ASD diagnosis but for some children we could only rely on their mothers' statement. Second, the two matched groups were rather small, and we could not perform a multigroup confirmatory factor analysis to check whether the factor structure of the questionnaire is comparable across groups of mothers with a child with ASD and mothers with a typically developing child. In the future, data of a different and lager group of both mothers and fathers with a child with ASD are needed to evaluate the scale properly.

Further research on the relationship with other children or parent variables and with observations of parenting behavior would be very interesting. As we mentioned in Introduction, many parents of preschoolers with ASD experience high levels of stress [3]. It would be interesting to study the relationship between parenting behavior and parental stress. Furthermore, it might be important to include a measure of the parents' social responsiveness because of the heritability of the disorder, which may influence their parenting behavior. Amongst other child variables, problem behavior and communication problems can play a significant role. Children with ASD, including very young children, have a relatively high chance of developing problem behavior [35] and parenting behavior can function as a risk factor as well as a protective factor in this area [26]. Additionally, communication problems are often related to problem behavior in children with ASD [36, 37].

Finally, after meeting the limitations mentioned before and doing more analyses on data from a larger ASD group, this instrument could be useful in practice. We think that it is important to have an instrument to screen parenting behavior among parents of young children with ASD in different domains. In contrast with observations of parenting behavior, a self-report questionnaire gives insight into the perspective of the parents concerning a variety of behaviors across a wide range of situations in a time efficient way. As we mentioned earlier, this can be a useful starting point for a conversation about parenting and for planning intervention in that context. Furthermore, this kind of instrument can also be used to evaluate interventions which focused on parenting behavior and to evaluate parenting as a moderator or mediator of treatment.

Ethical Approval

This study was reviewed and approved by the ethical committee of the KU Leuven.

Acknowledgments

The authors would like to thank all the parents who contributed to this study and the participating schools, centers, and associations. Furthermore, they would like to thank all Bachelor's and Master's students and researchers, in particular Dr. Kirstin Greaves-Lord and M.S. Geerte Slappendel from the Erasmus MC in Rotterdam, for their help in participant recruitment and data collection. This research was funded by the Marguerite-Marie Delacroix Support Fund, the Research Fund KU Leuven, and the Research Foundation Flanders.

References

[1] M. M. Bristol and E. Schopler, "A development perspective on stress and coping in families of autistic children," in *Severely Handicapped Children and their Families*, J. Blacher, Ed., pp. 91–141, Academic Press, New York, NY, USA, 1984.

[2] J. E. Dumas, L. C. Wolf, S. N. Fisman, and A. Culligan, "Parenting stress, child behavior problems, and dysphoria in parents of children with autism, Down syndrome, behavior disorders, and normal development," *Exceptionality*, vol. 2, no. 2, pp. 97–110, 1991.

[3] R. P. Hastings and E. Johnson, "Stress in UK families conducting intensive home-based behavioral intervention for their young child with autism," *Journal of Autism and Developmental Disorders*, vol. 31, no. 3, pp. 327–336, 2001.

[4] J. S. Karst and A. V. van Hecke, "Parent and family impact of autism spectrum disorders: a review and proposed model for intervention evaluation," *Clinical Child and Family Psychology Review*, vol. 15, no. 3, pp. 247–277, 2012.

[5] L. A. Osborne and P. Reed, "Stress and self-perceived parenting behaviors of parents of children with autistic spectrum conditions," *Research in Autism Spectrum Disorders*, vol. 4, no. 3, pp. 405–414, 2010.

[6] N. O. Davis and A. S. Carter, "Parenting stress in mothers and fathers of toddlers with autism spectrum disorders: associations with child characteristics," *Journal of Autism and Developmental Disorders*, vol. 38, no. 7, pp. 1278–1291, 2008.

[7] A. Zaidman-Zait, P. Mirenda, E. Duku et al., "Examination of bidirectional relationships between parent stress and two types of problem behavior in children with autism spectrum disorder," *Journal of Autism and Developmental Disorders*, vol. 44, no. 8, pp. 1908–1917, 2014.

[8] K. Wachtel and A. S. Carter, "Reaction to diagnosis and parenting styles among mothers of young children with ASDs," *Autism*, vol. 12, no. 5, pp. 575–594, 2008.

[9] M. H. van Ijzendoorn, A. H. Rutgers, M. J. Bakermans-Kranenburg et al., "Parental sensitivity and attachment in children with autism spectrum disorder: comparison with children with mental retardation, with language delays, and with typical development," *Child Development*, vol. 78, no. 2, pp. 597–608, 2007.

[10] M. D. S. Ainsworth, M. C. Blehar, E. Waters, and S. Wall, *Patterns of Attachment: A Psychological Study of the Strange Situation*, Lawrence Erlbaum Associates, Hillsdale, NJ, USA, 1978.

[11] Z. Biringen, J. L. Robinson, and R. N. Emde, "Appendix B: the emotional availability scales (3rd ed.; an abridged infancy/early childhood version)," *Attachment & Human Development*, vol. 2, no. 2, pp. 256–270, 2000.

[12] J. E. Grusec and M. Davidov, "Integrating different perspectives on socialization theory and research: a domain-specific approach," *Child Development*, vol. 81, no. 3, pp. 687–709, 2010.

[13] E. E. Maccoby and J. A. Martin, "Socialization in the context of the family: parent-child interaction," in *Handbook of Child Psychology: Socialization, Personality, and Social Development*, P. H. Mussen, Ed., vol. 4, pp. 1–101, Wiley, New York, NY, USA, 1983.

[14] S. A. Kelley, C. A. Brownell, and S. B. Campbell, "Mastery motivation and self-evaluative affect in toddlers: longitudinal relations with maternal behavior," *Child Development*, vol. 71, no. 4, pp. 1061–1071, 2000.

[15] B. Soenens, M. Vansteenkiste, W. Lens et al., "Conceptualizing parental autonomy support: adolescent perceptions of promotion of independence versus promotion of volitional functioning," *Developmental Psychology*, vol. 43, no. 3, pp. 633–646, 2007.

[16] C. Kasari, M. Sigman, P. Mundy, and N. Yirmiya, "Caregiver interactions with autistic children," *Journal of Abnormal Child Psychology*, vol. 16, no. 1, pp. 45–56, 1988.

[17] L. R. Watson, "Following the child's lead: mothers' interactions with children with autism," *Journal of Autism and Developmental Disorders*, vol. 28, no. 1, pp. 51–59, 1998.

[18] J. K. Baker, D. S. Messinger, K. K. Lyons, and C. J. Grantz, "A pilot study of maternal sensitivity in the context of emergent autism," *Journal of Autism and Developmental Disorders*, vol. 40, no. 8, pp. 988–999, 2010.

[19] K. L. Lemanek, W. L. Stone, and P. T. Fishel, "Parent-child interactions in handicapped preschoolers: the relation between parent behaviors and compliance," *Journal of Clinical Child Psychology*, vol. 22, no. 1, pp. 68–77, 1993.

[20] M. W. Wan, J. Green, M. Elsabbagh, M. Johnson, T. Charman, and F. Plummer, "Parent–infant interaction in infant siblings at risk of autism," *Research in Developmental Disabilities*, vol. 33, no. 3, pp. 924–932, 2012.

[21] M. Meirsschaut, H. Roeyers, and P. Warreyn, "The social interactive behaviour of young children with autism spectrum disorder and their mothers: is there an effect of familiarity of the interaction partner?" *Autism*, vol. 15, no. 1, pp. 43–64, 2011.

[22] J. Blacher, B. L. Baker, and A. Kaladjian, "Syndrome specificity and mother-child interactions: examining positive and negative parenting across contexts and time," *Journal of Autism and Developmental Disorders*, vol. 43, no. 4, pp. 761–774, 2013.

[23] A. H. Rutgers, M. H. van IJzendoorn, M. J. Bakermans-Kranenburg et al., "Autism, attachment and parenting: a comparison of children with autism spectrum disorder, mental retardation, language disorder, and non-clinical children," *Journal of Abnormal Child Psychology*, vol. 35, no. 5, pp. 859–870, 2007.

[24] G. Lambrechts, K. Van Leeuwen, H. Boonen, B. Maes, and I. Noens, "Parenting behaviour among parents of children with autism spectrum disorder," *Research in Autism Spectrum Disorders*, vol. 5, no. 3, pp. 1143–1152, 2011.

[25] K. Van Leeuwen, S. Rousseau, K. Hoppenbrouwers, R. Wiersema, and A. Desoete, *JOnG! Opvoedings—En Gezinsvariabelen bij de Vlaamse Geboortecohorte 0-Jarigen (Rapport 24)*, Steunpunt Welzijn, Volksgezondheid en Gezin (SWVG), Leuven, Belgium, 2011.

[26] K. G. Van Leeuwen and A. A. Vermulst, "Some psychometric properties of the ghent parental behavior scale," *European Journal of Psychological Assessment*, vol. 20, no. 4, pp. 283–298, 2004.

[27] K. Van Leeuwen and I. Noens, *Parental Behavior Scale for Autism Spectrum Disorders*, KU Leuven, Leuven, Belgium, 2013.

[28] A. Field, *Discovering Statistics Using SPSS*, SAGE Publications, London, UK, 2nd edition, 2005.

[29] J. Cohen, *Statistical Power Analysis for the Behavioural Sciences*, Lawrence Erlbaum Associates, New York, NY, USA, 2nd edition, 1988.

[30] R. B. Cattell, "The scree test for the number of factors," *Multivariate Behavioral Research*, vol. 1, no. 2, pp. 245–276, 1966.

[31] J. Maljaars, H. Boonen, G. Lambrechts, K. Van Leeuwen, and I. Noens, "Maternal parenting behavior and child behavior problems in families of children and adolescents with autism spectrum disorder," *Journal of Autism and Developmental Disorders*, vol. 44, no. 3, pp. 501–512, 2014.

[32] L. E. Berk, "Emotional and social development in early childhood," in *Development through the Lifespan*, L. E. Berk, Ed., pp. 245–275, Allyn & Bacon, Boston, Mass, USA, 1998.

[33] K. Chawarska and F. R. Volkmar, "Autism in infancy and early childhood," in *Handbook of Autism and Pervasive Developmental Disorders*, vol. 1 of *Diagnosis, Development, Neurobiology, and Behavior*, pp. 223–246, John Wiley & Sons, Hoboken, NJ, USA, 3rd edition, 2005.

[34] P. R. Hobson and J. A. Hobson, "Autism: self and others," in *Understanding Other Minds: Perspectives from Developmental Social Neuroscience*, S. Baron-Cohen, H. Tager-Flusberg, and M. V. Lombardo, Eds., pp. 397–412, Oxford University Press, New York, NY, USA, 2013.

[35] S. L. Hartley, D. M. Sikora, and R. McCoy, "Prevalence and risk factors of maladaptive behaviour in young children with autistic disorder," *Journal of Intellectual Disability Research*, vol. 52, no. 10, pp. 819–829, 2008.

[36] T. Charman, J. Ricketts, J. E. Dockrell, G. Lindsay, and O. Palikara, "Emotional and behavioural problems in children with language impairments and children with autism spectrum disorders," *International Journal of Language and Communication Disorders*, vol. 50, no. 1, pp. 84–93, 2015.

[37] C. J. Park, G. W. Yelland, J. R. Taffe, and K. M. Gray, "Brief report: the relationship between language skills, adaptive behavior, and emotional and behavior problems in pre-schoolers with autism," *Journal of Autism and Developmental Disorders*, vol. 42, no. 12, pp. 2761–2766, 2012.

7

About Face: Evaluating and Managing Tactile Impairment at the Time of Autism Diagnosis

Louisa M. T. Silva,[1] Mark Schalock,[2] and Kristen R. Gabrielsen[1]

[1] *Teaching Research Institute, Western Oregon University, Post Office Box 92, McMinnville, OR 97128, USA*
[2] *Teaching Research Institute, Western Oregon University, 345 N. Monmouth Avenue, Monmouth, OR 97361, USA*

Correspondence should be addressed to Louisa M. T. Silva; lmtsilva@qsti.org

Academic Editor: Hansen Wang

Evaluation for sensory impairment is a routine part of autism diagnosis. Sensory impairment of hearing, vision, or touch results in developmental delay and must be addressed before delay can resolve. Recent studies confirm that tactile impairment is present in autism and can be effectively treated with a tactile stimulation protocol. The research suggests a change in management at the time of autism diagnosis to include evaluation and treatment of tactile impairment. Here we validate screening and management tool for tactile impairment, the Autism Touch and Self-Regulation Checklist, in 404 typical and autistic preschool children. The tool assesses tactile impairment by location and severity. Autistic children were distinguished by mixed pain and numbness on multiple areas including the face and mouth ($F = 412.1(1, 402)$; $p < .000$). Oral-facial tactile impairment interferes with the tactile stimulus to orienting. We hypothesized that oral-facial tactile impairment and difficulty orienting are predictive of ASD and that severity of tactile impairment is predictive of severity of ASD. Questions evaluating oral-facial and orienting responses correctly predicted 91% of the autism group. Severity of tactile impairment correctly predicted 81% of mild versus severe ASD. Results underscore the importance of evaluating and treating tactile impairment at the time of autism diagnosis.

1. Introduction

The evaluation for sensory impairment is a routine part of the autism diagnosis. Sensory impairment of hearing, vision, or touch results in developmental delay and must be treated before normal development can resume. The inclusion of sensory problems in the diagnosis of autism in 2013 [1] leads to the recognition that although tactile abnormalities are universal and markedly severe in children with autism, the sense of touch has not been fully evaluated and cannot be presumed to be intact [2–4].

Recent studies confirm that tactile impairment is universally present in children with autism and describe a distinguishing clinical presentation characterized by mixed pain and numbness on multiple areas of skin including the face, mouth, hands, and feet [5, 6]. Tactile impairment is severe compared with other developmental disabilities and associated with delay of early self-regulation milestones [5]. The presentation is typical of early-onset sensory neuropathy [7].

A number of studies report that tactile impairment in children with autism can be reduced with a tactile stimulation protocol stimulating circulation to small sensory nerves in the skin: normalization of tactile symptoms by 50% is reported following five months of daily treatment [8–11]. Treatment also normalized autistic behavior by one-third and increased social/language development. In 2015, a large study replicated the results and confirmed that treatment was effective in high- and low-functioning children [12]. This was a breakthrough in treatment for autism.

The research suggests a change in management at the time of autism diagnosis to include evaluation and treatment of tactile impairment. To this end, clinicians require screening and management tool for tactile abnormalities that identifies signs of tactile impairment by severity and location and measures response to treatment. Only one such management tool is currently available.

The Autism Touch and Self-Regulation Checklist (ATSC) is a 59-item tool for managing tactile impairment in children

TABLE 1: Validation group demographics.

	ASD (N = 199)	Typically developing children (N = 205)
Gender		
Male	170	103
Female	29	102
Age		
Mean	3.83 years	3.80 years
Standard deviation	1.10	.98
Range	2–6 years	2–6 years

Note: N = number of children.

with autism (see http://qsti.org/ATSC.pdf). The checklist assesses tactile symptoms by severity and location and seeks confirmation of severity of tactile impairment by simultaneously assessing effects on touch-dependent, early self-regulation milestones (e.g., orientation-attention, self-soothing, and sleep) [6]. Since its being developed as a research tool, the ATSC has been refined for use by clinicians and is available free of charge at http://qsti.org/ATSC.pdf.

In this paper, we present updated validation data for the ATSC and investigate two hypotheses. The first is that the presence of tactile impairment on the face and mouth is predictive of ASD. We note that tactile impairment of the face and mouth would disrupt tactile stimulation of the orienting reflex and reduce face-to-face orienting and social attention on that basis [13]. The second is that severity of tactile impairment is predictive of severity of autism. We analyze the ASD data pool to determine whether we can distinguish between severely and mildly affected children on that basis.

The research questions are as follows:

(1) Is the Autism Touch and Self-Regulation Checklist a valid instrument for screening for and managing signs of tactile impairment in autism?

(2) To what extent do location of tactile signs on the face and mouth and failure to orient correctly identify the children with autism in the group?

(3) To what extent does severity of tactile impairment distinguish between children with severe autism and those with mild autism?

2. Materials and Methods

2.1. Participants. Data from 404 children aged 24 to 72 months were collected for this study: 199 children with Autism Spectrum Disorder (ASD) and 205 typically developing children. All informants were primary caregivers for the children concerned. Table 1 provides demographic information for each group.

2.2. Measures. Initially the ATSC was organized into individual sensory and self-regulatory domains. The choice of self-regulatory questions reflects disturbances commonly reported by parents in the main self-regulatory milestones in the first 3 years of life: orientation-attention, self-soothing, sleep, digestion, toilet training, and emotional and behavioral self-regulation.

The individual items were developed and selected through an iterative process by conducting a review of more than 100 interviews of parents with young autistic children in which parents were asked open-ended questions about their child's sensory and self-regulatory responses to ordinary, daily-life situations. As it became evident from parent interviews that sensory responses to both injurious and noninjurious stimuli were grossly abnormal, we created six sensory subdomains: touch-pain, auditory, visual, taste-smell, hyperreactive to noninjurious stimuli, and hyporeactive to injurious stimuli. The hyperreactive and hyporeactive subdomains do not have their own separate item. The hyperreactive subdomain was drawn from all sensory subdomains, and the hyporeactive subdomain is drawn from the oral-tactile subdomain only.

We created an additional category for analysis when we realized that parents were reporting abnormal touch-pain responses in multiple areas of the body, including the face, head, fingers, toes, skin, and diaper area. The ATSC labels touch-pain items by their respective body area; for example, "difficulty with haircuts" is assigned to the head and "difficulty cutting fingernails" is assigned to the fingers. Information regarding the number of areas involved was extracted from the sensory domain and analyzed separately.

Over an initial five-year period, we submitted the ATSC to an ongoing development and refinement process in which items were evaluated for inclusion, exclusion, and clarification of terminology. The ATSC caregiver report is suitable for use by caregivers who have an elementary school education and is available in English, Spanish, Portuguese, and Chinese. The results of this initial validation effort were published previously [6].

The ATSC has been refined since its initial design eight years ago in three ways. First, items in the oral domain reflecting responses to texture and pressure in the mouth have been moved, and a single oral-tactile domain was created. Second, a toilet training domain was added to assess self-regulation of toilet training, and several items that failed to differentiate between ASD and typical and other developmental delays groups have been deleted. Finally, the original checklist contained 56 items across 10 sensory and self-regulation domains. The revised checklist contains 59 items assessing nine domains.

Table 2 lists all ATSC items according to our revised organization by oral-tactile and self-regulatory domain and identifies the additional items related to the sensory domains of vision, hearing, and smell that can be used for clinical purposes if needed. Items are rated *never* (0), *rarely* (1), *sometimes* (2), or *often* (3). Domain scores are obtained by summing the individual items. Table 2 also shows the prevalence of responses scored *sometimes* or *often* across the three groups of children.

2.3. Data Collection. We collected ATSC data on children with autism from several research projects completed over the past seven years with Western Oregon University

Table 2: Item description and prevalence in children with autism.

Item	Autism spectrum disorder	Typically developing children
Oral-tactile domain		
Face-mouth		
Avoids foods with certain textures	78.9%	41.5%
Face washing is difficult	73.8%	20.0%
Tooth brushing is difficult	68.8%	18.0%
Eats very few foods	63.3%	16.6%
Mouths or chews objects	63.3%	18.1%
Head-hands-feet-skin-diaper		
Haircuts are difficult	72.3%	21.4%
Does not notice if the diaper is wet or dirty	60.3%	12.7%
Avoids wearing gloves	61.8%	16.6%
Cutting toenails is difficult	62.3%	24.4%
Does not cry tears when hurt	64.3%	14.6%
Refuses to wear a hat	56.2%	22.9%
Cutting fingernails is difficult	55.8%	23.9%
Head-bangs on soft surface	38.2%	2.0%
Will only wear certain footwear	36.7%	20.5%
Will only wear certain clothes	43.2%	24.4%
Cries tears when he or she falls, scrapes skin, or gets hurt	45.7%	56.6%
Head-bangs on a hard surface	28.2%	1.0%
Prefers to wear the same clothes day after day	29.7%	13.1%
Orienting-attending		
Stares off into space	73.9%	31.3%
Seems not to notice when spoken to in a normal voice	79.4%	18.0%
Does not respond to his or her name	72.8%	9.8%
Has to be prompted to make eye contact when spoken to	67.9%	25.4%
Seems unaware when others are hurt	73.4%	9.8%
Does not roll over onto back when asked	52.2%	1.0%
Does not notice or react when tapped on the back	43.2%	3.0%
Self-regulation domain		
Awakens very early and stays awake	65.8%	25.4%
Has difficulty falling asleep at bedtime	62.3%	33.7%
Has difficulty falling back asleep when he or she awakens during the night	64.4%	15.1%
Has difficulty awakening in morning	31.7%	14.6%
Will only eat familiar foods	83.9%	52.7%
Bowels are loose	51.2%	20.0%
Does not seem to be interested in food	50.7%	17.1%
Has difficulty calming when upset	87.4%	40.9%
Tantrums or meltdowns	80.4%	51.2%
Gets upset or tantrums when asked to make a transition	82.4%	29.8%
Cries easily when frustrated	71.9%	35.1%
Diaper is wet in the morning	69.9%	33.7%
Wears a diaper during the day	62.3%	13.2%
Is dry at night	52.5%	78.1%
Is toilet trained	46.2%	91.7%
Hits or kicks others	58.7%	35.1%
Throws things at others	18.1%	19.6%
Scratches or pulls others' hair	37.2%	10.3%
Bites others	29.2%	3.9%

TABLE 2: Continued.

Item	Autism spectrum disorder	Typically developing children
Gets aggressive or hyper with exposure to certain smells	15.1%	1.0%
Hits self	28.2%	2.9%
Bites self	21.6%	0.0%
Pulls own hair	18.1%	1.5%
Other sensory domains		
Reacts strongly when others cry loudly or scream	59.8%	20.5%
Is startled by sudden noises	59.8%	34.2%
Covers ears with certain sounds	61.8%	32.2%
Reacts poorly to certain everyday noises	44.85	6.4%
Looks at objects out of sides of eyes	51.7%	24.4%
Is bothered by certain lights	48.85	13.2%
Gags with certain smells	27.2%	7.8%
Constipation		
Bowel movement is hard and dry	32.6%	14.2%
Bowel movements are often green	20.6%	3.9%
Bowel movements are twice a week	18.5%	9.3%
Bowel movement is once a week	14.0%	5.4%
Requires regular use of laxative to avoid constipation	13.5%	4.0%

Institutional Review Board approval. Inclusion criteria for the children with autism were as follows: age less than six years, receiving state-sponsored early childhood special education services for autism, absence of other severe disabilities such as cerebral palsy, and taking no psychotropic medication. Children *with a preexisting autism diagnosis from an autism evaluation center or developmental pediatrician* were recruited from six regional autism programs across Oregon. The diagnostic evaluations were reviewed and autism diagnosis was confirmed by DSM-IV criteria prior to final acceptance into the study [14]. All data from these groups were collected prior to random assignment into treatment and control groups associated with specific studies conducted by the authors from 2008 to 2014.

We recruited parents of typically developing children to complete the surveys from one child care center, three mother support groups, and one toddler drop-in play center in Oregon. Parents completed the surveys on convenience basis. Inclusionary criteria for the children included the following: ages 3–6; no educational or medical diagnosis of autism; absence of developmental delays (DD) or previous assessment for DD; and absence of chronic medical conditions.

While ages of children in the typically developing and autism groups are similar, gender distribution is highly unequal. Given that the prevalence of Autism Spectrum Disorder is much higher in boys than girls, analyses were conducted to assess whether boys and girls in the typically developing group differed on the ATSC. To determine whether this influences the results, two sets of analyses were conducted. First, analyses were conducted to determine whether there are differences on measures by gender in the typically developing group.

Chi-square analyses were conducted to determine whether the prevalence of abnormal sensory responses differed by boys and girls on oral-tactile, vision, hearing, smell domains and the number of senses involved. Chi-square values ranged from .024 on hearing to 2.47 on oral-tactile domain. Associated p values ranged from .877 to .116. Consequently, there does not appear to be a significant difference between boys and girls on the prevalence of sensory issues.

Additionally, ANOVA/MANOVA was conducted comparing boys and girls on the outcome measures presented in Table 5. No significant differences were found. F values ranged from .002 for face-mouth to 2.00 for constipation. Associated p values ranged from .960 to .158.

To further test whether the unequal distribution was problematic, the analyses in Table 5 and the ROC curve analyses were replicated comparing only boys from the typically developing and ASD groups. F values ranged from 404.1 for face-mouth and orientation and attention to 23.3 for constipation. All F values were significant beyond the .000 level. AUC values decrease very little (usually by .001) and sensitivity and specificity scores typically increase by less than .025.

While the distribution in gender was unequal between the typically developing and Autism Spectrum Disorder groups, this did not overly influence the results presented here.

2.4. Data Analysis. To determine the prevalence of oral-tactile and self-regulatory symptoms in children with autism and typical development, simple frequency analyses were conducted on each item. The percentage of responses of *sometimes* or *often* was computed for each group.

We also investigated the ATSC's ability to discriminate between children with ASD and those typically developing on the basis of the number of senses involved and the number of areas of body involvement by analyzing frequency distributions using χ^2 analyses and the median test. To determine the prevalence of abnormal sensory responses and self-regulatory delay, we set the criterion as the mean score for typically developing children plus 1 standard deviation [15]. We conducted a parallel analysis on areas of the body affected.

To determine reliability, we calculated internal consistency estimates (Cronbach's alpha) for the total ATSC score, the sensory and self-regulation domain, and the individual subdomains for each population. We also calculated test-retest stability on a subsample of children in the control condition over a four-month time interval.

The ATSC's ability to differentiate between children with autism and typically developing children was evaluated with multivariate analysis of variance (MANOVA). In addition, response operator characteristic (ROC) curve analysis was conducted to determine the overall adequacy of the ATSC and various domains and subdomain composite scores as a screening tool for autism and levels of sensitivity and specificity at various cut-off scores.

The above set of analyses was replicated to determine whether the ATSC could effectively differentiate between severe and mild levels of severity of autism, as determined by a composite of measures. The ROC curve analyses were conducted to determine the overall adequacy of the ATSC and various domains and subdomain composite scores as a screening tool for severe versus mild autism and levels of sensitivity and specificity at various cut-off scores.

To create a composite severity of autism score we combined scores from the Pervasive Developmental Disorders Behavior Inventory Parent Version [16], the Autism Behavior Checklist [17], the Vineland Adaptive Behavior Scales [18], the Childhood Autism Rating Scale [19], and the Preschool Language Scale 5th Edition [20]. This composite score was evaluated to determine where each child performed from mild autism to severe autism. Three groups were identified: severe ($n = 43$), moderate ($n = 86$), and mild ($n = 49$). Language development was determined by total score on the Preschool Language Scale 5th Edition.

3. Results

3.1. Prevalence. At the item level, results from the ATSC indicate high and widespread prevalence of abnormal tactile and other sensory responses as well as self-regulatory delay in children with autism. As can be seen in Table 2, oral-tactile prevalence is significantly higher than that for typically developing children (on a magnitude of two to four times) for the face and mouth areas. Prevalence patterns vary across the areas of the body, though they generally hold to the same pattern as with the face-mouth areas.

Consistent patterns of prevalence between the groups also emerge for several of the domains of self-regulatory delay. For example, in the areas of orientation-attending, self-soothing, sleep, and behavior, children with autism exhibit much higher prevalence of delay than do typically developing children. This pattern is not as strong in the areas of appetite-digestion and toileting.

Table 3 presents data on the percentage of children experiencing abnormal sensory responses and the areas of the body impacted by abnormal tactile response. These data represent the percent of children scoring at the mean plus one standard deviation of typically developing children in the study. Results are shown both for children with differing levels of severity of autism and for typically developing children. As can be seen here, children with differing levels of severity of autism experience higher levels of abnormal sensory response than do typically developing children, and children with severe autism experience higher levels of abnormal sensory response than do children with moderate or mild autism (except for smell). χ^2 analyses were conducted on the four sensory domains and the number of domains affected. All tests between the three levels of autism presented here and typically developing children were significant at the .0001 level. χ^2 values ranged from 187.9 for oral-tactile domain to 26.8 for smell (with 3 d.f.). Total number of senses affected was significant as well with $\chi^2 = 190.9$ (d.f. = 12).

Parallel analyses were conducted on the areas of the body experiencing abnormal tactile response. Results were similar. All of the tests comparing children with differing levels of severity of autism to typically developing children were significant, with χ^2 values ranging from 171.6 for the mouth to 24.9 for the skin. The number of areas of the body affected was also significant with χ^2 value of 251.8 (d.f. = 21).

These results with a larger population and redesigned ATSC confirm previous reports that children with autism are distinguished by mixed pain and numbness of multiple areas of skin as well as global delay of early self-regulation milestones.

3.2. Reliability. Both internal consistency and test-retest estimates of reliability were calculated. We calculated internal consistency estimates (Cronbach's alpha) for the oral-tactile, orientation-attention, self-regulation, and other sensory domains and constipation and overall scores and a composite of face-mouth and orientation-attention. These results are shown in Table 4. Overall scale estimates were .873 for children with ASD and .899 for typically developing children. In the oral-tactile domain estimates of internal consistency were .708 for ASD and .791 for typically developing children. For the self-regulation domain, estimates were .769 for ASD and .794 for typically developing children. Subdomain scores demonstrated varying levels of internal consistency. The internal consistency of the composite for face-mouth and orientation-attention (a suggested set of items for screening purposes) is .764 for ASD and .763 for typically developing children.

Test-retest stability was estimated from a subsample of children in control group condition over a four-month time interval. Coefficients ranged from .763 for self-regulation to .806 for oral-tactile to .826 for the overall scale.

3.3. Discriminating between Populations. To test for the ability of the ATSC to discriminate between populations both MANOVA and ROC curve analyses were conducted. Table 5 contains the post hoc MANOVA results comparing children with autism and typically developing children. MANOVA results indicate that overall population means are

TABLE 3: Prevalence, number of impaired senses, and number of involved body areas by severity of autism.

(a)

Group	Sensory domain impaired, %			
	Oral/tactile	Visual	Auditory	Smell
Typically developing children	17.6%	17.6%	17.1%	7.8%
Severe autism	100%	67.4%	72.1%	23.3%
Moderate autism	88.4%	66.3%	61.6%	25.6%
Mild autism	79.6%	38.8%	63.3%	18.4%

(b)

Group	Number of senses impaired				
	4	3	2	1	0
Typically developing children	3.4%	5.9%	17.1%	29.8%	43.9%
Severe autism	37.2%	39.5%	14.0%	9.3%	0%
Moderate autism	30.2%	31.4%	24.4%	10.5%	3.5%
Mild autism	6.1%	36.7%	32.7%	20.4%	4.1%

(c)

Group	Areas of the body affected						
	Face	Mouth	Head	Hands	Feet	Skin	Diaper
Typically developing children	20.0%	16.1%	13.2%	21.0%	21.0%	18.0%	12.7%
Severe autism	83.7%	95.3%	95.3%	79.1%	74.4%	37.2%	79.1%
Moderate autism	77.9%	81.4%	75.6%	70.9%	53.5%	45.3%	62.8%
Mild autism	67.3%	71.4%	61.2%	61.2%	59.2%	30.6%	40.8%

(d)

Group	Number of areas of the body affected							
	7	6	5	4	3	2	1	0
Typically developing children	0%	1.0%	4.4%	3.9%	10.7%	10.2%	25.9%	43.9%
Severe autism	14.0%	41.9%	30.2%	7.0%	4.7%	0%	2.3%	0%
Moderate autism	9.3%	25.6%	26.7%	15.1%	10.5%	10.5%	2.3%	0%
Mild autism	0%	20.4%	26.5%	10.2%	24.5%	8.2%	6.1%	4.1%

TABLE 4: Internal consistencies of domains by group.

Domain	Cronbach's alpha		Number of items
	Autism total	Typically developing children	
Oral-tactile	.708	.791	17
Face-mouth	.625	.592	5
Head-hands-feet-skin-diaper	.607	.569	12
Orientation and attention	.760	.719	7
Self-regulation domains (sleep, appetite/digestion, self-soothing, toileting, and behavior)	.769	.794	23
Total oral-tactile, orientation and attention, and self-regulation	.864	.886	47
Other sensory domains (vision, hearing, and smell)	.694	.740	7
Constipation	.707	.599	5
Total scale	.873	.899	59
Face-mouth + orientation-attention	.764	.793	12

Table 5: Post hoc population comparisons.

	Autism $N = 199$	Typically developing children $N = 205$	F (d.f.)	p value
Oral-tactile				
M	27.60	10.66	525.1	<.000
SD	7.91	6.93	(1, 402)	
Face-mouth				
M	10.06	3.74	412.1	<.000
SD	3.43	2.81	(1, 402)	
Hands-feet-head-skin-diaper				
M	17.54	6.92	368.6	<.000
SD	6.08	5.00	(1, 402)	
Orientation and attention				
M	12.58	3.99	522.6	<.000
SD	4.40	3.05	(1, 402)	
Self-regulation total				
M	35.72	17.28	439.0	<.000
SD	9.75	7.86	(1, 402)	
Oral-tactile, orientation-attention, and self-regulation				
M	75.90	31.93	685.1	<.000
SD	18.47	15.18	(1, 402)	
Other sensory domains				
M	10.41	4.89	193.7	<.000
SD	4.32	3.63	(1, 402)	
Constipation				
M	3.23	1.60	36.6	<.000
SD	3.21	2.13	(1, 402)	
Total scale				
M	89.54	38.41	677.7	<.000
SD	21.35	18.03	(1, 402)	
Face-mouth + orientation-attention				
M	22.64	7.73	663.0	<.000
SD	6.50	5.07	(1, 402)	

Note: M = mean; SD = standard deviation; d.f. = degrees of freedom.

significantly different across all domains and subdomains on the ATSC: overall, $F = 123.3(6, 397)$, $p \leq .000$ with an effect size estimate of .651 (Partial eta^2).

Post hoc analyses show that population means differ significantly across all domains and subdomains. Mean scores for children with autism are significantly different from mean scores for typically developing children.

ROC curve analysis was conducted to determine the sensitivity and specificity of the ATSC in accurately identifying children with autism. For the primary checklist of 47 items (oral-tactile, orientation-attention plus self-regulation) the area under the curve (AUC) is .961. A score of 49 produces sensitivity of 91.0 and specificity of 84.9. Oral-tactile scores (17 items) have an AUC of .935. A score of 17 produces sensitivity of 91.0 and specificity of 82.9. Orientation-attention scores (7 items) have an AUC of .933. A score of 7 produces sensitivity of 86.4 and specificity of 85.6. All of these are adequate to screen for autism, but require large numbers of items. Combining face-mouth and orientation-attention (12 items) produces an AUC of .953 and with a score of 13 produce sensitivity of .910 and specificity of .847. This combination of items powerfully and efficiently distinguishes between children with autism and typically developing children. The ATSC clearly distinguishes children with autism from typically developing children across all domains.

3.4. Discriminating between Levels of Autism. Parallel analyses were conducted comparing two levels of autism: severe and mild as determined by a composite of scores. Table 6 contains the MANOVA post hoc results comparing children with different levels of autism. Overall MANOVA results indicate overall population means are significantly different between

Table 6: Post hoc levels of autism comparisons.

	Severe autism $n = 43$	Mild autism $n = 49$	F (d.f.)	p value
Oral-tactile				
M	32.49	24.02	42.72	<.000
SD	5.19	6.97	(1, 90)	
Face-mouth				
M	11.70	9.47	11.26	.001
SD	2.51	3.63	(1, 90)	
Hands-feet-head-skin-diaper				
M	20.79	14.55	39.05	<.000
SD	4.03	5.35	(1, 90)	
Orientation and attention				
M	15.47	9.94	55.24	<.000
SD	2.92	4.03	(1, 90)	
Self-regulation total				
M	41.84	29.24	52.05	<.000
SD	7.14	9.29	(1, 90)	
Oral-tactile, orientation-attention, and self-regulation				
M	89.87	63.20	91.58	<.000
SD	10.49	15.34	(1, 90)	
Other sensory domains				
M	11.63	9.20	7.66	.007
SD	4.59	3.81	(1, 90)	
Constipation				
M	2.84	2.57	0.25	.662
SD	2.62	2.53	(1, 90)	
Total scale				
M	104.26	74.98	79.05	<.000
SD	13.55	17.46	(1, 90)	
Face-mouth + orientation-attention				
M	27.16	19.41	58.86	<.000
SD	4.03	5.45	(1, 90)	

Note: M = mean; SD = standard deviation; d.f. = degrees of freedom.

children with severe and mild autism, $F = 17.32$ $(6, 85)$, $p < .000$ with an effect size estimate of .550 (Partial eta^2).

Post hoc analyses show only one domain (constipation) where specific population means do not differ significantly. Mean scores for severe and mild autism differ significantly on all other domains, with Fs ranging from 7.66 to 91.58.

ROC curve analysis was conducted to determine the sensitivity and specificity of the ATSC in accurately distinguishing between children with severe autism and those with mild autism. For the primary checklist of 47 items (oral-tactile, orientation-attention plus self-regulation) the area under the curve (AUC) is .918. A score of 76 produces sensitivity of 93.0 and specificity of 81.6. Both the total scale (59 items) and the composite of face-mouth and orientation-attention provide adequate sensitivity and specificity. Other domains do not. The overall scale has AUC of .908. A score of 90 produces sensitivity of 90.7 and specificity of 81.6. Combining face-mouth and orientation-attention (12 items) produces AUC of .884 and, with a score of 23, produces a sensitivity of 81.4 and specificity of 81.6. This combination of items provides an adequate and efficient screening tool to distinguish between children with autism and typically developing children. The ATSC is also able to distinguish between children with severe and mild autism.

4. Discussion

This study introduces clinicians to the Autism Touch and Self-Regulation Checklist and demonstrates that it is a reliable instrument with which to screen and manage tactile abnormalities in children with autism. The checklist assesses signs of peripheral tactile impairment by location and severity and has the additional benefit of confirming severity by measuring developmental impacts on early self-regulation. Existing sensory questionnaires are based on a sensory processing disorder model that does not distinguish between central and peripheral etiology of tactile symptoms [3, 4]. A central etiology for sensory problems cannot account for the high prevalence of tactile than other sensory abnormalities, the varying prevalence of tactile abnormalities on different areas of skin, or the findings of mixed pain and numbness reported in children with autism. In contrast, these are typical presenting signs of peripheral tactile impairment due to small fiber neuropathy [21, 22].

The first iteration of the ATSC explored whether symptoms were localized or generalized and mild or severe. Analysis indicated there was involvement of multiple areas of skin and the range of severity was more than twice that seen in typically developing children. Severity was confirmed by the finding of global delay of early touch-dependent, self-regulation milestones relative to orientation/attention, self-soothing, sleep, and digestion [6]. Thus, the evidence pointed to generalized tactile impairment that was severe enough to pose a barrier to parent/caregiver touch, resulting in self-regulatory delay. A subsequent outcome study showing improvement of self-regulatory delay following treatment of tactile abnormalities provided confirmation of a barrier to touch [11].

The hallmark of autism is social delay and it is argued that the search for the neurological basis of autism should focus on the social deficits [23]. An explanation for the early social deficits in autism has never been found. In our view, the search for the basis of social delay should focus on whether sensation is intact on the face. Social interaction in its earliest form is face-to-face interaction, and early damage to the sense of touch on the face would profoundly disrupt social development from the start. In Research Question #2 we screened the data pool for a direct relationship between evidence of damage to the sense of touch on the face and mouth and presence of social delay, that is, diagnosis of autism.

It was remarkable that five questions about touch/pain responses on the face and mouth should correctly identify 83% of the children with autism from typically developing children, especially since the questions bore little resemblance to the usual social and behavioral questions used to screen for autism. But intact oral-facial sensation is required for the orienting reflex to function. When we widened the net to include questions about failure to orient, 91% of the children with autism were correctly identified. This was an extraordinarily high yield, well above the usual yields from autism screening by parent questionnaire [24].

Oral-facial tactile impairment explains many things about social delay, especially the lack of attention to face seen in young children with autism [25]. Our results suggest that if the developmental hallmark of autism is social delay, then the physical hallmark of autism is tactile impairment of the face and mouth. And the connecting link between the two is failure of the orienting reflex to support early orientation to face and face-to-face attention.

One of the mysteries of autism is the spectrum of severity that it presents, as well as the basis on which the spectrum occurs. In using a tool designed to evaluate signs of tactile impairment, we hoped to identify a physical basis for that spectrum of severity. Our data described a spectrum of severity of tactile abnormalities ranging from mild withdrawal responses from texture of food in the mouth and trimming fingernails to mixed signs of pain and numbness on multiple areas of skin. In Research Question #3, we explored whether tactile impairment could provide physical basis for autism severity by seeking to differentiate severe from mild ASD on the basis of severity of tactile signs.

Over 80% of children with severe ASD were correctly identified from a pool of children with severe and mild ASD by severity of tactile scores. Given that the distinction is usually made on verbal and cognitive differences [26], it was perhaps astonishing that the two ends of the spectrum could be neatly identified without asking a single question about verbal or cognitive ability. But when the results were interpreted in light of what is known about early sensory impairment and development, they were similar to what would be expected from a range of hearing or vision impairment and exactly what would be expected from a range of tactile impairment. The conclusion is supported by treatment outcome research showing that reduction of severity of tactile abnormalities reduces severity of autism [12].

5. Conclusion

This paper presents data validating the reliability and usefulness of the Autism Touch and Self-Regulation Checklist to evaluate and manage tactile impairment in children with autism. The utility of identifying severity and location of tactile abnormalities is confirmed by finding that severity of tactile abnormalities was powerfully related to severity of autism, and location of impairment on the face and mouth efficiently screened the children with autism from the data pool. The finding that 91% of the children with autism could be correctly identified by signs of oral-facial tactile impairment and failure to orient illuminates the importance of the failure of the orienting reflex for the emergence of social delay in autism. Altogether, the findings add to mounting evidence of the importance of evaluating and managing tactile impairment at the time of autism diagnosis.

Acknowledgment

This study was supported in part by Grant R40 MC 24945 from the Maternal and Child Health Research Program, Maternal and Child Health Bureau, Health Resources and Services Administration, Department of Health and Human Services.

References

[1] American Psychiatric Association, *Diagnostic and Statistical Manual of Mental Disorders*, American Psychiatric Publishing, Washington, DC, USA, 5th edition, 2013.

[2] J. H. Foss-Feig, J. L. Heacock, and C. J. Cascio, "Tactile responsiveness patterns and their association with core features in autism spectrum disorders," *Research in Autism Spectrum Disorders*, vol. 6, no. 1, pp. 337–344, 2012.

[3] W. Dunn, *The Sensory Profile: Examiner's Manual*, Psychological Corporation, San Antonio, Tex, USA, 1999.

[4] G. T. Baranek, F. J. David, M. D. Poe, W. L. Stone, and L. R. Watson, "Sensory experiences questionnaire: discriminating sensory features in young children with autism, developmental

delays, and typical development," *The Journal of Child Psychology and Psychiatry*, vol. 47, no. 6, pp. 591–601, 2006.

[5] L. Silva and M. Schalock, "Prevalence and significance of abnormal tactile responses in young children with autism," *North American Journal of Medicine and Science*, vol. 6, no. 3, pp. 121–127, 2013.

[6] L. M. T. Silva and M. Schalock, "Sense and Self-regulation Checklist, a measure of comorbid autism symptoms: initial psychometric evidence," *The American Journal of Occupational Therapy*, vol. 66, no. 2, pp. 177–186, 2012.

[7] Neuromuscular Disease Center, *Childhood Onset Polyneuropathies*, Washington University, St. Louis, Mo, USA, 2015, http://neuromuscular.wustl.edu/time/child.html.

[8] L. M. Silva, M. Schalock, and K. Gabrielsen, "Early intervention for autism with a parent-delivered qigong massage program: a randomized controlled trial," *The American Journal of Occupational Therapy*, vol. 65, no. 5, pp. 550–559, 2011.

[9] L. M. T. Silva, M. Schalock, R. Ayres, C. Bunse, and S. Budden, "Qigong massage treatment for sensory and self-regulation problems in young children with autism: a randomized controlled trial," *American Journal of Occupational Therapy*, vol. 63, no. 4, pp. 423–432, 2009.

[10] L. M. T. Silva, R. Ayres, and M. Schalock, "Outcomes of a pilot training program in a Qigong massage intervention for young children with autism," *American Journal of Occupational Therapy*, vol. 62, no. 5, pp. 538–546, 2008.

[11] L. Silva and M. Schalock, "Treatment of tactile impairment in young children with autism: results with qigong massage," *International Journal of Therapeutic Massage & Bodywork*, vol. 6, no. 4, pp. 12–20, 2013.

[12] L. M. Silva, M. Schalock, K. R. Gabrielsen, S. S. Budden, M. Buenrostro, and G. Horton, "Early intervention with a parent-delivered massage protocol directed at tactile abnormalities decreases severity of autism and improves child-to-parent interactions: a replication study," *Autism Research and Treatment*, vol. 2015, Article ID 904585, 16 pages, 2015.

[13] E. N. Sokolov, "Higher nervous functions; the orienting reflex," *Annual Review of Physiology*, vol. 25, pp. 545–580, 1963.

[14] American Psychiatric Association, *Diagnostic and Statistical Manual of Mental Disorders*, American Psychiatric Association, Washington, DC, USA, 4th edition, 2000.

[15] G. T. Baranek, F. J. David, M. D. Poe, W. L. Stone, and L. R. Watson, "Sensory Experiences Questionnaire: discriminating sensory features in young children with autism, developmental delays, and typical development," *Journal of Child Psychology and Psychiatry and Allied Disciplines*, vol. 47, no. 6, pp. 591–601, 2006.

[16] I. Cohen and V. Sudhalter, *PDD Behavior Inventory*, Psychological Assessment Resources, Lutz, Fla, USA, 2005.

[17] D. Krug, J. Arick, and P. Almond, *Autism Screening Instrument for Educational Planning*, PRO-ED, Austin, Tex, USA, 1993.

[18] S. Sparrow, D. Cicchetti, and D. Balla, *Vineland Adaptive Behavior Scales: Interview Edition*, American Guidance Service, Circle Pines, Minn, USA, 2005.

[19] E. Schopler, R. Reichler, and B. Renner, *Childhood Autism Rating Scale, Standard Version*, Western Psychological Services, Los Angeles, Calif, USA, 2nd edition, 2013.

[20] I. Zimmerman, V. Steiner, and R. Pond, *Preschool Language Scale*, Pearson Education, San Antonio, Tex, USA, 5th edition, 2011.

[21] G. Devigili, V. Tugnoli, P. Penza et al., "The diagnostic criteria for small fibre neuropathy: from symptoms to neuropathology," *Brain*, vol. 131, no. 7, pp. 1912–1925, 2008.

[22] G. Lauria, A. Majorana, M. Borgna et al., "Trigeminal small-fiber sensory neuropathy causes burning mouth syndrome," *Pain*, vol. 115, no. 3, pp. 332–337, 2005.

[23] R. T. Schultz, "Developmental deficits in social perception in autism: the role of the amygdala and fusiform face area," *International Journal of Developmental Neuroscience*, vol. 23, no. 2-3, pp. 125–141, 2005.

[24] P. García-Primo, A. Hellendoorn, T. Charman et al., "Screening for autism spectrum disorders: state of the art in Europe," *European Child & Adolescent Psychiatry*, vol. 23, no. 11, pp. 1005–1021, 2014.

[25] J. S. Nomi and L. Q. Uddin, "Face processing in autism spectrum disorders: from brain regions to brain networks," *Neuropsychologia*, vol. 71, pp. 201–216, 2015.

[26] Autism Speaks, *Measuring Severity in Autism Spectrum Disorders*, Autism Speaks, New York, NY, USA, 2015, https://www.autismspeaks.org/science/grants/measuring-severity-autism-spectrum-disorders.

8

The Relationship between Comprehension of Figurative Language by Japanese Children with High Functioning Autism Spectrum Disorders and College Freshmen's Assessment of its Conventionality of usage

Manabu Oi,[1] Sanae Tanaka,[1] and Harue Ohoka[2]

[1] *Research Center for Child Mental Development, United Graduate School of Child Development, Kanazawa University, B-b43, 13-1 Takaramachi, Kanazawa 920-8640, Japan*
[2] *Nihon Fukushi University Chuo College of Social Services, 3-27-11 Chiyoda, Naka-ku, Nagoya 460-0012, Japan*

Correspondence should be addressed to Manabu Oi; oimanabu@ed.kanazawa-u.ac.jp

Academic Editor: Manuel F. Casanova

Unlike their English-speaking counterparts, Japanese children with high-functioning autism spectrum disorders (HFASDs) perform as well as typically developing (TD) children in comprehending metaphor, despite lacking 1st order theory of mind (ToM) reasoning. Additionally, although Japanese sarcasm and "indirect reproach" appear theoretically to need 2nd order ToM reasoning, HFASD children without this comprehended these forms of language as well as TD children. To attempt to explain this contradiction, we asked college freshmen to evaluate the strangeness (unconventionality) of these types of figurative language. We aimed to test the hypothesis that metaphor, sarcasm, and "indirect reproach" might be evaluated as more conventional than irony, which children with HFASDs do not comprehend as well as those with attention deficit hyperactivity disorder. The results for irony, metaphor, and "indirect reproach" supported the hypothesis, while those for sarcasm did not. Sarcasm is comprehended by HFASDs children as well as by TD children despite being evaluated as highly unconventional. This contradiction is discussed from a self-in-relation-to-other perspective. We postulate that a new explanation of disabilities of figurative language comprehension in children with HFASDs is needed instead of relying on a single cognitive process.

1. Introduction

As Norbury and Sparks [1] have suggested, autism spectrum disorders (ASDs) might be better understood when examined from a cultural point of view. Cross-cultural studies might also help to refine cognitive theories of disorder that have been derived exclusively from North American and European investigations. This is the case for the comprehension of figurative language in autism [2–9], which seems to vary greatly between cultures in terms of ways of using metaphorical expression and saying something disagreeable. For example, in Japanese, metaphors are more fluid than in English [10]. Moreover, while irony is regarded as conveying not just a negative meaning but also humor in English, few studies have attempted to investigate any positive role irony has to play in Japanese conversation [11]. Moreover, Japanese has many varieties of sarcasm [12]. The average Japanese person would find it hard to distinguish between the English terms "irony" and "sarcasm." Even among professionals, the Japanese *hiniku* is translated not only as "irony" but occasionally as "sarcasm," as by Adachi et al. [13]. In the present study, irony was defined as "the expression of one's meaning by using words of the opposite meaning in order to make one's remarks forceful." Sarcasm was defined as "the expression of one's meaning by using words of the opposite meaning in order to taunt the hearer."

Additionally, in addition to irony and sarcasm, Japanese researchers have coined the phrase "indirect reproach" [14], an expression intended to mitigate a face-threatening act toward the hearer by avoiding direct expression of anger or irritation. "Indirect reproach" has been defined as "criticizing the hearer by referring to any contextual information that relates to the speaker's intention." English does not contain a counterpart for this type of phrase. Investigating how these Japanese figurative language styles are comprehended in children with high-functioning autism spectrum disorders (HFASDs) seems beneficial for understanding autism from a cross-cultural point of view.

English-speaking children with HFASDs find irony more difficult to comprehend than metaphor [2, 3]. The same appears true for Japanese speakers. Adachi et al. [13] showed that Japanese children with Asperger syndrome (AS), ranging in age from 7 to 14 years, comprehended irony less well than children with attention deficit hyperactivity disorder (ADHD) matched for IQ and age, while there was no intergroup difference in metaphor comprehension. However, these studies differ in terms of theory of mind (ToM) development in the participants. Unlike the studies of Happé [2, 3], Adachi et al.'s study [13] did not test 2nd order ToM reasoning. Among the latter participants, those who passed 1st order ToM tests performed better in comprehending irony than those who failed such tests [13]. It is probable that the participants of Adachi et al.'s [13] study did not achieve 2nd order ToM reasoning. If this is the case, Adachi et al.'s results might differ from those of Happé [3] with respect to the relationship between ToM and irony comprehension. As for metaphor, Japanese AS children who failed 1st order ToM tests comprehended metaphor well [13], unlike their counterparts in Happé's study [3], which reported that adolescents who did not pass 1st order ToM tests also failed to comprehend metaphor. These differences suggest that, at least in Japanese children with HFASDs, 2nd order ToM reasoning is not necessary for irony comprehension, and that 1st order reasoning is not necessary for metaphor comprehension. This suggests that a factor other than ToM reasoning might influence figurative language comprehension, accounting for the differences between Japanese and English in this respect.

What about figurative language other than metaphor and irony in Japanese? In terms of understanding sarcasm and "indirect reproach," Yata and Oi [14] investigated children with HFASDs, ranging in age from 8 to 15 years, and typically developing (TD) children matched for age and receptive vocabulary. When these children were presented with five sentences for each type of language (i.e., 10 sentences in total) in the written form, no differences in comprehension were evident between the two groups. In addition to this, Taguchi et al. [15] investigated children with HFASDs, ranging in age from 8 to 16 years, and age-matched TD children. That study had similar findings regarding sarcasm and "indirect reproach" comprehension.

Oi and Tanaka [16] compared children with HFASDs (ranging in grade from 2nd to 6th) and grade-matched TD children with regard to comprehending ambiguous sentences including metaphor and sarcasm but not irony. They found intergroup differences for only 10 of 50 sentences. These 10 sentences included one metaphor (Appendix) and nine grammatically, lexically, or contextually ambiguous sentences. Of the 10 metaphors, no group difference in understanding was found for nine, and the two examples of sarcasm were understood equally well by the TD and HFASD children. Children with HFASDs showed literalness in only four of the 50 sentences. The most interesting finding was that HFASD children showed overnonliteral comprehension compared with TD children for six contextually or grammatically ambiguous sentences.

In terms of the reason why children with HFASDs fail to comprehend figurative language, Happé [3] postulated that without 1st order ToM reasoning they could not understand metaphor, and without 2nd order reasoning they would fail to comprehend irony. So how do Japanese forms of sarcasm and "indirect reproach" compare in this regard? These two forms of language appear similar to irony in terms of requiring some metacognitive ability for comprehension. Awareness of thought might be required on the part of children, meaning that they would need 2nd order ToM reasoning to comprehend these two types of language. An example of a sarcasm task given by Yata and Oi [14] was to choose a response describing the mother's opinion of the child for the following scenario: a mother said, "You're a genius, aren't you?" to a child who got a very bad mark in an exam (see Appendix for detail). An example of an "indirect reproach" task given by Yata and Oi [14] was to choose a response describing the boy's opinion of his friend in the following scenario: a boy said, "Are you leaving without tidying up?" to his friend who was getting ready to go, leaving a mess behind (see Appendix for detail). In addition, Japanese metaphors were again comprehended by children who failed to demonstrate 1st order ToM reasoning in this study [14] while English ones were not understood by their English-speaking counterparts in Happé's study [3].

Why were English ironic phrases not understood by children with ASD while Japanese sarcasm and "indirect reproaches" were, despite the fact that these three forms of figurative phrase appear to equally need 2nd order ToM reasoning? Of 20 children with HFASDs investigated by Yata and Oi [14], nine failed the 2nd order ToM task and three failed even the 1st order ToM task. Why were these children without 2nd order ToM reasoning able to comprehend sarcasm and "indirect reproach"? Additionally, why could Japanese metaphors be comprehended by those showing no 1st order TOM reasoning, while English ones were not understood by their English-speaking counterparts? Japanese and English seem to differ greatly from each other in terms of figurative language comprehension from the viewpoint of ToM. This reminds us of the theory by Hinds [17] that Japanese is a listener-responsible language while English is a speaker-responsible language. With less responsibility to make the message as clear as possible for the hearer, speakers of Japanese could rely more on figurative language than those of English. This might uniquely influence the development of figurative language comprehension in Japanese children with and without HFASDs when compared with their English-speaking counterparts.

Thus, another explanation for these differences should be sought other than the development of ToM reasoning. One possible factor is the role of conventionality or salience [8] in comprehending figurative language. The most suitable example of this in English comes from Ozonoff and Miller [4].

In investigating humor, inference, and indirect request comprehension in adults with autism and preserved intelligence quotient, they showed that "Can you ...?" type questions were comprehended more nonliterally by adults with autism than by matched controls. They argued that individuals with autism have overlearned the rule that questions beginning with "Can you ..." should be interpreted in a nonliteral way. In everyday situations, such syntactic forms are more likely to be polite requests for action than inquiries about ability. Ozonoff and Miller [4] assumed that individuals with autism may be less able to use context to determine when this rule should not be applied, due to difficulty inhibiting familiar or overlearned responses. This might relate to a deficit in executive function.

In any case, it is worth evaluating figurative language tasks in terms of their conventionality in order to better explain why Japanese sarcasm, "indirect reproach," and metaphor were successfully comprehended by children with HFASDs, irrespective of the level of ToM achieved. Statements in these three categories might be evaluated as more conventional when compared with irony. This hypothesis is plausible because Giora et al. [8] showed that "the graded salience hypothesis" could explain why their participants with AS responded to metaphorical and literal language in a similar way to that of controls. According to their study, both the AS group and controls performed worse on novel expressions than on familiar ones, whether literal or metaphorical. The novelty and familiarity of expressions were defined operationally by the authors. In the present study, we instead determined the degree of novelty of figurative language by having it evaluated by college freshmen, like Oi and Tanaka [18] did in showing that the comprehension of ambiguous language tasks in children with HFASDs was highly correlated with the evaluation of the sentences in terms of conventionality by college freshmen. The correlation (r) between children's mean literal-nonliteral preference magnitude (comprehension) and freshmen's mean strangeness rating (unconventionality) was -0.65 ($P < 0.001$) for children with HFASDs and -0.67 ($P < 0.001$) for TD children. The two r values did not differ significantly from each other.

The present study tested the abovementioned hypothesis that metaphor, sarcasm, and "indirect reproach" would be evaluated as more conventional than "irony" by asking college students to evaluate from the viewpoint of conventionality examples of these forms of language previously given to children with and without HFASDs. We compared the conventionality evaluation among these four categories of figurative language.

2. Materials and Methods

2.1. Participants. University freshmen were recruited in random order. Participants were 98 male freshmen (mean age = 19.50 years, SD = 0.74) and 96 female freshmen (mean age = 19.19 years, SD = 0.64).

None of the freshmen were evaluated for autistic personality traits. They were asked to rate the strangeness (unconventionality) of figurative language assigned to children. The study was conducted in accordance with Declaration of Helsinki (1964).

First, the freshmen were asked to rate the strangeness of 10 combinations of a written sentence and written scenario in which the sentence was embedded; these had previously been used in Adachi et al.'s study [13] (see Appendix). Of the 10 sentences, five were ironic phrases and the remaining five were metaphors, all of which had been presented to 123 children. These children were diagnosed according to the Diagnostic and Statistical Manual of Mental Disorders, Fourth Edition (DSM-IV), as having AS (n = 66, 57 boys and nine girls, mean age = 9.8 years, and SD = 2.0), high-functioning autism (HFA) (n = 20, 17 boys and three girls, mean age = 9.4 years, and SD = 2.0), or ADHD (n = 37, 33 boys and four girls, mean age = 9.4 years, and SD = 1.8). Mean full-scale IQ as measured by the third edition of the Wechsler Intelligence Scale was 98.6 (SD = 14.0), 93.4 (SD = 12.8), and 98.2 (SD = 14.7), respectively, for each group. The written sentences were presented to the children who read them and were then asked to choose one of five answers to a question based on the sentences. The answers consisted of literal, nonliteral, irrelevant, and situational responses as well as a response indicating that the child had not understood the question.

Second, the freshmen were asked to rate the strangeness of another 10 combinations of the written sentences and scenarios given by Yata and Oi [14] (see Appendix) in which the sentence was embedded. Of these 10 sentences, five were sarcastic phrases and the remaining five were "indirect reproaches." They had been presented to 20 children with HFASDs diagnosed according to DSM-VI criteria (17 boys and three girls, mean age = 11.99 years, and SD = 2.08) and 20 TD children (13 boys and seven girls, mean age = 11.35 years, and SD = 2.71). These were matched for raw scores in the Picture Vocabulary Test, for which the mean score for HFASDs children was 61.7 (SD = 6.0) and that for TD children was 59.0 (SD = 7.4). There was no intergroup difference in either age or raw score of the test. These HFASD children ranged in full-scale IQ from 71 to 129 (mean = 93.9, SD = 13.4), when assessed using the third edition of the Wechsler Intelligence Scale within a year before the data collection. Children were asked to read the sarcasm and "indirect reproach" scenarios and to answer a question based on these scenarios by choosing one of three options consisting of literal, nonliteral, and situational answers. In addition to this, 10 more combinations of the written sentences and scenarios given by Taguchi et al. [15] were rated by the freshmen. Similarly, of the 10, five were sarcastic phrases and the rest were "indirect reproaches." These had been presented to 17 children with HFASDs (14 boys and 3 girls, ranging in age from 8.67 to 16.08 years; the mean and SD were not obtained) and 15 TD children (13 boys and 2 girls, ranging in age from 7.08 to 16.33 years; mean and SD were not obtained).

Third, the freshmen were asked to rate the degree of strangeness of 20 combinations of a sentence and a cartoon picture representing the nonliteral and literal interpretations of the sentence (see Appendix). These sentences were all metaphors. These had been given by Oi and Tanaka [16] to 2nd to 6th graders with HFASDs (40 boys and five girls, mean grade = 4.29, and SD = 1.27) and 45 TD children matched exactly for grade and gender who were extracted in random order from 666 2nd to 6th graders at an elementary school. The TD children all attended regular classes, received no special educational services, and had no sensory or motor impairments. All the HFASD children were assessed by psychiatrists or pediatricians as fulfilling the criteria for at least one of the pervasive developmental disorders of DSM-IV-text revision (TR). They also all attended regular classes. All HFASDs children were assessed using the third edition of the Wechsler Intelligence Scale within a year before the data were collected: full-scale IQ ranged from 79 to 129 (M = 97.56, SD = 17.54) and verbal-IQ from 80 to 136 (M = 98.87, SD = 17.81). No standardized intelligence scale was administered to TD children, because this is not normal practice among typical council elementary schools in Japan. Children were asked to use a five-point scale to indicate whether they agreed with the literal or nonliteral interpretation of the cartoon. A summary of the abovementioned studies is shown in Table 1.

2.2. Procedures. The freshmen rated all the figurative language phrases listed above on a five-point scale.

The strangest (most unconventional) was assigned a score of 5 and the least strange (most conventional) a score of 1. First, we compared strangeness (unconventionality) values among ironic phrases, metaphors (from Adachi et al. [13]), sarcasm, and "indirect reproach" (from Yata and Oi [14] and Taguchi et al. [15]) using the Wilcoxon Signed Ranks test. For this comparison, and that described below, the test was two-tailed, with Z values used to calculate P values. Second, for Oi and Tanaka's [16] data, we made a comparison between one metaphor (Appendix), in which children with HFASDs preferred the literal interpretation more frequently than did TD children, and the remaining nine metaphors in which no intergroup difference was found. The freshmen's strangeness evaluation of the former metaphor was compared to that of the latter metaphors using the Wilcoxon Signed Ranks test.

Direct associations between freshmen's strangeness evaluation and children's interpretation of each figurative phrase could not be assessed as the authors of the present study did not have access to the full data of Adachi et al. [13]. Therefore, in the present study, indirect associations between freshmen's strangeness evaluation and children's ability to interpret figurative phrases were analyzed.

3. Results

As shown in Figure 1, ironic statements were rated as stranger (less conventional) than metaphors (Wilcoxon Signed Ranks test: Z scores were applied to calculate P; $z = -11.812$, $P < 0.001$) and "indirect reproaches" ($z = -11.829$, $P < 0.001$). Sarcastic phrases were rated as stranger (less conventional) than metaphors ($z = -12.047$, $P < 0.001$), "indirect reproaches" ($z = -12.048$, $P < 0.001$), and ironic statements ($z = -5.290$, $P < 0.001$). No difference was found between metaphors and "indirect reproaches." For the 10 metaphors from Okamoto [11], the one in which children with HFASD

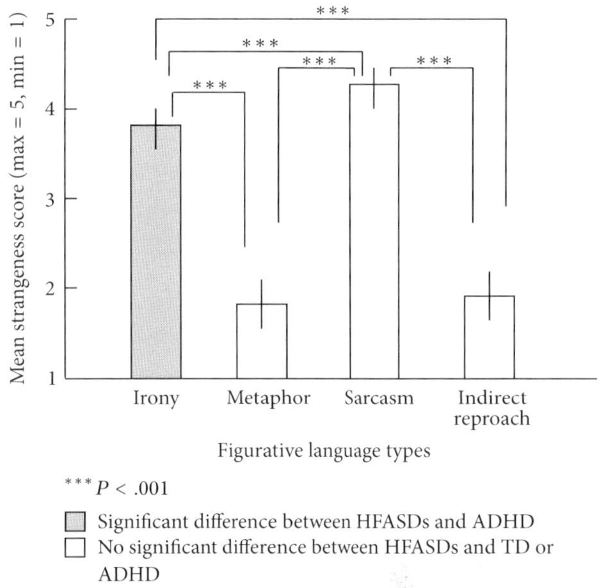

FIGURE 1: Mean evaluation values of strangeness (unconventionality) by college freshmen for each figurative language type.

preferred a literal meaning more frequently than did TD children was not rated differently from the remaining nine metaphors.

4. Discussion

The results did not fully support the hypothesis that the less strange a figurative language statement was rated, the more easily it would be comprehended by children with HFASD. The results for the ironic statements support the hypothesis as these statements were evaluated as highly strange by college freshmen and were more difficult for children with HFASDs than for those with ADHD to comprehend [13]. The findings for metaphor and "indirect reproach" also supported the hypothesis as both types of statements were evaluated as less strange and were comprehended as well by children with HFASDs as by their TD counterparts [14, 15]. The exception was sarcasm. Although sarcastic phrases were evaluated by the college students as the most strange among the four types of figurative language, these phrases were comprehended as well by children with HFASDs as by TD children, despite the lack of the 2nd order ToM reasoning in nearly half of the children with HFASDs [14].

Two questions arise here. The first is why only irony was poorly understood by Japanese children with HFASDs while the other three types of language were comprehended. The ironic statements investigated in the present study were evaluated as highly strange (far less conventional than typical statements). Giora et al. [8] postulate that conventionality can be seen as a major determinant influencing figurative language comprehension both in children with HFASDs and in TD children. They contend that making sense of nonliteral language relies on the salience of that language. According to their graded salience hypothesis, novelty (in other words,

Table 1: Summary of the studies by Adachi et al. [13], Yata and Oi [14], Taguchi et al. [15], and Oi and Tanaka [16].

	Number of children	ToM 1st	ToM 2nd	Tasks	Results
Adachi et al. [13]	66 AS children 20 HFASD children 37 ADHD children	15 failed 7 failed 4 failed	— — —	5 ironic statements 5 metaphors	Difference between AS and ADHD in comprehension of irony
Yata and Oi [14]	20 HFA children 20 TD children	3 failed 1 failed	9 failed 8 failed	5 sarcastic statements 5 indirect reproaches 5 indirect requests	No intergroup difference in comprehension of sarcasm, indirect reproaches, or indirect requests
Taguchi et al. [15]	17 HFASD children 15 TD children	— —	— —	5 sarcastic statements 5 indirect reproaches 5 indirect requests	No intergroup difference in comprehension of sarcasm, indirect reproaches, or indirect requests
Oi and Tanaka [16]	53 HFASD children 50 TD children	— —	— —	10 metaphors	Intergroup difference in comprehension of 1 metaphor

unconventionality) matters rather than nonliterality. This appears to hold true regarding the high degree of strangeness of ironic statements in the present study,r which were poorly understood by children with HFASDs, and it is also borne out by the low degree of strangeness of metaphors and "indirect reproaches," both of which were understood by children with HFASDs.

The present findings regarding sarcasm, however, do not support the graded salience hypothesis at all. We need an explanation that applies to both failure to understand ironic statements and ability to comprehend sarcastic ones. A closer look at the ironic statements used by Adachi et al. [13] might lend some insight into this. Of the five ironic statements investigated, four are not addressed directly from one character to the other in the scenario. Rather these were told in the form of a soliloquy with a humorous feel. In addition to this, in the remaining ironic statement, the child was asked to assume he or she was directly given the statement from another character in the scenario. In contrast, all the sarcastic statements investigated were addressed from one character to the other in the scenario. To succeed in comprehending these five ironic statements, children had to put themselves in the shoes of the character that made the statement or received the statement, while such a need did not exist for the sarcastic statements to be comprehended. In this regard, the metaphors and "indirect reproaches" investigated were similar to the sarcastic statements in that the children did not need to put themselves in the place of the listener or speaker. Hence, in metaphor, sarcasm, and "indirect reproach," it seems that the child would have understood the statement when he or she could observe correctly what the scenario depicted.

The second question to be addressed is whether or not sarcasm and "indirect reproach" are of sufficient difficulty as to require 2nd order ToM reasoning to be understood. Happé [19] suggested this was the case, as she, based on the findings of Sperber and Wilson [20], made a distinction between an utterance that requires elucidation of "an interpretation of an attributed thought or a desirable thought" and one that requires interpretation of "a description of an actual state of affairs or a desirable state of affairs." She stated that the former type of utterance includes ironic statements and interrogatives, and the latter includes ordinary assertions and basic imperatives. Happé [19] predicted that the former requires 2nd order metarepresentation while the latter requires only 1st order metarepresentation. The sarcastic statements and "indirect reproaches" investigated here seem to demand the child to interpret the speaker's thoughts regarding the hearer in the scenario. If this is true, how can we explain the finding that nearly half of the participants of the studies of Yata and Oi [14] failed the 2nd order ToM task?

One plausible explanation is again the absence of a need for the child to put her/himself in the shoes of another character to comprehend the statement. Hence, without requiring 2nd order ToM reasoning, children could comprehend sarcasm by logical computations such as those postulated by Oi and Tanaka [18] in learning to recognize situations where people "do not mean what they say." To do this, children would use simple rules such as literally false or puzzling speech + smile = joke, or literally false or puzzling speech + frown = sarcasm. The sarcastic phrases investigated in the present study were exchanged between third parties for the child. The child could accordingly behave as just an observer of the scenario who computes the meaning of the figurative language. If children had not achieved 2nd order ToM reasoning and sarcasm was not very familiar to them, they could comprehend these scenarios "correctly" by the sort of computation mentioned above, rather than "appropriately" by putting themselves in the place of the character in the scenario. However, children who had achieved 2nd order ToM reasoning could of course use this rather than the more difficult computation. On the other hand, as suggested by the present findings, "indirect reproach" might be more familiar than sarcasm, so that the child has the choice of relying on retrieving the memory of the meaning of "indirect reproach" as well as computation regarding the third parties, instead of using 2nd order ToM reasoning for comprehension.

Taguchi et al. [15] found, although not for the four categories of figurative language investigated here, that children with HFASDs failed to respond to indirect requests appropriately when these were directly addressed to them from adults, yet they succeeded when asked to choose an appropriate response from three types of responses when an indirect request scenario was written or played on a screen. This indicates that the difficulty relates to self-awareness,

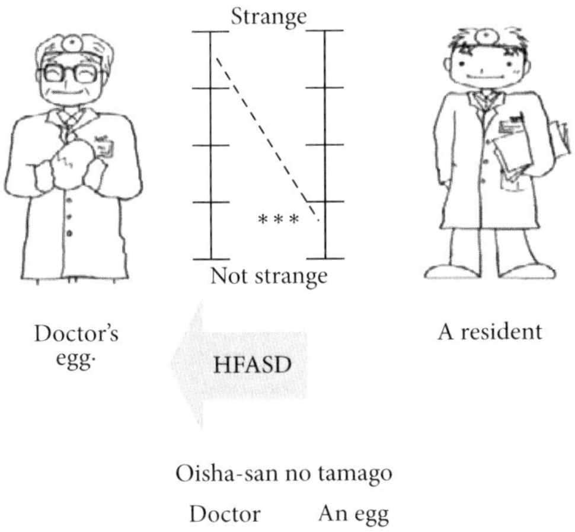

FIGURE 2

particularly the need to put oneself in another's place in the scenarios with embedded ironic statements. In responding appropriately to indirect requests such as "Is your mother there?" (meaning "Call your mother") via telephone, children have to put themselves in the shoes of the speaker. Children with HFASDs, indeed, failed this task [16]. We should therefore take a self-in-relation-to-other perspective [9] when investigating figurative language comprehension in autism, as well as considering ToM, conventionality (salience), weak central coherence, or executive dysfunction (the latter two factors were not discussed in the present study).

Comprehension of figurative language does not consist of a single cognitive process, but should instead be thought of as a product of complex activities of various sociocognitive processes.

5. Conclusion

Findings of studies on Japanese children with HFASDs suggest that the development of ToM reasoning is not the sole determinant of figurative language comprehension. The conventionality of figurative language also seems to influence comprehension. The conventionality of figurative language can be measured by having college freshmen evaluate its strangeness (unconventionality). Our findings suggest that Japanese ironic statements were difficult for children with HFASDs to comprehend as these were evaluated as far more strange than metaphors and "indirect reproaches." In addition to this, Japanese ironic statements seem to require children to put themselves in the position of a character in the scenario. The combination of this with high strangeness may explain why such statements were difficult to comprehend for children with HFASDs. For Japanese sarcastic phrases alone, conventionality did not appear to matter, as these were well comprehended by children with HFASDs despite (like ironic statements) being evaluated as far more strange than metaphors, "indirect reproaches," or ironic statements. This can be explained by neither the developmental level of ToM reasoning nor the degree of strangeness (unconventionality), but from the fact that the sarcastic phrases were exchanged between third parties. This might help children observe the figurative language and the scenario in which the language is embedded, leading to correct computation of the meaning. When comparing Japanese and English in terms of figurative language comprehension, we require a new way of explaining disabilities in figurative language comprehension as emergent products of complex interactions among sociocognitive activities [21].

The findings of the present study merit further investigation that directly examines the relationship between children's comprehension and freshmen's evaluation of strangeness of figurative language.

Appendices

A. Examples from Adachi et al. [13]

A.1. Irony. When Jiro's mother got home, she saw clothes left on the floor of Jiro's room. As she looked at this, she said, "Jiro always leaves his room in a tidy state." Does the mother think of Jiro as

(a) a boy who is organized,

(b) being messy,

(c) being a boy,

(d) taking a bath,

(e) I do not know.

A.2. Metaphor. A boy called Goro always wins sprint races. Taro, another boy, while watching Goro leaving the other runners behind, said, "Look, Goro looks like a cheetah!." Taro thinks of Goro as

(a) being a cheetah,

(b) being handsome,

(c) being a fast runner,

(d) leaving other runners behind,

(e) I do not know.

B. Examples from Yata and Oi [14] and Taguchi et al. [15]

B.1. Sarcasm. When a boy got a very bad mark in an exam, the mother told him, "You're a genius, aren't you?", while looking at the exam paper. What did the mother actually want to communicate?

(a) Her son is a genius.

(b) Her son is not a genius at all.

(c) Her son got a bad mark in an exam.

B.2. Indirect Reproach. When a friend of a boy was about to leave a mess behind after having played with many toys, the boy told his friend, "Are you leaving without tidying up?" What did the boy actually want to communicate?

(a) His friend is leaving now.

(b) His friend has a very bad attitude.

(c) They have played with many toys.

C. An Example from Oi and Tanaka [18]

See Figure 2.

Acknowledgments

This research was supported by a Grant (Grant-in-Aid for Scientific Research no. 23653184) from the Japan Society for the Promotion of Science. The authors thank Ms. Yumi Azuma for her assistance with data collection.

References

[1] C. F. Norbury and A. Sparks, "Difference or disorder? Cultural issues in understanding neurodevelopmental disorders," *Developmental Psychology*, vol. 49, no. 1, pp. 45–58, 2013.

[2] F. G. E. Happé, "Understanding minds and metaphors: Insights from the study of figurative language in autism," *Metaphor and Symbolic Activity*, vol. 10, no. 4, pp. 275–295, 1993.

[3] F. G. E. Happé, "Communicative competence and theory of mind in autism: a test of relevance theory," *Cognition*, vol. 48, no. 2, pp. 101–119, 1993.

[4] S. Ozonoff and J. N. Miller, "An exploration of right-hemisphere contributions to the pragmatic impairments of autism," *Brain and Language*, vol. 52, no. 3, pp. 411–434, 1996.

[5] G. MacKay and A. Shaw, "A comparative study of figurative language in children with autistic spectrum disorders," *Child Language Teaching and Therapy*, vol. 20, no. 1, pp. 13–32, 2004.

[6] G. Rundblad and D. Annaz, "The atypical development of metaphor and metonymy comprehension in children with autism," *Autism*, vol. 14, no. 1, pp. 29–46, 2010.

[7] S. Melogno, C. D'Ardia, M. A. Pinto, and G. Levi, "Metaphor comprehension in autistic spectrum disorders: case studies of two high-functioning children," *Child Language Teaching and Therapy*, vol. 28, no. 2, pp. 177–188, 2012.

[8] R. Giora, O. Gazal, I. Goldstein, O. Fein, and A. Stringaris, "Salience and context: interpretation of metaphorical and literal language by young adults diagnosed with Asperger 's syndrome," *Metaphor and Symbol*, vol. 27, no. 1, pp. 22–54, 2012.

[9] R. P. Hobson, "Autism, literal language and concrete thinking: some developmental considerations," *Metaphor and Symbol*, vol. 27, no. 1, pp. 4–21, 2012.

[10] M. Nomura, "The ubiquity of the fluid metaphor in Japanese: a case study," *Poetica*, vol. 46, pp. 41–75, 1996.

[11] S. Okamoto, "Politeness and the perception of irony: honorifics in Japanese," *Metaphor and Symbol*, vol. 17, no. 2, pp. 119–139, 2002.

[12] T. Adachi, "Sarcasm in Japanese," *Studies in Language*, vol. 20, pp. 1–36, 1996.

[13] T. Adachi, S. Hirabayashi, M. Shiota et al., "The study of situational recognition of attention deficit/hyperactivity disorders, Asperger's disorder and high functioning autism with the metaphor and sarcasm scenario test (MSST)," *No To Hattatsu*, vol. 38, no. 3, pp. 177–181, 2006.

[14] A. Yata and M. Oi, "Comprehension of indirect speech in children with high-functioning pervasive developmental disorders," *Japanese Journal of Learning Disabilities*, vol. 18, no. 2, pp. 128–137, 2009.

[15] A. Taguchi, M. Oi, and K. Takahashi, "Comprehension of indirect speech in children with high functioning pervasive developmental disorders under different task conditions," *Japanese Journal of Communication Disorders*, vol. 27, no. 3, pp. 168–177, 2010.

[16] M. Oi and S. Tanaka, "Comprehension of ambiguous language in children with high-functioning autism spectrum disorder," *The Japanese Journal of Communication Disorders*, vol. 27, no. 1, pp. 10–18, 2010.

[17] J. Hinds, "Reader versus writer responsibility: a new typology," in *Writing Across Languages: Analysis of L2 Text*, U. Connor and B. Kaplan, Eds., pp. 141–152, Addison-Wesley, Jacob Way Reading, MA, USA, 1987.

[18] M. Oi and S. Tanaka, "When do Japanese children with autism spectrum disorder comprehend ambiguous language overliterally or overnonliterally?" *Asia Pacific Journal of Speech, Language, and Hearing*, vol. 14, no. 1, pp. 1–12, 2011.

[19] F. G. E. Happé, "The autobiographical writings of three Asperger syndrome adults: problems of interpretation and implication for theory," in *Autism and Asperger Syndrome*, U. Frith, Ed., pp. 207–242, Cambridge University Press, Cambridge, UK, 1991.

[20] D. Sperber and A. Wilson, *Relevance: Communication and Cognition*, Blackwell, Oxford, UK, 1986.

[21] M. Perkins, *Pragmatic Impairment*, Cambridge University Press, Cambridge, UK, 2007.

9

Sensory Response Patterns in Nonverbal Children with ASD

Elena Patten,[1] Karla K. Ausderau,[2] Linda R. Watson,[3] and Grace T. Baranek[4]

[1] *Department of Communication Sciences and Disorders, The University of North Carolina, Greensboro, 300 Ferguson Building, Greensboro, NC 27412, USA*
[2] *The University of Wisconsin-Madison, 3195 Medical Sciences Center, 1300 University Avenue, Madison, WI 53706, USA*
[3] *Division of Speech & Hearing Sciences, The University of North Carolina at Chapel Hill, CB No. 7190 Chapel Hill, NC 27599, USA*
[4] *Division of Occupational Science & Occupational Therapy, The University of North Carolina at Chapel Hill, CB No. 7122 Chapel Hill, NC 27599, USA*

Correspondence should be addressed to Elena Patten; e_patten@uncg.edu

Academic Editor: Herbert Roeyers

We sought to examine concurrent and longitudinal associations between sensory response patterns (i.e., hyperresponsiveness, hyporesponsiveness, and sensory seeking) and verbal status of young children with autism spectrum disorder (ASD) as a potential factor influencing the development of verbal communication. Seventy-nine children with ASD (verbal, $n = 29$; nonverbal, $n = 50$) were assessed using cross-sectional analyses (Study 1), and 14 children with ASD (verbal, $n = 6$; nonverbal, $n = 8$) were assessed using prospective longitudinal analyses (Study 2). Data were collected regarding sensory response patterns and verbal ability. Hyporesponsiveness and sensory seeking behaviors were associated with verbal status in both cross-sectional and longitudinal analyses; nonverbal children were more likely to demonstrate higher hyporesponsive and sensory seeking patterns. Hyperresponsiveness did not significantly differ between verbal and nonverbal groups in either design. Sensory hyporesponsiveness and seeking behaviors may be important factors hindering the development of functional verbal communication in children with ASD. Unusual sensory responsiveness can often be observed before the onset of speech and may yield important prognostic capabilities as well as inform early interventions targeting verbal communication or alternative communication options in young children with ASD.

1. Introduction

Approximately 25–50% of children with autism spectrum disorder (ASD) do not develop functional verbal communication [1–3], and functional verbal communication rarely develops after age of five in children with ASD [4]. These nonverbal children have significantly poorer outcomes compared to children with ASD who do develop functional verbal communication; development of speech prior to this age predicts educational achievement, employment, the ability to live independently, and social relationships [5, 6]. Variability exists regarding terminology defining expressive communication in children with ASD, particularly regarding the term "functional verbal communication" [7]. For purposes of this paper, we conceptualize functional verbal communication based on discussions by Baghdadli et al. [1] and Tager-Flusberg et al. [7] as *spoken language that is spontaneous and meaningful and includes multiword utterances.*

Although nonverbal children with ASD comprise a substantial portion of the population and outcomes are poor for them, limited research elucidating potential explanatory factors for the failure of some children with ASD to acquire meaningful expressive language or examining treatments that may improve long-term outcomes is available for individuals who remain nonverbal into the school-age years. To address this issue, the National Institutes of Health (NIH) conducted a workshop to discuss the state of the science and to generate research priorities regarding nonverbal children with ASD [8]. One research priority identified by participants in this workshop was to identify mechanisms underlying the lack of development of functional verbal communication that occurs in some children with ASD. If auditory and visual information provided by communication models are not adequately processed, verbal communication may not develop normally [9]. Abnormal sensory processing of environmental stimuli may be one mechanism underlying both sensory features and impaired development of functional verbal communication in children with autism. Thus, we are interested in evaluating sensory response patterns that are manifest and observable early in life that may be associated with the development of functional verbal communication.

The ability to accurately process environmental stimuli, particularly early in development, is necessary for typical development of a number of early social and communication skills. Impairments in sensory processing are commonly associated with ASD; a meta-analysis by Ben-Sasson and colleagues [10] suggested that, to some degree, sensory processing disturbances may be universal in ASD. Increased frequency of unusual sensory features in individuals with ASD has been documented through self-reports [11] as well as through numerous empirical studies (e.g., [12–15]). More importantly, severity of sensory features in children with ASD has been found to predict various adaptive and maladaptive behaviors such as communication [9], socialization [16], and stereotyped behaviors [17].

The ability to process and respond to sensory stimuli has been conceptualized in the literature and tested in a variety of ways. Although in natural environments stimuli are multimodal, experimental studies often test single sensory modalities (e.g., vision, audition, and touch) (e.g., [18–20]). Some research teams have shown utility for categorizing responses to sensory stimuli across multiple modalities as reflecting at least three broad patterns or constructs: hyporesponsive, hyperresponsive, and sensory seeking [17, 21–24]. Each sensory response pattern is thought to represent a continuum related to the frequency or intensity with which sensory features characteristic of that pattern are observed. Hyporesponsiveness is characterized by delayed, absent, or more attenuated responses to stimuli than expected (e.g., child requires multiple or intense auditory cues to elicit an orienting response) [17, 21–24]. Hyperresponsiveness is characterized by an exaggerated, often negative, response to stimuli (e.g., child attempts to avoid stimulation, such as covering ears to filter certain sounds, or shows an aversive response to tactile stimuli that would not bother others) [17, 21–24]. Sensory seeking encompasses behaviors that appear to reflect a fascination with or craving of sensory stimulation that is intense or unusual and may be repetitive in nature (e.g., child uses peripheral vision to sight objects, repeatedly rubs a texture, or sniffs objects) [17, 21–24]. These sensory response patterns are evident across sensory modalities, and they often coexist within individuals with ASD [12, 23].

No studies found in the literature specifically address the potential for sensory response patterns to be a factor constraining the development of verbal communication (i.e., by grouping participants based on the presence or absence of verbal communication) in children with ASD. That is, although the impact of sensory processing problems on verbal communication has been hypothesized (e.g., [9, 25]), previous studies have not examined this question by grouping participants based on the presence or absence of verbal communication. Sensory responsiveness and communication may be associated in children from very early infant development. Both prospective and retrospective studies have shown that social-communication impairments and sensory-motor abnormalities coexist in infants who later developed ASD [26, 27]. Early in development, poor orienting to a communication partner may be a manifestation of unusual sensory processing [27]. A finding that has been replicated in the literature is that infants with ASD exhibit decreased orienting to social stimuli (e.g., [27, 28]). An inability to adequately orient to a communication partner and engage in dyadic attention precludes or at least hinders participation in further social and communicative interaction. Clifford and Dissanayake [29] suggest that dyadic attention, also impaired in ASD, requires both orienting and sustaining attention to social stimuli and plays a role in the development of joint attention. Joint attention (i.e., shared attention between two communication partners and an object or third person) is a robust predictor of language development in typically developing children as well as in children with ASD, with impairments frequently found in children with ASD [30–33]. Poor sensory responsiveness exhibited through decreased orienting is potentially the first observable measure of hyporesponsiveness that negatively impacts joint attention and later development of language [25, 34].

In preschool samples, empirical evidence indicates that hyporesponsiveness to environmental stimuli, including social stimuli, is concurrently associated with poor communication in children with ASD. Using cluster analysis, Liss et al. [23] found one cluster of individuals with ASD characterized by high levels of hyporesponsiveness and sensory seeking behaviors along with poor communication. Hilton et al. [16] found that three sensory response patterns (hyporesponsiveness, hyperresponsiveness, and sensory seeking) were associated with social-communicative symptom severity. Similarly, Watson et al. [9] found that hyporesponsiveness and sensory seeking, but not hyperresponsiveness, were negatively correlated with language and social-communication adaptive skills and positively correlated with social-communication symptoms of autism. In partial contrast, Lane et al. [35] used a stepwise multiple regression analysis with 54 children with ASD and found that sensory response patterns explained 24.5% of the variance in communication scores. This finding was largely accounted for by two of the seven subscales on the short sensory profile McIntosh et al., [36] predicting in opposite directions—specifically, "underresponsive/seeks sensation" was associated with lower communication adaptive skills, whereas "low energy/weak" was associated with higher communication adaptive skills.

In sum, unusual sensory features are highly prevalent and often observable at very young ages in children with ASD, and, in several studies by different research groups, sensory response patterns have been found to be related to communication in children with ASD.

Due to the substantial portion of children with autism who remain nonverbal and the associated poor prognoses for their long-term outcomes, research directed at understanding

TABLE 1: Demographic information for cross-sectional dataset.

	Nonverbal (N = 29)	Verbal (N = 50)	Total (N = 79)
Male	24 (30%)	43 (54%)	67 (85%)
Hispanic	1 (1%)	3 (4%)	4 (5%)
race*,+			
Asian	1 (3%)	0 (0%)	1 (1%)
Black	7 (24%)	2 (4%)	9 (11%)
White	16 (55%)	46 (92%)	62 (79%)
Multiple races	5 (17%)	2 (4%)	7 (9%)
Chronological age**,+	43.5 (12.74) mos	57.9 (16.35) mos	
IQ (proxy)***,+	33.8 (12.38)	73.5 (25.28)	
Maternal education****,++			
Partial high school	0 (0%)	1 (2%)	1 (1%)
High school/GED	8 (28%)	7 (14%)	15 (19%)
Associate/partial college	11 (38%)	8 (16%)	19 (24%)
Bachelor	8 (28%)	22 (44%)	30 (38%)
Masters/doctorate	2 (7%)	12 (24%)	14 (18%)
Household income*****,+			
<$20000	0 (0%)	1 (2%)	1 (1%)
$20000–59999	19 (66%)	15 (30%)	34 (43%)
$60000–99999	9 (31%)	20 (40%)	29 (37%)
>$100000	1 (3%)	14 (28%)	15 (19%)

+Significant differences based on verbal/nonverbal status at $P < .01$.
++Significant differences based on verbal/nonverbal status at $P < .05$.
*Verbal children were more likely to be white $X^2(3, N = 79) = 15.06, P = .002$.
**Verbal children were older $t(77) = -4.56, P < .001$.
***Verbal children had higher IQs $t(77) = -7.90, P < .001$.
****Mothers of verbal children tended to have more education $X^2(4, N = 79) = 10.37, P = .04$.
*****Verbal children tended to come from households with higher income $X^2(3, N = 79) = 12.19, P = .007$.

why some children with autism develop functional verbal communication and others do not is a current national priority [8]. With some inconsistencies in results, previous research has provided evidence of associations between communication and sensory response patterns, especially hyporesponsiveness and sensory seeking. The need to understand early behavioral features that may manifest in lack of spoken language by five years of age is of particular importance, due to indications that any spoken language by that age is predictive of eventual development of functional verbal communication. Aiming to examine the extent to which sensory response patterns are associated with the verbal status of young children with ASD, our research questions were as follows: (1) to what extent do sensory response patterns differ between verbal and nonverbal children with ASD and (2) to what extent are early sensory response patterns related to later verbal status in young children with ASD? Based on previous research, we hypothesized that two sensory response patterns, sensory hyporesponsiveness and sensory seeking, would be concurrently and predictively associated with verbal status (i.e., verbal versus nonverbal).

2. Method

We examined two extant datasets to address our research questions. The first study (Study 1) used data from all children with ASD who had been originally recruited as part of a larger study examining the development, functional impact, and cause of various sensory features in children with ASD, developmental delay, and/or typical development. The second dataset from which we derived Study 2 involved a subset of children from Study 1 of young, initially low verbal or nonverbal children; we included all participants from the second dataset for our Study 2 analyses. Study 1 included substantially more participants with data available for cross-sectional analyses; Study 2 participants were evaluated at two different time points and thus provided data for longitudinal analyses.

2.1. Participants. Children were recruited into Study 1 from a university-based research subject registry, developmental clinics, other research groups, parent support groups, local public schools, and the project website. A total of 79 children with a diagnosis of ASD (74 with autism, 5 with broader autism spectrum disorder) ranging from 25 to 89 months (M = 53; SD = 16.57) were included in this study. The participants with ASD largely overlapped with those in another study [9]. See Table 1 for participant and family descriptive and demographic information. The families received a monetary incentive ($75) for participation in the study and children received a small toy or book. The university's institutional review board approved the research, and a parent provided an informed consent for their child's participation. Participants had a diagnosis of ASD confirmed by the research staff through both the *Autism Diagnostic Interview—Revised* (ADI-R [37]) and *Autism Diagnostic Observation Schedule* (ADOS [38]). Participants were also required to have normal or corrected-to-normal hearing and vision as confirmed by screenings performed prior to assessment. Children were excluded if they presented with MA < 6 months, cerebral palsy, seizure disorder, or genetic conditions associated with a high risk of autism (e.g., fragile X, tuberous sclerosis), or were currently receiving psychopharmacological treatments as indicated by parents or from medical records.

ADOS Module 1, item A.1, was used for Study 1 to assign participants to either the verbal or nonverbal group, as in previous research [39], because it specifically quantifies the level of nonechoed language. Nonverbal status was assigned if the participant received a score of three (at least one word or word approximation but fewer than five words used during the session) or a score of eight (no words or word approximations). A child was considered verbal if she/he received a score of 0, 1, or 2 indicating at least 5 single, meaningful, and nonimitative words during the session. ADOS Module 1 is reserved for children who are preverbal or only produce single words. Some children in the verbal group received ADOS Module 2, used with children who use some multiword phrases but are not verbally fluent (i.e., expressive language level below that of a typical four years old); however, the majority of children from the Study 1 dataset ($n = 51$) received Module 1.

A subset of 14 children from Study 1, ranging from 28 to 42 months at entry (M = 35.79; SD = 4.34), were seen longitudinally in Study 2. Inclusion in Study 2 was restricted to children defined as having low verbal ability (i.e., no multiword utterances) at study entrance as determined by ADOS Module 1, item A.1 (overall level of nonechoed language). At the second time point, eight months later, 6 children were classified as verbal while 8 children maintained a nonverbal status based on ADOS results. For Study 2, parents received $25 and the children received a small toy or book for their contributions both for the entry assessments and the follow-up assessments.

2.2. Measures

2.2.1. Nonverbal Cognitive Measures. An estimate of nonverbal mental age was obtained from either the *Mullen Scales of Early Learning* (MSEL [40]) or the Stanford-Binet Intelligence Scales Fifth Edition (SB-5 [41]), depending on the child's age/ability level; 76 participants received the MSEL, and three participants received the SB-5. The MSEL is a standardized, examiner-administered measure of cognitive functioning for children from birth to 68 months of age. The SB-5 is a standardized, examiner-administered measure of cognitive functioning for individuals of ages 2 to 85 years. Nonverbal mental ages were used to avoid conflation with verbal ability. An IQ proxy was computed by dividing the nonverbal mental age from each assessment by the child's chronological age and multiplying by 100, as an estimate of cognitive functioning. We computed these IQ proxy scores due to the large number of children who scored at the lowest possible standard score on the MSEL or SB-5; thus, using the standard scores would have introduced floor effects and constrained variability in the analysis.

2.2.2. Sensory Measures. The *Sensory Experiences Questionnaire, version 2.1* (SEQ 2.1 [11, 42, 43]) is a 42-item caregiver questionnaire that assesses sensory responsiveness (hyporesponsiveness, hyperresponsiveness, and sensory seeking) across modalities (e.g., visual, tactile, and auditory) for children of ages from 6 months to 12 years. The SEQ has good psychometric properties: internal consistency ($\alpha = .800$) and test-retest reliability (ICC = .92) [43]. The *Sensory Profile* (SP [44, 45]) is a commonly used 125-item caregiver questionnaire for children of aged from 3 to 10 designed to assess sensory processing across modalities in a variety of clinical populations including children with autism [45]. The *Sensory Processing Assessment for Young Children* (SPA [25, 46, 47]) is a 20-minute clinically administered observational measure assessing sensory processing across modalities for children ages 9 months to 6 years. This protocol is semistructured and play based, providing behavioral presses to elicit various sensory responses in the tactile, auditory, and visual modalities. Intraclass correlation coefficients ranged from .91 to .99, indicating good reliability for scales. The *Tactile Defensiveness and Discrimination Test-Revised* (TDDT-R [48, 49]) is clinically administered and assesses tactile processing, specifically hyperresponsiveness and discrimination in preschool and school-age children. Presses are in the tactile modality and include touch stimuli applied to the participant's skin (e.g., finger puppet/cotton swab; sticker) and exploration of various tactile materials (e.g., sand, lotion, vibration, carpet, dried noodles, etc.).

A multitrait, multimethod approach (in this case, both parent report and observational methods) has been recommended in the measurement of psychological constructs [50, 51]. Consistent with such recommendations, this study utilized a factor analytic model created from these four sensory processing assessments, yielding standardized factor scores for each participant for each of the three sensory construct scores: hyperresponsiveness (HYPER), hyporesponsiveness (HYPO), and sensory seeking (SEEK). We created a measurement model in MPLUS (version 5) that had 5 latent constructs (observational measures, parent measures, HYPO, HYPER, and SEEK) and 11 manifest variables (each sensory pattern represented in each of the four sensory assessments; the TDDT-R only contributed HYPER and SEEK items, whereas the SEQ, SP, and SPA each contributed HYPO, HYPER, and SEEK items). The factor analytic model allowed for correction of rater effect (error variance) attributable to parent reporting in two instruments versus observational measurement in two other instruments. The measurement model had good fit, as shown by a nonsignificant chi-square, χ^2 (1, $N = 110$) = 32.4, $P = .40$; a comparative fit index (CFI) near 1 (CFI = 0.997); and a root-mean-square error of approximation (RMSEA) <.08 (RMSEA = .021).

TABLE 2: Language assessment means and standard deviations for the longitudinal sample at study initiation.

Language assessment	Status at T2 (nonverbal $n = 8$) (verbal $n = 6$)	Mean	SD
PLS total AE*	Nonverbal	7.25	3.11
	Verbal	16.33	5.85
PLS AC, AE	Nonverbal	6.25	5.12
	Verbal	16.50	7.48
PLS EC, AE*	Nonverbal	9.38	2.97
	Verbal	18.00	6.13
MCDI, EG	Nonverbal	7.71	3.60
	Verbal	11.50	4.09
MCDI, LG*	Nonverbal	9.71	7.04
	Verbal	22.50	2.74
Number of gestures used*	Nonverbal	17.43	10.26
	Verbal	34.00	6.20

*$P < .05$.
PLS: Preschool Language Scale, version 4.
AE: age equivalent (AE used due to floor effects with standard scores).
AC: auditory comprehension.
EC: expressive communication.
MCDI: MacArthur-Bates Communicative Development Inventories.
EG: early gestures.
LG: late gestures.

3. Results

Results from chi-square analyses and t-tests revealed several demographic characteristics that differed between the verbal and nonverbal groups in the Study 1 cross-sectional data. Verbal children were more likely to be white and older, have higher IQ proxy scores, have mothers with higher education, and have families with higher incomes. Verbal status was not associated with gender or ethnicity. See Table 1 for results. Demographic analyses (sex, ethnicity, race, chronological age, IQ, maternal education, household income) for our Study 2 longitudinal data did not show statistically significant differences between children who were verbal versus children who remained nonverbalwere not, which is not surprising given the small sample size. Additionally, our criteria that children who entered Study 2 have low verbal status may have resulted in more homogeneity within the sample. Language measures were obtained for children in Study 2 (longitudinal), and children who became verbal at the second time point had better receptive and expressive language at the first time point, including more gestures, than children who remained nonverbal. Thus, although all children met the criteria for low verbal status at study entry, differences in communication abilities were already evident. See Table 2 for results. The number of hours of participation in speech language therapy between study entry and eight months later was compared between groups and yielded no significant differences (P = .61).

Research Question 1: To What Extent Do Sensory Response Patterns Differ between Verbal and Nonverbal Children with ASD? Sensory patterns of verbal and nonverbal children from Study 1 (cross-sectional) were contrasted using a mixed ANOVA. The within subjects variable was the type of sensory response pattern (HYPO, SEEK, and HYPER) and the between subjects variable was verbal status (verbal versus nonverbal). This design allowed us to examine differences in performance across the three sensory response patterns, overall differences between verbal status across sensory patterns, and the sensory pattern versus verbal status interaction. The analyses were conducted with SPSS (PASW Statistics 18). Means are presented in Figure 1. The mixed ANOVA results indicated that there were nosignificant differences across the three sensory patterns, $F(2, 77) = 1.05$, $P = .31$. However, there was a significant main effect for verbal status, $F(1, 77) = 10.59$, $P = .002$, and a significant verbal status by sensory response pattern interaction; $F(2, 77) = 7.59$, $P = .001$. The nature of this interaction was examined using planned interaction contrasts [52]. These results indicate that the nonverbal group was significantly higher than the verbal group on HYPO ($P = .008$) and SEEK ($P < .001$) but not significantly different on HYPER, $P = .61$. Effect sizes for both HYPO and SEEK were large based on Cohen's d (Cohen, 1988), HYPO ($d = .56$); SEEK ($d = .62$). The effect size for HYPER was small ($d = .11$).

Research Question 2: To What Extent Are Early Sensory Features Related to Later Verbal Status in Preschool Children with ASD? Using the same analyses as above, we examined longitudinal data for 14 children from our Study 2 dataset who each met the criteria for low verbal status at study entry. The children were assigned to either the verbal or the nonverbal group based upon the ADOS assessment administered one year after the sensory measures were taken. Means for sensory scores are presented in Figure 2. The mixed ANOVA results indicated no significant differences

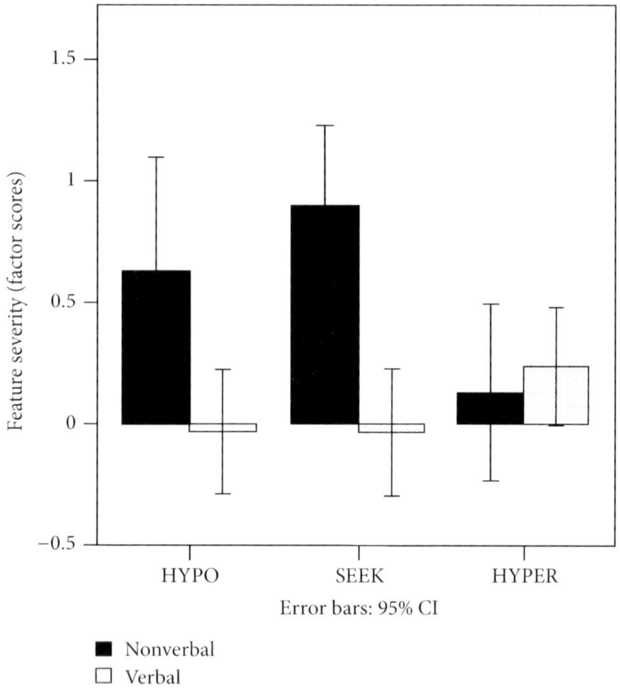

Figure 1: Level of severity of sensory response patterns for verbal and nonverbal subgroups in the cross-sectional sample.

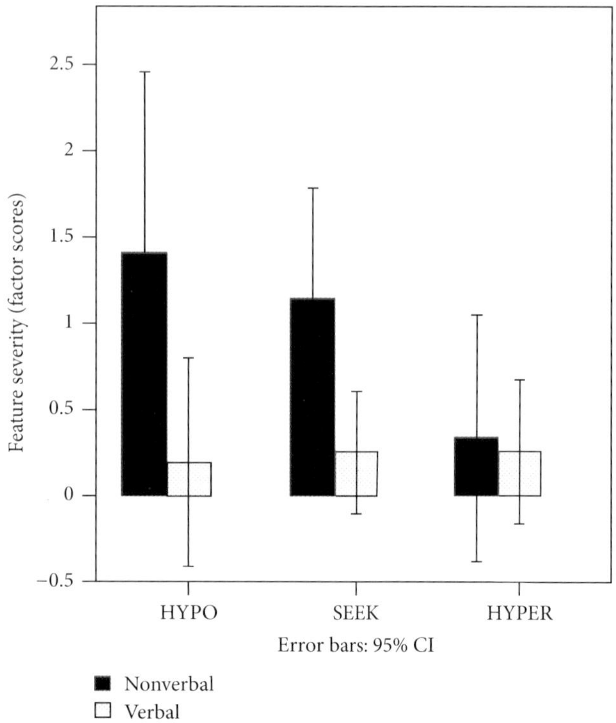

Figure 2: Level of severity of sensory response patterns for verbal and nonverbal subgroups in the longitudinal sample.

across the three sensory response patterns, $F(2, 12) = .09$, $P = .77$. There was a significant main effect for verbal status across the three sensory response patterns, $F(1, 12) = 7.43$, $P = .018$; however, there was no significant verbal status by sensory response pattern interaction, $F(2, 24) = 1.94$, $P = .17$. Pairwise comparisons were used to examine group differences. These results indicate that the nonverbal group was significantly higher than the verbal group on HYPO ($P = .05$) and SEEK ($P = .02$) but not significantly different on HYPER, $P = .84$. Effect sizes were calculated using Hedge's g to account for small sample sizes and were large for both HYPO and SEEK: HYPO ($g = 1.47$), SEEK ($g = 1.16$). The effect size for HYPER was small ($g = .12$).

4. Discussion

We examined associations between sensory response patterns and verbal status in children with ASD. Our cross-sectional and longitudinal data demonstrated that higher levels of sensory hyporesponsiveness and sensory seeking were both concurrently and predictively associated with nonverbal status, as we initially predicted. Sensory hyperresponsiveness did not differentiate children who were verbal from children who were nonverbal in either the cross-sectional or the longitudinal data. Our findings support those of other research teams indicating that both sensory hyporesponsiveness and sensory seeking behaviors are inversely associated with language development [9, 16, 23, 34]. Also, the current studies confirm and elaborate on our previously reported findings on many of these same participants [9, 25] by explicitly examining the association of sensory response patterns with verbal versus nonverbal status and demonstrating for the first time that hyporesponsiveness and sensory seeking patterns also predict longitudinally later verbal or nonverbal status. Both hyporesponsiveness and sensory seeking patterns may reflect established deficits in attention orienting and shifting in children with ASD (e.g., [34, 53, 54]) that may constrain communication development. Measures of hyporesponsiveness are not clearly separable from attention orienting, in that failure to look toward the source of a novel sound can be labeled as both poor attention orienting as well as hyporesponsiveness to sensory stimuli. Attention orienting is a necessary gateway to the larger construct of attention that involves sustaining and shifting attention and allows for deeper processing of information. Likewise, sensory seeking behaviors that involve an intense focus on stimuli preferred by the child may preclude attention orienting to other important stimuli (e.g., conventional toys and/or stimuli being referenced in language directed to the child) and in essence have the same result as hyporesponsiveness. It may be that unusual sensory responses result in some of the communication symptoms associated with autism, but a separate underlying factor may result in both unusual sensory responses and communication symptoms; thus the two may not be causally related.

Neural deficits in early stages of sensory processing may result in behavioral patterns of sensory hyporesponsiveness and contribute to inadequate attention to environmental stimuli, thus hindering the ability to process and learn from both ambient social-communication as well as direct bids for interaction. Early in development, caregiver-generated stimuli are laden with social and communicative elements. Typically developing infants are drawn to such dyadic interactions, but infants with ASD demonstrate impairments in dyadic attention [29]. Thus, early sensory processing deficits could contribute to the lack of attention to dyadic interactions as well as other environmental stimuli. Sensory seeking behavior (e.g., fixation on light patterns) also may constrain social and communication learning opportunities due to over-focused attention to nonsocial stimuli. Thus, both of these sensory response patterns may adversely impact a child's ability to take advantage of important social and communicative learning opportunities.

Our findings regarding demographic differences between verbal and nonverbal children indicate that verbal children come from families who are white, with higher education and income. Although this is a sample of convenience rather than an epidemiological sample, these findings may reflect disparities in services that are related to demographic variables. For example, in an analysis of service utilization, in which the sample largely overlapped that in the current study, higher parental education was related to more intervention services obtained [55].

4.1. Clinical Implications. This study adds to the growing body of research linking sensory hyporesponsiveness and sensory seeking patterns to poorer communication outcomes in children with ASD [9, 16, 23]. Because sensory hyporesponsiveness may be observable in infancy, these findings have implications for early detection and intervention and suggest that children with autism may benefit from techniques to enhance capture of attention to salient social and communicative stimuli perhaps through enhancements of perceptual elements and/or motivational systems. Many available clinical interventions incorporate techniques to enhance attention (e.g., audio-visual pairings such as a pointing gesture with a verbal command, "look" [56]). For a review of additional attention enhancing techniques, see [57]. Therapeutic interventions to enhance sensory processing functions are popular in the treatment of ASD [58], but the efficacy of these treatments is mixed and debated among researchers [59–61]; thus more research is needed particularly with respect to communication outcomes.

4.2. Limitations and Future Direction. This study was based on two extant databases that were not specifically designed to address the impact of sensory features on verbal status. Our longitudinal dataset was small ($n = 14$) but provided unique information regarding the predictive nature of early sensory features. Future studies should examine trajectories of attainment of verbal status, at a variety of age ranges, as a function of sensory features both concurrently and predictively in larger samples.

Our assessments were all behavioral measures relying on observation or parent report. Sensory processing and language development may share some neurobiological mechanisms that require bio-physiological measures to adequately assess them. Therefore, future studies should include more direct measures of potential underlying neurological mechanisms.

Our analyses revealed significant demographic differences between verbal and nonverbal children with autism. Future studies should explore the stability of these findings and why the differences exist. Further, factors such as access to services should be included as potential mediators between demographic differences (e.g., income disparity) and developmental outcomes.

Acknowledgments

This research was made possible through a grant from the National Institute for Child Health and Human Development (R01-HD42168), a grant from the National Alliance for Autism Research/Autism Speaks (no. 681), and the University of North Carolina at Chapel Hill research subject registry (supported by the Intellectual and Developmental Disabilities Research Center; P30HD03110). The authors thank the families whose participation made this study possible and the staff who collected and processed data for this project.

References

[1] A. Baghdadli, B. Assouline, S. Sonié et al., "Developmental trajectories of adaptive behaviors from early childhood to adolescence in a cohort of 152 children with autism spectrum disorders," *Journal of Autism and Developmental Disorders*, vol. 42, no. 7, pp. 1314–1325, 2012.

[2] C. Lord, S. Risi, and A. Pickles, "Trajectory of language development in autistic spectrum disorders," in *Developmental Language Disorders: From Phenotypes to Etiologies*, M. L. Rice and S. F. Warren, Eds., pp. 7–29, Lawrence Erlbaum Associates, Mahwah, NJ, USA, 2004.

[3] M. Sigman and C. W. McGovern, "Improvement in cognitive and language skills from preschool to adolescence in autism," *Journal of Autism and Developmental Disorders*, vol. 35, no. 1, pp. 15–23, 2005.

[4] E. Pickett, O. Pullara, J. O'Grady, and B. Gordon, "Speech acquisition in older nonverbal individuals with autism: a review of features, methods, and prognosis," *Cognitive and Behavioral Neurology*, vol. 22, no. 1, pp. 1–21, 2009.

[5] R. Kobayashi, T. Murata, and K. Yoshinaga, "A follow-up study of 201 children with autism in Kyushu and Yamaguchi areas, Japan," *Journal of Autism and Developmental Disorders*, vol. 22, no. 3, pp. 395–411, 1992.

[6] A. Venter, C. Lord, and E. Schopler, "A follow-up study of high-functioning autistic children," *Journal of Child Psychology and Psychiatry and Allied Disciplines*, vol. 33, no. 3, pp. 489–507, 1992.

[7] H. Tager-Flusberg, S. Rogers, J. Cooper et al., "Defining spoken language benchmarks and selecting measures of expressive language development for young children with autism spectrum disorders," *Journal of Speech, Language, and Hearing Research*, vol. 52, no. 3, pp. 643–652, 2009.

[8] L. Gilotty, "Meeting summary. *NIH workshop on nonverbal school-aged children with autism*," Rockville, Md, USA, April, 2010, http://www.nimh.nih.gov/research-funding/

scientific-meetings/2010/nih-workshop-on-nonverbal-school-aged-children-with-autism/nih-workshop-on-nonverbal-school-school-aged-children-with-autism.shtml.

[9] L. R. Watson, E. Patten, G. T. Baranek et al., "Differential associations between sensory response patterns and language, social, and communication measures in children with autism or other developmental disabilities," *Journal of Speech, Language, and Hearing Research*, vol. 54, no. 6, pp. 1562–1576, 2011.

[10] A. Ben-Sasson, L. Hen, R. Fluss, S. A. Cermak, B. Engel-Yeger, and E. Gal, "A meta-analysis of sensory modulation symptoms in individuals with autism spectrum disorders," *Journal of Autism and Developmental Disorders*, vol. 39, no. 1, pp. 1–11, 2009.

[11] L. Cesaroni and M. Garber, "Exploring the experience of autism through firsthand accounts," *Journal of Autism and Developmental Disorders*, vol. 21, no. 3, pp. 303–313, 1991.

[12] G. T. Baranek, F. J. David, M. D. Poe, W. L. Stone, and L. R. Watson, "Sensory experiences questionnaire: discriminating sensory features in young children with autism, developmental delays, and typical development," *Journal of Child Psychology and Psychiatry and Allied Disciplines*, vol. 47, no. 6, pp. 591–601, 2006.

[13] C. Lord, M. Rutter, and A. L. Couteur, "Autism diagnostic interview-revised: a revised version of a diagnostic interview for caregivers of individuals with possible pervasive developmental disorders," *Journal of Autism and Developmental Disorders*, vol. 24, no. 5, pp. 659–685, 1994.

[14] S. J. Rogers, S. Hepburn, and E. Wehner, "Parent reports of sensory symptoms in toddlers with autism and those with other developmental disorders," *Journal of Autism and Developmental Disorders*, vol. 33, no. 6, pp. 631–642, 2003.

[15] L. D. Wiggins, D. L. Robins, R. Bakeman, and L. B. Adamson, "Breif report: sensory abnormalities as distinguishing symptoms of autism spectrum disorders in young children," *Journal of Autism and Developmental Disorders*, vol. 39, no. 7, pp. 1087–1091, 2009.

[16] C. Hilton, K. Graver, and P. LaVesser, "Relationship between social competence and sensory processing in children with high functioning autism spectrum disorders," *Research in Autism Spectrum Disorders*, vol. 1, no. 2, pp. 164–173, 2007.

[17] B. A. Boyd, G. T. Baranek, J. Sideris et al., "Sensory features and repetitive behaviors in children with autism and developmental delays," *Autism Research*, vol. 3, no. 2, pp. 78–87, 2010.

[18] J. H. Foss-Feig, J. L. Heacock, and C. J. Cascio, "Tactile responsiveness patterns and their association with core features in autism spectrum disorders," *Research in Autism Spectrum Disorders*, vol. 6, no. 1, pp. 337–344, 2012.

[19] N. Neumann, A. M. Dubischar-Krivec, F. Poustka, N. Birbaumer, S. Bölte, and C. Braun, "Electromagnetic evidence of altered visual processing in autism," *Neuropsychologia*, vol. 49, no. 11, pp. 3011–3017, 2011.

[20] K. O'Connor, "Auditory processing in autism spectrum disorder: a review," *Neuroscience and Biobehavioral Reviews*, vol. 36, no. 2, pp. 836–854, 2012.

[21] J. Ashburner, J. Ziviani, and S. Rodger, "Sensory processing and classroom emotional, behavioral, and educational outcomes in children with autism spectrum disorder," *American Journal of Occupational Therapy*, vol. 62, no. 5, pp. 564–573, 2008.

[22] A. Ben-Sasson, S. A. Cermak, G. I. Orsmond, H. Tager-Flusberg, M. B. Kadlec, and A. S. Carter, "Sensory clusters of toddlers with autism spectrum disorders: differences in affective symptoms," *Journal of Child Psychology and Psychiatry and Allied Disciplines*, vol. 49, no. 8, pp. 817–825, 2008.

[23] M. Liss, C. Saulnier, D. Fein, and M. Kinsbourne, "Sensory and attention abnormalities in autistic spectrum disorders," *Autism*, vol. 10, no. 2, pp. 155–172, 2006.

[24] S. D. Tomchek and W. Dunn, "Sensory processing in children with and without autism: a comparative study using the short sensory profile," *American Journal of Occupational Therapy*, vol. 61, no. 2, pp. 190–200, 2007.

[25] G. T. Baranek, L. R. Watson, B. A. Boyd, M. D. Poe, F. J. David, and L. Mcguire, "Hyporesponsiveness to social and nonsocial sensory stimuli in children with autism, children with developmental delays, and typically developing children," *Development and Psychopathology*, vol. 25, no. 2, pp. 307–320, 2013.

[26] S. E. Bryson, L. Zwaigenbaum, J. Brian et al., "A prospective case series of high-risk infants who developed autism," *Journal of Autism and Developmental Disorders*, vol. 37, no. 1, pp. 12–24, 2007.

[27] G. T. Baranek, "Autism during infancy: a retrospective video analysis of sensory-motor and social behaviors at 9–12 months of age," *Journal of Autism and Developmental Disorders*, vol. 29, no. 3, pp. 213–224, 1999.

[28] E. Werner, G. Dawson, J. Osterling, and N. Dinno, "Brief report: recognition of autism spectrum disorder before one year of age: a retrospective study based on home videotapes," *Journal of Autism and Developmental Disorders*, vol. 30, no. 2, pp. 157–162, 2000.

[29] S. M. Clifford and C. Dissanayake, "The early development of joint attention in infants with autistic disorder using home video observations and parental interview," *Journal of Autism and Developmental Disorders*, vol. 38, no. 5, pp. 791–805, 2008.

[30] M. Carpenter, K. Nagell, and M. Tomasello, "Social cognition, joint attention, and communicative competence from 9 to 15 months of age," *Monographs of the Society for Research in Child Development*, vol. 63, no. 4, pp. 1–143, 1998.

[31] T. Charman, J. Swettenham, S. Baron-Cohen, A. Cox, G. Baird, and A. Drew, "Infants with autism: an investigation of empathy, pretend play, joint attention, and imitation," *Developmental psychology*, vol. 33, no. 5, pp. 781–789, 1997.

[32] S. R. Leekam, B. López, and C. Moore, "Attention and joint attention in preschool children with autism," *Developmental Psychology*, vol. 36, no. 2, pp. 261–273, 2000.

[33] D. McArthur and L. B. Adamson, "Joint attention in preverbal children: autism and developmental language disorder," *Journal of Autism and Developmental Disorders*, vol. 26, no. 5, pp. 481–496, 1996.

[34] G. Dawson, K. Toth, R. Abbott et al., "Early social attention impairments in autism: social orienting, joint attention, and attention to distress," *Developmental Psychology*, vol. 40, no. 2, pp. 271–283, 2004.

[35] A. E. Lane, R. L. Young, A. E. Z. Baker, and M. T. Angley, "Sensory processing subtypes in autism: association with adaptive behavior," *Journal of Autism and Developmental Disorders*, vol. 40, no. 1, pp. 112–122, 2010.

[36] D. N. McIntosh, L. J. Miller, V. Shyu, and W. Dunn, "Overview of the short sensory profile," in *The SenSory Profile Examiner's Manual*, W. Dunn, Ed., pp. 59–73, The Psychological Corporation, San Antonio, Tex, USA, 1999.

[37] A. le Couteur, C. Lord, and M. Rutter, *Autism Diagnostic Interview-Revised (ADI-R)*, Western Psychological Corporation, Los Angeles, Calif, USA, 2003.

[38] C. Lord, M. Rutter, P. Dilavore, and S. Risi, *The Autism Diagnostic Observation Schedule (ADOS)*, Western Psychological Corporation, Los Angeles, Calif, USA, 1999.

[39] K. Gordon, G. Pasco, F. McElduff, A. Wade, P. Howlin, and T. Charman, "A communication-based intervention for nonverbal children with autism: What changes? Who benefits?" *Journal of Consulting and Clinical Psychology*, vol. 79, no. 4, pp. 447–457, 2011.

[40] E. M. Mullen, *Scales of Early Learning (AGS Edition)*, Western Psychological Services, Los Angeles, Calif, USA, 1995.

[41] G. H. Roid, ,*Stanford Binet Intelligence Scales*, Riverside Publishing, Rolling Meadows, Ill, USA, 5th edition, 2003.

[42] G. T. Baranek, *Sensory Experiences Questionnaire (SEQ)*, University of North Carolina, Chapel Hill, NC, USA, 1999.

[43] L. M. Little, A. C. Freuler, M. B. Houser et al., "Psychometric validation of the sensory experiences questionnaire," *American Journal of Occupational Therapy*, vol. 65, no. 2, pp. 207–210, 2011.

[44] W. Dunn, *Sensory Profile*, Psychological Corporation, San Antonio, Tex, USA, 1999.

[45] M. A. Kientz and W. Dunn, "A comparison of the performance of children with and without autism on the sensory profile," *American Journal of Occupational Therapy*, vol. 51, no. 7, pp. 530–537, 1997.

[46] G. T. Baranek, *Sensory Processing Assessment for Young Children (SPA)*, University of North Carolina, Chapel Hill, NC, USA, 1999.

[47] G. T. Baranek, B. A. Boyd, M. D. Poe, F. J. David, and L. R. Watson, "Hyperresponsive sensory patterns in young children with autism, developmental delay, and typical development," *American Journal on Mental Retardation*, vol. 112, no. 4, pp. 233–308, 2007.

[48] G. T. Baranek, *Tactile Defensiveness and Discrimination Test: Revised*, University of North Carolina, Chapel Hill, NC, USA, 1998.

[49] G. T. Baranek and G. Berkson, "Tactile defensiveness in children with developmental disabilities: responsiveness and habituation," *Journal of Autism and Developmental Disorders*, vol. 24, no. 4, pp. 457–471, 1994.

[50] M. Eid, F. W. Nussbeck, C. Geiser, D. A. Cole, M. Gollwitzer, and T. Lischetzke, "Structural equation modeling of multitrait-multimethod data: different models for different types of methods," *Psychological Methods*, vol. 13, no. 3, pp. 230–253, 2008.

[51] O. P. John and V. Benet-Martinez, "Measurement: reliability, construct validation, and scale construction," in *Handbook of Research Methods in Social and Personality Psychology*, H. T. Reis and C. M. Judd, Eds., pp. 339–369, Cambridge University Press, New York, NY, USA, 2000.

[52] G. Keppel and S. Zedeck, *Data Analysis For Research Designs: Analysis of Variance and Multiple Regression/Correlation Approaches*, W. H. Freeman; Times Books; Henry Holt, New York, NY, USA, 1989.

[53] R. Landry and S. E. Bryson, "Impaired disengagement ofattention in young children with austism," *Journal of Child Psychology and Psychiatry and Allied Disciplines*, vol. 45, no. 6, pp. 1115–1122, 2004.

[54] J. Swettenham, S. Baron-Cohen, A. Cox et al., "The frequency and distribution of spontaneous attention shifts between social and nonsocial stimuli in autistic, typically developing, and nonautistic developmentally delayed infants," *Journal of Child Psychology and Psychiatry and Allied Disciplines*, vol. 39, no. 5, pp. 747–753, 1998.

[55] E. Patten, G. T. Baranek, L. R. Watson, and B. S. Schultz, "Child and family characteristics influencing intervention choices in autism spectrum disorders," *Focus on Autism and Other Developmental Disabilities*, 2012.

[56] S. R. Leekam, E. Hunnisett, and C. Moore, "Targets and cues: gaze-following in children with autism," *Journal of Child Psychology and Psychiatry and Allied Disciplines*, vol. 39, no. 7, pp. 951–962, 1998.

[57] E. Patten and L. R. Watson, "Interventions targeting attention in young children with autism," *American Journal of Speech-Language Pathology*, vol. 20, no. 1, pp. 60–69, 2011.

[58] S. Hodgetts and W. Hodgetts, "Somatosensory stimulation interventions for children with autism: Literature review and clinical considerations," *Canadian Journal of Occupational Therapy*, vol. 74, no. 5, pp. 393–400, 2007.

[59] G. T. Baranek, "Efficacy of sensory and motor interventions for children with autism," *Journal of Autism and Developmental Disorders*, vol. 32, no. 5, pp. 397–422, 2002.

[60] R. Lang, M. O'Reilly, O. Healy et al., "Sensory integration therapy for autism spectrum disorders: a systematic review," *Research in Autism Spectrum Disorders*, vol. 6, no. 3, pp. 1004–1018, 2012.

[61] National Autism Center, *National Standards Report: Addressing the Need for Evidence-Based Practice Guidelines for Autism Spectrum Disorders*, National Autism Center, Randolph, Mass, USA, 2009.

10

Gait Deviations in Children with Autism Spectrum Disorders

Deirdre Kindregan,[1] Louise Gallagher,[2] and John Gormley[1]

[1] *Discipline of Physiotherapy, School of Medicine, Trinity College Dublin, Dublin, Ireland*
[2] *Discipline of Psychiatry, School of Medicine, Trinity College Dublin, Dublin, Ireland*

Correspondence should be addressed to Deirdre Kindregan; kindregd@tcd.ie

Academic Editor: Robert F. Berman

In recent years, it has become clear that children with autism spectrum disorders (ASDs) have difficulty with gross motor function and coordination, factors which influence gait. Knowledge of gait abnormalities may be useful for assessment and treatment planning. This paper reviews the literature assessing gait deviations in children with ASD. Five online databases were searched using keywords "gait" and "autism," and 11 studies were found which examined gait in childhood ASD. Children with ASD tend to augment their walking stability with a reduced stride length, increased step width and therefore wider base of support, and increased time in the stance phase. Children with ASD have reduced range of motion at the ankle and knee during gait, with increased hip flexion. Decreased peak hip flexor and ankle plantar flexor moments in children with ASD may imply weakness around these joints, which is further exhibited by a reduction in ground reaction forces at toe-off in children with ASD. Children with ASD have altered gait patterns to healthy controls, widened base of support, and reduced range of motion. Several studies refer to cerebellar and basal ganglia involvement as the patterns described suggest alterations in those areas of the brain. Further research should compare children with ASD to other clinical groups to improve assessment and treatment planning.

1. Introduction

Autism is a developmental disorder which presents before three years of age [1]. It is a spectrum of pervasive developmental disorders and is found across all ethnic cultures and economic groups. From 2013, all children with autism, Asperger's syndrome, or other pervasive developmental disorders will receive one umbrella diagnosis of autism spectrum disorder (ASD) [2]. There has been a steady increase in the prevalence of ASD over the last twenty years [3, 4]. This may however be due to increased access to diagnostic services or increasing awareness of the condition. Children with ASD have difficulty with social interaction, communication, and language skills with many children demonstrating restrictive and repetitive behaviour [5, 6]. These kinds of behaviour may include rocking, finger flicking, or arm flapping [7]. Motor stereotypies are defined as "involuntary, coordinated, patterned, repetitive, rhythmic, and purposeless but seemingly purposeful movements" [8]. Children with ASD have been found to demonstrate numerous gait stereotypies such as pacing, jumping, hopping, skipping, and spinning and it has been suggested that these may also be considered restrictive and repetitive behaviour [9]. Gait abnormality can be simply defined as a deviation from normal walking pattern and may include, but is not limited to, the above mentioned stereotypies.

The "manner or style of walking" or gait is described as a method of locomotion using reciprocal placement of the lower limbs to provide both propulsion and support by Levine et al. [10]. Alterations in movement patterns in children with ASD were noted as far back as 1943 by Kanner who found that those with ASD often demonstrated "clumsy" gait and gross motor patterns [11]. In more recent years, Ghaziuddin and Butler found that children with ASD demonstrated poorer coordination than those with Asperger's disorder [12]. Many studies have subsequently examined motor coordination in children with ASD and a recent review, by Fournier et al., provided further evidence that children diagnosed with ASD may be "less coordinated and show fewer motor capabilities" [13]. This may therefore suggest that gait disturbances may be common among children with ASD. For example, it has been observed that children with ASD are more prone to idiopathic toe walking than age-matched healthy controls [14, 15]. This, however, is only evident in children under six years of age.

The motor deficits reported in association with ASD, that is, impaired vestibular control and fine and gross motor abnormalities, have been likened to patients with known cerebellar deficits [16]. Deficits in smooth pursuit and saccadic eye movements are reported in ASD and are suggestive of vermal dysfunction in the cerebellum [17, 18]. Neuroimaging studies in children with ASD show reduced ipsilateral activation of the cerebellum during gross motor movement and more diffuse activation in lobules VI-VII [19, 20]. Cerebellar deficits are widely reported in ASD, reduced Purkinje and granule cells, and vermal hypo- and hyperplasia have been reported and both pre- and postnatal processes have been implicated [21–25]. The cerebellum has been implicated in the motor deficits in ASD via connections with the parietal lobe and wide ranging connections with cortical and subcortical brain regions serve to modulate multiple brain functions that are impaired in ASD [26]. Deficits in postural control and gait in ASD have been linked to dysfunction in sensory integration to the cerebellum or to the basal ganglia due to similarities with gait abnormalities observed in Parkinson's disease [13, 27, 28]. Abnormalities in basal ganglia shape have also been associated with motor deficits in ASD [29].

In adults, the first study on kinematic and kinetic gait patterns in ASD was carried out by Hallett et al. [30]. Adults with ASD were found to demonstrate "mild clumsiness" during gait but the only significant abnormality was a reduced range of motion at the ankle joint. Following on from this, in the last twenty years, there have been several papers published which examined gait patterns in children with autism spectrum disorders. The objective of this review is to identify gait abnormalities that may be present in children with ASD. Identification of gait abnormalities may permit earlier diagnosis and better treatment planning.

2. Methods

2.1. Terminology. The terms kinematics and kinetics are used to describe gait. Kinematic analysis of gait describes the linear and angular displacement, velocities, and accelerations of motion. Inherent in kinematic analysis is the description of motion from a temporospatial perspective which describes, for example, step or stride lengths as well as cadence and gait velocity. Kinetics is the study of the forces that cause motion. In movement analysis, kinetic parameters define the forces causing the movement. The most common force acting on the body during gait is the ground reaction force (GRF), which is the force exerted by the ground on the foot [31]. Another kinetic parameter commonly described is the joint moment which is the turning effect of a force generated by a muscle across a joint.

2.2. Search Strategy. Articles included in this review were retrieved from five online databases (PubMed, EmBase, Medline, CINAHL, and Web of Science) by a single investigator. The following key terms were used: gait, autism. Reference lists of the articles retrieved in this search were then manually searched.

2.3. Selection Criteria. Studies which assessed the relationship between temporospatial, kinematic, or kinetic gait parameters and ASD in children aged between four and 18 years were selected for inclusion in this review. Studies written in English and published between January 1970 and February 2015 were included. Of 126 studies retrieved in the search, only 11 studies met the inclusion criteria and were therefore selected and included in this review. Table 1 shows the studies included for review.

3. Results

3.1. Temporospatial Parameters. Temporal and spatial parameters refer to gait parameters which are related to timing and displacement or distance. The temporospatial parameters that have been examined in children are stride length, step length, step width, cadence (steps per minute), velocity, stance time, and double support. Of the ten studies that examined stride/step length, five found that stride length/step length was significantly reduced in children with ASD compared to healthy controls [33, 37, 39–41], which is consistent with the study by Hallett et al. who found a reduced stride length in adults with ASD. The other five studies, however, found no significant differences in stride length between children with ASD and controls [28, 34–36, 38]. Step width was assessed in four studies and has been found to be significantly increased in children with ASD in two [32, 35, 37], but no significant differences were found by another [38].

Of the 11 studies, eight assessed cadence. Calhoun et al. [36] found that children with ASD had, on average, a higher cadence than the controls, contrasting with Weiss et al. [33] who found it to be reduced in the ASD group and the six studies which found no significant difference between groups [28, 34, 35, 37–39, 41]. Velocity was assessed by nine studies, but no significant differences between children with ASD and controls were found by six of them [28, 34–36, 38, 39]. Velocity was, however, found to be significantly reduced in the ASD in two studies [33, 40] and slightly reduced in a third [37]. In two studies, stance time was found to be significantly increased [33, 41] but no significant difference was found in four other studies [34, 36, 37, 39]. Double support was examined by six studies, but only one found significant differences. Weiss et al. [33] found that double support time was significantly increased in the ASD group when compared to controls.

The wide variation in temporospatial results between studies may be due to varying inclusion criteria such as age, gender, and IQ or differing gait analysis methods.

3.2. Kinematic Parameters. Kinematics is the study of motion without regard to the forces that cause it. In gait, kinematic

Table 1: Studies included in review.

Author	Year	Title	Sample size total (ASD)	Average age in sample (years)	Gait analysis method	Major findings
Shetreat-Klein et al. [32]	2014	Abnormalities of joint mobility and gait in children with autism spectrum disorders	76 (38)	4.58	Video Analysis	Gait with wide base of support common in ASD
Weiss et al. [33]	2013	Gait analysis of teenagers and young adults diagnosed with autism and severe verbal communication disorders	19 (9)	19	GAITRite	Reduced stride length and increased stance time in ASD
Chester and Calhoun [34]	2012	Gait symmetry in children with autism	36 (14)	6.06	8-Cam Vicon	No significant differences in mean temporospatial gait parameters
Nayate et al. [35]	2012	Differentiation of high-functioning autism and Asperger's disorder based on neuromotor behaviour	33 (11)	12.75	GAITRite	Increased step width in ASD; visual cues increased stride length variability in ASD
Calhoun et al. [36]	2011	Gait patterns in children with autism	34 (12)	6.06	8-Cam Vicon	Increased cadence, reduced peak ankle plantar flexion and hip flexion moments in ASD
Nobile et al. [37]	2011	Further evidence of complex motor dysfunction in drug naive children with autism using automatic motion analysis of gait	32 (16)	10.28	ELITE	Increased step width, reduced ankle plantar flexion and knee flexion-extension at toe-off, and a reduced hip range of motion in ASD
Rinehart et al. (a) [28]	2006	Gait function in high-functioning autism and Asperger's disorder: evidence for basal-ganglia and cerebellar involvement?	30 (10)	10.69	Clinical Stride Analyzer	Increased variability in stride length in ASD
Rinehart et al. (b) [38]	2006	Gait function in newly diagnosed children with autism: cerebellar and basal ganglia related motor disorder	22 (11)	5.79	GAITRite	Increased variability in stride length and stride time in ASD
Vernazza-Martin et al. [39]	2005	Goal directed locomotion and balance control in autistic children	15 (9)	5	ELITE	Reduced step length in ASD
Ambrosini et al. [40]	1998	Motion analysis of patients with infantile autism	8 (8)	10.8	5 Cam Vicon	Reduced stride length, increased step width, and reduced ground reaction forces during terminal stance in ASD
Vilensky et al. [41]	1981	Gait disturbances in patients with autistic behavior: a preliminary study	41 (21)	7.73	Video Analysis	Reduced stride length and increased stance time in ASD. Reduced ankle dorsiflexion and knee extension at initial contact and increased hip flexion at toe-off in ASD

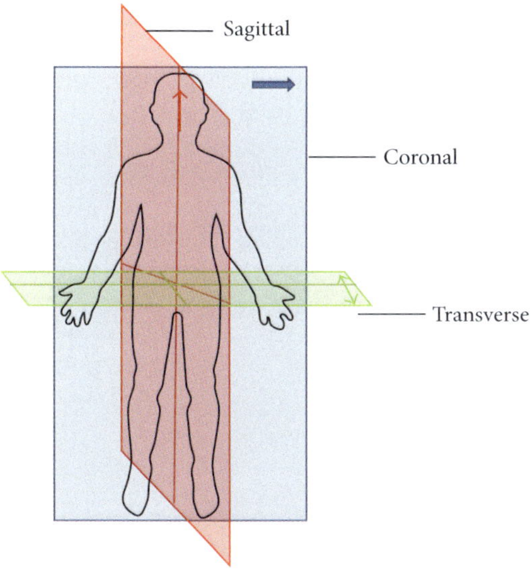

FIGURE 1: Anatomical planes of the body.

parameters refer to joint motions and angles at specific points in the gait cycle. These motions occur within three planes: the sagittal plane, the coronal plane, and the transverse plane (Figure 1). The sagittal plane is the plane through which most of the motion of gait occurs. As such it is the plane that splits the human body into right and left and the plane through which forward/backward motion occurs, for example, flexion/extension of the hip. The results will be discussed by joint in order of ankle, knee, and hip.

Children with ASD were found by Vilensky et al. [41] to have reduced dorsiflexion of the ankle joint at ground contact but found other ankle joint angles to be within normal limits [41]. At toe-off, significantly reduced plantar flexion was detected by Nobile et al. in children with ASD compared to controls [37]. Children with ASD had overall reduced range of motion at the ankle joint [40]. Ambrosini et al. [40] found that children with ASD had slightly, but not significantly, increased dorsiflexion during midstance and toe-off. This may be interpreted to mean they had reduced plantar flexion at toe-off, as found by Nobile et al. [37].

At the knee, children with ASD were found to have significantly reduced ROM with a decreased flexion-extension angle at toe-off when compared to healthy controls [37]. Significantly reduced knee extension in children with ASD was also found by Vilensky et al. [41] only this time at initial contact. At the hip joint there is no consensus with Nobile et al. [37] finding a significantly reduced range of motion at the hip but Vilensky et al. [41] found that the children with ASD had increased hip flexion at toe-off.

3.3. Kinetic Parameters. Kinetic gait parameters are those which are concerned with the forces involved in the production of movement. Calhoun et al. [36] and Ambrosini et al. [40] are the only studies to investigate kinetic gait parameters in children with ASD. Children with ASD were found to have reduced peak plantar flexion moments at the ankle but all other ankle kinetics were within normal ranges [36]. No significant differences were found in knee joint kinetics, but one significant difference was found in hip joint kinetics between groups. The children with ASD had decreased peak hip flexor moments compared to the control group [36]. Ground reaction forces are the forces exerted by the ground on an object or body in contact with it. Children with ASD were found to have relatively normal ground reaction forces, with the exception, being the second vertical peak which was reduced in children with ASD when compared to normative data [40]. The second vertical peak refers to the ground reaction force during the period of terminal stance, which ends with toe-off.

3.4. Variability in Gait. Three studies investigated the effect of external factors on the variability of gait in children with ASD. One study [35] examined the effect of self-determined speed on the temporal spatial gait patterns of children with ASD. They asked the children to walk at their normal pace and then asked them to walk at faster and slower rates and found that the children with ASD widened their base of support while walking at increased speed. They also studied the effect of cueing and concurrent tasks on gait in children with ASD. Their results showed that visual cues significantly increased stride length variability in children with ASD, but effects of dual tasks, tapping while walking (motor task) and counting while walking (cognitive task), were not statistically significant. Some studies found that children with ASD had significantly increased variability in their stride lengths [28, 38], walking velocities, and stride times [38]. One study found that children with ASD demonstrated an unusual cadence-stride length relationship in their gait pattern, with an increased stride length at a given cadence compared to controls [35].

In summary, between-group gait parameter varied across the different studies. Stride/step length was found to be increased in ASD in half of the studies that examined it. Step width was assessed in two studies and was found to be increased in both. Cadence was found to be increased in children with ASD in one study but decreased in another, and no significant differences were found by six other studies. Stance time has been found to be increased in ASD in two studies, but other studies found no differences. Joint ranges of motion were found to be significantly different in children with ASD compared to controls in all studies that presented kinematic data. However the joints affected and the periods of the gait cycle in question varied between studies. Two studies assessed kinetic gait parameters. The ASD groups demonstrated altered joint moments at the ankle and the hip in one study and ground reaction forces were found to be reduced in another.

4. Discussion

Although there are few studies completed in the area of gait analysis in children with ASD, some emerging commonalities were identified. Some studies have found differences in temporal and spatial gait parameters between children diagnosed with ASD and healthy controls. The most common deviations found are an increased step width and, debatably, a decreased step length and stride length. Nayate et al. [35] revealed an increase in stride length at a given cadence when compared to controls, which may account for the disagreement in results between studies, as this may not have been taken into account [35]. Cadence was found to be increased in children with ASD in one study, and since the children were found to take smaller steps in many studies, this is not surprising. An increased step width gives the children a wider base of support, and reduced step and stride lengths allow them to keep their centre of gravity firmly within this base of support. This, combined with reduced velocity and increased time in the stance phase of gait, suggests a tendency to augment their stability during walking. This may be due to issues with balance [42], proprioception [43], or behavioural anxiety [44].

Of the studies in this review, three which studied kinematic parameters have found reduced range of motion during gait in children with ASD, especially ankle dorsiflexion. Nobile et al. [37] and Ambrosini et al. [40] found that there was increased ankle dorsiflexion (i.e., decreased plantar flexion) at toe-off. Vilensky et al. [41] found that children with ASD had reduced dorsiflexion at heel strike but did not find any significant differences at toe-off. It is not possible therefore to draw a conclusive picture of changes at the ankle joint during gait in children with ASD. At the knee, children with ASD were observed to have reduced ROM in two studies [37, 41], but there was no agreement at the hip joint with one study stating that children with ASD had reduced hip ROM [37] but another suggesting an increase in hip flexion in children with ASD [41]. An increase in hip flexion would fit in with the above findings of reduced plantar flexion at toe-off as increased hip flexion would compensate for the reduced propulsive force and aid in foot clearance as the ipsilateral limb enters the swing phase.

Overall, the kinematic findings of these studies are sparse and often contradict each other. There is a lack in comparability in results as analysis differs. For example, Vilensky et al. [41] concentrate on the angles at initial contact, whereas Nobile et al. [37] focus on those at toe-off. These possibly suggest that there is a general reduction in range of motion at the joints of the lower limbs in children with ASD during gait. However, little research has been done solely on joint mobility in ASD so it is unclear whether children with ASD have reduced range of motion or simply have a more rigid gait pattern than healthy controls. This would fit in with the aforementioned idea that children with ASD seek to stabilise their gait. Further research in the area should aim to clarify this.

Only two studies investigated kinetic gait parameters and yielded few results of significance. The only significant differences in joint moments between children with ASD and healthy controls were in peak ankle plantar flexion moments and peak hip flexor moments. The children with ASD had reduced peak plantar flexion moments, meaning that the forces acting around the ankle joint during flexion were reduced when compared to controls. Since children with ASD have been shown to have reduced plantar flexion at toe-off [41], it makes sense that the forces generated would also be reduced [41]. This finding may imply a weakness of the plantar flexor muscles or may be due to the group's reduced peak plantar flexion angles as less force is required to generate a smaller movement in the joint. The author suggested that it may also be caused by hypotonia, which was confirmed in one-third of the children diagnosed with ASD. Children with ASD were also found to have reduced peak hip flexor moments but had increased hip flexion angles. This may imply weakness in the hip flexor muscles as they are unable to generate the same amount of force as those that healthy controls can, and the increased angles may imply weakness or a lack of control of the hip flexor muscles.

The findings of many studies in children with ASD concluded that gait abnormalities observed are indicative of widespread dysfunction in cerebellar and frontostriatal basal ganglia circuitry [28, 32, 33, 35, 37–41]. This is in agreement with Hallett et al., who found that adults with ASD had a gait pattern similar to patients with Parkinson's disease and suggested cerebellar involvement. A study compared brain images of children with ASD to healthy controls and showed abnormal cerebellar maturation in the ASD group [44]. The kinematic gait pattern exhibited by children with ASD shares common characteristics with "crouch gait," a pattern commonly elicited in Parkinson's disorder which involves changes to the cerebellum. As referenced previously a wide range of studies point towards cerebellar deficits in ASD based on postmortem histopathological studies, structural and functional imaging. It has been argued that cerebellar dysfunction may explain the heterogeneous deficits observed in ASD, both sensory-motor and cognitive [45].

However, the increased variability of gait parameters exhibited by children with ASD, as examined by three studies, may suggest an association with extensive neurobiological dysfunction which is unlike adult-onset disorders such as Parkinson's disorder [28, 35, 38]. Furthermore, the lack of improvement with visual cues as well as increase in variability of gait parameters with dual-task observed in children with ASD lends strength to the argument for ASD to be viewed as a "disorder of complex information processing" as initially proposed by Minshew and Goldstein [46].

Velocity has been shown to affect gait patterns [47–49]. No study examining gait in children with ASD has controlled for velocity, which may lead to velocity being a confounding factor. Although no study found velocity to be significantly reduced in children with ASD, this does not mean that each child walked at the same velocity. It is very difficult to impose a standard velocity across groups but this may lead to deviations in gait patterns becoming more apparent.

There are also study-design considerations in relation to the studies reviewed here. Sample sizes in all studies were quite small with the cohort studied by Shetreat-Klein et al. [32] being by far the largest at 76 including 38 children diagnosed with ASD. By definition, ASD is a spectrum rather than one specific condition with differing subtypes and varying levels of severity. These high levels of variability in this group, combined with small sample groups, may lead to between-group differences to be obscured. Several studies cited this as a limitation to their research and recommended that future studies include a larger cohort [34–36, 40].

Furthermore ASDs frequently are accompanied by a range of comorbid conditions such as attention deficit hyperactivity disorder (ADHD), developmental coordination disorder (DCD), and anxiety disorders. The *Fifth Edition of the Diagnostic and Statistical Manual of Mental Disorders* [2] by the American Psychiatric Association now permits the diagnosis of comorbid ADHD and DCD with ASD. The extent to which gait abnormalities in ASD are unique or associated with other comorbid conditions remains unclear and existing studies have not addressed this issue. This is a question therefore for future study.

Overall, the studies reviewed had significant differences in terms of methodology, thus reducing comparability of their results. This may explain some of the inconsistencies found; for example, Vilensky et al. [41] found that the ASD group had increased time in stance phase whereas Rinehart et al. [28] found no significant difference in the same parameter, the split opinion on stride/step length. These may be accounted for by the differing inclusion criteria such as age: the mean age of the children with ASD in the study by Vilensky et al. [41] was 6.1 years, with the youngest being just three, compared to the group studied by Rinehart et al. [28] which had a mean age of 10.7 years and the youngest was six years old. Gait patterns develop as a child grows so patterns will be different with differing age ranges, making it very difficult to compare the gait patterns observed. There were also differences in IQ between the groups of both studies, with Rinehart et al. [28] only including "normally intelligent" children, but Vilensky et al. [41] had seven children who were classed as "severely retarded" which may influence movement patterns, and the two studies used different gait analysis systems so differences in detection of patterns may arise.

Many children with ASD are prescribed antipsychotic medications, which may have effects on certain parts of the brain responsible for the control of movement such as the cerebellum. Only Nobile et al. [37] specified that all the children included in the study were drug naïve. Nayate et al. [35] cited this as a limitation to their research as three children in the study were on a mood-altering drug called sodium valproate which, at high doses, may have clinical effects on the cerebellum [50], which in turn may affect gross motor control and, therefore, movement patterns.

The temporospatial patterns exhibited by children with ASD were similar to the gait of children with obesity, with a wide base of support and shorter strides [51]. None of the studies reviewed examined the effects of BMI or body weight as a confounding factor. To date, no study has been published which compares gait patterns in children with ASD to healthy controls and also to children with obesity. It may also be of clinical importance to compare gait patterns in children with ASD to children with obesity as it has been shown that children with ASD have, by temporospatial parameters, a similar gait to children with obesity and have, on average, a significantly higher body fat percentage and lower lean tissue masses than healthy controls [52].

There are several factors that may affect research in this area such as intellectual ability, behavioural problems, and severity of the condition. Most studies in the area examined gait patterns in children with high-functioning ASD. This means that the current research cannot provide an overall picture of gait deviations in children across the autism spectrum disorders. The question of whether changes in gait patterns become more obvious with increasing severity of the disorder was raised by Weiss et al. [33]. They suggested that future research should be carried out including more low-functioning individuals.

The studies reviewed are helping to provide clinical practitioners, across a variety of disciplines, with a description of physical characteristics of ASD. The knowledge and understanding of this aspect of ASD may increase routine referral to services, such as physiotherapy, and allow for better intervention and treatment planning. Since children with ASD were found to have reduced range of motion during gait [37, 40, 41], there may be underlying weakness within muscles of the lower limb and the wider base of support found [32, 35, 37, 40] may imply issues with balance and/or proprioception. An assessment-based individually tailored exercise programme including gait reeducation, lower limb strengthening and balance, and proprioceptive training may improve gait patterns and coordination, with the overall aim of increasing physical activity and quality of life for children with ASD.

5. Conclusion

In conclusion, the overall findings of the studies conducted in the area are inconclusive, due to a number of confounding factors as discussed; however, some results suggest an emerging pattern. The current perspective on gait patterns in children with ASD is that there are a number of deviations present in terms of temporospatial, kinematic, and kinetic parameters and that gait, along with other movement pattern changes, may be used to allow for earlier diagnosis of ASD. There is, however, some consensus regarding the involvement of the cerebellum and basal ganglia in children with ASD and the relationship with observed motor deficits. Several limitations have been acknowledged and future research will need to address these more rigorously. More research should be done comparing children with ASD to other diagnostic groups to determine the degree of specificity of deficits and whether observed deficits influence treatment planning.

Abbreviation

ASD: Autism spectrum disorder.

Authors' Contribution

Ms. Kindregan carried out the literature search, chose the articles that met selection criteria and critically reviewed them, drafted the initial paper, and approved the final paper as submitted. Professor Gallagher and Dr. Gormley reviewed and revised the paper and approved the final paper as submitted.

References

[1] S. J. Rogers, "Interventions that facilitate socialization in children with autism," *Journal of Autism and Developmental Disorders*, vol. 30, no. 5, pp. 399–409, 2000.

[2] American Psychiatric Association, *Diagnostic and Statistical Manual of Mental Disorders (DSM-5)*, American Psychiatric Publishing, Washington, DC, USA, 5th edition, 2013.

[3] E. Fombonne, "Epidemiology of pervasive developmental disorders," *Pediatric Research*, vol. 65, no. 6, pp. 591–598, 2009.

[4] P. Lenoir, C. Bodier, H. Desombre et al., "Prevalence of pervasive developmental disorders. A review," *Encephale*, vol. 35, no. 1, pp. 36–42, 2009.

[5] American Psychiatric Publishing, *Diagnostic and Statistical Manual of Mental Disorders*, Text Revision (DSM-IV-TR), American Psychiatric Publishing, Washington, DC, USA, 4th edition, 2000.

[6] X. Ming, M. Brimacombe, and G. C. Wagner, "Prevalence of motor impairment in autism spectrum disorders," *Brain & Development*, vol. 29, no. 9, pp. 565–570, 2007.

[7] C. Lord and R. M. Jones, "Annual research review: Re-thinking the classification of autism spectrum disorders," *Journal of Child Psychology and Psychiatry*, vol. 53, no. 5, pp. 490–509, 2012.

[8] C. D. Marsden and S. Fahn, Eds., *Movement Disorders*, Butterworth-Heinemann, London, UK, 3rd edition, 1994.

[9] S. Goldman, C. Wang, M. W. Salgado, P. E. Greene, M. Kim, and I. Rapin, "Motor stereotypies in children with autism and other developmental disorders," *Developmental Medicine and Child Neurology*, vol. 51, no. 1, pp. 30–38, 2009.

[10] D. Levine, J. Richards, and M. W. Whittle, Eds., *Whittle's Gait Analysis*, Churchill Livingstone, Philadelphia, Pa, USA, 5th edition, 2012.

[11] L. Kanner, "Autistic disturbances of affective contact," *Acta Paedopsychiatrica*, vol. 35, no. 4, pp. 100–136, 1968.

[12] M. Ghaziuddin and E. Butler, "Clumsiness in autism and Asperger syndrome: a further report," *Journal of Intellectual Disability Research*, vol. 42, no. 1, pp. 43–48, 1998.

[13] K. A. Fournier, C. J. Hass, S. K. Naik, N. Lodha, and J. H. Cauraugh, "Motor coordination in autism spectrum disorders: a synthesis and meta-analysis," *Journal of Autism and Developmental Disorders*, vol. 40, no. 10, pp. 1227–1240, 2010.

[14] W. J. Barrow, M. Jaworski, and P. J. Accardo, "Persistent toe walking in autism," *Journal of Child Neurology*, vol. 26, no. 5, pp. 619–621, 2011.

[15] A. Marcus, B. Sinnott, S. Bradley, and I. Grey, "Treatment of idiopathic toe-walking in children with autism using GaitSpot Auditory Speakers and simplified habit reversal," *Research in Autism Spectrum Disorders*, vol. 4, no. 2, pp. 260–267, 2010.

[16] C. M. Freitag, C. Kleser, M. Schneider, and A. von Gontard, "Quantitative assessment of neuromotor function in adolescents with high functioning autism and Asperger syndrome," *Journal of Autism and Developmental Disorders*, vol. 37, no. 5, pp. 948–959, 2007.

[17] Y. Takarae, N. J. Minshew, B. Luna, C. M. Krisky, and J. A. Sweeney, "Pursuit eye movement deficits in autism," *Brain*, vol. 127, no. 12, pp. 2584–2594, 2004.

[18] Y. Takarae, N. J. Minshew, B. Luna, and J. A. Sweeney, "Oculomotor abnormalities parallel cerebellar histopathology in autism," *Journal of Neurology, Neurosurgery and Psychiatry*, vol. 75, no. 9, pp. 1359–1361, 2004.

[19] S. H. Mostofsky, S. K. Powell, D. J. Simmonds, M. C. Goldberg, B. Caffo, and J. J. Pekar, "Decreased connectivity and cerebellar activity in autism during motor task performance," *Brain*, vol. 132, no. 9, pp. 2413–2425, 2009.

[20] G. Allen and E. Courchesne, "Differential effects of developmental cerebellar abnormality on cognitive and motor functions in the cerebellum: an fMRI study of autism," *The American Journal of Psychiatry*, vol. 160, no. 2, pp. 262–273, 2003.

[21] D. M. Arin, M. L. Bauman, and T. L. Kemper, "The distribution of Purkinje cell loss in the cerebellum in autism," *Neurology*, vol. 41, supplement, p. 307, 1991.

[22] A. Bailey, P. Luthert, A. Dean et al., "A clinicopathological study of autism," *Brain*, vol. 121, no. 5, pp. 889–905, 1998.

[23] M. L. Bauman and T. L. Kemper, Eds., *The Neurobiology of Autism*, Johns Hopkins University Press, Baltimore, Md, USA, 2005.

[24] E. R. Whitney, T. L. Kemper, M. L. Bauman, D. L. Rosene, and G. J. Blatt, "Cerebellar Purkinje cells are reduced in a subpopulation of autistic brains: a stereological experiment using calbindin-D28k," *Cerebellum*, vol. 7, no. 3, pp. 406–416, 2008.

[25] E. Courchesne, E. Redcay, J. T. Morgan, and D. P. Kennedy, "Autism at the beginning: microstructural and growth abnormalities underlying the cognitive and behavioral phenotype of autism," *Development and Psychopathology*, vol. 17, no. 3, pp. 577–597, 2005.

[26] J. D. Schmahmann, D. L. Rosene, and D. N. Pandya, "Motor projections to the basis pontis in rhesus monkey," *Journal of Comparative Neurology*, vol. 478, no. 3, pp. 248–268, 2004.

[27] N. J. Minshew, K. Sung, B. L. Jones, and J. M. Furman, "Underdevelopment of the postural control system in autism," *Neurology*, vol. 63, no. 11, pp. 2056–2061, 2004.

[28] N. J. Rinehart, B. J. Tonge, J. L. Bradshaw, R. Iansek, P. G. Enticott, and J. McGinley, "Gait function in high-functioning autism and Asperger's disorder: evidence for basal-ganglia and cerebellar involvement?" *European Child and Adolescent Psychiatry*, vol. 15, no. 5, pp. 256–264, 2006.

[29] A. Qiu, M. Adler, D. Crocetti, M. I. Miller, and S. H. Mostofsky, "Basal ganglia shapes predict social, communication, and motor dysfunctions in boys with autism spectrum disorder," *Journal of the American Academy of Child and Adolescent Psychiatry*, vol. 49, no. 6, pp. 539–551, 2010.

[30] M. Hallett, M. K. Lebiedowska, S. L. Thomas, S. J. Stanhope, M. B. Denckla, and J. Rumsey, "Locomotion of autistic adults," *Archives of Neurology*, vol. 50, no. 12, pp. 1304–1308, 1993.

[31] D. A. Winter, "Kinematic and kinetic patterns in human gait: variability and compensating effects," *Human Movement Science*, vol. 3, no. 1-2, pp. 51–76, 1984.

[32] M. Shetreat-Klein, S. Shinnar, and I. Rapin, "Abnormalities of joint mobility and gait in children with autism spectrum disorders," *Brain & Development*, vol. 36, no. 2, pp. 91–96, 2014.

[33] M. J. Weiss, M. F. Moran, M. E. Parker, and J. T. Foley, "Gait analysis of teenagers and young adults diagnosed with autism and severe verbal communication disorders," *Frontiers in Integrative Neuroscience*, vol. 7, article 33, 2013.

[34] V. L. Chester and M. Calhoun, "Gait symmetry in children with autism," *Autism Research and Treatment*, vol. 2012, Article ID 576478, 5 pages, 2012.

[35] A. Nayate, B. J. Tonge, J. L. Bradshaw, J. L. McGinley, R. Iansek, and N. J. Rinehart, "Differentiation of high-functioning autism and asperger's disorder based on neuromotor behaviour," *Journal of Autism and Developmental Disorders*, vol. 42, no. 5, pp. 707–717, 2012.

[36] M. Calhoun, M. Longworth, and V. L. Chester, "Gait patterns in children with autism," *Clinical Biomechanics*, vol. 26, no. 2, pp. 200–206, 2011.

[37] M. Nobile, P. Perego, L. Piccinini et al., "Further evidence of complex motor dysfunction in drug naïve children with autism using automatic motion analysis of gait," *Autism*, vol. 15, no. 3, pp. 263–283, 2011.

[38] N. J. Rinehart, B. J. Tonge, R. Iansek et al., "Gait function in newly diagnosed children with autism: cerebellar and basal ganglia related motor disorder," *Developmental Medicine and Child Neurology*, vol. 48, no. 10, pp. 819–824, 2006.

[39] S. Vernazza-Martin, N. Martin, A. Vernazza et al., "Goal directed locomotion and balance control in autistic children," *Journal of Autism and Developmental Disorders*, vol. 35, no. 1, pp. 91–102, 2005.

[40] D. Ambrosini, E. Courchesne, and K. Kaufman, "Motion analysis of patients with infantile autism," *Gait & Posture*, vol. 7, no. 2, p. 188, 1998.

[41] J. A. Vilensky, A. R. Damasio, and R. G. Maurer, "Gait disturbances in patients with autistic behavior. A preliminary study," *Archives of Neurology*, vol. 38, no. 10, pp. 646–649, 1981.

[42] C. P. Whyatt and C. M. Craig, "Motor skills in children aged 7-10 years, diagnosed with autism spectrum disorder," *Journal of Autism and Developmental Disorders*, vol. 42, no. 9, pp. 1799–1809, 2012.

[43] E. B. Torres, M. Brincker, R. W. Isenhower et al., "Autism: the micro-movement perspective," *Frontiers in Integrative Neuroscience*, vol. 7, article 32, 2013.

[44] N. J. Rinehart, J. L. Bradshaw, A. V. Brereton, and B. J. Tonge, "A clinical and neurobehavioural review of high-functioning autism and Asperger's disorder," *Australian & New Zealand Journal of Psychiatry*, vol. 36, no. 6, pp. 762–770, 2002.

[45] J. D. Schmahmann, *The Cerebellum and Cognition*, Academic Press, San Diego, Calif, USA, 1997.

[46] N. J. Minshew and G. Goldstein, "Autism as a disorder of complex information processing," *Mental Retardation and Developmental Disabilities Research Reviews*, vol. 4, no. 2, pp. 129–136, 1998.

[47] M. Bishop, D. Brunt, N. Pathare, and B. Patel, "The effect of velocity on the strategies used during gait termination," *Gait & Posture*, vol. 20, no. 2, pp. 134–139, 2004.

[48] M. U. McCulloch, D. Brunt, and D. Vander Linden, "The effect of foot orthotics and gait velocity on lower limb kinematics and temporal events of stance," *Journal of Orthopaedic & Sports Physical Therapy*, vol. 17, no. 1, pp. 2–10, 1993.

[49] R. D. Crowinshield, R. A. Brand, and R. C. Johnston, "The effects of walking velocity and age on hip kinematics and kinetics," *Clinical Orthopaedics and Related Research*, vol. 132, pp. 140–144, 1978.

[50] D. W. McCandless, G. K. Feussner, W. D. Lust, and J. V. Passonneau, "Metabolite levels in brain following experimental seizures: the effects of isoniazid and sodium valproate in cerebellar and cerebral cortical layers," *Journal of Neurochemistry*, vol. 32, no. 3, pp. 755–760, 1979.

[51] K. Sheehan and J. Gormley, "Gait and increased body weight (potential implications for musculoskeletal disease)," *Physical Therapy Reviews*, vol. 17, no. 2, pp. 91–98, 2012.

[52] Y. Roke, P. N. Van Harten, J. K. Buitelaar et al., "Bone mineral density in male adolescents with autism spectrum disorders and disruptive behavior disorder with or without antipsychotic treatment," *European Journal of Endocrinology*, vol. 167, no. 6, pp. 855–863, 2012.

11

Minor Physical Anomalies in Adults with Autism Spectrum Disorder and Healthy Controls

Irina Manouilenko,[1,2] Jonna M. Eriksson,[1] Mats B. Humble,[3] and Susanne Bejerot[1]

[1] *Department of Clinical Neuroscience, Karolinska Institutet, Stockholm, Sweden*
[2] *Järva Psychiatric Outpatient Clinic, Rinkebysvängen 70A, 4tr, 163 74 Spånga, Sweden*
[3] *School of Health and Medical Sciences, Psychiatric Research Center, Örebro University, Örebro, Sweden*

Correspondence should be addressed to Irina Manouilenko; irina.manouilenko@ki.se

Academic Editor: Klaus-Peter Ossenkopp

Minor Physical Anomalies (MPAs) are subtle abnormalities of the head, face, and limbs, without significant cosmetic or functional impact to the individual. They are assumed to represent external markers of developmental deviations during foetal life. MPAs have been suggested to indicate severity in mental illness and constitute external markers for atypical brain development. Higher frequencies of MPAs can be found in children with autism. The aims of the present study were to examine the prevalence and patterns of MPAs in adults with autism spectrum disorder (ASD) and to investigate whether MPAs are associated with symptom severity and overall functioning. Fifty adults with ASD and intelligence within the normal range and 53 healthy controls were examined with the Waldrop scale, an instrument for assessing MPAs. Face and feet were photographed enabling blinded assessment. Significant differences between the ASD and the control group were found on the MPA total scores, and also in the craniofacial region scores. Moreover, the shape of the ears was associated with autistic traits, in the ASD group. High MPA total scores were associated with poorer functioning. The findings suggest a link between MPAs, autistic traits, and level of functioning. Assessment of MPAs may assist in the diagnostic procedure of psychiatric disorders.

1. Introduction

Autism spectrum disorder (ASD) is a group of neurodevelopmental disorders, characterized by atypical development, impairment in reciprocal social interaction and communication, and restricted repetitive and stereotyped patterns of behavior, interests, and activities. ASD includes autistic disorder, Asperger disorder, and pervasive developmental disorders not otherwise specified [1] and occurs in nearly 2% of the population [2]. Males are more affected than females with a sex ratio at about 4 : 1 [3]. ASD is remarkably heterogeneous and includes people with intelligence levels ranging from severe intellectual disability to very high IQ. Since no specific biological markers for ASD have been identified, the diagnosis of ASD is based on expert evaluation of cognitive, language, social, and emotional functioning along with developmental progress. In twin studies a strong evidence of genetic etiology of ASD has been shown [4–6]. Several prenatal and perinatal risk factors have also been suggested [7–10]. Furthermore, autistic traits can be measured at subthreshold level in the normal population, suggesting that the autism phenotype lies along a continuum of quantitative traits [11].

Minor Physical Anomalies (MPAs) are subtle morphological abnormalities of the craniofacial region and limbs, without significant cosmetic or functional impact to the individual. They are assumed to represent markers of deviant morphogenesis during the first or early second trimester of pregnancy and to have ectodermal embryonic origins in common with the developing brain. Genetic factors and prenatal events, such as maternal bleeding with subsequent fetal hypoxia, gestational diabetes, medication use, or toxemia, may contribute to MPAs [12, 13].

MPAs include minor malformations and phenogenetic variants that are stable over time [14]. *Minor malformations* are qualitative defects of embryogenesis arising during organogenesis and are true deviations from normal. *Phenogenetic variants* are quantitative defects arising after organogenesis representing equivalents of normal anthropometric variants [15, 16].

Higher frequencies of MPAs can be found in patients with schizophrenia, bipolar disorder, ADHD, and Tourette syndrome [17–21]. In addition, MPAs are suggested to be indicators of severity of the illness [22]. Taken together, MPAs are markers for aberrant development and may be used as markers of risk for certain psychiatric disorders [23, 24].

In studies of children with ASD, MPAs are suggested to be the external markers for atypical brain development and excessive MPAs have been found when compared to neurotypically developing children [25–28]. Hitherto, only one study has examined MPAs in adults with ASD and normal intelligence. In this study interorbital and interlens distances were measured using MRI scan and showed that hypotelorism (i.e., short interorbital length) may be present in a subgroup of individuals with autism and IQ within the normal lower range [29]. However, the use of advanced methodology such as MRI for this purpose seems inappropriate for clinical practice. Accordingly, MPAs other than orbital have not been reported regarding this group. Thus it seems relevant to investigate whether MPAs contribute to the assessment of adults with ASD and normal intelligence.

The aim of the present study was (1) to investigate the prevalence, (2) to investigate the topographical pattern of MPAs in adults with ASD in comparison to neurotypical controls, and (3) to investigate whether MPAs may support diagnosis of ASD and serve as markers of impairment.

We hypothesized that (1) adults with ASD would show higher rates of MPAs than neurotypical controls; (2) the pattern of topographical distribution of MPAs would differentiate individuals with ASD from neurotypical controls; and (3) the rates of MPAs would correlate with severity of symptoms and overall functioning.

2. Methods

2.1. Participants. A total of 103 Swedish adults, including 50 adults with ASD (24 females and 26 males; mean age 30 years; range 20–47) and 53 neurotypical controls (25 females and 28 males; mean age 30.4 years; range 20–46), participated in the study (Table 1). These subjects have also been included in a study on gender coherence [30].

Inclusion criteria for all participants were age between 18 and 50 years and Caucasian descent. Exclusion criteria were any neurological or genetic syndrome, diagnosed malformations, schizophrenia spectrum disorders, intellectual disability, or having attended special education in primary or secondary school. Normal intelligence was assumed by mainstream schooling and patient records. Additional exclusion criteria for the control group were ASD in a first-degree family member, current psychiatric or personality disorder, and use of psychotropic medication.

Table 1: Sample characteristics of the ASD group and the neurotypical controls.

	ASD (n = 50)	Controls (n = 53)
Age, years, mean (SD)	30.0 (7.3)	30.4 (7.5)
Sex, males, n (%)	26 (52)	28 (53)
Education, n		
≤9 years	8	1
≤12 years	18	7
University level	24	45
Cohabiting with partner, n (%)	9 (18)	26 (49)
Having children, n (%)	8 (16)	11 (21)
The Autism Spectrum Quotient, mean (SD)	29.4 (9.8)	11.2 (4.9)
GAF, past month, mean (SD)		
Symptoms	55.6 (6.5)	97.5 (4.4)
Functioning	55.0 (9.2)	97.6 (4.2)
ADOS, mean (SD)		
Soc-Com	8.3 (2.9)	—
Total	10.4 (3.3)	—

ASD: autism spectrum disorder; GAF: Global Assessment of Functioning; ADOS: Autism Diagnostic Observation Schedule; Soc-Com: combined social interaction-communication score.

2.2. Procedures and Materials. Participants were recruited between November 2006 and October 2010. Individuals with ASD and of normal intelligence were recruited through an outpatient tertiary psychiatric unit, a community-based center for adults with ASD, and also a website for people with ASD. All participants with ASD had been previously diagnosed according to the rigorous and extensive standard procedure for diagnosing ASD in Sweden at the time of the study (approximately 18 hours of assessments comprising diagnostic interviews, rating scales, neuropsychological assessments, and structured interviews with parents of the subjects) [31]. The diagnosis was further confirmed with Autism Diagnostic Observation Schedule module 4 (ADOS) [32], patient records, and a clinical interview performed by a psychiatrist experienced in ASD.

Neurotypical controls were recruited through advertisements towards a nonprofit keep-fit organization, university campuses, student residences, private companies, dentists and vaccination centers, employment agencies, and word of mouth. They were enrolled after the ASD group in order to be matched for sex and age.

Autistic traits were assessed in all participants with the Autism Spectrum Quotient (AQ): a self-report questionnaire that measures autistic traits in individuals with normal intelligence. The AQ consists of 50 items that cover abilities within social skills, communication, attention switching, attention to details, and imagination. The discriminant validity and screening properties are suggested to be satisfactory [11]. In the ASD group, the assessment of autistic traits also comprised observed traits as measured by the ADOS. The ADOS score consists of the combined communication and social interaction subscores.

Overall impairment in psychological, social, and occupational functioning was assessed with the DSM-IV Global Assessment of Functioning (GAF), shown to have good psychometric properties [1, 33]. The GAF score is a combined measure of symptom severity and level of functioning and ranges from 1 to 100. Low scores indicate severe symptoms and/or low functioning. In order to differentiate these two dimensions, severity of symptoms (GAF symptoms) and social, occupational, or school functioning (GAF-functioning) were assessed separately [34].

The study was approved by the Regional Ethical Review Board in Stockholm and written informed consents were obtained from all subjects.

2.3. Assessment of Minor Physical Anomalies (MPAs). The assessment of MPAs included being photographed in a standardized manner, standing against a white wall in an examination room, which was used throughout the study. The digital photos included face close-up photos, front and in profile. Feet were photographed from beneath and from above. The participants were requested to wear a shower hat to hide the hair, but not the ears. Excessive makeup and jewelry were removed before photographing.

The Waldrop Physical Anomaly Scale [35], consisting of 16 items with total scores ranging from 0 to 25 (total MPA score), was used to assess MPAs. Head circumference was measured with a measuring tape and then categorized by reference to population based normative values (as ≥1.5 and >2 standard deviations, resp.). All other items were assessed according to descriptive anchor points, scored 0-1 or 0–2, relating to severity. Eight items (epicanthus, hypertelorism (i.e., widely spaced eyes), low-settled ears, adherent ear lobe, malformed ears, relative toe lengths, partial syndactylia, and sandal gap between first and second toe) were assessed from photographs of face (front and in profile) and feet by two psychiatrists (Irina Manouilenko, Mats B. Humble), independently and blinded to diagnosis. If their ratings on any item differed, they reached a consensus after discussion. MPAs of mouth and hands and the item "fine electric hair" were examined by two unblinded assessors (Susanne Bejerot, Jonna M. Eriksson).

According to the Waldrop Physical Anomaly Scale, the MPAs are divided into six subscales that reflect anatomic body areas: head, eyes, ears, mouth, hands, and feet. These MPAs are further classified as either minor malformation or phenogenetic variants [16] (Table 2). In addition to the total MPA score, the craniofacial index (CF-MPA) was calculated from scores of the head, eyes, ears, and mouth subscales and the periphery index (P-MPA) from scores of hands and feet subscales.

2.4. Statistics. Since the MPA data was not normally distributed, comparisons between the ASD group and controls were made using Mann-Whitney U test for continuous variables and Pearson Chi-square distribution for categorical variables. Student's t-test was used for analyses of normally distributed variables. Differences between groups on the MPA total scores, the subscores from the six body areas, and the CF-MPA and P-MPA were analyzed with Mann-Whitney U test. Missing data, assumed to be random, were present for five participants with ASD and one of the controls.

Since total MPA scores of 5 or greater have been associated with various psychiatric conditions [18, 26, 36], the participants were split into a low-MPA group, defined as having a total MPA score below 5, and the high-MPA group, defined as having a total MPA score of 5 or greater. For both groups bivariate correlations were performed to examine the relationships between MPAs, autistic traits (AQ and ADOS), and severity of symptoms (GAF-s) and overall functioning (GAF-f). Due to skewness of AQ and MPA distributions, Spearman's rank correlation test was used.

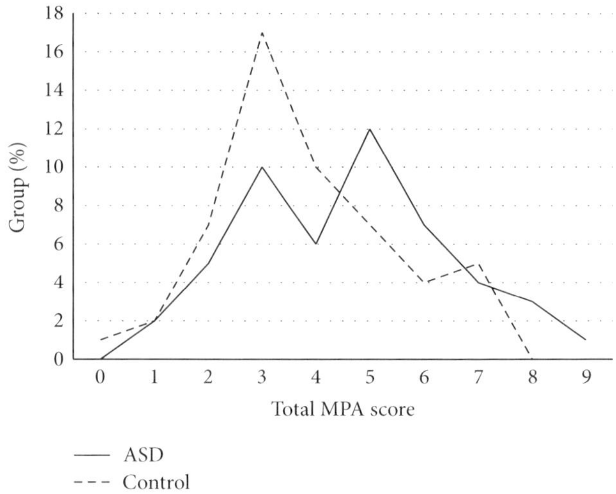

Figure 1: Frequency distribution of total Minor Physical Anomalies (MPA) scores in 50 individuals with autism spectrum disorder and 53 neurotypical controls.

3. Results

Comparisons between the ASD and control groups revealed, as expected, large differences in the three symptom-related measures tested in both groups (Table 1).

The total MPA scores ranged from 1 to 9 (median = 5) in the ASD group and from 0 to 7 (median = 3) in the neurotypical control group; thus all participants in the ASD group displayed at least one MPA. The distribution of the total MPA score in the ASD group was bimodal; the lower mode overlapped with the distribution of the controls whereas the higher mode only appeared in the ASD group (Figure 1).

In the ASD group, the CF-MPA index, head subscale score, and MPA total score were significantly higher in comparison with the control group (Table 3). When analysed by gender, differences only reached significance for the head subscale score, which was higher in the ASD women than in control women ($U = 191$, $P = 0.02$, $r = -0.33$).

When the sample was split into low- and high-MPA groups, 60 individuals were allocated to the low-MPA category and 43 individuals into the high-MPA group (14 women with ASD and 10 female controls and 13 men with ASD

TABLE 2: Comparison of MPA rates between the ASD and neurotypical control groups.

Minor Physical Anomalies	Score	MM/PV	ASD n (%)	NC n (%)	χ^2 (df)	P value
Head						
Head circumference		PV				
1.5–2 SD	1		23 (46)	27 (50.9)		
>2 SD	2		8 (16)	2 (3.8)		
Fine electric hair		MM			6.6 (2)	0.037*
Hair soon awry	1		12 (24)	4 (7.5)		
Hair unmanageable	2		1 (2)	—		
Eyes						
Epicanthus (the point of union where upper and lower lids join the nose)		PV				
Partly covered	1		8 (16)	7 (13.2)		
Deeply covered	2		1 (2)	2 (3.8)		
Intercanthal distance/hypertelorism (approximate distance between tear ducts)		PV				
Moderate	1		22 (44)	19 (35.8)		
Extensive	2		1 (2)	1 (1.9)		
Ears						
Seating ears—bottom of ears in line with		PV				
Area between mouth and nose	1		8 (16)	9 (17)		
Mouth (or lower)	2		—	—		
Adherent ear lobes		MM				
Lower edges of ears extend						
Moderate/Straight back toward rear of neck	1		16 (32)	14 (26.4)		
Extensive/Upward and back toward crown of head	2		18 (36)	14 (26.4)		
Asymmetrical ears	1	PV	10 (20)	3 (5.7)		
Malformed ears	1	MM	5 (10)	4 (7.5)		
Mouth						
High/steepled palate		PV				
Roof of mouth:						
Flat and narrow at the top	1		12 (24)	13 (24.5)		
Definitely steepled	2		—	3 (5.7)		
Furrowed tongue (one with deep ridges)	1	MM	7 (14)	4 (7.5)		
Hands						
Curved fifth finger:		MM			5.5 (1)	0.019[a]
Moderately curved	1		2 (4)	10 (18.9)		
Extensively curved	2		—	—		
Single transverse palmar crease	1	MM	7 (14)	—	78.0 (1)	0.005*
Fifth-finger stubbing	1	MM	1 (2)			
Feet						
Third toe:						
Equal in length to second	1	PV	2 (4)	—		
Definitely longer than second	2		—	—		
Partial syndactylia of second and third toes	1	MM	—	3 (5.7)		
Big gap between first and second toes	1	PV	36 (72)	40 (75.5)		

ASD: autism spectrum disorder; NC: neurotypical controls; MM: minor malformation; PV: phenogenetic variants; [a]Higher scores in controls; level of significance $^*P < 0.05$. Items are assessed according to descriptive anchor points (scored 0-1 or 0–2) depending on severity and "0" is defined as "no deviation".

TABLE 3: Comparison of MPA scores by Mann-Whitney U test.

	ASD (n = 50)		Neurotypical controls (n = 53)		U (z)	P	r
	Mean (SD)	Median	Mean (SD)	Median			
CF-MPA	3.64 (1.97)	4	2.69 (1.51)	3	990 (−2.2)	0.025	0.22
Head	1.06 (0.89)	1	0.66 (0.67)	1	1001 (−2.3)	0.022	0.23
Eyes	0.68 (0.77)	1	0.61 (0.82)	0	1213 (−0.6)	n.s.	
Ears	1.52 (1.27)	1.5	1.09 (1.07)	1	1069 (−1.8)	n.s.	
Mouth	0.38 (0.60)	0	0.43 (0.60)	0	1255 (−0.6)	n.s.	
P-MPA	0.95 (0.69)	1	1.0 (0.65)	1	1262 (−0.5)	n.s.	
Hands	0.19 (0.43)	0	0.19 (0.40)	0	1314 (−0.1)	n.s.	
Feet	0.76 (0.52)	1	0.81 (0.48)	1	1259 (−0.5)	n.s.	
Total MPA	**4.59 (1.91)**	**5**	**3.79 (1.67)**	**3**	**1010 (−2.1)**	**0.034**	**0.21**

ASD: autism spectrum disorder; MPA: Minor Physical Anomalies; CF-MPA: craniofacial MPAs including MPAs in head, eyes, ears, and mouth; P-MPA: periphery index including MPAs in hands and feet; U (z): Mann-Whitney U; r: Pearson effect size.

and 6 male controls). Significantly more ASD participants compared with the controls showed a high rate of MPAs (P = 0.014). The pattern of topographical distribution over the six body regions only showed differences between the groups in the head region (Figure 2). The single transverse palmar crease only appeared in the ASD group (P = 0.005); conversely the curved fifth finger was assessed as more common among the controls (P = 0.021), thus making the hand MPA score seemingly normal.

Testing the hypothesis that MPAs are related to functioning and autistic traits, the correlations between the MPA measures, that is, the total MPA score, CF-MPA index, and the MPA subscales, and GAF, AQ, and ADOS scores were calculated (Table 4). In the control group a pattern of correlation could only be observed between head MPA subscale and GAF-s in the high-MPA group (data not shown); thus, all other correlations presented here were derived from the ASD group alone.

In the high-MPA group, the number of MPAs correlated moderately negatively with overall functioning (GAF-f) and with severity of psychiatric symptoms (GAF-s). In the low-MPA group, moderate correlations could be observed between total MPA scores and both self-reported and observed autistic traits. In the entire ASD group, number of ear MPAs and CF-MPAs correlated weakly with the ADOS score and, negatively, with GAF-functioning. When the ASD group was analyzed for women and men separately, the above correlations could only be observed in the ASD men (Table 4). Amongst the ASD participants in the high- versus low-MPA groups no significant differences appeared in the AQ, ADOS, or GAF score. However, numerically the high-MPA group was assessed with more autistic traits according to AQ median (quartiles) scores (33 [27, 37] versus 29.0 [19, 36]) and slightly lower functioning (data not shown) compared with the low-MPA group.

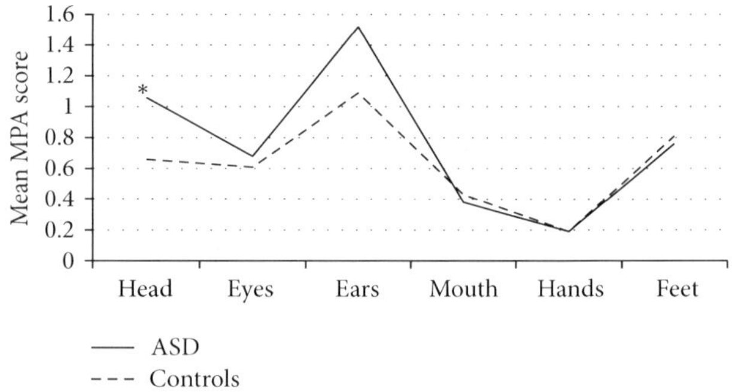

FIGURE 2: Topographical distributions of MPAs in ASD and controls. The graph shows the mean MPA score distributed on each of the six body regions in ASD and neurotypical controls, respectively.

4. Discussion

Adults with ASD and with intelligence within the normal range showed higher rates of MPAs compared with neurotypical controls. Differences between the groups were mostly found in the craniofacial region and in the hand. Higher rates of MPAs in the ASD participants were associated with somewhat lower level of functioning. Our findings are in line with earlier reports on children with ASD showing high rates of MPAs [26, 28] as well as correlations between facial phenotypes and clinical and behavioral characteristics [37]. For measuring MPAs we used the Waldrop Physical Anomaly Scale [35] with items originally developed in the midsixties for identifying children with schizophrenia. Plausibly if these children were to be assessed today, they would more likely be diagnosed with ASD.

Early in foetal morphogenesis, the development of structures in the craniofacial region occurs simultaneously with central structures of the brain implicated in the pathogenesis of, for example, ASD [38–40]. Possibly, in analogy with schizophrenia, early cerebrocraniofacial dysmorphogenesis reflects an early stage of pathogenesis that occurs before behavioral manifestations [41]. The nonspecificity of MPAs is comparable with the nonspecificity of the genetics implicated in schizophrenia, ADHD, ASD, and bipolar disorder [42] and supports the idea of biological markers transgressing the boundaries of categorical diagnoses [43]. The potential specificity of the MPAs, possibly distinguishing these disorders, has not been fully explored. Some MPAs were reported to

TABLE 4: Correlations between MPA total, ear MPA, CF-MPA, AQ, and GAF scores for the ASD group, by MPA level (high or low) and gender.

ASD individuals	n (%)		Ear index (ear MPA)	Craniofacial index (CF-MPA)	Total MPA
Low-MPA (total MPA < 5)	23 (46)	AQ	0.16	0.39	0.46*
		GAF-s	−0.04	−0.04	−0.05
		GAF-f	−0.29	−0.41	−0.14
		ADOS	0.30	0.56**	0.37
High-MPA (total MPA > 5)	27 (54)	AQ	0.10	−0.20	−0.08
		GAF-s	−0.25	−0.54**	−0.57**
		GAF-f	−0.30	−0.50**	−0.52**
		ADOS	0.43*	0.30	0.25
All	50 (100)	AQ	0.23	0.20	0.23
		GAF-s	−0.06	−0.12	−0.13
		GAF-f	−0.30*	−0.36*	−0.31*
		ADOS	0.30*	0.30*	0.23
Men	26 (52)	AQ	0.42*	0.38	0.35
		GAF-s	−0.002	−0.012	−0.05
		GAF-f	−0.40	−0.48*	−0.49*
		ADOS	0.49*	0.53**	0.50**
Women	24 (48)	AQ	0.070	0.031	0.12
		GAF-s	−.052	−0.18	−0.14
		GAF-f	−0.19	−0.20	−0.093
		ADOS	0.14	0.12	0.013

ASD: autism spectrum disorder; MPA: Minor Physical Anomalies; GAF-s: Global Assessment of Functioning-symptoms; GAF-f: Global Assessment of Functioning-functioning; AQ: the Autism Spectrum Quotient; ADOS: ADOS-4 social interaction-communications score. Significances of correlations (Spearman's rank correlation test) are denoted by $^{*}P < 0.05$, $^{**}P < 0.01$.

be common in bipolar disorder [17] while they were rare amongst our participants with ASD. In order to improve the understanding of the pathophysiological mechanisms linked to MPAs, future studies should include genetic information related to these disorders.

Self-report questionnaires in addition to clinical assessment of behavioral characteristics are widely used in diagnostic procedures. However, the mentalizing deficits that characterize ASD may impair the ability for self-assessment of autistic traits, especially in those with severe ASD. Additional examination of objective morphological markers may in such cases support biological underpinnings for the dysfunction. Especially MPAs in the ear region were associated with more observable autistic traits according to the ADOS in the high-MPA group. Both the craniofacial index and the ear index were associated with higher ADOS scores and lower functioning in the entire ASD group. External ear malformations, such as low-seated ears, adherent ear lobes, and posteriorly rotated ears, have been associated with autism in several studies [12, 25, 27, 44]. Also, a possible link between external and middle ear anomalies has been proposed in children with autism [45]. Probably, the developmental anomalies of ears occur during neural tube formation in the first month of gestation —a time point when the developing brain is particularly sensitive to various teratogenic factors [46, 47]. Consequently, assessment of ear MPAs is suggested to be of interest in diagnosis and in evaluation of functional impairment in adults with ASD. However, in contrast to previous studies of children, in which minor anomalies of the ears discriminated effectively children with autism (mostly with intellectual disability) from typically developing children [13, 25, 27], this was not the case in the present study. Plausibly, the difference is due to the normal intellectual functioning of the current participants. Nevertheless, it is of interest that ASD, also within the normal intelligence range, is associated with Minor Physical Anomalies.

Notably, a substantial subgroup of our neurotypical controls exhibited MPAs, but mostly in the lower range and comparable to scores shown in other neurotypical control groups [18, 26, 28, 48, 49]. Moreover, whereas the ASD group was almost equally distributed between having high and low total MPA scores, most of the controls (70%) fell into the low-MPA group.

4.1. MPAs as a Method to Differentiate ASD from Neurotypical Controls. Only two out of the 16 MPAs measured with Waldrop Physical Anomaly Scale differed between ASD and controls, the minor malformations "fine electric hair" and "single palmar crease." Although the presence of a single palmar crease is a straightforward finding, the assessment of fine electrical hair tends to be subjective and should be interpreted with caution [22, 50].

The palmar flexion creases develop during early fetal life and arise due to interaction between genetic and environmental factors, as well as movement of the developing hand in the fetus [51]. Since the flexion movements of the hands are closely associated with joint formation and muscular function, deviations in development of the palmar creases reflect either anatomical or functional alterations of the developing hand [52, 53]. In consequence, alterations may indicate intrauterine insults early in pregnancy and may be of predictive value for developmental disorders or genetic syndromes [54]. However, as alterations in palmar creases were observed in only 14% of the individuals with ASD, a single palmar crease alone is a poor predictor.

Another possibility to differentiate the groups appeared when MPAs were combined into subscales by body region. Thus the head subscale differed between the ASD group and neurotypical controls, but none of the other five body region subscales (Figure 2, Table 3). In a study on children with ASD, increased head circumference was associated with a more severe social impairment [55]. This relationship was partially supported by our findings showing a positive association between MPAs in the craniofacial region and poorer functioning (Table 4).

4.2. Limitations. This study has several important limitations. First, the sample was relatively small which limits the power and increases risk for type II errors. On the other hand, we did not correct P values for multiple comparisons, increasing the risk for type I error. Thus, when interpreting the statistical significance of the results, these two factors should be taken into consideration. Second, some of the MPAs were not blindly assessed. However, the area where we found most associations with autistic traits and functioning, that is, the ears, was blindly assessed. The assessment from photographs by blinded psychiatrists is a strength and to our knowledge not previously utilized for this kind of assessment. Earlier studies have mostly been unblinded in the sense that people with ASD have visible social impairments that may reveal their diagnosis. Also, it could be stressful for people with ASD to undress and be examined by an unfamiliar clinician, which is avoided by using photographs. Hypothetically it is conceivable that different "subtypes" composition of the ASD sample may have somewhat different MPA profiles and different course, outcome, and, respectively, global functioning. Our participants were not "subtyped" beyond being of normal intelligence, which is another caveat of this study. But given the relatively small sample size, further subtyping was considered inappropriate. Finally, in this study only Caucasians were included because hair and shape of eyes and ears often vary between different ethnic groups. Thus, the present findings cannot be generalized to other ethnic groups. Future research should preferably include larger samples and include photographs of all body regions to enable blinded assessments.

5. Conclusions and Clinical Implication

In this study links were shown between MPAs, autistic traits, and level of functioning in adults with ASD. MPAs of head, ears, eyes, mouths, and hands can easily be assessed in the clinician's office. Information on MPAs may provide important information for the diagnostic process. In the current study, particularly the shape and seating of the ears are suggested to be associated with autistic traits. An association between MPA scores and severity of impairments was found. Thus more MPAs may suggest need for more supportive interventions. MPAs are suggested to serve as potential biological risk markers for psychiatric disorders, and careful examination of morphological features can be helpful in the estimation of psychological, social, and occupational functioning in psychiatric patients.

Authors' Contribution

Susanne Bejerot and Jonna M. Eriksson conducted the research interviews and examined and photographed the participants. Irina Manouilenko and Mats B. Humble rated the MPAs from the photographs. Irina Manouilenko drafted the paper and Irina Manouilenko, Jonna M. Eriksson, and Mats B. Humble performed the statistical analysis. All authors participated in writing the final paper.

Acknowledgments

This study was founded through the Swedish Medical Research Council (Grant no. 523-2011-3646), the St. Göran Foundation, the Swedish Society of Medicine, and Praktikertjänst Psykiatri AB. The authors want to express their gratitude towards all participants who agreed to sign up for the study.

References

[1] American Psychiatric Association, *Diagnostic and Statistical Manual of Mental Disorders*, American Psychiatric Association, Washington, DC, USA, 4th edition, 1994.

[2] M. Wingate, B. Mulvihill, R. S. Kirby, S. Pettygrove, C. Cunniff, and F. Meaney, "Prevalence of autism spectrum disorders—autism and developmental disabilities monitoring network, 14 sites, United States, 2008," *Morbidity and Mortality Weekly Report*, vol. 61, no. 3, pp. 1–19, 2012.

[3] E. Fombonne, "Epidemiology of pervasive developmental disorders," *Pediatric Research*, vol. 65, no. 6, pp. 591–598, 2009.

[4] A. Ronald, F. Happé, P. Bolton et al., "Genetic heterogeneity between the three components of the autism spectrum: a twin study," *Journal of the American Academy of Child and Adolescent Psychiatry*, vol. 45, no. 6, pp. 691–699, 2006.

[5] A. Bailey, A. Le Couteur, I. Gottesman et al., "Autism as a strongly genetic disorder: evidence from a British twin study," *Psychological Medicine*, vol. 25, no. 1, pp. 63–77, 1995.

[6] P. Lichtenstein, E. Carlström, M. Råstam, C. Gillberg, and H. Anckarsäter, "The genetics of autism spectrum disorders and related neuropsychiatric disorders in childhood," *The American Journal of Psychiatry*, vol. 167, no. 11, pp. 1357–1363, 2010.

[7] C. Gillberg, "Maternal age and infantile autism," *Journal of Autism and Developmental Disorders*, vol. 10, no. 3, pp. 293–297, 1980.

[8] K. M. Abel, C. Dalman, A. C. Svensson et al., "Deviance in fetal growth and risk of autism spectrum disorder," *American Journal of Psychiatry*, vol. 170, no. 4, pp. 391–398, 2013.

[9] H. O. Atladóttir, P. Thorsen, L. Østergaard et al., "Maternal infection requiring hospitalization during pregnancy and autism spectrum disorders," *Journal of Autism and Developmental Disorders*, vol. 40, no. 12, pp. 1423–1430, 2010.

[10] H. Gardener, D. Spiegelman, and S. L. Buka, "Prenatal risk factors for autism: comprehensive meta-analysis," *The British Journal of Psychiatry*, vol. 195, no. 1, pp. 7–14, 2009.

[11] S. Baron-Cohen, S. Wheelwright, R. Skinner, J. Martin, and E. Clubley, "The autism-spectrum quotient (AQ): evidence from asperger syndrome/high-functioning autism, males and females, scientists and mathematicians," *Journal of Autism and Developmental Disorders*, vol. 31, no. 1, pp. 5–17, 2001.

[12] K. Strömland, V. Nordin, M. Miller, B. Akerström, and C. Gillberg, "Autism in thalidomide embryopathy: a population study," *Developmental Medicine and Child Neurology*, vol. 36, no. 4, pp. 351–356, 1994.

[13] M. Campbell, B. Geller, A. M. Small, T. A. Petti, and S. H. Ferris, "Minor physical anomalies in young psychotic children," *The American Journal of Psychiatry*, vol. 135, no. 5, pp. 573–575, 1978.

[14] T. F. Mcneil and E. Cantor-Graae, "Minor physical anomalies and obstetric complications in schizophrenia," *The Australian and New Zealand Journal of Psychiatry*, vol. 34, supplement, pp. S65–S73, 2000.

[15] J. Spranger, K. Benirschke, J. G. Hall et al., "Errors of morphogenesis: concepts and terms recommendations of an international working group," *The Journal of Pediatrics*, vol. 100, no. 1, pp. 160–165, 1982.

[16] J. M. Opitz, "Heterogeneity and minor anomalies," *American Journal of Medical Genetics*, vol. 92, no. 5, pp. 373–375, 2000.

[17] V. Akabaliev, S. Sivkov, M. Mantarkov, and F. Ahmed-Popova, "Minor physical anomalies in patients with bipolar i disorder and normal controls," *Journal of Affective Disorders*, vol. 135, no. 1–3, pp. 193–200, 2011.

[18] M. Trixler, T. Tényi, G. Csábi, and R. Szabó, "Minor physical anomalies in schizophrenia and bipolar affective disorder," *Schizophrenia Research*, vol. 52, no. 3, pp. 195–201, 2001.

[19] G. Csábi, J. Gádoros, S. Jeges, E. Gyenge, M. Trixler, and T. Tényi, "Minor physical anomalies in Tourette syndrome," *European Journal of Psychiatry*, vol. 22, no. 3, pp. 173–180, 2008.

[20] B. Ismail, E. Cantor-Graae, and T. F. Mcneil, "Minor physical anomalies in schizophrenic patients and their siblings," *The American Journal of Psychiatry*, vol. 155, no. 12, pp. 1695–1702, 1998.

[21] M. Waldrop, R. Bell, B. Mclaughlin, and F. Halverson Jr., "New born minor physical anomalies predict short attention span, peer aggression, and impulsivity at age 3," *Science*, vol. 199, no. 4328, pp. 563–565, 1978.

[22] J. J. Mcgrath, J. van Os, C. Hoyos, P. B. Jones, I. Harvey, and R. M. Murray, "Minor physical anomalies in psychoses: associations with clinical and putative aetiological variables," *Schizophrenia Research*, vol. 18, no. 1, pp. 9–20, 1995.

[23] M. T. Compton and E. F. Walker, "Physical manifestations of neurodevelopmental disruption: are minor physical anomalies part of the syndrome of schizophrenia?" *Schizophrenia Bulletin*, vol. 35, no. 2, pp. 425–436, 2009.

[24] V. A. Mittal and E. F. Walker, "Minor physical anomalies and vulnerability in prodromal youth," *Schizophrenia Research*, vol. 129, no. 2-3, pp. 116–121, 2011.

[25] P. M. Rodier, S. E. Bryson, and J. P. Welch, "Minor malformations and physical measurements in autism: data from Nova Scotia," *Teratology*, vol. 55, no. 5, pp. 319–325, 1997.

[26] G. Tripi, S. Roux, T. Canziani, F. B. Brilhault, C. Barthélémy, and F. Canziani, "Minor physical anomalies in children with autism spectrum disorder," *Early Human Development*, vol. 84, no. 4, pp. 217–223, 2008.

[27] H. A. Walker, "Incidence of minor physical anomaly in autism," *Journal of Autism and Childhood Schizophrenia*, vol. 7, no. 2, pp. 165–176, 1977.

[28] H. Ozgen, G. S. Hellemann, R. K. Stellato et al., "Morphological features in children with autism spectrum disorders: a matched case—control study," *Journal of Autism and Developmental Disorders*, vol. 41, no. 1, pp. 23–31, 2011.

[29] A. Y. Hardan, M. S. Keshavan, S. Sreedhar, M. Vemulapalli, and N. J. Minshew, "An MRI study of minor physical anomalies in autism," *Journal of Autism and Developmental Disorders*, vol. 36, no. 5, pp. 607–611, 2006.

[30] S. Bejerot, J. M. Eriksson, S. Bonde, K. Carlström, M. B. Humble, and E. Eriksson, "The extreme male brain revisited: gender coherence in adults with autism spectrum disorder," *The British Journal of Psychiatry*, vol. 201, pp. 116–123, 2012.

[31] E. Rydén and S. Bejerot, "Autism spectrum disorders in an adult psychiatric population a naturalistic cross-sectional controlled study," *Clinical Neuropsychiatry*, vol. 5, no. 1, pp. 13–21, 2008.

[32] C. Lord, M. Rutter, P. Dilavore, and S. Risi, "Autism diagnostic observation schedule," ADOS Manual, Western Psychological Services, Los Angeles, Calif, USA, 2002.

[33] S. H. Jones, G. Thornicroft, M. Coffey, and G. Dunn, "A brief mental health outcome scale-reliability and validity of the Global Assessment of Functioning (GAF)," *The British Journal of Psychiatry*, vol. 166, no. 5, pp. 654–659, 1995.

[34] H. H. Goldman, A. E. Skodol, and T. R. Lave, "Revising axis V for DSM-IV: a review of measures of social functioning," *The American Journal of Psychiatry*, vol. 149, no. 9, pp. 1148–1156, 1992.

[35] M. F. Waldrop and J. D. Goering, "Hyperactivity and minor physical anomalies in elementary school children," *American Journal of Orthopsychiatry*, vol. 41, no. 4, pp. 602–607, 1971.

[36] J. D. Guy, L. V. Majorski, C. J. Wallace, and M. P. Guy, "The incidence of minor physical anomalies in adult male schizophrenics," *Schizophrenia Bulletin*, vol. 9, no. 4, pp. 571–582, 1983.

[37] K. Aldridge, I. D. George, K. K. Cole et al., "Facial phenotypes in subgroups of prepubertal boys with autism spectrum disorders are correlated with clinical phenotypes," *Molecular Autism*, vol. 2, no. 1, article 15, 2011.

[38] M. M. Haznedar, M. S. Buchsbaum, E. A. Hazlett, E. M. Licalzi, C. Cartwright, and E. Hollander, "Volumetric analysis and three-dimensional glucose metabolic mapping of the striatum

and thalamus in patients with autism spectrum disorders," *The American Journal of Psychiatry*, vol. 163, no. 7, pp. 1252–1263, 2006.

[39] L. D. Kwakye, J. H. Foss-Feig, C. J. Cascio, W. L. Stone, and M. T. Wallace, "Altered auditory and multisensory temporal processing in autism spectrum disorders," *Frontiers in Integrative Neuroscience*, vol. 4, article 129, 2011.

[40] U. Frith and C. D. Frith, "Development and neurophysiology of mentalizing," *Philosophical Transactions of the Royal Society B*, vol. 358, no. 1431, pp. 459–473, 2003.

[41] J. L. Waddington, A. Lane, C. Larkin, and E. O'Callaghan, "The neurodevelopmental basis of schizophrenia: clinical clues from cerebro-craniofacial dysmorphogenesis, and the roots of a lifetime trajectory of disease," *Biological Psychiatry*, vol. 46, no. 1, pp. 31–39, 1999.

[42] S. H. Lee, S. Ripke, B. M. Neale et al., "Identification of risk loci with shared effects on five major psychiatric disorders: a genome-wide analysis," *The Lancet*, vol. 381, no. 9875, pp. 1371–1379, 2013.

[43] B. N. Cuthbert and T. R. Insel, "Toward the future of psychiatric diagnosis: the seven pillars of RDoC," *BMC Medicine*, vol. 11, no. 126, 2013.

[44] A. L. Christianson, N. Chesler, and J. G. Kromberg, "Fetal valproate syndrome: clinical and neuro-developmental features in two sibling pairs," *Developmental Medicine and Child Neurology*, vol. 36, no. 4, pp. 361–369, 1994.

[45] M. M. Konstantareas and S. Homatidis, "Brief report: ear infections in autistic and normal children," *Journal of Autism and Developmental Disorders*, vol. 17, no. 4, pp. 585–594, 1987.

[46] S. Kösling, M. Omenzetter, and S. Bartel-Friedrich, "Congenital malformations of the external and middle ear," *European Journal of Radiology*, vol. 69, no. 2, pp. 269–279, 2009.

[47] M. T. Miller, "Thalidomide embryopathy: a model for the study of congenital incomitant horizontal strabismus," *Transactions of the American Ophthalmological Society*, vol. 89, pp. 623–674, 1991.

[48] M. F. Green, P. Satz, and C. Christenson, "Minor physical anomalies in schizophrenia patients, bipolar patients, and their siblings," *Schizophrenia Bulletin*, vol. 20, no. 3, pp. 433–440, 1994.

[49] S. T. Sivkov and V. H. Akabaliev, "Minor physical anomalies in mentally healthy subjects: internal consistency of the Waldrop Physical Anomaly Scale," *American Journal of Human Biology*, vol. 15, no. 1, pp. 61–67, 2003.

[50] J. P. Krouse and J. M. Kauffman, "Minor physical anomalies in exceptional children: a review and critique of research," *Journal of Abnormal Child Psychology*, vol. 10, no. 2, pp. 247–264, 1982.

[51] B. A. Schaumann and S. Kimura, "Palmar, plantar, and digital flexion creases: morphologic and clinical considerations," *Birth Defects Original Article Series*, vol. 27, no. 2, pp. 229–252, 1991.

[52] S. Kimura, "Embryologic development of flexion creases," *Birth Defects Original Article Series*, vol. 27, no. 2, pp. 113–129, 1991.

[53] G. A. Popich and D. W. Smith, "The genesis and significance of digital and palmar band creases: preliminary report," *The Journal of Pediatrics*, vol. 77, no. 6, pp. 1017–1023, 1970.

[54] J. S. Tay, "The genetics of palmar creases a study in the inheritance of liability estimated from the incidence among relatives," *Annals of Human Genetics*, vol. 42, no. 3, pp. 327–332, 1979.

[55] J. E. Lainhart, E. D. Bigler, M. Bocian et al., "Head circumference and height in autism: a study by the Collaborative Program of Excellence in Autism," *American Journal of Medical Genetics A*, vol. 140, no. 21, pp. 2257–2274, 2006.

12

Recognition of Emotion from Facial Expressions with Direct or Averted Eye Gaze and Varying Expression Intensities in Children with Autism Disorder and Typically Developing Children

Dina Tell,[1] Denise Davidson,[2] and Linda A. Camras[3]

[1] *Department of Health Promotion, Loyola University Chicago, Marcella Niehoff School of Nursing, 2160 S. First Avenue, Maywood, IL 60153, USA*
[2] *Department of Psychology, Loyola University Chicago, 1032 W. Sheridan Road, Chicago, IL 60660, USA*
[3] *Department of Psychology, DePaul University, 2219 N. Kenmore Avenue, Chicago, IL 60614, USA*

Correspondence should be addressed to Denise Davidson; ddavids@luc.edu

Academic Editor: Geraldine Dawson

Eye gaze direction and expression intensity effects on emotion recognition in children with autism disorder and typically developing children were investigated. Children with autism disorder and typically developing children identified happy and angry expressions equally well. Children with autism disorder, however, were less accurate in identifying fear expressions across intensities and eye gaze directions. Children with autism disorder rated expressions with direct eyes, and 50% expressions, as more intense than typically developing children. A trend was also found for sad expressions, as children with autism disorder were less accurate in recognizing sadness at 100% intensity with direct eyes than typically developing children. Although the present research showed that children with autism disorder are sensitive to eye gaze direction, impairments in the recognition of fear, and possibly sadness, exist. Furthermore, children with autism disorder and typically developing children perceive the intensity of emotional expressions differently.

1. Introduction

A number of studies have shown deficits in face, eye gaze, and emotion processing in individuals with autism disorder (see [1–5], for reviews). It has been suggested that the deficits found for face and eye processing may underlie impairments seen in the recognition of emotion by such individuals and subsequently may contribute to their social impairments [5]. Although some studies have shown that children and adults with autism disorder show reflexive orienting to eye gaze cues (see [4], for a review), other studies have shown that these individuals look less at the eye region of the face (e.g., [6, 7]), engage in less mutual eye gaze behavior (e.g., [8]), and show more deficits in gaze following behaviors (e.g., [9]) than neurotypical individuals.

A number of critical issues remain concerning the facilitative effects of eye gaze cues on emotion recognition in children with autism disorder as well as typically developing children. According to the "shared signal hypothesis" [10, 11], when eye gaze direction is combined with the intent communicated by an emotional expression, it should enhance the perception of that emotion. That is, direct eye gaze should facilitate the processing of facially communicated approach-oriented emotions (e.g., anger and joy), whereas averted eye gaze should facilitate the processing of facially communicated avoidance-oriented emotions (e.g., fear and sadness).

In support of the shared signal hypothesis, Adams and Kleck [10] found that happy and angry expressions were more quickly identified with direct than averted eye gaze, whereas fear and sadness were more quickly identified with averted than direct eye gaze, at least in neurotypical adults. Additional research with neurotypical adults has shown that angry faces are judged "more angry" with direct eye gaze than averted eye gaze (e.g., [12, 13]). Consistent with these findings, in a developmental study, Akechi and colleagues found that typically developing children were faster at detecting a facial expression accompanying a gaze direction with a congruent emotional expression: anger with a direct gaze and fear with an averted gaze [14].

In contrast, Akechi et al. [14] found that children with autism disorder did not show this pattern of responding: eye gaze direction did not affect their reaction times in detecting angry or fearful faces, although they were just as accurate as typically developing children. According to Akechi et al. [14], these results suggest that children with autism disorder are less likely than their typically developing peers to integrate communicative signals present in the eyes with their emotional quality. Akechi et al. [14] postulated that children with autism disorder may not spontaneously integrate eye gaze direction and its communicative intent, especially in connection to emotional expressions or within social contexts.

Still, although a number of studies have examined sensitivity to eye gaze cues in adolescents and adults with autism disorder (see [3, 4], for reviews) and emotion recognition in such individuals (see [1, 2, 5], for reviews), far fewer studies have examined the effects of eye gaze direction on emotion recognition in children with autism disorder. In the Akechi et al. [14] study, only two emotional expressions, anger and fear, were presented to children. A primary goal of the present research was to explore the effects of eye gaze direction on emotion recognition in children with autism disorder and typically developing children across a greater range of emotional expressions and expression intensities. In particular, children with autism disorder and typically developing children were shown happy, angry, sad, fearful, and neutral faces with direct or averted eye gaze directions at two expression intensities (50% and 100%).

One reason for presenting this range of emotions was because past studies have found that while emotion recognition in individuals with autism disorder may be on par with neurotypical individuals for happy expressions (e.g., [15–17]), several studies have demonstrated that such individuals may show impairment in the recognition of negative emotions, including anger (e.g., [18]), sadness (e.g., [16]), and fear (e.g., [17, 19]). These studies, however, were conducted primarily with adolescents and/or adults, and not children with autism disorder. Moreover, it is possible that the developmental trajectory for emotion recognition may differ between children with autism disorder and typically developing children. While emotion recognition appears to be correlated with age in typically developing children (e.g., [20–23]); not all studies have found similar developmental improvements in children with autism disorder (e.g., [24]).

Equally important, differences between children with autism disorder and typically developing children in recognizing emotions may be less prevalent when emotional expressions are depicted at stronger or greater intensities than when less intense expressions are presented. However, the intensity of emotional expressions has only occasionally been studied as a factor affecting children's recognition of emotion. When photographs of emotional expressions of varying intensity levels were shown to a sample of 4- to 15-year-old typically developing children, these children were more accurate in matching emotions when photographs were presented at 50% expression intensity than when they were presented at 25% expression intensity, at least for fear, sadness, anger, and happy expressions [25]. In a study of both typically developing children and children with autism disorder, Mazefsky and Oswald [26] found that high-functioning children with autism disorder were less accurate than both children with Asperger's syndrome and typically developing children in perceiving emotion from low intensity voice cues, but not with high intensity cues. In a similar vein, Law Smith et al. [27] found that high functioning adolescents with autism disorder were significantly worse than typically developing adolescents at detecting surprise, anger, and disgust using dynamic facial stimuli at lower, but not higher, intensities. Finally, Wallace and his colleagues showed that adolescents with autism disorder required more intense facial expressions for accurate emotion recognition than typically developing adolescents [28].

These are important differences given that in everyday settings emotional expressions are often subtle. Only by examining a range of different emotions using both highly intense and less intense facial displays can a more accurate picture of emotion recognition abilities in children with autism disorder and typically developing children be generated.

2. Overview of Present Research

In light of past findings, the present research examined the effects of eye gaze direction and expression intensity on emotion recognition in children with autism disorder and typically developing children between eight and twelve years of age. Using a photograph task, children's accuracy in recognizing facial expressions of happy, angry, sad, and fear emotional expressions, along with neutral expressions, was investigated. All emotional expressions were presented with computer-generated direct or averted eye gaze at 50% or 100% expression strength. While other intensities can be presented (e.g., 25% or 75%), these intensities were selected because fewer differences were expected between more closely matched intensity rates (e.g., 0% versus 25%; 75% versus 100%) than less closely matched intensity rates (50% versus 100%). Specific predictions for each emotional expression were as follows.

(1) Based on past studies that have shown that emotion recognition in individuals with autism disorder may be on par with neurotypical individuals for happy expressions (e.g., [15, 16]), it was predicted that children with autism disorder would be as accurate as typically developing children in recognizing happy expressions in all conditions (i.e., with direct and averted eye gaze and at 50% and 100% expression intensities).

(2) It was predicted that children with autism disorder would recognize angry expressions at full (100%) strength as well as typically developing children. At 50% expression strength, children with autism disorder should perform more poorly than typically developing children. These findings were expected

regardless of eye gaze direction and were based in part on the findings of Law Smith et al. [27], who showed that recognition of anger in adolescents with autism disorder was intact at 100% expression strength, but not at lower levels of intensity.

(3) It was predicted that children with autism disorder would recognize fear expressions less well than typically developing children, regardless of eye gaze direction or expression intensity, based on past findings showing a "fear recognition impairment" in individuals with autism disorder (e.g., [17, 19]). Averted eye gaze was expected to facilitate recognition of fear in typically developing children, especially at 50% expression intensity.

(4) Sad emotional expressions at 100% intensity and averted eyes were expected to be recognized equally well by children with autism disorder and typically developing children, based on the findings of Akechi et al. [14]. However, given that studies have shown that adults with autism disorder do not recognize sadness expressions as well as their neurotypical peers (e.g., [16]), children with autism disorder may not recognize expressions of sadness as well as typically developing children, especially at 50% intensity and regardless of eye gaze directions.

(5) Children with autism disorder would be more likely to label neutral (no emotion) expressions with an emotion label than typically developing children. This prediction was based on the results of Kuusikko et al. [29], who showed that children with autism disorder perceived ambiguous emotional stimuli as negative emotions, whereas typically developing children did not perceive them as emotional.

(6) Children with autism disorder would rate emotions with direct gaze as more intense and were expected to rate 50% emotional displays as more intense, than typically developing children. These predictions were based on the results of past studies that have shown that direct eye gaze can elicit arousing physiological effects in children with autism disorder and may even be too overstimulating for such children (e.g., [30]).

3. Method

3.1. Participants

3.1.1. Children with Autism Disorder. Twenty-eight children with autism disorder were identified and recruited through specialized schools and clinical centers in Chicago, IL. One child relocated before the investigators could complete the procedures, and five children were unable to participate due to various scheduling difficulties, resulting in a final sample of 22 children with autism disorder (mean age = 10.31; age range = 8–12). Seventeen were male and 5 were female. All children with autism disorder who participated in this study were recruited from organizations that serve exclusively students with a formal diagnosis of autism disorder.

Clinical diagnosis for all children was established by medical evaluation with a developmental pediatrician and/or by a licensed clinical psychologist in accordance with the *Diagnostic and Statistical Manual of Mental Disorders*-IV [31] and the criteria for autism as outlined by IDEA ("Individuals with Disabilities Education Improvement Act of 2004"). Almost all of the children ($n = 20$) were administered the Autism Diagnostic Observation Schedule (ADOS-G; [32]) and the Autism Diagnostic Interview Revised (ADI-R; [33]) as part of their evaluation by the organization that was providing their educational/therapeutic services. The records of two children noted that they had been administered the Childhood Autism Rating Scale (CARS; [34]) and the Vineland Adaptive Behavior Scales (Vineland II; [35]), although their scores from these measures were not included in their records. Moreover, we were not able to locate these children's ADOS-G or ADI-R scores or determine if they were available. However, because these two children were attending the same program as the other children with autism disorder and because these two children did not perform differently on any measures than the other children with autism disorder, the decision was made to include their data in our sample.

Children with autism disorder were eligible to participate if they had (1) a formal and clinical diagnosis of autism disorder without comorbid conditions including ADHD, ODD, bipolar disorder, and anxiety disorder; (2) a verbal mental age (VMA) at or above 5 years; (3) English as their primary language; and (4) an IQ performance score (PIQ) greater than 75. For the latter, all children with autism disorder had been administered the WISC-III by a licensed professional within a year or less of the present study. In our sample, children with autism disorder had PIQ scores in the average range ($M = 102.68$, $SD = 6.64$). Children with lower PIQ scores (and VM scores below 5 years) were not recruited because of the nature of our experimental task.

According to children's records, children met the cutoff for autism disorder in the social domain, ADOS (social + communication): $M = 11.00$, $SD = 4.66$; ADI-R (social interaction): $M = 20.00$, $SD = 6.11$; in the communication and language domain (ADI-R: $M = 12.33$, $SD = 4.67$); and in the repetitive/stereotyped behavior domain ADOS (stereotyped behavior): $M = 1.44$, $SD = 1.68$; ADI-R (restricted/repetitive behaviors): $M = 6.1$, $SD = 2.12$. As an additional measure of severity of symptoms, parents of children with autism disorder were asked to complete the Social Responsiveness Scale (SRS; [36]). The SRS is a 65-item questionnaire designed to assess social awareness, social information processing, capacity for reciprocal social communication, social anxiety/avoidance, and autistic preoccupations and traits. It has shown good reliability (median alpha = .85) and is conceptually appropriate as it measures severity of symptoms rather than the presence or absence of them, thus capturing the spectrum-like condition of the diagnosis [36]. On average, children with autism disorder were evaluated to have moderate to severe levels of social impairment, $M_{T\text{score}} = 109.25$, $SD = 8.49$, and range = 98–124. T-scores above 76 are strongly associated with a clinical diagnosis of autism

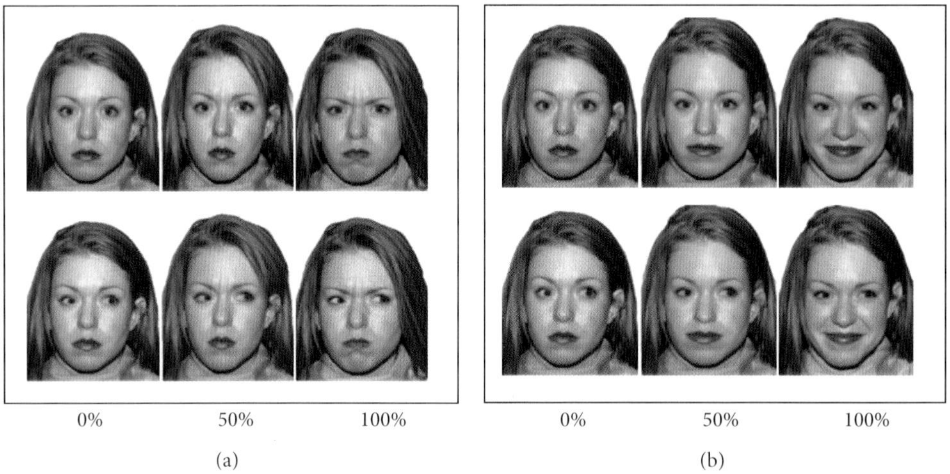

Figure 1: Examples of angry and happy expressions. Each emotional expression is presented as neutral, at 50% and 100% emotion intensity (from left to right) and with direct eye gaze (top) and averted eye gaze (bottom).

disorder and suggest severe interference in everyday social functioning.

3.1.2. Typically Developing Children. Typically developing children (TD; mean age = 9.8 years; age range = 8–12 years) were recruited through schools in the Chicago area in order to match children with autism disorder and typically developing children on sex, chronological age, and verbal mental age. Only typically developing children who were enrolled in normal, age-appropriate classrooms were considered. Of the typically developing children recruited, 22 children with autism disorder were matched to 22 typically developing children on sex (17 males, 5 females) and chronological age (±2 months). Group differences in verbal mental age could not be completely eliminated (AD: VMA = 9.32, SD = 1.69; TD: VMA = 10.64, SD = 1.67) and were statistically controlled for the analysis of covariance. Verbal mental age was obtained from age equivalent scores from the Peabody Picture Vocabulary Test (PPVT-III; [37]).

3.2. Measures and Procedure. Each participating child was tested individually in a quiet area outside of the classroom at a time specified by the school. A school professional (e.g., teacher, nurse, and teacher's aide) was present at each session for all children. The experimental procedure was divided into two 20-minute sessions to accommodate children's school schedules. The first session consisted of the Emotion Recognition Task and the Emotion Expression Intensity Rating Task, and the second session consisted of the Emotion Situation Task which provided data for another study not included here and the administration of the PPVT. The procedure for each experimental task is outlined below.

3.2.1. Emotion Recognition Task. Facial expressions of happy, angry, sad, fear, and neutral emotions of twelve adult Caucasian actors (6 males and 6 females) were selected from the MacBrain Face Stimulus Set [38]. These high-intensity expressions were considered to be at 100% strength. To create intermediate (i.e., 50% in-tensity) expressions, a procedure described in Calder et al. [39] was used. This process consisted of positioning 160 points manually on the anatomical landmarks in each neutral and intense emotional photograph of the same person and combining these images using Morph X software (http://www.norrkross.com/software/morphx/MorphX.php). This resulted in the morphed intermediate expression that represented a 50% deviation in the pattern of relevant muscle movements away from the neutral expression [39]. Each emotional expression was presented at 0% (or neutral), 50%, and 100% expression strength (see Figure 1). Utilizing Adobe Photoshop software, face stimuli with direct eye gaze were computer-altered to display averted eye gaze. Averted gaze shift (right or left) was randomly assigned for each averted gaze face. Photographs were printed in black and white scale approximately 20 cm × 24 cm (see Figure 1).

3.2.2. Emotion Photographs Validation Check. In order to present emotional stimuli with direct or averted eye gaze at varying expression intensities in the present study, we had to construct the stimuli ourselves, using the procedures outlined above, because none currently existed. To validate the photographic stimuli, a sample ($N = 40$) of undergraduates students at our university was asked to identify each emotional expression prior to the beginning of the study. Using frequency analysis, it was found that 98% of college students identified happy, anger, sad, and fear correctly at 100% expression strength with direct or averted eye gaze. At 50% expression strength, there was more variation: for sad and fear expressions, averted eye gaze expressions were identified correctly more often ($M = 81\%$) than expressions with direct eye gaze ($M = 70\%$). In contrast, happy and angry expressions were identified correctly 89%–98% of the time, respectively, regardless of eye gaze direction. Details about the validation procedure itself are available from the first author.

3.2.3. Emotion Recognition Task Procedure. During the emotion recognition task, each child was presented with a set of 60 photographs of facial expressions. Forty-eight photographs included happy, angry, sad, and fearful expressions at 50% and 100% expression strengths, each with direct or averted eye gaze, and 12 photographs showed neutral faces with direct or averted eye gaze. There were a total of 12 facial expressions per emotion. To control for possible order effects, four different sets were created. Within each set, the direction of the eye gaze and expression strength were counterbalanced such that photographs with direct and averted eye gaze and 50% and 100% expression strength did not appear back to back. Potential priming effect was controlled by organizing facial expressions such that a 50% photograph never followed a 100% photograph for the same emotional expression. Each set was rotated among the participating children as enrollment progressed.

A categorization procedure in which children indicated how the person in each picture felt was used. The task started with two practice items in order to assure that children understood the nature of the task. After successful practice trials, each child was presented with the rest of the set, one photograph at a time. Photographs remained visible for as long as the child needed to identify the emotion displayed. After presenting participants with a photograph, the researcher asked *"How do you think this person feels?"* followed by presentation of a response panel of schematic faces that included verbal labels that the experimenter pointed to while saying *"Does she/he feel happy, sad, angry, scared or just ok?"* The schematic faces were black and white line drawings (4 cm × 4 cm) adapted from past research [40, 41]. The display of schematic faces was counterbalanced in order to control for biases due to a preference for a particular position. The child was allowed to either point to a schematic face or verbally state the answer. All children, however, verbally stated their answers.

3.2.4. Emotion Intensity Rating Task and Procedure. A subset of 18 pictures was selected from the emotion recognition task. Two expressions (randomly selected) were used as practice items. Sixteen experimental stimuli included four emotional expressions (happy, angry, sad, and fear) at 50% and 100% of their expression strength, with direct and averted eye gaze. Using a 4-point scale, each participant was asked to judge the intensity of the emotion presented on the facial stimuli. Similar to the Hoffner and Badzinski [42] rating scale procedure, four circles increasing in size were labeled: *a little bit* (happy, angry, sad, and scared), *pretty* (happy, angry, sad, and scared), *very* (happy, angry, sad, and scared), and *very, very* (happy, angry, sad, and scared). Each picture was presented one at a time. Participants were given as much time as they needed to accomplish this task.

4. Results

4.1. Preliminary Analyses and Data Screening. Prior research suggests that the recognition of emotions might be related to overall development of verbal ability, as several studies have shown that when children with autism disorder and typically developing children were matched on verbal mental age (VMA) no differences on facial emotion recognition tasks were found [43, 44]. In the present research, VMA was obtained from age equivalent scores from the Peabody Picture Vocabulary Test (PPVT-III). An independent-samples t-test revealed that the difference in VMA between children with autism disorder and typically developing children was significant, $t(42) = 2.69$, $P < .05$. Therefore, in order to account for the effects of verbal ability, analysis of covariance (ANCOVA) was used with VMA as a covariate in all remaining analyses. An examination of the homogeneity of regression assumption necessary for the ANCOVA showed no violation, as evident by the nonsignificant diagnostic group (AD, TD) × VMA interactions ($Fs(1, 40) = .08–1.25$, $P \geq .41$).

4.2. Children's Ability to Recognize Facially Expressed Emotions: The Effects of Expression Intensity and Eye Gaze Direction. Children's mean percent accuracy scores for each emotion, across expression intensity and eye gaze directions, are shown in Table 1. To establish that children selected emotion labels for each facial expression at or above chance, goodness of fit χ^2 tests were utilized. Results indicated that children were not choosing emotions based on chance alone, χ^2 $(4, N = 44) = 13.50–113.27$, $P < .001$. A mixed 4 (emotion type: happy, angry, sad, fear) × 2 (expression intensity: 50%, 100%) × 2 (eye gaze direction: direct, averted) × 2 (diagnostic group: AD, TD) ANCOVA was performed on the accuracy scores. The Bonferroni approach was used with all post hoc pairwise comparisons in order to control for familywise error rate.

4.3. Recognition of Emotional Expressions: Between Group Effects at 100% and 50% Intensities. A significant diagnostic group × emotion type × expression strength × eye gaze direction four-way interaction, $\Lambda = .80$, $F(3, 39) = 3.34$, $P < .03$, and partial $\eta^2 = .21$ was found. Follow-up analyses revealed several between-group findings, as shown in Table 1. Children with autism disorder and typically developing children did not differ in their ability to correctly identify happy and angry emotional expressions at 100% and 50% strength with direct and averted eye gaze, $Fs(1, 41) = .45–2.37$, $P > .05$; see Table 1. In contrast, children with autism disorder were significantly less accurate than typically developing children at identifying fear across both levels of emotion intensity (i.e., 100% and 50%), and with direct and averted eye gaze, $Fs(1, 41) = 4.68–5.81$, $P < .05$; see Table 1. A trend toward significance ($F(1, 41) = 3.65$, $P < .06$) was also observed for sad emotional expressions at 100% strength with direct eye gaze, such that typically developing children were more accurate at identifying sadness than children with autism disorder.

TABLE 1: Mean percent correct values for happy, sad, angry, and fear emotional expressions as a function of expression strength and eye gaze direction.

	100% emotion strength		50% emotion strength	
	Direct	Averted	Direct	Averted
Typically developing children				
Happy	88.0 (3.6)	92.8 (4.4)	**58.0 (5.0)**	**79.5 (6.0)**
Sad	72.0 (7.2)	78.7 (7.2)	**20.9 (7.8)**	**47.1 (5.2)**
Angry	**78.0 (4.8)**	**96.3 (4.3)**	41.6 (4.9)	47.1 (4.6)
Fear	88.1 (6.6)*	74.7 (6.0)*	**57.4 (5.2)***	**71.7 (8.1)***
Children with autism disorder				
Happy	94.8 (3.6)	89.6 (4.4)	**50.1 (5.1)**	**86.2 (6.0)**
Sad	54.1 (6.4)	68.5 (7.1)	30.2 (5.1)	33.6 (5.2)
Angry	77.5 (4.2)	86.2 (4.7)	40.3 (5.4)	49.5 (4.6)
Fear	54.9 (5.6)*	54.5 (6.0)*	37.8 (5.9)*	58.5 (7.0)*

Adjusted group means as percent correct values are shown. Group means are adjusted for VMA. Standard deviations are in parentheses.
*Asterisks indicate significant between-group differences (typically developing versus with autism disorder), $P \leq .05$.
Bolded values indicate significant within-group differences (direct versus averted eye gaze), $P \leq .05$.

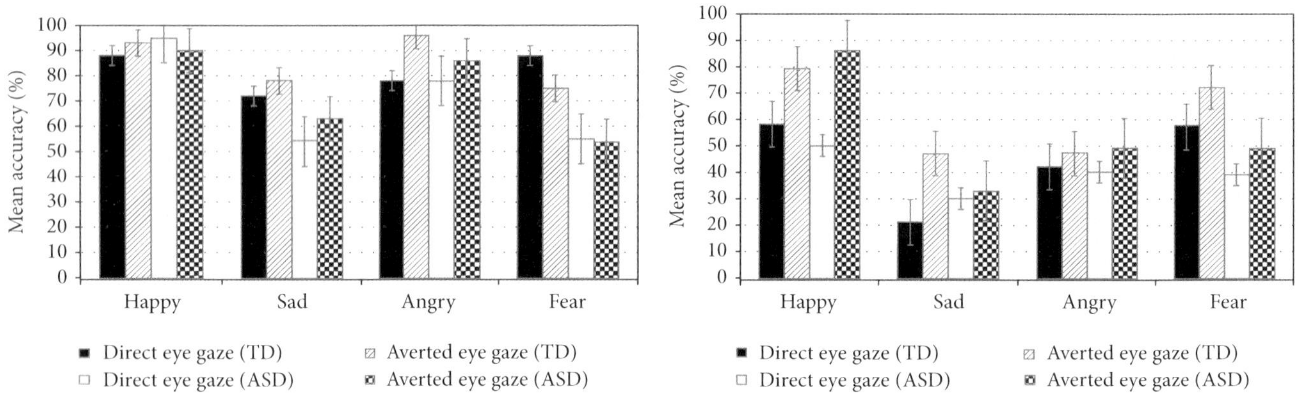

(a) 100% strength level

(b) 50% strength level

FIGURE 2: Mean percent accuracy scores for the effects of eye gaze direction on recognition of facial expressions at 100% and 50% expression strengths for children with autism disorder and typically developing children.

4.4. Recognition of Emotional Expressions: Within-Group Effects at 100% Emotion Intensity. Pairwise post hoc comparisons were also used to examine the within-group effects of eye gaze direction on children's accuracy in recognizing each of the four emotional expressions at each intensity (Table 1 and Figure 2). In a number of instances, a different pattern of within group findings emerged for children with autism disorder and typically developing children.

Although averted eye gaze enhanced recognition of fear expressions at 100% intensity in typically developing children, it did not enhance performance in children with autism disorder, $F(1, 39) = 5.52$, $P > .05$ (see Table 1 and Figure 2). Additionally, full expressions of anger were recognized significantly better when presented with averted versus direct eye gaze in typically developing children, $F(1, 41) = 13.88$, $P < .01$, although only a trend was observed for children with autism disorder, $F(1, 41) = 3.55$, $P < .06$; see Table 1. Finally, at 100% expression strength, eye gaze direction did not influence recognition of happy expressions, $Fs(1, 41) = .09–2.49$, $P > .05$, in typically developing children or children with autism disorder (see Figure 2).

4.5. Recognition of Emotional Expressions: Within-Group Effects at 50% Emotion Intensity. When emotional expressions were presented at 50% of their strength, typically developing children were better at recognizing expressions with averted eye gaze direction than direct eye gaze for happy, $F(1, 41) = 10.86$, $P < .001$, sad $F(1, 41) = 13.86$, $P < .001$, and fear $F(1, 41) = 5.32$, $P < .02$ expressions. Children with autism disorder benefited from averted eye gaze in the case of happy expressions, $F(1, 41) = 32.97$, $P < .001$.

4.6. The Effects of Emotion Type: Between and within-Group Effects. Finally, an interactive effect of diagnostic group × emotion type, $\Lambda = .79$, $F(3, 39) = 4.89$, $P < .04$, partial $\eta^2 = .18$, and two-way interaction was found for emotion type. Between-group pairwise comparisons with Bonferroni

TABLE 2: Mean percent correct values for happy, sad, angry, and fear emotional expressions for children with AD and typically developing children.

	Happy	Sad	Angry	Fear
Typically developing children	79.6 (4.7)	54.5 (6.9)	65.8 (4.7)	73.2 (6.4)[a]
Children with autism disorder	80.2 (4.8)	45.0 (5.9)	63.3 (4.9)	49.3 (7.1)[b]

Adjusted group means as percent correct values are shown. Group means are adjusted for VMA. Standard deviations are in parentheses.
[a, b]Superscripts indicate significant between-group differences, $P \leq .05$.

correction revealed that children with autism disorder were less accurate in their recognition of fear, $F(1, 39) = 7.20$, $P < .02$, than their typically developing peers. No group (AD, TD) differences were observed for happy, sad, or angry emotions, $Fs(1, 41) = .04–.28$, $P > .05$. Typically developing children identified happy expressions with significantly greater accuracy than sadness and anger, but not fear, $F(3, 37) = 11.65$, $P < .001$. Children with autism disorder were better at recognizing happy expressions than sad, angry, and fear expressions, $F(3, 37) = 25.04$, $P < .001$; see Table 2.

4.7. Children's Attributions of an Emotional State to Neutral Facial Expressions. A mixed 2 (diagnostic group: AD, TD) × 2 (eye gaze direction: direct, averted) ANCOVA was performed on children's accuracy in labeling neutral facial expressions as "no emotion." An interactive effect of diagnostic goup × eye gaze direction was found $F(1, 41) = 20.71$, $P < .05$, $\eta^2 = .25$. Children with autism disorder were less accurate at identifying neutral expressions as nonemotional when they included direct eye gaze direction ($M = 71\%$, SD = 5.1), than TD children ($M = 85\%$, SD = 5.2). Children with autism disorder were more likely to label a neutral facial photograph with an emotion than typically developing children (see error analysis below). No diagnostic group differences were observed for neutral expressions with averted eye gaze.

4.8. Error Analysis in Recognition of Facially Expressed Emotions. To examine the type of errors children made when identifying faces, emotional expressions were analyzed in terms of the frequency with which the target emotion was identified incorrectly using a 4 (error type: happy, angry, sad, fear) × 2 (expression intensity: 100%, 50%) × 2 (eye gaze direction: direct, averted) × 2 (diagnostic group: AD, TD) ANCOVAs, with diagnostic group as a between-subject factor and expression intensity, eye gaze direction, and error type as within-subject factors.

The analysis of errors revealed a significant error type × expression intensity × eye gaze direction interactions for the happy, angry, and fear emotions, $\Lambda s = .70–.79$, $Fs(3, 40) = 5.10–5.45$, $P < .01$, and partial $\eta^2 = .28$. Children with autism disorder and typically developing children were more likely to label happy, angry, sad, and fear expressions as neutral when faces were presented at 50% expression strength with direct eye gaze than when presented with averted eye gaze (all $Ps < .01$). Children with autism disorder mislabeled sad expressions at 50% expression strength with averted eye gaze as anger more often than typically developing children. A significant main effect of error type, $F(3, 117) = 3.98$, $P < .03$, partial $\eta^2 = .16$, was found when children were viewing neutral expressions. Children across both groups confused neutral expressions with fear more so than with any other emotion.

4.9. Children's Ratings of Emotional Intensity: The Effects of Expression Intensity and Eye Gaze Direction. It was predicted that averted eye gaze would increase emotional intensity ratings for expressions of sadness and fear, whereas direct eye gaze would increase intensity ratings for happy and angry expressions in at least typically developing children. Interactive effects of diagnostic group × expression strength, $\Lambda = .76$, $F(1, 41) = 14.82$, $P < .001$, partial $\eta^2 = .28$, and diagnostic group × eye gaze direction, $\Lambda = .88$, $F(1, 41) = 5.23$, $P < .02$, partial $\eta^2 = .11$, were found.

While both children with autism disorder and typically developing children rated 100% expressions as more emotionally intense than 50% expressions, $F(1, 41) = 83.45$, $P < .001$, $F(1, 41) = 12.11$, $P < .01$, respectively, children with autism disorder rated facial expressions presented at 50% as more emotionally intense than typically developing children, $F(1, 39) = 8.35$, $P < .001$. Children with autism disorder also gave higher emotion intensity ratings to expressions with direct eye gaze than typically developing children, $F(1, 41) = 10.68$, $P < .01$. Within-group comparisons revealed that children with autism disorder perceived facial expressions with direct eye gaze as more emotionally intense than those with averted eye gaze, $F(1, 41) = 22.39$, $P < .001$, whereas no differences in intensity ratings between direct and averted eye gaze expressions were observed for typically developing children (see Table 3).

Intensity ratings also varied across different emotional expressions, $\Lambda = .69$, $F(3, 39) = 5.77$, $P < .01$ partial $\eta^2 = .31$, for children with autism disorder and typically developing children. Children with autism disorder rated expressions of fear as more intense than typically developing children.

4.10. Relation between Recognition Accuracy and SRS Scores in Children with Autism Disorder. Linear regression analyses revealed a significant negative relation between the social communication subscale and recognition of fear, $\beta = -.64$, $P < .05$ in children with autism disorder: children with a more severe social communication impairment were less accurate at recognizing fear than children with autism disorder who showed less impairment. A similar trend emerged for recognition of sad expressions, $\beta = -.58$, $P < .07$, in children with autism disorder. No other relations between the remaining SRS subscales scores and recognition accuracy (or

TABLE 3: Mean intensity ratings for facial expressions by emotion strength and eye gaze direction in children with AD and typically developing children.

	Mean intensity ratings for facial expressions by emotion strength	
	100% emotion strength	50% emotion strength
Typically developing children	1.82 (.90)^{a*}	2.73 (.88)*
Children with autism disorder	2.38 (.80)^{b*}	2.73 (.89)*
	Mean intensity ratings of facial expressions by eye gaze direction	
	Direct eye gaze	Averted eye gaze
Typically developing children	2.36 (.08)^{a}	2.25 (.09)
Children with autism disorder	2.72 (.08)^{b*}	2.33 (.09)*

Intensity ratings ranged from 1 (least intense) to 4 (most intense). Standard deviations are in parentheses.
^{a,b}Superscripts indicate significant between-group differences (typically developing versus with autism disorder), $P \leq .05$.
*Asterisks indicate significant within-group differences, $P \leq .05$.

other DVs) were found, βs = .04–.13, *P*s >.05. PIQ scores, VMA scores and diagnostic scores were not significantly related to children's responses (*r*s = .07–.23, *P*s > .05).

5. Discussion

In the present research, a number of significant findings regarding recognition of emotional expressions in children with autism disorder and typically developing children were revealed. As predicted, children with autism disorder and typically developing children did not differ in their ability to correctly identify happy and angry emotional expressions at 50% or 100% intensity with direct or averted eye gaze. However, the ability to identify fear at 50% or 100% expression intensity with direct or averted eyes was significantly less accurate in children with autism disorder than typically developing children. A trend was also found for sadness expressions: children with autism disorder were less accurate in recognizing sadness at 100% intensity and direct eye gaze than typically developing children.

The lack of difference between children with autism disorder and typically developing children in recognizing happy expressions regardless of eye gaze direction and expression intensity is consistent with the assertion that recognition of positive emotion is relatively intact in children and adults with autism disorder (e.g., [19, 45, 46]). Happy expressions are characterized by a unique mouth pattern that alone could be sufficient to discriminate them from other emotions [47]. According to Gross [46], it is possible that a visual preference for the lower part of the face accounts for the superior performance found in their recognition of happiness in individuals with autism disorder, although this cannot be determined from our data.

Also consistent with our prediction, the present study demonstrated that children with autism disorder are able to recognize expressions of anger as well as their typically developing peers. However, the expected facilitative effects of direct eye gaze on the recognition of anger were not found in either group. In fact, in typically developing children, averted eye gaze enhanced recognition of anger expressions. However, while direct eye gaze may not have improved children's recognition of anger, all children *perceived* expressions with *direct* eye gaze as more intense than expressions with averted eye gaze. This is consistent with previous research that demonstrated greater ratings of intensity for angry faces that were coupled with direct eye gaze than averted eye gaze in neurotypical adults [48].

It is not clear why averted eyes resulted in better recognition of anger expressions, as this finding is inconsistent with the shared signal hypothesis. One possibility is that children pay more attention to emotional expressions such as anger when they include averted eye gaze because they find that the same expressions with direct eyes too stimulating. This hypothesis is consistent with our findings that children rated faces with direct eye gaze, including angry expressions, as more intense than faces with averted eye gaze. It may also be that while the shared signal hypothesis holds true for adults, there may be a developmental trajectory to this effect, such that younger children do not demonstrate it. Additional research is needed to assess this assertion.

The present findings also showed that children with autism disorder were not as accurate as typically developing children in recognizing fear, regardless of expression intensity or eye gaze direction. Our results add to the growing body of literature that has reported similar "fear recognition impairments" in adults with autism disorder (e.g., [45, 49]). A number of explanations have been given to explain this impairment in recognizing fear expressions, including atypical neurological functioning in individuals with autism disorder. For example, Ashwin et al. [15, 45] showed a differential pattern of neural activity in various "social" brain areas in adults with autism disorder, compared with typical adults, during the perception of fearful facial expressions. These differences included less activation in the left amygdala and left orbitofrontal cortex brain in adults with autism disorder than in neurotypical adults.

Deficits in the recognition of fear may also be due to the fact that fear is communicated primarily by the eye region of the face and that individuals with autism disorder may pay less attention to the eyes. Although all children in this study showed sensitivity to eye gaze direction (e.g., both rated expressions with direct eyes as more intense than expressions with averted eyes for fear), averted eye gaze facilitated recognition in typically developing but not children with autism disorder. As Wallace et al. [19] note, eyes may appear differently for individual emotions, and for fear, the eyes themselves may be negatively arousing and maybe even be over arousing, for the individual with autism disorder. In expressing fear, there is a large amount of sclera visible that may lead to "fearful" eyes being perceived as threatening to the individual with autism. Thus, less attention may be paid to them [19].

Finally, our trend finding ($P < .06$) for less accurate recognition of sadness in children with autism disorder is consistent with the results of Wallace et al. [28], whose research revealed a particularly diminished sensitivity to sad expressions in adolescents with autism disorder. It is also consistent with Boraston et al.'s [16] finding of less accurate recognition of sadness in adults with autism disorder. The present results provide evidence that difficulties in recognizing fear and sad expressions may begin early in individuals with autism disorder and thus warrant further investigation.

Interestingly, negative relations between the social communication subscale of the SRS and recognition of fear and sadness were found in the present study, with children with more severe social communication impairment being less accurate at recognizing these emotions than children who showed less impairment. These results are consistent with Bal et al. [50], who showed that more severe autism disorder symptoms identified through the SRS, especially the social communication subscale, were related to less accurate recognition of emotion from dynamic (video) stimuli. Nevertheless, it is unclear whether social communicative difficulties result in less accurate recognition of negative emotions such as fear and sadness or vice versa. It has been suggested that an understanding of certain emotions such as fear requires joint communication between parents (or other adults) and children [51]. That is, the capacity to communicate, coordinate, and share attention with a social partner regarding characteristics that underlie certain emotion situations, particularly those eliciting fear or sadness, are needed for adequate perception of those emotions. For example, learning through joint attention and communication with an adult or another individual may be required in order to develop an understanding that an expression of fear is a response to a potentially threatening object in the environment.

Finally, in the present research it was found that intensity ratings for emotional expressions at 100% strength were similar for children with autism disorder and typically developing children. Moreover, both groups rated expressions presented at 100% strength as more intense than expressions presented at 50% strength. Notably, children with autism disorder rated expressions with direct eye gaze as more intense than expressions with averted eye gaze. Children with autism disorder also rated and fear emotional expressions as more intense than their typically developing peers. Children with autism disorder were also more likely than typically developing children to label neutral (no emotion) photographs with direct eyes as representing an emotion. Consistent with Kuusikko et al. [29], when children with autism disorder and typically developing children labeled neutral facial expressions with an emotion, they almost always labeled it with a negative emotion.

Although we feel these are compelling findings, limitations of this study should be noted. Firstly, we were not able to match typically developing and children with autism disorder on both chronological age and verbal mental age (VMA). However, when used as a covariate, VMA did not reveal any additional findings. Secondly, while evidence was found that children with autism disorder were sensitive to eye gaze direction, given the extensive number of manipulations in the present study, we were unable to present more than three examples per emotion of averted and direct eye gaze directions. Thirdly, while we were able to recruit all of our children with autism disorder from classrooms or programs designed to serve children with autism disorder exclusively, and ADOS-G and ADI-R scores were included in most (over 90%) children's records, we did not administer these tests ourselves. We were also not able to include a range of children on the spectrum because of the makeup of the children in the classrooms. We acknowledge that this limits the generalizability of our findings.

Finally, some have suggested that static photographical images are not ecologically valid, as emotion in everyday life is often expressed quickly and dynamically. Although static photographs may be ecologically limited, there are several reasons why the use of such stimuli in a study has value. Children's ability to recognize emotion from static images often eliminates the difficulty, and resultant floor effects, in their ability to recognize emotion from dynamic images. Additionally, emotion recognition training for children with autism disorder is often completed with static photographs of emotion. In fact, we purposely began this study before any emotion training began that year in the classroom, although we acknowledge that the children in our sample may have received emotion training in prior years. More careful inspection of the emotion training children received in a classroom or program prior to the start of research studies should be considered in future research. In spite of these limitations, an important implication of the present results is that photographs of varying expression intensities and eye gaze directions are used in emotion training, with an emphasis on presenting subtle intensities of expressions. This would provide more ecological validity with real-world emotions, to the extent that subtle displays of emotional expressions are an integral part of everyday life.

6. Conclusions

To conclude by highlighting our key findings, the present study showed that eye gaze direction modulates emotion perception from facial expressions in both typically developing and children with autism disorder and that children with autism disorder are sensitive to gaze direction. However, children with autism disorder showed a more significant impairment in the recognition of fear expressions and a trend for sad expressions, rated happy and fear expressions as more intense, and rated most 50% strength expressions as more intense than typically developing children. These compelling findings merit further investigation. In future research, electrophysiological and neural imaging methods with our stimuli would be valuable in shedding light on the origins of these and other differences between children with autism disorder and typically developing children in their processing of emotional expressions.

Acknowledgments

The authors thank the children who participated in this study and the staff and administrators at their schools or programs for their assistance throughout the study. Portions of this research were presented at the biennial meetings of the Society for Research in Child Development (2011) and the International Society for Research on Emotion (2013).

References

[1] S. Begeer, H. M. Koot, C. Rieffe, M. Meerum Terwogt, and H. Stegge, "Emotional competence in children with autism: diagnostic criteria and empirical evidence," *Developmental Review*, vol. 28, no. 3, pp. 342–369, 2008.

[2] M. B. Harms, A. Martin, and G. L. Wallace, "Facial emotion recognition in autism spectrum disorders: a review of behavioral and neuroimaging studies," *Neuropsychology Review*, vol. 20, no. 3, pp. 290–322, 2010.

[3] R. J. Itier and M. Batty, "Neural bases of eye and gaze processing: the core of social cognition," *Neuroscience and Biobehavioral Reviews*, vol. 33, no. 6, pp. 843–863, 2009.

[4] K. Nation and S. Penny, "Sensitivity to eye gaze in autism: is it normal? Is it automatic? Is it social?" *Development and Psychopathology*, vol. 20, no. 1, pp. 79–97, 2008.

[5] M. Uljarevic and A. Hamilton, "Recognition of emotions in autism: a formal meta-analysis," *Journal of Autism and Developmental Disorders*, vol. 43, no. 7, pp. 1517–1526, 2013.

[6] K. M. Dalton, B. M. Nacewicz, T. Johnstone et al., "Gaze fixation and the neural circuitry of face processing in autism," *Nature Neuroscience*, vol. 8, no. 4, pp. 519–526, 2005.

[7] A. Klin, W. Jones, R. Schultz, F. Volkmar, and D. Cohen, "Visual fixation patterns during viewing of naturalistic social situations as predictors of social competence in individuals with autism," *Archives of General Psychiatry*, vol. 59, no. 9, pp. 809–816, 2002.

[8] F. R. Volkmar and L. C. Mayes, "Gaze behavior in autism," *Development and Psychopathology*, vol. 2, pp. 61–69, 1990.

[9] S. R. Leekam, B. López, and C. Moore, "Attention and joint attention in preschool children with autism," *Developmental Psychology*, vol. 36, no. 2, pp. 261–273, 2000.

[10] R. B. Adams Jr. and R. E. Kleck, "Perceived Gaze direction and the processing of facial displays of emotion," *Psychological Science*, vol. 14, no. 6, pp. 644–647, 2003.

[11] R. B. Adams Jr. and R. E. Kleck, "Effects of direct and averted gaze on the perception of facially communicated emotion," *Emotion*, vol. 5, no. 1, pp. 3–11, 2005.

[12] R. Graham and K. S. LaBar, "Garner interference reveals dependencies between emotional expression and gaze in face perception," *Emotion*, vol. 7, no. 2, pp. 296–313, 2007.

[13] D. Sander, D. Grandjean, S. Kaiser, T. Wehrle, and K. R. Scherer, "Interaction effects of perceived gaze direction and dynamic facial expression: evidence for appraisal theories of emotion," *European Journal of Cognitive Psychology*, vol. 19, no. 3, pp. 470–480, 2007.

[14] H. Akechi, A. Senju, Y. Kikuchi, Y. Tojo, H. Osanai, and T. Hasegawa, "Does gaze direction modulate facial expression processing in children with autism spectrum disorder?" *Child Development*, vol. 80, no. 4, pp. 1134–1146, 2009.

[15] C. Ashwin, E. Chapman, L. Colle, and S. Baron-Cohen, "Impaired recognition of negative basic emotions in autism: a test of the amygdala theory," *Social Neuroscience*, vol. 1, pp. 349–363, 2006.

[16] Z. Boraston, S.-J. Blakemore, R. Chilvers, and D. Skuse, "Impaired sadness recognition is linked to social interaction deficit in autism," *Neuropsychologia*, vol. 45, no. 7, pp. 1501–1510, 2007.

[17] K. A. Pelphrey, N. J. Sasson, J. S. Reznick, G. Paul, B. D. Goldman, and J. Piven, "Visual scanning of faces in autism," *Journal of Autism and Developmental Disorders*, vol. 32, no. 4, pp. 249–261, 2002.

[18] J. L. Lindner and L. A. Rosén, "Decoding of emotion through facial expression, prosody and verbal content in children and adolescents with Asperger's syndrome," *Journal of Autism and Developmental Disorders*, vol. 36, no. 6, pp. 769–777, 2006.

[19] S. Wallace, M. Coleman, and A. Bailey, "An investigation of basic facial expression recognition in autism spectrum disorders," *Cognition and Emotion*, vol. 22, no. 7, pp. 1353–1380, 2008.

[20] L. A. Camras and K. Allison, "Children's understanding of emotional facial expressions and verbal labels," *Journal of Nonverbal Behavior*, vol. 9, no. 2, pp. 84–94, 1985.

[21] D. Davidson, "The role of basic, self-conscious and self-conscious evaluative emotions in children's memory and understanding of emotion," *Motivation and Emotion*, vol. 30, no. 3, pp. 232–242, 2006.

[22] E. R. Tuminello and D. Davidson, "What the face and body reveal: in-group emotion effects and stereotyping of emotion in African American and European American children," *Journal of Experimental Child Psychology*, vol. 110, no. 2, pp. 258–274, 2011.

[23] S. C. Widen and J. A. Russell, "A closer look at preschoolers' freely produced labels for facial expressions," *Developmental Psychology*, vol. 39, no. 1, pp. 114–128, 2003.

[24] K. O'Connor, J. P. Hamm, and I. J. Kirk, "The neurophysiological correlates of face processing in adults and children with Asperger's syndrome," *Brain and Cognition*, vol. 59, pp. 82–95, 2005.

[25] C. M. Herba, S. Landau, T. Russell, C. Ecker, and M. L. Phillips, "The development of emotion-processing in children: effects of age, emotion, and intensity," *Journal of Child Psychology and Psychiatry and Allied Disciplines*, vol. 47, no. 11, pp. 1098–1106, 2006.

[26] C. A. Mazefsky and D. P. Oswald, "Emotion perception in Asperger's syndrome and high-functioning autism: the importance of diagnostic criteria and cue intensity," *Journal of Autism and Developmental Disorders*, vol. 37, no. 6, pp. 1086–1095, 2007.

[27] M. J. Law Smith, B. Montagne, D. I. Perrett, M. Gill, and L. Gallagher, "Detecting subtle facial emotion recognition deficits in high-functioning Autism using dynamic stimuli of varying intensities," *Neuropsychologia*, vol. 48, no. 9, pp. 2777–2781, 2010.

[28] G. L. Wallace, L. K. Case, M. B. Harms, J. A. Silvers, L. Kenworthy, and A. Martin, "Diminished sensitivity to sad facial expressions in high functioning autism spectrum disorders is associated with symptomatology and adaptive functioning," *Journal of Autism and Developmental Disorders*, vol. 41, no. 11, pp. 1475–1486, 2011.

[29] S. Kuusikko, H. Haapsamo, E. Jansson-Verkasalo et al., "Emotion recognition in children and adolescents with autism spectrum disorders," *Journal of Autism and Developmental Disorders*, vol. 39, no. 6, pp. 938–945, 2009.

[30] A. Senju, K. Yaguchi, Y. Tojo, and T. Hasegawa, "Eye contact does not facilitate detection in children with autism," *Cognition*, vol. 89, no. 1, pp. B43–B51, 2003.

[31] American Psychiatric Association, *Diagnostic and Statistical Manual of Mental Disorders*, Arthur, Washington, DC, USA, 4th edition, 2000.

[32] C. Lord, S. Risi, L. Lambrecht et al., "The autism diagnostic observation schedule-generic: a standard measure of social and communication deficits associated with the spectrum of autism," *Journal of Autism and Developmental Disorders*, vol. 30, no. 3, pp. 205–223, 2000.

[33] C. Lord, M. Rutter, and A. L. Couteur, "Autism diagnostic interview-revised: a revised version of a diagnostic interview for caregivers of individuals with possible pervasive developmental disorders," *Journal of Autism and Developmental Disorders*, vol. 24, no. 5, pp. 659–685, 1994.

[34] E. Schopler, R. J. Reichier, and B. R. Renner, *The Childhood Autism Rating Scale (CARS)*, Western Psychological Services, Los Angeles, Calif, USA, 1993.

[35] S. Sparrow, D. V. Cicchetti, and D. A. Balla, *Vineland Adaptive Behavior Scales*, American Guidance Service, Circle Pines, Minn, USA, 2nd edition, 2005.

[36] J. N. Constantino and C. P. Gruber, *Social Responsiveness Scale (SRS) Manual*, Western Psychological Services, Los Angeles, Calif, USA, 2005.

[37] L. M. Dunn and L. M. Dunn, *Peabody Picture Vocabulary Test-Third Edition*, American Guidance Service, Circle Pines, Minn, USA, 1997.

[38] N. Tottenham, J. W. Tanaka, A. C. Leon et al., "The NimStim set of facial expressions: judgments from untrained research participants," *Psychiatry Research*, vol. 168, no. 3, pp. 242–249, 2009.

[39] A. J. Calder, A. W. Young, D. I. Perrett, N. L. Etcoff, and D. Rowland, "Categorical perception of morphed facial expressions," *Visual Cognition*, vol. 3, no. 2, pp. 81–117, 1996.

[40] G. Green, "Early behavioral intervention for autism: what does research tell us?" in *Behavioral Interventions for Young Children with Autism*, C. Maurice, G. Green, and S. Luce, Eds., pp. 29–44, Pro Ed, Austin, Tex, USA, 1996.

[41] S. Thayer and W. Schiff, "Stimulus factors in observer judgment of social interaction: facial expression and motion pattern," *The American Journal of Psychology*, vol. 82, no. 1, pp. 73–85, 1969.

[42] C. Hoffner and D. M. Badzinski, "Children's integration of facial and situational cues to emotion," *Child Development*, vol. 60, no. 2, pp. 411–422, 1989.

[43] F. Castelli, "Understanding emotions from standardized facial expressions in autism and normal development," *Autism*, vol. 9, no. 4, pp. 428–449, 2005.

[44] K. Loveland and B. Tunali-Kotoski, "The school-aged child with autism," in *The Handbook of Autism and Pervasive Developmental Disorders*, F. R. Volkmar, A. Klin, and R. Paul, Eds., pp. 247–287, Wiley, New York, NY, USA, 3rd edition, 2005.

[45] C. Ashwin, S. Baron-Cohen, S. Wheelwright, M. O'Riordan, and E. T. Bullmore, "Differential activation of the amygdala and the "social brain" during fearful face-processing in Asperger Syndrome," *Neuropsychologia*, vol. 45, no. 1, pp. 2–14, 2007.

[46] T. F. Gross, "The perception of four basic emotions in human and nonhuman faces by children with autism and other developmental disabilities," *Journal of Abnormal Child Psychology*, vol. 32, no. 5, pp. 469–480, 2004.

[47] P. Ekman, "Are there basic emotions?" *Psychological Review*, vol. 99, no. 3, pp. 550–553, 1992.

[48] W. Sato, T. Kochiyama, S. Yoshikawa, E. Naito, and M. Matsumura, "Enhanced neural activity in response to dynamic facial expressions of emotion: an fMRI study," *Cognitive Brain Research*, vol. 20, no. 1, pp. 81–91, 2004.

[49] K. Humphreys, N. Minshew, G. L. Leonard, and M. Behrmann, "A fine-grained analysis of facial expression processing in high-functioning adults with autism," *Neuropsychologia*, vol. 45, no. 4, pp. 685–695, 2007.

[50] E. Bal, E. Harden, D. Lamb, A. V. Van Hecke, J. W. Denver, and S. W. Porges, "Emotion recognition in children with autism spectrum disorders: relations to eye gaze and autonomic state," *Journal of Autism and Developmental Disorders*, vol. 40, no. 3, pp. 358–370, 2010.

[51] P. Mundy and C. Burnetter, "Joint attention and neurodevelopment," in *Handbook of Autism and Pervasive Developmental Disorders*, F. R. Volkmar, A. Klin, and R. Paul, Eds., pp. 650–681, John Wiley, Hoboken, NJ, USA, 3rd edition, 2005.

13

Parasympathetic Response Profiles Related to Social Functioning in Young Children with Autistic Disorder

Stephen J. Sheinkopf,[1,2,3] A. Rebecca Neal-Beevers,[4] Todd P. Levine,[1,3] Cynthia Miller-Loncar,[1,2,3] and Barry Lester[1,2,3]

[1] *Department of Psychiatry and Human Behavior, Warren Alpert Medical School of Brown University, Providence, RI 02912, USA*
[2] *Department of Pediatrics, Warren Alpert Medical School of Brown University, Providence, RI 02912, USA*
[3] *Brown Center for the Study of Children at Risk, Women & Infants Hospital, 101 Dudley Street, Providence, RI 02905, USA*
[4] *Department of Psychology, University of Texas at Austin, 108 E. Dean Keeton Street, Austin, TX 78712, USA*

Correspondence should be addressed to Stephen J. Sheinkopf; stephen_sheinkopf@brown.edu

Academic Editor: Jean-Louis Adrien

Psychophysiology studies of heart rate and heart rate variability can be employed to study regulatory processes in children with autism. The objective of this study was to test for differences in respiratory sinus arrhythmia (RSA; a measure of heart rate variability) and to examine the relationship between physiologic responses and measures of social behavior. Participants included 2- to 6-year-old children with Autistic Disorder and children without autism. Heart rate and RSA were derived from ECG recordings made during a baseline period and then a stranger approach paradigm. Social and adaptive behavior was assessed by parent report. Groups did not differ in mean heart rate or RSA at baseline or in response to social challenge. However, children with autism were more likely to show a physiologic response to intrusive portions of the stranger approach than to less intrusive portions of this procedure. Nonautistic children were equally likely to respond to intrusive and less intrusive social events. Within the autistic group, physiologic response to the intrusive stranger approach corresponded to higher ratings of social adaptive behaviors. These results suggest that physiologic responses to social challenge may help understand differences in social behavioral outcomes in children with autism.

1. Introduction

Past research has suggested that children with autism show disruptions in autonomic responses to environmental stressors [1–5]. However, research has varied in terms of the ages of children included in studies, the nature of stimuli that constituted the observational protocols, and the resulting findings of physiologic responses in comparison to nonautistic individuals. Moreover, while some studies have examined relations between autonomic measures and measures of social and behavioral functioning (e.g., [5]), relatively little research has compared individual differences in physiologic and behavioral characteristics. Examinations of responses in relation to behavioral markers of symptom presentation, syndrome severity, and other aspects of behavioral functioning may help to reconcile some of the inconsistencies found in prior research and has potential implications for developing and refining assessments and treatments of autism.

Cardiorespiratory measures, including heart rate, respiratory sinus arrhythmia (RSA), and more general measures of heart rate variability (HRV), have been widely used in studies of child psychopathology, including some research on autism. RSA, a phenomenon defined as periodic variation in heart rate due to respiratory activity, reflects central nervous system influences on heart rate. RSA is mediated by inhibitory signals to the sinoatrial node from brainstem nuclei via the vagus and reflects parasympathetic nervous system (PNS) influences on heart rate variability. Higher baseline RSA is thought to indicate a readiness to engage with or respond to environmental demands, including aspects of the social environment. On the other hand, changes in RSA in response to environmental challenge are thought to indicate active engagement with and attention to stimuli [6]. Decreases in RSA during social stressors may indicate adaptive attention to social information and thus may be related to positive social behavior and adaptation to social environmental demands.

Two studies have investigated changes in HRV, during cognitive tasks. Althaus and colleagues [7] examined HRV during a cognitive challenge in children with autism. They found that children with autism and typically developing children did not differ on measures of baseline heart rate or baseline HRV. However, the children with autism failed to show task-associated decreases in HRV in comparison to nonautistic children. These response patterns did not differentiate autistic children with and without hyperactivity, but changes in HRV from baseline did correlate with measures of behavioral inflexibility in the children with autism. Toichi and Kamio [4] also reported that adolescents with autism failed to show decreases in HRV during a cognitive task. All individuals in the control sample showed task-related decreases in HRV. In contrast, the autistic group showed a variable response, with some children showing decreases in HRV and others showing an unexpected increase in HRV. The authors argued that this finding was indicative of hyperarousal and that some individuals with autism may have found the baseline condition more stressful than the condition where they were engaged in a task. An additional relevant interpretation of this observation is that focusing on the average levels of physiologic responses may mask important and potentially meaningful individual differences.

Few studies have examined RSA or other measures of HRV in response to social events and stimuli. Althaus and colleagues [8] demonstrated qualitative differences between 8–12-year-old children with and without a diagnosis of Pervasive Developmental Disorder Not Otherwise Specified (PDD-NOS) on parasympathetic-related changes in HRV, but not on components of HRV modeled as sympathetic influences. Furthermore, the magnitude of these differences was greatest for a subgroup of children with PDD-NOS and comorbid hyperactivity and attention problems. In another study of higher functioning children with autism, Levine et al. [3] found no difference in RSA between autistic and nonautistic children during the Trier Social Stress Test [9]. There were also no differences at baseline and following the task. Bal et al. [10] found that 7–17-year-old children with autism without significant cognitive deficits had lower RSA when compared to controls at baseline. Within the autism group, those with higher RSA showed more rapid recognition of facial emotions than those with lower RSA.

An additional and notable aspect of prior research is that there have been limited studies of autonomic measures of response and regulation in young children with autism. Corona et al. [11] reported that 3–5-year-old children with autism failed to show a heart rate response to the feigned distress of an examiner, as compared to a matched sample of children with developmental delays that showed an overall decrease in heart rate in response to the examiner's distress display. In related work, Sigman and colleagues [12] reported that both young children with autism and a matched group of children with developmental delays showed decreased heart rate when viewing a video of babies laughing or crying. While these studies did not examine measures of HRV such as RSA, they do suggest experimental design will affect the intensity, salience, or other aspects of the stimuli that can account for between-study discrepancies in findings. More recently, Patriquin et al. [13] reported a positive association between baseline RSA and both receptive language and children's sharing behaviors during play in a relatively high functioning sample of 4- to 7- year-old children with autism spectrum disorders.

With these issues in mind, the goal of the present pilot study was to investigate group and individual differences in autonomic responses to graded social stimuli in young, relatively lower functioning children with autism and to determine whether individual differences in autonomic responses would be related to behavioral measures of competence. To this end, we recorded electrocardiograph (ECG) signals during a standardized stranger approach paradigm, during which a female examiner entered the room and progressively approached and interacted with the child. We hypothesized that children with autism would show a diminished or delayed RSA response to stranger approach compared to a matched comparison sample, and children who showed greater RSA responses to the social approach of the stranger (i.e., decreases in RSA) would have higher ratings of social behavioral competence.

2. Materials and Methods

2.1. Participants. Participants included children with Autistic Disorder (AUT; $n = 15$) and children without autism (non-AUT; $n = 8$), group-matched on chronological age and nonverbal IQ. Autism diagnoses were determined by clinician best estimate diagnosis confirmed by above-threshold scores on the Autism Diagnostic Observation Schedule [14]. Participants ranged in age from 30 to 79 months and had variable levels of cognitive and language functioning. Cognitive developmental abilities were assessed by either the Differential Ability Scales (DAS) [15] or the Bayley Scales of Infant and Toddler Development, second edition [16], as was developmentally appropriate. In order to allow for some comparability of cognitive scores across children who received different measures, we group-matched participants on the basis of the DAS nonverbal IQ score or the Bayley Mental Development Index (MDI). Adaptive functioning, including social behavioral skills, was assessed using the Vineland Adaptive Behavior Scales [17]. The AUT group had lower Vineland Composite scores, as well as lower Daily Living and Socialization scores, than the non-AUT group. The variability in level of functioning in the children with autism is consistent with what is seen in the general population of children with autism spectrum disorders. Roughly half (47%) had cognitive standard scores (from the Bayley Scales or DAS) less than 75, and 80% had Communication standard scores on the Vineland less than 75 (i.e., more than 1.5 standard deviations below the normative sample means). The comparison group included some children with general developmental cognitive delays (63% with cognitive standard scores less than 75; 87% with Vineland Communication standard scores less than 75). There were no comparison children with developmental delays of known etiology (i.e., there were no children with Down Syndrome, fragile X, or other known genetic conditions).

Groups did not differ in other demographic characteristics. Descriptive data are presented in Table 1. Parents provided informed consent for study participation, and the research was approved by the hospital Institutional Review Board that provided oversight for the ethical treatment of human participants.

2.2. Procedure. We recorded ECG data from a 5-minute baseline period during which children were engaged in a quiet and nonchallenging tabletop activity (determined with consultation with the child's parent). This was followed by a stranger approach procedure similar to methods used in prior developmental research [18]. With the child seated at the table and his or her parent seated behind and slightly to the side, a female experimenter, unfamiliar to the child entered the room and then approached the child in two stages, each lasting 2 minutes. This resulted in an overall stranger approach procedure that was similar in length to the baseline. The comparison of a somewhat longer baseline to shorter stimulus conditions (i.e., 5 min. baseline versus 2 min. stages of the stranger approach) is consistent with prior psychophysiology research in this and other populations (e.g., [11]).

During the procedure, children remained seated at a small table facing towards the door to the room. A developmentally appropriate set toys were on the table during the stranger approach procedure. At the first stage, that we will call the distal stranger approach, the examiner stood near the door to the room while talking with the child's parent (60 seconds) and moved to a mark about half way to the child and continued to chat with the parent (60 seconds; strangers were instructed to participate in "small talk" with the parent, and the parent was briefed beforehand so as to expect this). At the second stage, that we will call the proximal stranger approach, the examiner sat down diagonally across the table from the child and started to talk to the child in a friendly voice (60 seconds) and then leaned in toward the child, gently touching the child on the arms, while talking in a friendly but intrusive manner (60 seconds). The order of these events (baseline, distal stranger, proximal stranger) was the same for all participants. The overall intent of this behavioral assay was to present a friendly but increasingly intrusive social approach of a stranger.

2.3. ECG Acquisition and Processing. ECG data were acquired via three electrodes placed on the child's chest and abdomen. The ECG raw data were recorded, digitized, and stored on a computer hard drive using a system designed to coordinate the collection of physiologic data with video recordings in real time [19]. This system included a Hewlett Packard ECG monitor that recorded R-wave peaks to the nearest millisecond. The ECG monitor output included a set of second by second HR estimates and a separate set of R-R interval data that was used to calculate RSA.

Table 1: Characteristics of the children in the autistic (AUT) and nonautistic (non-AUT) groups.

	AUT	non-AUT	P
Age—mean (SD)	4.3 (1.2)	3.6 (1.0)	ns
Gender (n)			ns
Male	12	7	
Female	3	1	
Race/ethnicity (n)			ns
White	15	7	
Black	0	1	
SES-Hollingshead (n)			ns
Mid/high (levels I–III)	15	7	
Low (levels IV-V)	0	1	
Vineland scores—mean (SD)			
Communication	64.1 (14.6)	73.4 (16.9)	ns
Daily living	56.6 (5.2)	71.4 (10.9)	<.01
Socialization	57.4 (5.1)	74.4 (12.9)	<.01
Motor	66.2 (11.5)	76.4 (15.6)	ns
Vineland composite	56.3 (6.1)	69.3 (14.8)	<.01
IQ estimate—mean (SD)	71.9 (28.7)	75.0 (18.7)	ns

Further offline processing of the ECG signal involved data cleaning and calculation of RSA. Artifact detection and correction was performed using a series of automated algorithms. A moving confidence interval was used to detect RR intervals outside of expected values. Missed or spurious R-waves were in this way detected, flagged, and corrected by linear interpolation. Subsequent processing employed a time-series analysis and a moving polynomial filter to remove low frequency trends in the HR signal. This process removes periodicities in the ECG signal that are outside the frequency range of the respiratory cycle. The resulting measure is one of HRV in the frequency range of respiratory rate. The natural logarithm of heart period variance in this frequency range is a measure of RSA. The computations for RSA utilized the time-series analysis and calculations developed by Porges et al. [20].

2.4. Statistical Analysis. Using these methods, we summarized the mean heart rate (HR) and RSA values for the baseline and stranger approach conditions. We also calculated percent change values for RSA from baseline to distal and proximal stranger approach stages. Moreover, based on our hypotheses, we grouped children into those showing a decrease in RSA from baseline to the distal and proximal stranger conditions and those who did not show a change in RSA or who showed an increase in RSA (i.e., a change score ≥ 0). Changes in RSA were calculated as a percentage change from baseline. t-tests of means were used to compare groups of children on dependent measures of physiology and adaptive behaviors. Tests of the likelihood of children to show physiologic responses to the study conditions were examined with Chi-square tests and McNemar tests of within-subject likelihood of responses.

3. Results

3.1. HR and RSA Differences by Condition. The AUT and non-AUT groups did not differ in mean HR or mean RSA at baseline or during distal or proximal stranger approach conditions. In addition, groups did not differ significantly on the percent change of RSA from baseline to the distal or proximal stranger conditions. These results are reported in Table 2. Individual HR and RSA data points are presented in Table 3. There was one participant in AUT group with high levels of artifact in the RSA signal during stranger approach. The data from this procedure for this child was excluded. Artifactual HR data were found for 3 AUT group children and 2 non-AUT group children. These data points were also excluded from analyses.

3.2. Differences in Likelihood to Show an RSA Response. While the groups did not differ in the mean levels of RSA or percent RSA change, there were individual differences in responses across participants. Within the AUT group, 3 of 14 children with RSA stranger approach data (21%) showed an RSA decrease in response to the distal stranger condition, whereas 9 of these 14 children (64%) showed an RSA decrease in response to the proximal stranger condition. Within the non AUT group, 3 of 8 children (38%) showed an RSA decrease in response to the distal stranger condition, whereas 4 of these 8 children (50%) showed an RSA decrease in response to the proximal stranger condition. Chi square tests of likelihood for responses by group were not significant for either the distal or proximal conditions (Fishers exact tests). However, when comparing likelihood of response across the conditions but within each group, the AUT group was found to be more likely to show an RSA decrease in response to the proximal stranger approach than to the distal stranger approach (McNemar test, $P = .03$). Specifically, 6 of the 11 (55%) AUT children who did not show a response to the distal stranger approach showed an RSA decrease to the proximal stranger approach, and all 3 AUT children who showed an RSA decrease to the distal stranger also showed a proximal stranger-related RSA decrease. This difference in likelihood of response between conditions was not found in the non AUT group.

3.3. Comparison of Responders versus Nonresponders. We classified the AUT subjects into RSA responders versus nonresponders on the basis of RSA decreases from baseline to the proximal stranger condition (i.e., a "responder" was a child whose RSA was lower during the stranger approach than that during baseline). These groups were compared on Vineland Scales standard scores. One subject had missing Vineland data. Therefore, there were 9 responders and 5 non-responders included in these comparisons. AUT children classified as responders had higher Vineland Socialization standard scores than non-responders, $t\ (11) = 2.4$, $P = .03$. Responders did not differ from non-responders on the other Vineland domain scores. These results are reported in Table 4.

TABLE 2: Descriptive data for heart rate (HR) and respiratory sinus arrhythmia (RSA) measures for the autistic (AUT) and nonautistic (non-AUT) groups.

Measure	AUT Mean (SD)	non-AUT Mean (SD)	Effect size $\|d\|$	P
HR				
Baseline	108.93 (13.96)	109.88 (15.43)	0.06	ns
Distal stranger	108.32 (15.34)	109.92 (13.34)	0.11	ns
Proximal stranger	106.06 (16.87)	106.71 (12.87)	0.04	ns
RSA				
Baseline	4.87 (1.55)	4.87 (0.92)	<0.01	ns
Distal stranger	5.33 (1.35)	4.87 (1.07)	0.37	ns
Proximal stranger	4.96 (1.24)	4.76 (1.11)	0.17	ns

4. Discussion

This study revealed differences in patterns of RSA responses to social events of varying degrees of intensity in children with autism compared to controls. Specifically, children with autism were more likely to show a response (a decrease in RSA from baseline) during the intrusive "proximal" stranger approach than during the initial and less intrusive entry of the stranger into the room. This difference in likelihood of response was not seen in the nonautistic group. Because decreases in RSA reflect active response and engagement with the environment, this finding suggests that an increased level of intensity of stimulation or a degree of vigor of interaction is needed to elicit normative physiologic responses in children with autism. Importantly, and consistent with prior work [11], we did not see evidence for heart rate increases in the autistic versus nonautistic group in response to the intrusive stranger approach. Thus, where RSA responses are elicited, they do not appear to be indicative of a "fight-or-flight" sympathetic response to social stimuli.

Individual differences in responses to intrusive social events were associated with social functioning in the children with autism. Autistic children who were physiologically responsive to the proximal stranger approach had better social functioning as measured by the Vineland scales, a parent-report instrument. It is noteworthy that in the group of children with autism, responders and non-responders did not differ on other sections of the Vineland scales. This provides discriminant validity to our findings and suggests that patterns of autonomic responses specifically to people are indicative of levels of social attention that support social behavioral functioning in children with autism. Physiologic responses to social events may be related to behavioral functioning, but the nature of the observational context will affect whether meaningful individual differences are observed. This finding has implications for individualizing educational and behavioral strategies for subgroups of children with autism who are less reactive to the environment as indicated by attenuated RSA responses to social presses. For example, it may be beneficial to individually tailor the degree to which therapeutic interactions vigorously attempt to elicit social responses from children. A relevant question

TABLE 3: Individual data values for RSA and HR for AUT and non-AUT participants.

Subject	RSA values			HR values		
	Baseline	Distal stranger	Proximal stranger	Baseline	Distal stranger	Proximal stranger
AUT group						
AUT1	4.83	5.05	4.58*	118.93	123.58	122.75
AUT2	8.19	8.51	8.19	90.91	86.02	91.01
AUT3	5.31	5.66	4.66*	97.35	99.35	102.49
AUT4	5.86	5.96	4.70*	100.62	97.33	86.74
AUT5	5.74	6.01	6.36	92.23	96.15	92.28
AUT6	6.46	5.99*	5.03*	88.88	90.88	77.99
AUT7	5.72	5.83	5.25*	112.27	110.73	111.47
AUT8	3.12	5.91	5.14	115.67	120.95	118.02
AUT9	3.64	4.26	4.81	124.57	117.79	112.85
AUT10	3.56	3.54	3.35*	125.99	122.55	124.45
AUT11	3.20	a	a	118.871	a	a
AUT12	4.64	4.38*	4.06*	120.92	125.87	124.44
AUT13	5.81	5.63*	5.65*	m	90.16	89.14
AUT14	2.13	2.89	3.22	m	126.87	125.13
AUT15	4.87	5.01	4.38*	m	m	m
non-AUT group						
Non-AUT1	4.65	4.37*	4.79	m	112.62	104.86
Non-AUT2	5.88	6.12	6.20	99.20	96.73	95.69
Non-AUT3	5.01	4.54*	4.30*	114.47	123.51	117.69
Non-AUT4	5.43	3.65*	3.96*	m	113.40	110.16
Non-AUT5	5.40	5.58	5.20*	99.77	103.61	96.41
Non-AUT6	5.59	6.52	6.26	91.80	86.34	87.59
Non-AUT7	3.59	4.30	4.43	131.40	121.38	125.30
Non-AUT8	3.41	3.85	2.97*	122.65	121.80	115.94

*indicates subjects categorized as having an RSA response defined as a decrease in RSA versus baseline.
a indicates missing values due to artifact in the ECG signal.
m indicates missing HR data during technical problem with the HR calculation for this subject.

TABLE 4: Adaptive behavior standard scores for AUT group participants classified as RSA responders versus non-responders to proximal stranger approach.

Vineland domain	Responders Mean (SD)	Nonresponders Mean (SD)	Effect size $\|d\|$	P
Communication	66.63 (15.81)	59.20 (14.36)	0.48	ns
Daily living skills	57.38 (5.78)	54.00 (2.45)	0.70	ns
Socialization skills	59.50 (4.90)	53.40 (3.51)	1.37	.03
Composite score	57.25 (5.95)	54.40 (7.30)	0.44	ns

raised by these results is whether research on physiologic responses can be utilized to validate behavioral indicators, or whether physiologic monitoring can itself augment such individual treatment strategies. This can be seen as consistent with clinical approaches that include attention to managing arousal during treatment [21].

Young children with autism, however, did not differ in their level of RSA during a baseline condition and did not differ in RSA response during an increasingly intrusive stranger approach observation. This negative finding is perhaps related to the small sample size in this study. However, the small effect sizes of group differences and the variability of responses to stranger approach suggest that putative differences in RSA and similar measures of autonomic functioning may be relatively small for children with autism when compared to children matched on age and cognitive abilities. Interestingly, in terms of RSA differences, the largest effect size, although relatively small and statistically nonsignificant, was for the comparison of RSA during the initial distal stranger approach. Here, the children with autism showed a modest RSA increase from baseline, whereas the comparison group showed a modest decrease in RSA from baseline. This could suggest that novel social events, such as initial entry of a new person, are more salient for nonautistic children than for autistic children, although larger samples are needed to determine if such differences are statistically reliable. Some prior studies have found differences between older groups of children with autism and comparison subjects on measures of baseline and task-related heart rate variability. Thus, an additional explanation for our finding of no group difference is that the children observed in this study were fairly young. Because baseline RSA can be expected to increase with age in the early childhood years, group differences in levels of RSA may not be evident until this system matures and RSA approaches adult-like levels [22]. It is also noted that whereas some children showed decreases in RSA relative to baseline, others showed increases in RSA. The interpretation of such increases is unclear, but it is possible that the increases in RSA during tasks or experimental conditions could be attributable to individual differences in how children responded to initial baseline conditions as much as their parasympathetic response to challenge.

These results are preliminary in nature, and there are several limitations to this study that should be discussed. The sample size in this study was small, limiting our statistical power to detect significant differences between groups. A related challenge to this work is the difficulties, both practical and conceptual in nature, in matching on key characteristics. Subject matching in autism research is a common but challenging practice [23]. One of the emerging complexities with subject matching is the heterogeneity of individuals with autism. In the present study, we matched the groups on age and IQ. However, the variability in these characteristics, while similar in the two groups, may add measurement error. Thus, future research may yield different results with more homogenous groupings on age and level of functioning.

5. Conclusions

In this study we report on individual differences in RSA responses to social events in relation to parent-reported social adaptive functioning in children with autism. While children with autism did not differ from controls in RSA reactivity to a social approach paradigm, they were more likely to demonstrate decreased RSA in response to more proximal social interactions. This reactivity to proximal social interactions was related to better social functioning, indicating that individual differences in social competence, along with intensity of a social interaction can discriminate subgroups of children with autism who may show differential responses to graded social interactions. Findings such as these have implications for treatment and suggest that individual differences in thresholds for social responses may indicate therapeutic strategies matched to such characteristics. Clearly, replication and extension of these findings are needed, and future research should also focus on the stability of such response styles within individuals. More generally, and in conclusion, this pilot research suggests that a focus on individual differences in psychophysiologic responses may help to clarify inconsistencies in prior research and would have implications for understanding individual differences in treatment outcomes in this population.

Acknowledgments

The authors wish to thank the families who participated in this study. Portions of the results described in this paper were presented at the International Meeting for Autism Research, Philadelphia, PA, May 2010. This research was supported by the National Alliance for Autism Research (now Autism Speaks) and by NIMH, 1-R03-MH072856-01.

References

[1] W. Hirstein, P. Iversen, and V. S. Ramachandran, "Autonomic responses of autistic children to people and objects," *Proceedings of the Royal Society B*, vol. 268, no. 1479, pp. 1883–1888, 2001.

[2] A. Kylliäinen and J. K. Hietanen, "Skin conductance responses to another person's gaze in children with autism," *Journal of Autism and Developmental Disorders*, vol. 36, no. 4, pp. 517–525, 2006.

[3] T. P. Levine, S. J. Sheinkopf, M. Pescosolido, A. Rodino, G. Elia, and B. Lester, "Physiologic arousal to social stress in children with Autism Spectrum Disorders: a pilot study," *Research in Autism Spectrum Disorders*, vol. 6, no. 1, pp. 177–183, 2012.

[4] M. Toichi and Y. Kamio, "Paradoxical autonomic response to mental tasks in autism," *Journal of Autism and Developmental Disorders*, vol. 33, no. 4, pp. 417–426, 2003.

[5] A. V. Van Hecke, J. Lebow, E. Bal et al., "Electroencephalogram and heart rate regulation to familiar and unfamiliar people in children with autism spectrum disorders," *Child Development*, vol. 80, no. 4, pp. 1118–1133, 2009.

[6] S. W. Porges, "The polyvagal theory: phylogenetic substrates of a social nervous system," *International Journal of Psychophysiology*, vol. 42, no. 2, pp. 123–146, 2001.

[7] M. Althaus, L. J. M. Mulder, G. Mulder, C. C. Aarnoudse, and R. B. Minderaa, "Cardiac adaptivity to attention-demanding tasks in children with a pervasive developmental disorder not otherwise specified (PDD-NOS)," *Biological Psychiatry*, vol. 46, no. 6, pp. 799–809, 1999.

[8] M. Althaus, A. M. Van Roon, L. J. M. Mulder, G. Mulder, C. C. Aarnoudse, and R. B. Minderaa, "Autonomic response patterns observed during the performance of an attention-demanding task in two groups of children with autistic-type difficulties in social adjustment," *Psychophysiology*, vol. 41, no. 6, pp. 893–904, 2004.

[9] C. Kirschbaum, K.-M. Pirke, and D. H. Hellhammer, "The "Trier social stress test"—a tool for investigating psychobiological stress responses in a laboratory setting," *Neuropsychobiology*, vol. 28, no. 1-2, pp. 76–81, 1993.

[10] E. Bal, E. Harden, D. Lamb, A. V. Van Hecke, J. W. Denver, and S. W. Porges, "Emotion recognition in children with autism spectrum disorders: relations to eye gaze and autonomic state," *Journal of Autism and Developmental Disorders*, vol. 40, no. 3, pp. 358–370, 2010.

[11] R. Corona, C. Dissanayake, S. Arbelle, P. Wellington, and M. Sigman, "Is affect aversive to young children with autism? Behavioral and cardiac responses to experimenter distress," *Child Development*, vol. 69, no. 6, pp. 1494–1502, 1998.

[12] M. Sigman, C. Dissanayake, R. Corona, and M. Espinosa, "Social and cardiac responses of young children with autism," *Autism*, vol. 7, no. 2, pp. 205–216, 2003.

[13] M. A. Patriquin, A. Scarpa, B. H. Friedman, and S. W. Porges, "Respiratory sinus arrhythmia: a marker for positive social functioning and receptive language skills in children with autism spectrum disorders," *Developmental Psychobiology*, vol. 55, pp. 101–112, 2013.

[14] C. Lord, S. Risi, L. Lambrecht et al., "The Autism Diagnostic Observation Schedule-Generic: a standard measure of social and communication deficits associated with the spectrum of

autism," *Journal of Autism and Developmental Disorders*, vol. 30, no. 3, pp. 205–223, 2000.

[15] C. D. Elliott, *Differential Ability Scales*, Psychological Corporation, San Antonio, Tex, USA, 1990.

[16] N. Bayley, *Bayley Scales of Infant Development*, Psychological Corporation, San Antonio, Tex, USA, 2nd edition, 1993.

[17] S. S. Sparrow, D. A. Balla, and D. V. Cicchetti, *Vineland Adaptive Behavior Scales*, American Guidance Service, Circle Pines, Minn, USA, 1984.

[18] G. Bohlin and B. Hagekull, "Stranger wariness and sociability in the early years," *Infant Behavior and Development*, vol. 16, no. 1, pp. 53–67, 1993.

[19] B. M. Lester and M. Peucker, "New technology helps scientists study interface of behavior and physiologal activity," *Hewlett-Packard: Advances for Medicine*, vol. 13, pp. 4–6, 1994.

[20] S. W. Porges, "Respiratory sinus arrhythmia: physiological basis, quantitative methods, and clinical implications," in *Cardiorespiratory and Cardiosomatic Psychophysiology*, P. Grossman, K. Janssen, and D. Vaitl, Eds., pp. 101–115, Plenum Press, New York, NY, USA, 1986.

[21] B. M. Prizant, A. M. Wetherby, E. Rubin, A. C. Laurent, and P. J. Rydell, *The SCERTS Model*, Paul H. Brookes, Baltimore, Md, USA, 2006.

[22] M. H. Bornstein and P. E. Suess, "Child and mother cardiac vagal tone: continuity, stability, and concordance across the first 5 years," *Developmental Psychology*, vol. 36, no. 1, pp. 54–65, 2000.

[23] C. B. Mervis and B. P. Klein-Tasman, "Methodological issues in group-matching designs: α levels for control variable comparisons and measurement characteristics of control and target variables," *Journal of Autism and Developmental Disorders*, vol. 34, no. 1, pp. 7–17, 2004.

14

Awareness of Autism in Primary School Teachers

Muhammad Mustafa Arif, Ayesha Niazy, Bilal Hassan, and Farah Ahmed

Department of Community Health Sciences, Ziauddin University, 4/B, Shahrah-e-Ghalib, Block 6, Clifton, Karachi 75600, Pakistan

Correspondence should be addressed to Muhammad Mustafa Arif; mustafa_arif@hotmail.com

Academic Editor: Mikhail V. Pletnikov

Objective. To assess the knowledge and perception of primary school teachers regarding autism in private and public schools of Karachi, Pakistan. *Methods.* A cross-sectional survey was conducted on primary school teachers in different districts of Karachi. A sample size of 170 teachers was selected by purposive sampling. Primary data was collected using self-administered questionnaires. These questions assessed the teacher's knowledge and perception of Autism. Data was entered on SPSS version 20. Frequencies and percentages were taken out for categorical variables. *Results.* Of the total 170 teachers, 85 were from the Private and 85 from Public sector schools. 55% ($n = 94$) of the teachers knew about Autism through the media and only 9% ($n = 15$) had formal training through workshops on Autism. 62% ($n = 105$) of the teachers were of the opinion that Autism is treatable. Majority of the teachers (57%) said that proper training is required for teaching autistic children. *Conclusion.* The knowledge related to Autism in our existing sample has mostly come from the media. Although we cannot undermine the role of media, there is a need to give formal training to teachers regarding the differentiating features of Autism, which in turn will aid in early diagnosis of the disease.

1. Introduction

Autism is a disorder of neural development, characterized by impaired social interaction, communication, and by restricted, repetitive behavior [1]. This condition begins at birth or within the first two-and-a-half years of life. The children affected are perfectly normal in appearance, but they spend their time engaged in puzzling and disturbing behaviors which are markedly different from those of typical children [2].

The cause of autism is not known [3, 4]. Studies suggest that there is a strong genetic basis, but it cannot be traced to a Mendelian (single-gene) mutation or to a single chromosome abnormality [5, 6]. Risk factors for autism include gender, males are three to four times more likely than females to get autism, family history, parents' age, and other disorders such as fragile **x** syndrome, tuberous sclerosis, Tourette's syndrome, and epilepsy [7]. Apart from these, the use of drugs during pregnancy has also been identified as a risk factor. This was evident by a retrospective case study, which showed that maternal valproic acid used during pregnancy caused autism in the newborn [8]. Studies have even suggested the association of congenital rubella with autism [9, 10]. Another relatively frequent medical condition is cerebral palsy [11], in which the rates of children getting autism are high.

People with autism can have very different features or symptoms; thus, health care providers think of autism as a spectrum disorder [3]. Some children with autism make no eye contact and seem aloof, while others may show intermittent engagement with the environment and may make inconsistent eye contact, smile, and hug. Children may also exhibit varying verbal abilities, ranging from being nonverbal to having advanced speech.

Intellectual functioning can vary from mental retardation to superior intellectual functioning in selected areas. Some children with autism showed typical development in certain skills and even showed strengths in specific areas, such as puzzles, art, and music. However, in general, an Autistic child is often withdrawn and spends hours in solitary play [12].

Several screening tools have been developed to aid in early detection of children with autism Spectrum Disorder. The Checklist for autism in Toddlers (CHAT) is a screening tool designed for 18-month-old children in primary care settings. The Modified Checklist for autism in Toddlers (M-CHAT) is a twenty-three-item parent questionnaire for screening children between 16 and 30 months of age to assess their risk for autism spectrum disorder. The pervasive developmental disorder screening test (PDDST) is a parent completed survey that targets children from birth to three years of age [12].

Studies in Asia, Europe, and North America have identified individuals with an autism spectrum disorder with an approximate prevalence of 0.6%–1% of the newborn population [13]. A study conducted in the 50 states in the USA checked the differences amongst them, in terms of identification of autism spectrum disorders [14]. It was concluded that states with better educational and healthcare expenditures were more apt in the diagnosis of autism.

According to Pakistan's country report on autism, the prevalence of the disease in children is reported to be approximately 1 in 120 [15]. The actual reported prevalence of autism is much lower in Pakistan than that in the western world, due to the lack of awareness about it. The general public is unaware of the severity of the disease and how to diagnose it. The object of this study is to determine the level of awareness of autism in Primary school teachers. The results of this study will help schools and organizations increase the awareness levels related to autism, so it can be diagnosed at an early age and intervention can be started accordingly.

2. Materials and Methods

This was a cross-sectional study conducted on Primary School Teachers in different districts of Karachi.

Sample size was calculated to be 160 by keeping confidence interval at 95%, precision at 5%, and prevalence at 1%. Wastage was added and the sample size was inflated to increase the validity of the study. A total of 170 teachers were selected by simple random sampling (SRS). Only the teachers teaching students form grades 1 to 5, with at least three years of teaching experience, were included in the study. Primary data was collected from teachers through questionnaires which assessed the teacher's knowledge of autism.

The questionnaire was designed to assess different aspects of their knowledge such as diagnosis, symptoms, and treatment. Questions regarding symptomalogy of autism were based on the diagnostic criteria by the American Psychiatric Association Diagnostic and Statistical Manual for Mental Disorders, Fourth Edition. After the questionnaires were filled, the data was analyzed using SPSS 20. The teachers were divided into two categories (i.e., private and nonprivate). Frequencies and percentages were taken out for each category. Chi-square test was applied to find out differences between the two categories and P value less than 0.05 was taken as significant.

An average value of the number of correct responses amongst the teachers from both sectors was taken out. These values were then compared using Chi-square test and Fisher exact test, where applicable.

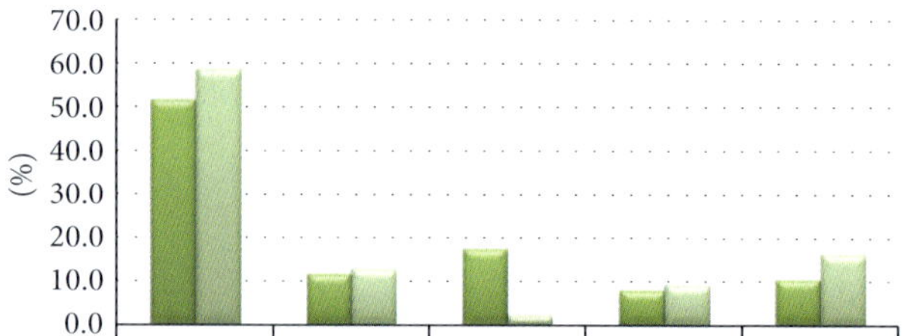

	Media	Personal experience	Workshop	Formal training	Other
Private	51.8%	11.8%	17.6%	8.2%	10.6%
Nonprivate	58.8%	12.9%	2.4%	9.4%	16.5%

FIGURE 1: Source of awareness of autism according to institution type.

3. Results

Data from 170 teachers from private and nonprivate sectors was analyzed. It was determined that 55% ($n = 94$) of the sample had acquired their knowledge of autism through media (see Figure 1). Only 10% ($n = 17$) of the sample had attended formal training whereas 8.8% ($n = 15$) had attended a workshop regarding autism. The source of information regarding autism in the rest of the sample was either from personal experiences or other sources.

The education level of both the private and nonprivate samples was also compared. 33% ($n = 28$) of the sample in the nonprivate sector had an M.S. degree, whereas the remaining had a B.S. degree. Comparing this to the education level of the teachers teaching in the private sector, it was determined that 31% ($n = 26$) had M.S. degree, 60% ($n = 51$) had a B.S. degree, and 9% ($n = 8$) just had a college education.

The questionnaire had 16 questions regarding basic knowledge and perception of autism. The first 13 questions tested the teacher's basic knowledge about autism (see Table 1). Only 22% ($n = 19$) of the teachers in the Private sector and 28% ($n = 24$) of the teachers in the nonprivate sector were aware that autism is an inherited disorder. When inquiring about what type of disorder autism is, 48% ($n = 41$) of the teachers in the Private sector and 46% ($n = 39$) of the teachers in the nonprivate sector recognized the fact that autism is both a learning and a mental disorder.

On comparing responses regarding the knowledge of autism in both categories, we found that there was no statistical significance, except in two categories: communication skills of an Autistic child (P value $= 0.002$) and emotional temperament of an Autistic child (P value $= 0.002$) (see Table 1). Regarding the communication skills of an Autistic child, we saw that teachers in the public sector were better aware that an Autistic child has poor communication skills and cannot express himself. When we analyzed the results of emotional status of an Autistic child, we found out that teachers in the private sector were better aware of autism and recognized the fact that an autistic child throws frequent bouts of rage.

On investigating the perception of autism in both categories (see Figure 2), we found out that P values were significant when teachers were questioned regarding the

TABLE 1: Percentage of correct responses according to the type of institution.

	Private		Nonprivate		*P* value
	n	%	*n*	%	
Autism is an inherited disorder	19	22	24	28	.585
Autism is a learning and mental disorder	41	48	39	46	.954
Signs of Autism show between 0 and 3 years	30	35.3	35	41.2	.104
An autistic child is not social	47	55	57	67	.255
An autistic child has poor communication skills and cannot express himself	45	53	64	75.3	.002
Verbally, an autistic child will have a hard time phrasing a sentence	32	38	51	60	.012
Nonverbally, an autistic child does repetitive gestures to express himself	34	40	26	31	.512
The attention span of an autistic child is deficient	59	69	58	68	.443
General interests of an autistic child are restricted	37	44	43	51	.401
An autistic child maintains minimal eye contact with others	58	68	69	81	.112
General eating habits of an autistic child are normal	22	26	22	26	.081
An autistic child is resistant to change	42	49	53	62	.366
An autistic child throws frequent bouts of anger	45	53	28	33	.002

TABLE 2: Table comparing correct responses among private and nonprivate teachers.

	Total no. of questions (total no. of responses)	Total no. of correct responses *n* (%)	Average no. of correct responses per subject (mean ± SD)	Median no. of correct responses	*P* Value
		Comparison of knowledge			
Private	13 (1105)	496 (44.9%)	5.84 ± 2.75	6	0.058
Non-Private	13 (1105)	563 (51%)	6.62 ± 2.63	7	
Total	**13 (2210)**	**1059 (47.9%)**	**6.23 ± 2.71**	**6.5**	
		Comparison of perception			
Private	3 (255)	86 (33.7%)	1.01 ± 0.764	1	0.058
Non-Private	3 (255)	107 (42%)	1.26 ± 0.915	1	
Total	**6 (510)**	**193 (37.8%)**	**1.14 ± 0.849**	**1**	
		Comparison of knowledge and perception combined			
Private	16 (1360)	582 (42.8%)	6.85 ± 2.89	7	0.029
Non-Private	16 (1360)	670 (49.3%)	7.88 ± 3.23	8	
Total	**16 (2720)**	**1252 (46%)**	**7.36 ± 3.10**	**7**	

treatment of autism using, solely, medication (*P* value = 0.005). Participants in the nonprivate sector had a better perception of the treatment of autism and were aware that it is a condition that is not managed by medication alone, but a combination of medication and different behavioral and cognitive therapies. All the other responses regarding perception of autism had insignificant *P* values.

We then compared the correct responses in both categories (see Table 2). Responses from the 16 questions on knowledge and perception were combined into two categories (i.e., right and wrong) (see Table 2). In the private sector, average no. of correct answers by a participant was 6.85 with a standard deviation of 2.89. This was considerably smaller when compared to the nonprivate sector, where average no. of correct answer per subject was 7.88 with a standard deviation of 3.23. The knowledge and perception scores were then compared using independent sample test

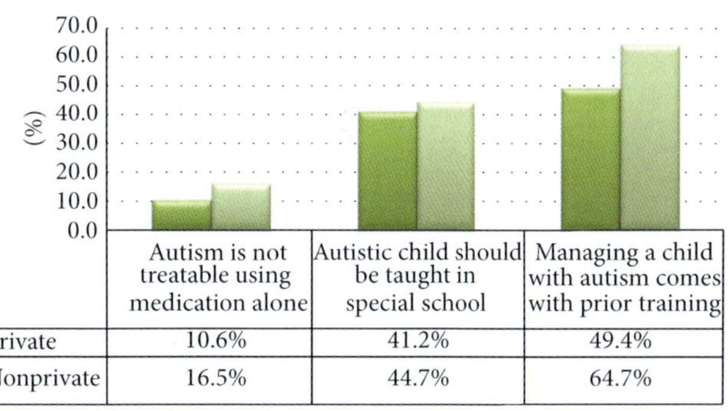

	Autism is not treatable using medication alone	Autistic child should be taught in special school	Managing a child with autism comes with prior training
Private	10.6%	41.2%	49.4%
Nonprivate	16.5%	44.7%	64.7%

FIGURE 2: Perception of autism according to institution type.

which showed significant (*P* value = 0.029) difference. Thus, we concluded that the teachers in the nonprivate sector had better knowledge and perception regarding autism when compared with their counterparts in the private sector.

4. Discussion

Autism is currently diagnosed in approximately 1 out of every 150 children [13]. With increasing prevalence of this condition, more awareness is needed amongst the population to diagnose it at an early age so that therapy can be initiated.

A study conducted in Singapore [16], amongst 503 preschool teachers, displayed the deficiency of teachers regarding knowledge, attitudes, and practices on childhood developmental and behavioral disorders. Similarly, in our study, we saw that, out of all the responses on knowledge, only 47.9% of the responses were correct. This clearly displayed the fact that majority of the population is not aware of the basic facts about autism.

Diagnosis of autism at an early age is highly beneficial in the intellectual development of the child. Early diagnosis of the disease enables initiation of appropriate therapy in children, aiding in their development. Teachers play a vital role in interaction with a child during the early years of life. Their ability to pick out Autistic children in the classroom will be beneficial on the long term.

Management of autism includes a combination of medication plus behavioral and cognitive therapies [17]. A clinical trial conducted by Ghanizadeh and Moghimi-Sarani [18] concluded that risperidone and acetylcysteine, in combination, decreased irritability in children with autism but had no effect on the core symptoms of autism. Similarly, in a systemic review of medications commonly used to treat autism, it was seen that although medications are commonly used for treatment of autism, there is little evidence of effectiveness of these treatments [19].

A catalogue published by the Illinois Weselan University [20] in 2005 greatly emphasizes the role of teacher training in management of autism Spectrum Disorders in infancy. In our study, even though 57% ($n = 91$) of the teachers realized the importance of getting prior training when dealing with children with autism, only 8% ($n = 7$) of teachers in the private sector and 9% ($n = 8$) of the teachers in the nonprivate sector had attended formal training on autism. This clearly displays the lack of training opportunities regarding autism for teachers.

The Ministry of Education, British Columbia [21] published a resource book for teachers dealing with autism in 2000. Multiple tools were given to help teachers when facing Autistic children. When the tool was used by teachers on Autistic children, they showed marked intellectual improvement and coped up well with the school work. A few of the kids also started attending a normal school later. This again emphasizes the fact that through proper training of teachers we can greatly improve the quality of education of autistic children and improve their intellectual ability.

Eldevik et al. [22], in 2012, reported favorable outcomes in children undergoing behavioral interventions in mainstream preschool settings compared to children who were receiving normal treatments. He reported that students in preschool settings had better IQ scores and better adaptive techniques.

5. Conclusion

Our research clearly elaborates the lack of awareness amongst teachers regarding autism. We suggest that schools implement proper training programs for teachers to train them in diagnosing Autistic children and then teach them accordingly.

References

[1] American Psychiatric Association, *Diagnostic and Statistical Manual of Mental Disorders*, 4th edition, 2000.

[2] "Is it autism?" Autism Research institute, http://www.autism.com/index.php/is_it_autism.

[3] Autism: Mediline Plus, http://www.nlm.nih.gov/medlineplus/autism.html.

[4] C. J. Newschaffer, L. A. Croen, J. Daniels et al., "The epidemiology of autism spectrum disorders," *Annual Review of Public Health*, vol. 28, pp. 235–258, 2007.

[5] B. S. Abrahams and D. H. Geschwind, "Advances in autism genetics: on the threshold of a new neurobiology," *Nature Reviews Genetics*, vol. 9, no. 5, pp. 341–355, 2008.

[6] R. Muhle, S. V. Trentacoste, and I. Rapin, "The genetics of autism," *Pediatrics*, vol. 113, no. 5, pp. e472–e486, 2004.

[7] Mayo Clinic, mayoclinic.com/health/autism/DS00348/DSECTION=symptoms.

[8] G. Williams, J. King, M. Cunningham, M. Stephan, B. Kerr, and J. H. Hersh, "Fetal valproate syndrome and autism: additional evidence of an association," *Developmental Medicine and Child Neurology*, vol. 43, no. 3, pp. 202–206, 2001.

[9] S. Chess, P. Fernandez, and S. Korn, "Behavioral consequences of congenital rubella," *Journal of Pediatrics*, vol. 93, no. 4, pp. 699–703, 1978.

[10] B. E. Berger, A. M. Navar-Boggan, and S. B. Omer, "Congenital rubella syndrome and autism spectrum disorder prevented by rubella vaccination—United States, 2001-2010," *BMC Public Health*, vol. 11, article 340, 2011.

[11] E. Fombonne, "The prevalence of autism," *Journal of the American Medical Association*, vol. 289, no. 1, pp. 87–89, 2003.

[12] R. M. Kliegman, R. E. Beahrman, H. B. Jenson, and B. M. D. Stanton, *Nelson Textbook of Paedriatics*, vol. 1, 2007.

[13] CDC—Data and Statistics, "Autism spectrum disorders," http://www.cdc.gov/ncbddd/autism/data.html.

[14] D. S. Mandell and R. Palmer, "Differences among states in the identification of autistic spectrum disorders," *Archives of Pediatrics and Adolescent Medicine*, vol. 159, no. 3, pp. 266–269, 2005.

[15] M. A. Khan, Pakistan Country Report-Autism.

[16] W. B. Lian, S. H. K. Ying, S. C. H. Tean, D. C. K. Lin, Y. C. Lian, and H. L. Yun, "Pre-school teachers' knowledge, attitudes and practices on childhood developmental and behavioural disorders in Singapore," *Journal of Paediatrics and Child Health*, vol. 44, no. 4, pp. 187–194, 2008.

[17] S. M. Myers, C. P. Johnson, P. H. Lipkin et al., "Management of children with autism spectrum disorders," *Pediatrics*, vol. 120, no. 5, pp. 1162–1182, 2007.

[18] A. Ghanizadeh and E. Moghimi-Sarani, "A randomized double blind placebo controlled clinical trial of N-Acetylcysteine added to risperidone for treating autistic disorders," *BMC Psychiatry*, vol. 13, article 196, 2013.

[19] M. L. McPheeters, Z. Warren, N. Sathe et al., "A systematic review of medical treatments for children with autism spectrum disorders," *Pediatrics*, vol. 127, no. 5, pp. e1312–e1321, 2011.

[20] Amber Hays, "Parent-teacher collaboration for students with autism spectrum disorders: the role of teacher training," Honors Projects, Paper 9, 2005, http://digitalcommons.iwu.edu/psych_honproj/9.

[21] *Teaching Students with Autism—A Resource Guide for Schools*, Special Programs Branch, Ministry Of Education, British Columbia, 2000.

[22] S. Eldevik, R. P. Hastings, E. Jahr, and J. C. Hughes, "Outcomes of behavioral intervention for children with autism in mainstream pre-school settings," *Journal of Autism and Developmental Disorders*, vol. 42, no. 2, pp. 210–220, 2012.

15

Disability Identification and Self-Efficacy among College Students on the Autism Spectrum

Paul T. Shattuck,[1] Jessica Steinberg,[2] Jennifer Yu,[3] Xin Wei,[3] Benjamin P. Cooper,[2] Lynn Newman,[3] and Anne M. Roux[1]

[1] *A. J. Drexel Autism Institute, Drexel University, 3020 Market Street, Suite 560, Philadelphia, PA 19104, USA*
[2] *Washington University, One Brookings Drive, St. Louis, MO 63130, USA*
[3] *SRI International, 333 Ravenswood Avenue, BS169, Menlo Park, CA 94025-3493, USA*

Correspondence should be addressed to Paul T. Shattuck; pts33@drexel.edu

Academic Editor: Geraldine Dawson

The number of youth on the autism spectrum approaching young adulthood and attending college is growing. Very little is known about the subjective experience of these college students. Disability identification and self-efficacy are two subjective factors that are critical for the developmental and logistical tasks associated with emerging adulthood. This study uses data from the National Longitudinal Transition Study 2 to examine the prevalence and correlates of disability identification and self-efficacy among college students on the autism spectrum. Results indicate nearly one-third of these students do not report seeing themselves as disabled or having a special need. Black race was associated with lower likelihood of both disability identification and self-efficacy.

1. Introduction

Approximately 50,000 youth on the autism spectrum turn 18 years old each year, a proxy indicator for the number entering adulthood. About 35%, or 17,500 youth on the autism spectrum per year, go on to attend college within the first six years after high school [1]. Of the youth on the autism spectrum who attend college, about 34% choose a major in science, technology, engineering, or math (STEM). This rate of STEM majoring is significantly higher than that seen in any other disability category and also higher than the 23% rate seen in the general population [2, 3]. In the broader context of a competitive global economy, the subset of students who pursue STEM majors are especially important to consider.

Some research has documented how the core challenges of autism spectrum disorder (ASD)—difficulty maintaining the reciprocal interaction essential to learning, poor nonverbal communication, and a limited ability to understand and use the rules of social behavior—may limit success in college [4–6]. However, very few studies have examined subjective perceptions of self among postsecondary college students on the autism spectrum. This fact is at odds with the current federal priority to promote ASD research that emphasizes understanding the insights, personal experiences, and perspectives of people on the autism spectrum [7].

Two important components of self-perception that are central to the developmental challenges of transitioning from adolescence to emerging adulthood are identity formation and self-efficacy [8–10]. Identity refers to one's self-image and has multiple facets including racial and ethnic identity, gender identity, and disability identity. Identity formation is a dynamic, nuanced, multidimensional, and lifelong process that takes on particular importance during emerging adulthood when questions about life purpose and direction move to the foreground [11, 12]. The emergent sense of identity during this period has ramifications for decision making related to college majors, persistence to degree completion, career choices, and relationship formation.

Particularly salient for emerging adults on the autism spectrum is disability identity. The literature regarding disability and identity includes complex definitions and debates about the social versus medical model of disability and what it truly means to be "disabled" [13–15]. Clearly, identity formation is a highly nuanced topic. For the purposes of this exploratory paper, we rely on a self-report measure of seeing oneself as having a disability or special need. We argue that this singular dimension of disability identity is more appropriately referred to as "disability identification." We were not able to find studies focusing on disability identity or identification exclusively among college students on the autism spectrum. We did find one report that described rates of disability identification among a sample of postsecondary youth (a mix of college students and nonstudents) with a variety of disability types [16]. Approximately three-quarters (76.1%) of youth on the autism spectrum in that study considered themselves individuals with a disability, but this rate was not broken out for college students.

Self-efficacy refers to one's perceived ability to do things for one's self and be successful [8]. A strong sense of self-efficacy has been recognized in developmental research as a component of resilience and an asset that helps foster healthy development [10]. Studies have shown a connection between a student's sense of self-efficacy and positive postsecondary education outcomes, such as higher grade-point averages and persistence [17–20], and specifically for completion rates and grades in STEM fields [21–23]. Although these studies draw a clear connection between self-efficacy and postsecondary success, there are very few studies that look at the issue for students on the autism spectrum.

Prior research has found that self-efficacy beliefs among STEM students with disabilities are malleable and have a reciprocally influential relationship with academic success and persistence [24]. Exploring the association between STEM majoring and self-efficacy is an important step toward a better understanding of which factors might promote success in a segment of the ASD population who could be especially valuable contributors to the national economy.

Study Aims. This exploratory study is one of the first of its kind to consider the subjective experiences of college students on the autism spectrum by examining disability identification and self-efficacy. In this study we use data from a large national survey to examine two questions. First, what are the distributions of disability identification and self-efficacy in college students on the autism spectrum? Second, what are the correlates of disability identification and self-efficacy in this group?

Given the lack of prior research on these topics among college students on the autism spectrum, we opted to examine a small set of correlates that were available in this secondary data set and are known to be significantly associated with a range of postsecondary outcomes for young adults on the autism spectrum: sex, race, household income, functional skills, and STEM major [1, 25–28]. Difficulty with social communication, another covariate in this study, is a defining feature of ASDs and is a consistently strong predictor of variability in adult outcomes [29].

2. Methods

2.1. Ethics Statement. Use of these data is governed by a data use agreement with the US Department of Education and was deemed exempt by the Drexel University Institutional Review Board.

2.2. Study Sample. Data for this study came from the National Longitudinal Transition Study 2 (NLTS2) conducted by SRI International under contract with the U.S. Department of Education. The NLTS2 was conducted over 5 waves, each 2 years apart, from 2001 to 2009. At baseline, all youth were ages 13–16 years old and receiving special education services. The NLTS2 began with over 11,000 students, including 920 in the autism special education category.

The NLTS2 used a nationally representative two-stage sampling design. Local education agencies (LEAs) were sampled first followed by selection of students from special education enrollment rosters. Weighted estimates generalize to the national population of youth who had been receiving special education services at baseline [30]. Full details of the sampling strategy for NLTS2 were previously published [31]. The dependent variables for the current study are from the youth survey at wave 5, collected in 2009. This wave of NLTS2 had the largest number of postsecondary youth available for analysis. Unweighted sample numbers in this report were rounded to the nearest ten, as required by the US Department of Education.

For the sake of official special education enrollment reports, each student is counted only once in a primary disability category. Autism is one of twelve primary disabilities reporting categories mandated by the Individuals with Disabilities Education Act (IDEA) and included in the NLTS2. Each student's eligibility for special education services was determined by the school district from whose roster the student was sampled. Population-based research in the US has consistently found that the vast majority (>95%) of children receiving special education services in the autism category also meet *DSM-IV*-based case criteria for an ASD [32, 33].

There were approximately 660 participants identified in the autism category at the beginning of the NLTS2 who remained as participants at wave 5. Approximately 190 of these 660 youth had attended either a 2-year or 4-year college at some point since exiting high school. The total number of college attendees with valid values on all dependent measures was approximately 120—the total N for this study. Some only attended a 4-year college (13.9%). The rest either only attended a 2-year college (42.0%) or attended both 2- and 4-year colleges (44.1%) during the first eight years after high school. They ranged in age from 21 to 25 years old.

2.3. Dependent Measures

Disability Identification. The NLTS2 Youth Survey included a yes/no question about disability identification—"Some people have a disability or special need that makes it hard for them to do some things. Do you consider yourself to have any kind of disability or special need?"

Self-Efficacy. Valid self-efficacy questions should be phrased in ways that ask about a person's perceived capability—what they believe they can do or know how to do [34]. We carefully reviewed all NLTS2 Youth Survey questions to find items that were either worded very similarly to items from validated self-efficacy scales or had high face validity based on Bandura's guidelines for the construction of self-efficacy measures [34]. We found three questions asking youth how well each statement described him/herself: (1) "You can handle most things that come your way," (2) "You know how to get information you need," and (3) "You can get school staff and other adults to listen to you." For each statement, the ordinal responses were (1) not at all like me, (2) a little like me, and (3) very much like me. Question 1 is nearly identical to an item from Schwarzer's widely used Generalized Self-Efficacy scale: "I can usually handle whatever comes my way" [35]. Asking about perceived ability to obtain needed information is commonly used in measures of self-efficacy among patients and students [34, 36]. Asking about perceived ability to be assertive and communicate effectively with teachers and adults is also common in measures of student self-efficacy [34].

2.4. Covariates. College major was split into STEM and not-STEM. STEM majors included computer science/information technology, engineering, mathematics, and other hard sciences such as biology, physics, and chemistry. Demographic covariates included sex, race, and household income. The income variable was collapsed into 4 ordinal categories for stratifying the descriptive point estimates and then rescaled to increments of $10,000 for the regression models to make odds ratios and coefficients interpretable as the estimated unit change in each dependent variable per $10,000 change in income. A 3-category, parent-report ordinal variable measured how well each youth can carry on a conversation: (1) "Does not carry on a conversation at all" or "Has a lot of trouble carrying conversation," (2) "Has a little trouble carrying conversation," and (3) "Has no trouble carrying conversation." A functional skills scale was constructed by summing eight 4-category (not at all well, not very well, pretty well, and very well) parent-report questions about how well a youth could do the following tasks without help: tell time on an analog clock, read and understand common signs, count change, look up telephone numbers and use a telephone, get to places outside the home, use public transportation, buy own clothes at a store, and arrange a plane or train trip (Cronbach's alpha = 0.85 in the ASD group).

2.5. Data Analysis. Rates of missing data per covariate ranged from 0% to 15%, with two variables missing more than 10% (functional skills scale 11%; income 15%). Missing covariates were imputed using sequential regression in IVEware (version 0.1) to create 50 sets of data with no missing values [37, 38].

All reported estimates were weighted and variances adjusted to account for the complex sampling and the multiple imputations using the "mi svy" procedures available in Stata v12 which uses standard methods for combining estimates in the analysis of multiply imputed data [39]. Univariate point estimates and 95% confidence intervals were computed for describing the independent and dependent variables (Table 1). A logistic regression model estimated the adjusted association between correlates and the disability identification indicator (Table 2). Linear regression models estimated the adjusted associations with each ordinal self-efficacy item. We also estimated these models using an ordinal logistic method and found no differences in which covariates were found to be significantly associated with outcomes. We chose to report the linear regression findings for ease of interpretation.

Table 1: Characteristics of college students on the autism spectrum.

Variable	Percentages (95% confidence interval)
Male	85.2 (65.0, 94.7)
Race	
White	83.3 (70.0, 91.5)
Black	8.8 (4.4, 16.6)
Other race	7.9 (2.4, 22.6)
Parent or guardian household income	
Up to $25,000	7.7 (3.7, 15.3)
$25,001–$50,000	16.3 (7.9, 30.2)
$50,001–$75,000	38.7 (25.7, 53.5)
More than $75,000	37.3 (22.2, 55.3)
How well youth converses	
No ability/lot of trouble	7.7 (4.0, 14.3)
Little trouble	66.2 (52.9, 77.3)
No trouble	26.2 (16.1, 39.5)
Had a STEM major	40.8 (25.8, 57.9)
Dependent measures	
Disability identification (youth considers self to have a disability or special need)	69.4 (57.6, 79.1)
Self-efficacy indicators	
(1) "You can handle most things that come your way"	
Not at all like me	4.3 (2.1, 8.5)
A little like me	54.8 (42.1, 66.9)
Very much like me	40.9 (29.8, 53.1)
(2) "You know how to get information you need"	
Not at all like me	2.7 (1.2, 6.1)
A little like me	25.2 (14.9, 39.3)
Very much like me	72.1 (58.4, 82.7)
(3) "You can get school staff and other adults to listen to you"	
Not at all like me	5.5 (2.8, 10.6)
A little like me	22.8 (14.4, 34.0)
Very much like me	71.7 (60.1, 81.0)

Source: National Longitudinal Transition Study 2.
Notes: number of multiply imputed data sets = 50. Weighted to population levels. Variances adjusted for sampling method.

TABLE 2: Regression model results.

Covariate	Disability identification (logistic regression odds ratios)	Self-efficacy (linear regression coefficients)		
		"You can handle most things that come your way"	"You know how to get information you need"	"You can get school staff and other adults to listen to you"
STEM major	0.7	-0.3^{*}	0.1	0.0
Male	0.5	$0.4^{!}$	-0.3^{*}	−0.1
Race				
White	Reference	Reference	Reference	Reference
Black	0.1^{*}	−0.1	−0.1	-0.5^{**}
Other race	0.9	−0.2	−0.3	−0.1
Parent or guardian household income ($10 K increments)	1.0	0	0	0
Conversation ability	0.6	0.3^{*}	0.3^{**}	0.1
Functional skills scale	$0.9^{!}$	0.0	0.0	0.0
"You can handle most things that come your way"	0.6			
"You know how to get information you need"	0.5			
"You can get school staff and other adults to listen to you"	1.9			
Disability identification		−0.1	−0.1	0.1

$^{!}P < 0.10$, $^{*}P < 0.05$, $^{**}P < 0.01$.
Source: National Longitudinal Transition Study 2.
Notes: number of multiply imputed data sets = 50. Weighted to population levels. Variances adjusted for sampling method.

Given the small sample size and the exploratory nature of our research aims we chose an alpha level of 0.10 for indicating statistical significance in tables. This choice decreases the likelihood of making a Type II Error (i.e., determining there is no effect in the population when there really is) while increasing the likelihood of making a Type I Error (i.e., determining there is an effect in the population when there really is not). Readers should interpret findings of statistical significance with caution.

3. Results

Reviewing the characteristics of the population of youth on the autism spectrum who attended either a 2-year or 4-year college or university since leaving high school (Table 1), these youth were more likely to be male (85.2%) and were concentrated in the higher income categories (38.7% with income $50,001–$75,000 and 37.3% with family income >$75,000).

Approximately two-thirds (69.4%) of youth on the autism spectrum considered themselves to have a disability or special need. Overall, college students on the autism spectrum reported a high level of confidence in their ability to "get information they needed" and "getting school staff and other adults to listen to them" (approximately 72% reported these statements described them "very much"), but lower confidence for "can handle most things that come their way" with only 40.9% reporting "very much."

Regression model results (Table 2) revealed that the odds of disability identification were significantly lower among blacks and those with higher functional skills. Believing "one can handle most things that come their way" was significantly lower among STEM majors but higher among males and those with better conversation ability. Belief in being able to get needed information was lower in males but higher among those with better conversation ability. Belief in being able to get people to listen was lower among blacks (versus whites). Identity and self-efficacy measures were not significantly associated with each other in these models.

4. Discussion

Several important findings emerged from this study. Approximately one-third of college students on the autism spectrum do not consider themselves to have a disability or special need. Some colleges are now offering support programs targeted at students on the autism spectrum [40, 41]. If students are required to self-identify as being on the autism spectrum before qualifying for services then this may unintentionally exclude a large proportion of those in need. Colleges might consider options for reducing stigma by creating services to support social and academic success that are marketed to all students without requiring students to "out" themselves with respect to disability status. This is already done at many colleges for general academic tutoring and help with writing.

There can be both costs and benefits to accepting or rejecting disability identity. Lower rates of mental health problems have been associated with rejecting disability identity [42]. However, to succeed in college, many students on the autism spectrum will need supportive services and accommodations [43], and college students generally need to disclose and document their disability in order to receive accommodations and services through a college's disability services program. Strategically presenting one's disability is a key factor in obtaining disability services at postsecondary institutions [44, 45]. The transition planning process during high school needs to include a clear exploration of the potential pros and cons of disability disclosure on an individualized basis.

Less than half of college students on the autism spectrum expressed a high degree of global expectancy that they could "handle most things that come their way." However, self-efficacy was higher on measures of getting information needs met and getting people to listen. Controlling for other factors, better conversation ability was significantly associated with higher self-efficacy on two measures: handling most things and getting needed information. Blacks had a lower likelihood of seeing themselves as disabled and a lower self-efficacy rating related to getting others to listen. This particular finding underscores the importance of examining racial disparities, a topic that has frequently been ignored by research on outcomes and services for adults on the autism spectrum [46]. Together, these findings suggest the need for interventions to improve self-efficacy and an understanding of disability identification, especially among blacks and those with more severe impairments.

Students with STEM majors reported lower self-efficacy on the measure of being able to "handle most things that come their way." At first glance, this might seem to suggest STEM majors on the autism spectrum need to be targeted for supportive assistance. However, a recent study found that ASD students in STEM majors who only attended a 2-year college had a higher likelihood of persisting compared with their non-STEM ASD peers [2]. This counter-intuitive finding about self-efficacy and college persistence among STEM majors deserves further investigation. It could be that there are aspects of participating in a STEM major that buffer the impact of lower self-efficacy. It is also possible that STEM majoring presents students with greater challenges than non-STEM majoring, thereby lowering the sense of self-efficacy.

Future research should examine whether the students who do not self-report having a disability truly believe they have no disability or simply do not wish to acknowledge their disability in the context of a survey. Furthermore, there needs to be a careful examination of the link between disability identification and the formal disability disclosure and self-advocacy required to receive needed supports and accommodations during college.

We acknowledge several limitations of these findings. Self-efficacy has been measured many different ways in past research. As noted, we carefully selected three questions based on face validity and consistency with questions from validated instruments. However, we cannot tell with absolute certainty the degree to which they correspond with validated measures of self-efficacy. Our results cannot directly support a directional causal conclusion about the relationship between communication skills and self-efficacy. Additionally, disability identification was measured at one point in time. However, self-report of having a disability may not be temporally stable. The analysis plan was constrained by the list of covariates available in the data set—an inherent challenge when working with secondary data. Finally, the NLTS2 sampling approach made it impossible to examine the experiences of youth on the autism spectrum who did not participate in special education during high school compared to who did so but under a different reporting category than autism.

Strengths of this study include the nationally representative nature of the data, yielding population-level results reflective of the socioeconomic diversity of college students with ASD. A unique strength of this report is the use of self-report data to learn more about the subjective experience of this population.

Disclaimer

This paper's contents are solely the responsibility of the authors and do not represent the views of the National Institute of Mental Health, the Institute for Educational Sciences, or other funders.

Acknowledgments

This work was supported by funding to Dr. Shattuck from the Emch Foundation, Autism Speaks, the National Science Foundation (HRD-1130088), and the National Institute of Mental Health (R01 MH086489), and to Dr. Newman from the Institute for Educational Sciences (R305A120300).

References

[1] P. T. Shattuck, S. C. Narendorf, B. Cooper, P. R. Sterzing, M. Wagner, and J. L. Taylor, "Postsecondary education and employment among youth with an autism spectrum disorder," *Pediatrics*, vol. 129, no. 6, pp. 1042–1049, 2012.

[2] X. Wei, E. R. A. Christiano, J. W. Yu, J. Blackorby, P. Shattuck, and L. A. Newman, "Postsecondary pathways and persistence for STEM versus non-STEM majors: among college students with an Autism Spectrum Disorder," *Journal of Autism and Developmental Disorders* , 2013.

[3] S. Baron-Cohen, S. Wheelwright, A. Burtenshaw, and E. Hobson, "Mathematical talent is linked to autism," *Human Nature*, vol. 18, no. 2, pp. 125–131, 2007.

[4] D. R. Banda and R. M. J. Kubina, "Increasing academic compliance with mathematics tasks using the high-preference strategy with a student with autism," *Preventing School Failure*, vol. 54, no. 2, pp. 81–85, 2010.

[5] D. R. Banda, J. T. Neisworth, and D. L. Lee, "High-probability request sequences and young children: enhancing compliance," *Child and Family Behavior Therapy*, vol. 25, no. 2, pp. 17–29, 2003.

[6] J. B. Donaldson and D. Zager, "Mathematics interventions for students with high functioning Autism/Asperger's Syndrome," *TEACHING Exceptional Children*, vol. 42, no. 6, pp. 40–46, 2010.

[7] Interagency Autism Coordinating Committee, "Strategic plan for autism spectrum disorder research," Department

of Health and Human Services Interagency Autism Coordinating Committee, 2011, http://iacc.hhs.gov/strategic-plan/2011/index.shtml.

[8] A. Bandura, *Self-Efficacy: The Exercise of Control*, Worth, New York, NY, USA, 1997.

[9] E. Erikson, *Identity: Youth and Crisis*, W.W. Norton & Company, New York, NY, USA, 1968.

[10] N. Zarrett and J. Eccles, "The passage to adulthood: challenges of late adolescence," *New Directions for Youth Development*, vol. 2006, no. 111, pp. 13–28, 2006.

[11] J. J. Arnett, "Emerging adulthood: a theory of development from the late teens through the twenties," *American Psychologist*, vol. 55, no. 5, pp. 469–480, 2000.

[12] J. J. Arnett, *Emerging Adulthood: The Winding Road from the Late Teens through the Twenties*, Oxford University Press, New York, NY, USA, 2004.

[13] M. Oliver, "Defining impairment and disability: issues at stake. Exploring the divide: illness and disability," 1996, http://www.disability.co.uk/sites/default/files/resources/ex%20div%20ch3.pdf.

[14] T. Shakespeare and N. Watson, "The social model of disability: an outdated ideology?" *Research in Social Science and Disability*, vol. 2, pp. 9–28, 2001.

[15] N. Watson, "Well, I know this is going to sound very strange to you, but I don't see myself as a disabled person: identity and disability," *Disability & Society*, vol. 17, no. 5, pp. 509–527, 2002.

[16] L. Newman, M. Wagner, A.-M. Knokey et al., "The post-high school outcomes of young adults with disabilities up to 8 years after high school: a report from the National Longitudinal Transition Study-2 (NLTS2)," NCSER 2011-3005, National Center for Special Education Research, 2011.

[17] S. J. Dewitz, M. L. Woolsey, and W. B. Walsh, "College student retention: an exploration of the relationship between self-efficacy beliefs and purpose in life among college students," *Journal of College Student Development*, vol. 50, no. 1, pp. 19–34, 2009.

[18] M. Vuong, S. Brown-Welty, and S. Tracz, "The effects of self-efficacy on academic success of first-generation college sophomore students," *Journal of College Student Development*, vol. 51, no. 1, pp. 50–64, 2010.

[19] A. Zajacova, S. M. Lynch, and T. J. Espenshade, "Self-efficacy, stress, and academic success in college," *Research in Higher Education*, vol. 46, no. 6, pp. 677–706, 2005.

[20] P. A. Gore Jr., "Academic self-efficacy as a predictor of college outcomes: two incremental validity studies," *Journal of Career Assessment*, vol. 14, no. 1, pp. 92–115, 2006.

[21] S. Larose, C. F. Ratelle, F. Guay, C. Senécal, and M. Harvey, "Trajectories of science self-efficacy beliefs during the college transition and academic and vocational adjustment in science and technology programs," *Educational Research and Evaluation*, vol. 12, no. 4, pp. 373–393, 2006.

[22] M. Soldner, H. Rowan-Kenyon, K. K. Inkelas, J. Garvey, and C. Robbins, "Supporting students' intentions to persist in STEM disciplines: the role of living-learning programs among other social-cognitive factors," *The Journal of Higher Education*, vol. 83, no. 3, pp. 311–336, 2012.

[23] M. K. Di Benedetto and H. Bembenutty, "Within the pipeline: self-regulated learning, self-efficacy, and socialization among college students in science courses," *Learning and Individual Differences*, vol. 23, pp. 218–224, 2013.

[24] R. J. Jenson, A. N. Petri, A. D. Day, K. Z. Truman, and K. Duffy, "Perceptions of self-efficacy among STEM students with disabilities," *Journal of Postsecondary Education and Disability*, vol. 24, no. 4, pp. 269–283, 2011.

[25] P. T. Shattuck, M. Wagner, S. Narendorf, P. Sterzing, and M. Hensley, "Post-high school service use among young adults with an autism spectrum disorder," *Archives of Pediatrics and Adolescent Medicine*, vol. 165, no. 2, pp. 141–146, 2011.

[26] G. I. Orsmond, P. T. Shattuck, B. P. Cooper, P. R. Sterzing, and K. A. Anderson, "Social participation among young adults with an autism spectrum disorder," *Journal of Autism and Developmental Disorders*, vol. 43, no. 11, pp. 2710–2719, 2013.

[27] A. M. Roux, P. T. Shattuck, B. P. Cooper, K. A. Anderson, M. Wagner, and S. C. Narendorf, "Postsecondary employment experiences among young adults with an autism spectrum disorder," *Journal of the American Academy of Child and Adolescent Psychiatry*, vol. 52, no. 9, pp. 931–939, 2013.

[28] K. A. Anderson, P. T. Shattuck, B. P. Cooper, A. M. Roux, and M. Wagner, "Prevalence and correlates of postsecondary residential status among young adults with an autism spectrum disorder," *Autism*.

[29] P. Howlin and P. Moss, "Adults with autism spectrum disorders," *Canadian Journal of Psychiatry*, vol. 57, no. 5, pp. 275–283, 2012.

[30] "National Longitudinal Transition Study II," (NLTS2) Sampling Plan, SRI International, Menlo Park, Calif, USA, 2000.

[31] M. Wagner, K. Kutash, A. J. Duchnowski, and M. H. Epstein, "The special education elementary longitudinal study and the national longitudinal transition study: study designs and implications for children and youth with emotional disturbance," *Journal of Emotional & Behavioral Disorders*, vol. 13, no. 1, pp. 25–41, 2005.

[32] J. Bertrand, A. Mars, C. Boyle, F. Bove, M. Yeargin-Allsopp, and P. Decoufle, "Prevalence of autism in a United States population: the Brick Township, New Jersey, investigation," *Pediatrics*, vol. 108, no. 5, pp. 1155–1161, 2001.

[33] M. Yeargin-Allsopp, C. Rice, T. Karapurkar, N. Doernberg, C. Boyle, and C. Murphy, "Prevalence of autism in a US metropolitan area," *Journal of the American Medical Association*, vol. 289, no. 1, pp. 49–55, 2003.

[34] A. Bandura, *Guide for Constructing Self-Efficacy Scales. Self-Efficacy Beliefs of Adolescents*, Information Age Publishing, Charlotte, NC, USA, 2006.

[35] R. Schwarzer and M. Jerusalem, "Generalized Self-Efficacy scale," in *Measures in Health Psychology: A User's Portfolio. Causal and Control Beliefs*, J. Weinman, S. Wright, and M. Johnston, Eds., Windsor, UK, 1995.

[36] K. Lorig, P. Stewart, V. González, D. Laurent, and J. Lynch, *Outcome Measures for Health Education and Other Health Care Interventions*, Sage, Thousand Oaks, Calif, USA, 1996.

[37] T. Raghunathan, J. Lepkowski, J. Van Hoewyk, and P. Solenberger, "A multivariate technique for multiply imputing missing values using a sequence of regression models," *Survey Methodology*, vol. 27, no. 1, pp. 85–95, 2001.

[38] "IVEware: Imputation and Variance Estimation Software," Survey Methodology Program, Survey Research Center, Institute for Social Research, University of Michigan, Ann Arbor, Mich, USA, 2002.

[39] D. Rubin, *Multiple Imputation for Nonresponse in Surveys*, John Wiley & Sons, New York, NY, USA, 1987.

[40] Drexel University, "Drexel Autism Support Program," http://www.pages.drexel.edu/~fdh23/.

[41] Marshall University, "The college program for students with Autism Spectrum Disorder," http://www.marshall.edu/college-program/.

[42] M. F. Olney, K. F. Brockelman, J. Kennedy, and M. A. Newsom, "Do you have a disability? A population-based test of acceptance, denial, and adjustment among adults with disabilities in the U.S," *Journal of Rehabilitation*, vol. 70, no. 1, pp. 4–9, 2004.

[43] D. R. Hendricks and P. Wehman, "Transition from school to adulthood for youth with autism spectrum disorders: review and recommendations," *Focus on Autism and Other Developmental Disabilities*, vol. 24, no. 2, pp. 77–88, 2009.

[44] L. Marshak, T. Van Wieren, D. R. Ferrell, L. Swiss, and C. Dugan, "Exploring barriers to college student use of disability services and accommodations," *Journal of Postsecondary Education and Disability*, vol. 22, no. 3, pp. 151–165, 2010.

[45] J. Trammell, "Red-shirting college students with disabilities," *Learning Assistance Review*, vol. 14, no. 2, pp. 21–31, 2009.

[46] P. T. Shattuck, A. M. Roux, L. E. Hudson, T. J. Lounds, M. J. Maenner, and J.-F. Trani, "Services for adults with an autism spectrum disorder," *Canadian Journal of Psychiatry*, vol. 57, no. 5, pp. 284–291, 2012.

16

Temporal Synchrony Detection and Associations with Language in Young Children with ASD

Elena Patten,[1] Linda R. Watson,[2] and Grace T. Baranek[3]

[1]*Department of Audiology and Speech Pathology, University of Tennessee Health Science Center, 434 South Stadium Hall, Knoxville, TN 37996, USA*
[2]*Division of Speech & Hearing Sciences, CB No. 7190, University of North Carolina at Chapel Hill, Chapel Hill, NC 27599, USA*
[3]*Division of Occupational Sciences, CB No. 7122, University of North Carolina at Chapel Hill, Chapel Hill, NC 27599, USA*

Correspondence should be addressed to Elena Patten; epattenl@uthsc.edu

Academic Editor: Mikhail V. Pletnikov

Temporally synchronous audio-visual stimuli serve to recruit attention and enhance learning, including language learning in infants. Although few studies have examined this effect on children with autism, it appears that the ability to detect temporal synchrony between auditory and visual stimuli may be impaired, particularly given social-linguistic stimuli delivered via oral movement and spoken language pairings. However, children with autism can detect audio-visual synchrony given nonsocial stimuli (objects dropping and their corresponding sounds). We tested whether preschool children with autism could detect audio-visual synchrony given video recordings of linguistic stimuli paired with movement of related toys in the absence of faces. As a group, children with autism demonstrated the ability to detect audio-visual synchrony. Further, the amount of time they attended to the synchronous condition was positively correlated with receptive language. Findings suggest that object manipulations may enhance multisensory processing in linguistic contexts. Moreover, associations between synchrony detection and language development suggest that better processing of multisensory stimuli may guide and direct attention to communicative events thus enhancing linguistic development.

1. Introduction

Communication impairment is a hallmark feature of autism spectrum disorder (ASD) [1]. Identifying latent behaviors necessary for communication to develop normally could provide early diagnostic and prognostic indicators, suggest mechanisms underlying impairments, and inform the development of novel habilitative interventions. The ability to detect and benefit from multisensory auditory-visual stimulation early in development may be one of the latent prelinguistic behaviors which is critical for communication to develop normally; in autism, early impairments in multisensory processing could place the developing child on a trajectory that yields increasingly abnormal attention and communication.

Bahrick and Lickliter's [2, 3] *Intersensory Redundancy Hypothesis* proposes that an infant's ability to detect intersensory redundancy (i.e., stimulation across senses from a unitary event) guides perceptual development such that global amodal properties (i.e., not specific to a single sensory modality, such as periodicity) are processed before local unisensory details. Auditory-visual temporal synchrony, for example, is a form of intersensory redundancy and is a condition of stimulation that leads to the binding of multisensory information. This phenomenon allows properties of an event to "pop out," allowing further processing of the unitary event while preventing incorrect binding of either auditory or visual stimuli with unrelated adjacent stimuli. For example, attention is directed at the temporally synchronous presentation of a mouth moving and the speech of a person in a crowd while other auditory and visual stimuli fade into the background. In fact, by two months of age, infants are able to match speech and lip movement pairings [4]. This facilitating effect of temporal synchrony on attention is present in infancy and engages infants in important communication and social events, providing fertile ground for language to develop [2, 3].

Infant directed speech is heavily laden with auditory and visual cues that draw attention to the most salient aspects of the communication stream and includes synchronized and exaggerated voice and facial expression (for review, see Ratner, 2013 [5]). Moreover, there is evidence that caregivers consciously or subconsciously take advantage of temporal synchrony during interactions. Smith and Strader (2014), for example, found that caregivers temporally align their voice and head movements when communicating with their infants [6].

Research on children with ASD, on the other hand, suggests that they do not show the same degree of preference for infant directed speech as do typically developing children [7]. Thus, the benefits of intersensory redundancy may be reduced in children with ASD in that their attention may not be drawn to the most important aspects of communication. Evidence that this may be the case comes from research suggesting that children with ASD are more likely to incorrectly link a spoken label with an object [8].

Intersensory redundancy has been studied in several different contexts, both linguistic and nonlinguistic, as well as natural and artificial. Linguistic stimuli use speech sounds (phonemes, true words, or speech streams), whereas nonlinguistic stimuli are environmental sounds such as one object striking another. The sight of an object accompanied by the sound it makes (e.g., keys dropping) creates intersensory redundancy as does the sight of moving lips accompanied by speech sounds. These examples are natural and draw attention; thus, the observer is repeatedly exposed to intersensory invariance (i.e., stable, predictable patterns or regularities). Since children prefer intersensory redundancy and since linguistic patterns tend by nature to be intersensorily redundant, they may be a critical form of input during language development and may encourage infants to tune in to the most salient aspects of spoken language [9] (for a broader view of perceptual learning, see Gibson, 1969 [10]).

Intersensory redundancy can also be manufactured such as when an object is moved in synchrony with a verbalization. Unlike natural intersensory redundancy, artificial intersensory redundancy can be manipulated and is potentially useful for teaching. This type of stimulation, sometimes referred to as "multimodal motherese," is linked to better lexical learning in infants [11]. Further, it is preferred by infants over communication without additional cues [12] and appears to heighten and draw attention to the communicative event [13, 14]. It may be that the temporal redundancy created by the movement of an object paired with the spoken label is what triggers the infant to look at the object, thus encouraging joint attention [9], which is an important precursor to language [15]. In fact, infants engage in more joint attention with their mothers, demonstrate more attention to targets, and show better learning of new words when their mothers use more object-speech temporal synchrony in their communication (i.e., "multimodal motherese") [11]. Multiple studies have demonstrated improved attention and learning as a result of presenting object-speech temporal synchrony [16–20]. For example, seven-month-olds are able to learn to associate a speech sound with an object only when the auditory and moving visual stimuli are temporally aligned [17] and two-month-olds can detect changes in syllable-object pairings when temporal synchrony is present [19].

Such findings suggest that the ability to detect synchrony may be important for early learning. Rader and Goldring-Zukow (2010) found that moving an object in synchrony with the label drew infants' attention from the speaker's face to the object and, more importantly, was associated with better word learning [21]. It may be that children with ASD can detect synchrony under certain conditions (e.g., artificial versus natural) and glean associated benefits. To date, the effects of infusing artificial intersensory redundancy into language learning in language disabled populations have not been studied. However, a recent study by Gogate et al. (2014) found that preterm infants are less sensitive to multimodal synchrony compared to term infants, which may be causally related to word mapping delays in this group [22]. This finding suggests that early impairments in synchrony detection could negatively impact language development in populations with disabilities.

Difficulty with intersensory processing is well established in autism (for reviews, see [23, 24]); however, the nature of the deficit, particularly the impact on language development, is far less studied. Bahrick and Todd [25] have described ways in which early impairments in detection of intersensory redundancy, including detection of temporal synchrony, may trigger a cascade of disordered developments that yield symptoms of autism. The Intersensory Redundancy Hypothesis describes a hierarchical ordering of attention based on salience of perceptual information. Information that is redundantly specified (e.g., the sound and lip movement of a speaker) is prioritized over nonredundantly specified information (e.g., the color of the speaker's shirt) within the same event. It may be that intersensory redundancy does not cue this prioritized processing in children with ASD. Overall stimulus perception might not be organized from global to local but rather as a disjointed percept, possibly giving the impression of preference for local processing at the expense of global processing (e.g., [26, 27]).

Although there is a fair amount of evidence for impairments in intersensory processing in children with autism, some studies show intact intersensory processing. For example, when given a simple discrimination task such as matching the sound of keys with a visual image of keys, intersensory processing appears to be intact [28]. This may be cognitively mediated, indicating that the child knows the sound of keys regardless of the temporal construction. Findings in children with autism are limited and mixed regarding detection of audio-visual temporal synchrony when the visual stimuli to be matched with the sound are identical with the exception of onset time. Evidence both for and against audio-visual temporal synchrony detection in natural, nonlinguistic contexts has been found. Bebko and colleagues found children with ASD detected audio-visual synchrony in a nonlinguistic, natural context [29], while Bahrick et al. [30] did not. Neither study found evidence that children with autism discriminate between temporally synchronous and asynchronous events in linguistic audio-visual contexts. These studies featuring linguistic stimuli used paradigms that displayed only faces as the visual stimuli [29, 30], such that the temporal synchrony, both natural and linguistic, occurred between the lips moving and the words spoken. This lack of discrimination in face-voice contexts may suggest an underlying impairment in intersensory processing of complex stimuli or, alternatively, perhaps difficulties in face processing negatively impact synchrony discrimination for children with autism (e.g., [31, 32]). Although research demonstrates that typically developing children benefit in terms of attention and language given temporal synchrony between object-speech stimuli independent of the presence of faces and moving lips [16–20], it is unknown whether or not children with autism can detect temporal synchrony between object movement and speech stimuli (artificial, linguistic synchrony). Some of the previously mentioned studies demonstrate that children with ASD can detect temporal synchrony while other studies have found they cannot. If children with ASD demonstrate attention to object-speech synchrony, they may be better positioned to take advantage of lexical training [16–20]. That is, the benefits of synchrony detection may be just powerful with object-speech stimuli as with mouth-speech stimuli, in light of findings by Yu and Smith (2012) who found that typically developing toddlers look mainly at their mother's hand during object naming as opposed to her face [33]. However, even if children with autism are able to detect object-speech temporal synchrony in this context, it would be important to determine if this ability is associated with any developmental skills, such as language, adaptive, or social skills.

We examined children with autism to determine if they could detect temporal synchrony in a linguistic context featuring object movement and verbal labels as described in Gogate et al. [34]. Additionally, we examined the extent to which the amount of time they spent looking toward temporally synchronous audio-visual displays was associated with their language skills.

2. Methods

2.1. Participants and Settings. A total of 23 children with autism (19 males; 4 females) were recruited to participate in this study through flyers distributed to existing research projects and preschools in North and South Carolina. Inclusion criteria were (a) an age between 3 years and 5 years, 11 months, (b) a clinical diagnosis of autism, and (c) meeting criteria for autism on the *Autism Diagnostic Observation Schedule* (*ADOS*) [35] previously administered by public school system psychologists or other research groups. All children displayed symptoms consistent with an autism diagnosis during their participation in this study, based on informal observation. Children were excluded if they had concomitant genetic diagnoses (fragile X syndrome, tuberous sclerosis, etc.). Vision and hearing were required to be within normal limits or to be corrected to within normal limits, as confirmed by record review and/or parent report.

Participants were seen during a single visit lasting less than one hour. The testing environments were child-friendly settings that were quiet and away from distraction of other activities, either in a lab or a separate room in the child's preschool.

2.2. Measures. To gauge the overall severity of symptoms of social relatedness in autism, the *Social Responsiveness Scale-Preschool for Three-Year-Olds* (*SRS-P*) [36], a validated 65-item parent questionnaire, was completed by each child's caregiver. The SRS-P is based upon the original version, the *Social Responsiveness Scale* (SRS) [37], and is only slightly different from the original version, with changes in wording of some items to make them more appropriate for younger children. Due to these minimal differences, the SRS-P for 3-year-olds was used for the entire sample. The SRS uses a rating scale from zero to three for each item. A score of 60 or greater is associated with an autism spectrum disorder [38].

The Auditory Comprehension portion of the *Preschool Language Scale-4* (*PLS-4*) [39] was administered to measure receptive language. The *PLS-4* is a standardized test of expressive and receptive language skills designed for use with children from birth to 6 years, 11 months.

2.3. Design and Apparatus. We used a two-choice intermodal preferential looking paradigm [40], with the two competing stimuli being displayed on separate video monitors. It was selected for the current study because preferential looking toward synchrony is thought to reflect intersensory matching (perceiving multisensory stimuli as a cohesive unit) and integration by requiring that the participant detect and discriminate the intersensory relationship and then select an explicit response [41]. Benefits of temporal synchrony can only be derived given those conditions.

Two 19-inch computer monitors were placed side by side with a six-inch gap between them. A Canon VIXIA HF R100 camcorder, used to record looking behaviors, was placed behind and above the two monitors, centered between them, and a speaker to broadcast the auditory stimuli was placed in between the monitors with the volume set at a comfortable listening level similar to conversation. Video clips were held on a Macintosh minicomputer and stored in i-Tunes.

2.4. Stimuli. Four 30-second video clips featured four different dolls, each paired with a different name and different play set. Four generic dolls (two males and two females) were selected in order to decrease the likelihood that children would already be familiar with the dolls. The dolls were called "Kiku," "Pilou," "Nuwa," and "Barra," names selected because they were not likely to be familiar to the child, and their bisyllabic structure readily allowed for movement of the dolls in synchrony with speaking the dolls' names.

The midportion of the investigator's trunk was recorded as she held each doll and vertically bounced the doll in synchrony with the doll's name each time she uttered the name. Each video clip segment contained five statements about the play activity and included the doll's name once per statement. Therefore, each doll's name was presented a total of five times during each segment. The name of the doll was uttered with movement of the doll in synchrony with the double syllables resulting in a "double bounce." The bounce was always done vertically and spanned approximately 6 inches. For example, the investigator said, "Kiku likes milk" while moving the doll during the production of "Kiku" and then demonstrating the doll drinking milk. Deliberate movement paired with auditory stimuli only occurred on screen during production of the doll's name. The doll drinking milk occurred after the statement was complete. The doll's name paired with movement was evident in only the synchronous version. The name of the doll came at the beginning of the sentence in 14 of 16 opportunities. The researcher inserted a slight pause after the name of the doll was uttered, which a llowed the movement in the asynchronous video to occur before the initiation of the rest of the utterances. For 2 of the 16 utterances, the name of the doll was embedded in the utterance: "Let's put lotion on Kiku's feet" and "Let's clean Nuwa's booboo." In the asynchronous version, movement occurred during the production of the word "feet" but did not follow the synchronous two-syllable movement pattern. The word "booboo" was produced with movement of the doll in the asynchronous video. This unintended synchrony was not felt to invalidate the segment because adults viewing the segment were immediately able to tell which condition was synchronized, as was the case in a similar design by Bahrick [42].

The investigator held the doll and materials at chest level and her face was not captured on tape. This prevented confounds of sound and lip movement synchrony, as the target linguistic event was the pairing of the referent (doll) with the speech cue (name) and not the mouth with the speech cue. In addition, this intentional avoidance of the investigator's face removed the need for face processing, a known deficit for children with autism (e.g., [43]). Each video monitor featured identical recordings, but on one monitor, the video was delayed by 700 milliseconds in order to provide the same auditory and visual stimuli with only temporal synchrony being manipulated. A 700-millisecond delay was selected because typically developing infants are able to identify nonspeech auditory and visual stimuli as asynchronous at 350 milliseconds [44] and speech stimuli at 633 milliseconds [45]. Stimuli presented with gaps greater than 700 milliseconds were considered independent events rather than asynchronous in Gogate et al. [34]. At the neurophysiological level, temporal binding of synchronous multisensory stimuli is essential for the perception of the stimuli as a single event and may be disrupted in autism [46]. According to findings in school-age children and adolescents with autism, temporal-binding windows are framed within ±300 milliseconds [47], and young children with autism might have even larger temporal-binding windows because the temporal-binding window is larger in infancy and gradually decreases with age in typical development [48]. Therefore, based on prior research from several sources, the 700-millisecond delay was assumed to allow for adequate detection of asynchronies among this sample.

2.5. Procedure. Each child was centered between the two monitors, at a comfortable viewing distance (25 inches away) with the monitors at eye-level. A brief intermission (30 seconds) occurred between each of the four 30-second video segments. Attention was cued between the monitors to serve as a fixation point prior to the commencement of each of the four segments. For each trial, the sound-synchronous version of the video segment played on one monitor while the sound-asynchronous version of the same video segment played on the other monitor. Counterbalancing occurred with order of doll presentation and side of synchrony (i.e., two segments were created for each doll—one with synchrony on the right and one with synchrony on the left). Each condition (synchronous and asynchronous) was presented twice on each side.

Occasionally, a child required cues to remain in his or her seat. This was accomplished by gently physically cuing him or her around the waist. No incidents of extreme fussiness occurred. No child was ever coaxed to look at one or another monitor.

2.6. Data Collection Methods and Coding. We used the first 15 seconds of each video segment for coding in order to be more consistent with existing methods on preferential looking paradigms (e.g., [18, 29]). The attention of infants during intermodal preferential looking tasks tends to be distributed in an increasingly random manner as time progresses in a trial [49, 50], so the first fifteen seconds of each trial were coded to mitigate effects of decreasing participation in the task and to obtain the most reliable measure. Using digital video manipulation, the first frame of each 500-millisecond segment was captured, yielding two freeze-frames per second. Trained research assistants coded the frames as directed toward (a) right monitor, (b) left monitor, and (c) neither screen. This yielded a frequency count for each type of looking direction for each 15-second segment. Although a saccade (rapid simultaneous movement of both eyes) can be as fast as 300 milliseconds in typically developing preschoolers [51], coding 500-millisecond frames was sufficient because there were no examples of rapid saccades back and forth between screens that would potentially change the results; that is, participants tended to look at a screen for several seconds before shifting attention either off screen or to the other screen. In addition, data from five randomly selected participants, each with four 15-second video recordings, were coded using a frame-by-frame (30 frames per second) method. This resulted in Pearson correlation of .991, $P = .001$, with the data coded for 500-millisecond frames. Coding fidelity was checked on 4 of the 23 participants by the first author yielding 97% agreement. Coders were blind to the stimulus conditions (synchronous or asynchronous) on each monitor. The four segments for each participant were matched to condition (synchronous/asynchronous) after all coding was completed. The PLS-4 was administered to examine language skills. The receptive language age-equivalent (A-E) scores were used to compute a receptive language ratio score (receptive language A-E/child's chronological age) rather than using a standard score due to 8 of the 23 children having standard scores at the floor for the PLS-4 (i.e., a score of 50 or below). Table 1 summarizes the characteristics of the sample.

3. Results

3.1. Synchrony Detection. Preferential looking to (1) a synchronous display condition and (2) an asynchronous display condition and (3) off-screen was evaluated in twenty-three preschool children with autism. Out of a total of 60 seconds

TABLE 1: Sample characteristics.

Participant characteristics	Mean (SD)	Range
Chronological age (mos)	55.45 (7.54)	42–69
PLS-4 receptive language A-E	38.05 (15.30)	17–75
Receptive language ratio*	.69 (.06)	.31–1.21
Social responsiveness scale-P	83.32 (29.56)	19–122

* Receptive language ratio = PLS-4 receptive language A-E/chronological age.

of available looking time to synchrony and to asynchrony or off-screen, synchronous looking time ranged from a total of 15 to 40 seconds with a mean of 28.8 seconds (SD = 8.08). Asynchronous looking time ranged from a total of 15 to 31.50 seconds with a mean of 22.24 seconds (SD = 4.65). Off-screen looking time ranged from a total of .50 to 29.50 seconds with a mean of 8.93 (SD = 8.84) (see Figure 1). There were no significant side preferences $t(22) = 1.37$, $P > .05$, and no significant difference between time spent looking to synchrony for the first 7.5 seconds compared to the last 7.5 seconds $t(22) = 1.54$, $P > .05$. In addition, the condition to which the child first looked (4 opportunities per child) was coded to ensure that children were not simply directing attention to the object that moved first. Thirty-nine of 92 opportunities were first to the synchronous display (where the object moved first), 32 were to the asynchronous display, and 21 were off screen; thus, less than half of the first looks were to the synchronous display.

We used a percent of looking time to the synchronous display based on the first 15 seconds of recorded looking behavior (i.e., synchronous looking/[synchronous + asynchronous looking]; not including off-screen looking). Our sample looked to synchrony 55.75% of the time (see above for mean and standard deviations in seconds) and to asynchrony 44.25% of the time, as a proportion of total looking time to one screen or the other. Based upon a one-sample t-test against chance looking (50%), looking to synchrony occurred significantly longer than chance, $t(22) = 3.14$, $P = .005$. The percent of total looking to synchrony is the proportional inverse of total looking to asynchrony; therefore, the significant difference in looking to synchrony reflects the same significant difference in looking to asynchrony.

3.2. Associations with Language. A Pearson correlation revealed a strong, positive association between time looking to synchrony and language ratio scores, $r(23) = .54$, $P = .008$. Additionally, a Pearson correlation showed a negative association between off-screen looking and receptive language score, $r(23) = .54$, $P = .007$. See Figure 2.

4. Discussion

Twenty-three preschool children with autism were evaluated to determine (1) their ability to detect audio-visual temporal synchrony of objects paired with linguistic stimuli through a preferential looking paradigm and (2) the extent to which preferential looking to synchrony was associated with language skills. Our sample demonstrated preferential looking toward the visual presentation that was synchronous to the sound source as opposed to the visual display that was slightly out of synchrony with the sound source. An important methodological difference between the previous studies that found children with autism did not demonstrate preferential looking to synchrony using linguistic auditory stimuli and the present study is that the visual stimuli in the present study did not include faces but rather a person moving objects in synchrony with linguistic stimuli. This difference in findings could reflect difficulty with face processing or an overarching sensory processing deficit. The fine-grained movements associated with lip postures for speech may not have been salient enough to capture attention but the larger and simpler movement of an object bouncing could be more easily processed. Future studies should assess differences between synchrony detection with and without faces present as well as with high and low visual complexity in the same sample to determine the extent to which faces potentially interrupt audio-visual sensory processing in children with autism. If complexity does not impact synchrony detection like the presence of faces, it may be that attention is not being appropriately trained to prioritize the highly social nature of face stimuli, thus diminishing social motivation (for a review of the social motivation theory of autism, see Chevallier et al., 2012 [52]). Similarly, the question of whether or not synchronized object-voice stimulation is powerful enough to draw attention to objects being labeled, as is the case with typically developing children [28], requires further study.

Our sample demonstrated that more time spent looking to the temporally synchronized object-speech stimuli was significantly associated with higher language skills. Although our study does not determine causality, the association is in line with previous studies on typically developing infants and toddlers that show synchrony detection is associated with better attention to language and better language learning [16–20]. It is likely that development of synchrony detection precedes language development and guides attention to the most important aspects of communication. We might conclude that children with ASD who detect synchrony better are at

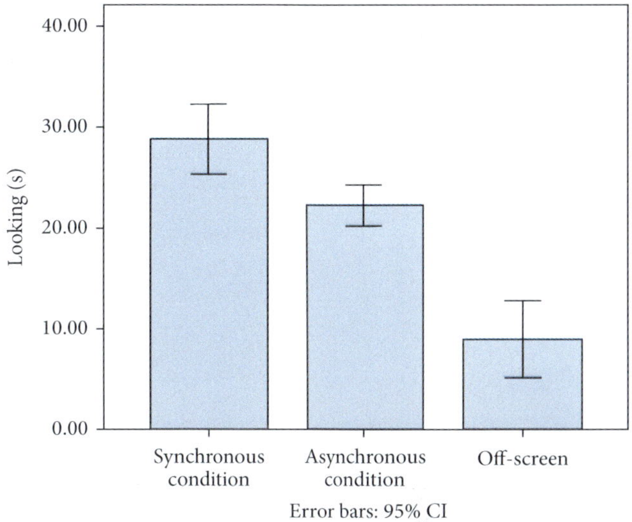

FIGURE 1: Preferential looking by stimulus condition.

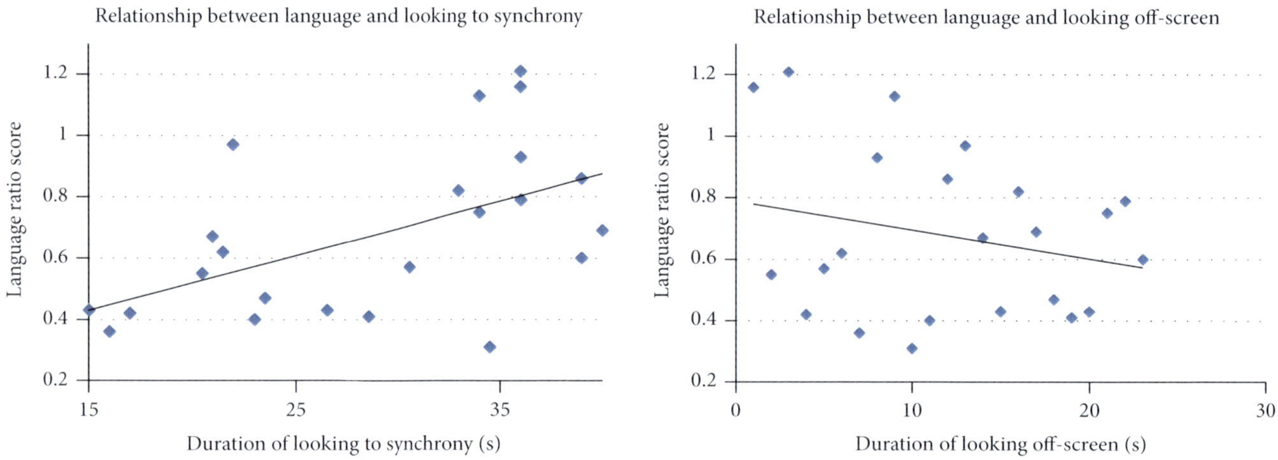

FIGURE 2: Language as a function of looking behavior.

an advantage in directing attention to linguistic content and are less likely to succumb to the ambiguity inherent in attempting to connect two unrelated stimuli (words with referents). As mentioned earlier, Gogate and colleagues suggested that delays in language development in preterm infants might be a result of early attenuations in synchrony detection [22]. Future studies should investigate a variety of populations with known delays in language development to elucidate potential underlying mechanisms of early lexical acquisition based on intersensory processing in various contexts. In addition, specific areas of language (e.g., phonology and pragmatics) should be teased out to determine if they are differentially associated with poorer intersensory processing.

The more time children spent looking off-screen, the worse their language skills became. Again, the direction of causality is unclear; it is possible that children with poorer language skills have less interest in looking to language-based video vignettes or that children with less interest in language-based stimuli learn language more slowly.

5. Conclusions

These findings demonstrate that children with autism can discriminate audio-visual temporal synchrony in certain contexts and may suggest that exaggerated multisensory stimuli aid in synchrony detection for these children. It should be noted that our experimental task purposefully obscured the actors face in the videos which may have improved attention to the multimodal stimuli; however, the findings underscore the potential clinical benefits of using exaggerated multisensory cues (i.e., moving objects in synchrony with auditory stimuli). Harnessing the benefits of intersensory redundancy may support better joint attention, language learning, and memory [53].

The correlational nature of this study precludes causal interpretations; thus, future longitudinal studies are needed to determine the extent to which synchrony detection impacts later language skills. Moreover, measures of intersensory processing may have diagnostic utility when applied to samples with infants at risk for ASD.

Acknowledgment

This paper is based on the Elena Patten's doctoral dissertation from the University of North Carolina at Chapel Hill.

References

[1] American Psychiatric Association, *Diagnostic and Statistical Manual of Mental Disorders*, American Psychiatric Association, Washington, DC, USA, 5th edition, 2013.

[2] L. E. Bahrick and R. Lickliter, "Intersensory redundancy guides early perceptual and cognitive development," in *Advances in Child Development and Behavior*, R. Kail, Ed., vol. 30, pp. 153–187, Academic Press, New York, NY, USA, 2002.

[3] L. E. Bahrick and R. Lickliter, "The role of intersensory redundancy in early perceptual, cognitive, and social development," in *Multisensory Development*, A. Bremner, D. J. Lewkowicz, and C. Spence, Eds., pp. 183–205, University Press, Oxford, UK, 2012.

[4] M. L. Patterson and J. F. Werker, "Two-month-old infants match phonetic information in lips and voice," *Developmental Science*, vol. 6, no. 2, pp. 191–196, 2003.

[5] N. B. Ratner, "Why talk with children matters: clinical implications of infant- and child-directed speech research," *Seminars in Speech and Language*, vol. 34, no. 4, pp. 203–214, 2013.

[6] N. A. Smith and H. L. Strader, "Infant-directed visual prosody: Mothers' head movements and speech acoustics," *Interaction Studies: Social Behaviour and Communication in Biological and Artificial Systems*, vol. 15, no. 1, pp. 38–54, 2014.

[7] R. Paul, K. Chawarska, C. Fowler, D. Cicchetti, and F. Volkmar, ""Listen my children and you shall hear": auditory preferences in toddlers with autism spectrum disorders," *Journal of Speech, Language, and Hearing Research*, vol. 50, no. 5, pp. 1350–1364, 2007.

[8] S. Baron-Cohen, D. A. Baldwin, and M. Crowson, "Do children with autism use the speaker's direction of gaze strategy to crack the code of language?" *Child Development*, vol. 68, no. 1, pp. 48–57, 1997.

[9] L. J. Gogate and G. Hollich, "Invariance detection within an interactive system: a perceptual gateway to language development," *Psychological Review*, vol. 117, no. 2, pp. 496–516, 2010.

[10] E. J. Gibson, *Principles of Perceptual Learning and Development*, Appleton-Century-Crofts, East Norwalk, Conn, USA, 1969.

[11] L. J. Gogate, L. E. Bahrick, and J. D. Watson, "A study of multimodal motherese: the role of temporal synchrony between verbal labels and gestures," *Child Development*, vol. 71, no. 4, pp. 878–894, 2000.

[12] R. J. Brand and W. L. Shallcross, "Infants prefer motionese to adult-directed action," *Developmental Science*, vol. 11, no. 6, pp. 853–861, 2008.

[13] R. J. Brand, D. A. Baldwin, and L. A. Ashburn, "Evidence for "motionese": modifications in mothers' infant-directed action," *Developmental Science*, vol. 5, no. 1, pp. 72–83, 2002.

[14] E. A. Koterba and J. M. Iverson, "Investigating motionese: the effect of infant-directed action on infants' attention and object exploration," *Infant Behavior and Development*, vol. 32, no. 4, pp. 437–444, 2009.

[15] P. Mundy and A. Gomes, "Individual differences in joint attention skill development in the second year," *Infant Behavior and Development*, vol. 21, no. 3, pp. 469–482, 1998.

[16] L. J. Gogate, "Learning of syllable-object relations by preverbal infants: the role of temporal synchrony and syllable distinctiveness," *Journal of Experimental Child Psychology*, vol. 105, no. 3, pp. 178–197, 2010.

[17] L. J. Gogate and L. E. Bahrick, "Intersensory redundancy facilitates learning of arbitrary relations between vowel sounds and objects in seven-month-old infants," *Journal of Experimental Child Psychology*, vol. 69, no. 2, pp. 133–149, 1998.

[18] L. J. Gogate and L. E. Bahrick, " Intersensory redundancy and 7-month-old infants' memory for arbitrary syllable-object relations," *Infancy*, vol. 2, no. 2, pp. 219–231, 2001.

[19] L. J. Gogate, C. G. Prince, and D. J. Matatyaho, "Two-month-old infants' sensitivity to changes in arbitrary syllable-object pairings: the role of temporal synchrony," *Journal of Experimental Psychology: Human Perception and Performance*, vol. 35, no. 2, pp. 508–519, 2009.

[20] D. J. Matatyaho and L. J. Gogate, "Type of maternal object motion during synchronous naming predicts preverbal infants' learning of word-object relations," *Infancy*, vol. 13, no. 2, pp. 172–184, 2008.

[21] N. D. V. Rader and P. Goldring-Zukow, "How the hands control attention during early word learning," *Gesture*, vol. 10, no. 2-3, pp. 202–221, 2010.

[22] L. Gogate, M. Maganti, and A. Perenyi, "Preterm and term infants' perception of temporally coordinated syllable-object pairings: implications for lexical development," *Journal of Speech, Language, and Hearing Research*, vol. 57, no. 1, pp. 187–198, 2014.

[23] G. Iarocci and J. McDonald, "Sensory integration and the perceptual experience of persons with autism," *Journal of Autism and Developmental Disorders*, vol. 36, no. 1, pp. 77–90, 2006.

[24] E. J. Marco, L. Hinkley, S. S. Hill, and S. S. Nagarajan, "Sensory processing in autism: a review of neurophysiologic findings," *Pediatric Research*, vol. 69, pp. 48R–54R, 2011.

[25] L. E. Bahrick and J. T. Todd, "Multisensory processing in autism spectrum disorders: Intersensory processing disturbance as a basis for atypical development," in *The New Handbook of Multisensory Processes*, B. E. Stein, Ed., pp. 657–674, MIT Press, Cambridge, Mass, USA, 2012.

[26] F. Happé and U. Frith, "The weak coherence account: detail-focused cognitive style in autism spectrum disorders," *Journal of Autism and Developmental Disorders*, vol. 36, no. 1, pp. 5–25, 2006.

[27] S. Baron-Cohen, E. Ashwin, C. Ashwin, T. Tavassoli, and B. Chakrabarti, "Talent in autism: hyper-systemizing, hyper-attention to detail and sensory hypersensitivity," *Philosophical Transactions of the Royal Society B: Biological Sciences*, vol. 364, no. 1522, pp. 1377–1383, 2009.

[28] A. S. Walker-Andrews, J. M. Haviland, L. Huffman, and L. Toci, "Brief report: Preferential looking in intermodal perception by children with autism," *Journal of Autism and Developmental Disorders*, vol. 24, no. 1, pp. 99–107, 1994.

[29] J. M. Bebko, J. A. Weiss, J. L. Demark, and P. Gomez, "Discrimination of temporal synchrony in intermodal events by children with autism and children with developmental disabilities without autism," *Journal of Child Psychology and Psychiatry and Allied Disciplines*, vol. 47, no. 1, pp. 88–98, 2006.

[30] L. E. Bahrick, J. T. Todd, M. Vaillant-Molina, B. M. Sorondo, and C. H. Ronacher, "Impaired detection of temporal synchrony for social and nonsocial events in children with autism spectrum disorders," in *Proceedings of the International Meeting for Autism Research (IMFAR '10)*, 2010.

[31] G. Dawson, S. J. Webb, and J. McPartland, "Understanding the nature of face processing impairment in autism: insights from behavioral and electrophysiological studies," *Developmental Neuropsychology*, vol. 27, no. 3, pp. 403–424, 2005.

[32] S. J. Webb, G. Dawson, R. Bernier, and H. Panagiotides, "ERP evidence of atypical face processing in young children with autism," *Journal of Autism and Developmental Disorders*, vol. 36, no. 7, pp. 881–890, 2006.

[33] C. Yu and L. B. Smith, "Embodied attention and word learning by toddlers," *Cognition*, vol. 125, no. 2, pp. 244–262, 2012.

[34] L. J. Gogate, L. H. Bolzani, and E. A. Betancourt, "Attention to maternal multimodal naming by 6- to 8-month-old infants and learning of word-object relations," *Infancy*, vol. 9, no. 3, pp. 259–288, 2006.

[35] C. Lord, M. Rutter, P. Dilavore, and S. Risi, *The Autism Diagnostic Observation Schedule (ADOS)*, Western Psychological Corporation, Los Angeles, Calif, USA, 1999.

[36] E. Pine, J. Luby, A. Abbacchi, and J. N. Constantino, "Quantitative assessment of autistic symptomatology in preschoolers," *Autism*, vol. 10, no. 4, pp. 344–352, 2006.

[37] J. N. Constantino, *The Social Responsiveness Scale*, Western Psychological Services, Los Angeles, Calif, USA, 2002.

[38] J. N. Constantino, S. A. Davis, R. D. Todd et al., "Validation of a brief quantitative measure of autistic traits: comparison of the social responsiveness scale with the Autism Diagnostic Interview-Revised," *Journal of Autism and Developmental Disorders*, vol. 33, no. 4, pp. 427–433, 2003.

[39] I. Zimmerman, V. Steiner, and R. E. Pond, *Preschool Language Scale*, Harcourt, San Antonio, Tex, USA, 4th edition, 2002.

[40] E. Spelke, "Infants' intermodal perception of events," *Cognitive Psychology*, vol. 8, no. 4, pp. 553–560, 1976.

[41] D. J. Lewkowicz, "The development of intersensory temporal perception: an epigenetic systems/limitations view," *Psychological Bulletin*, vol. 126, no. 2, pp. 281–308, 2000.

[42] L. E. Bahrick, "Infants' perception of substance and temporal synchrony in multimodal events," *Infant Behavior and Development*, vol. 6, no. 4, pp. 429–451, 1983.

[43] C. S. Monk, S.-J. Weng, J. L. Wiggins et al., "Neural circuitry of emotional face processing in autism spectrum disorders," *Journal of Psychiatry and Neuroscience*, vol. 35, no. 2, pp. 105–114, 2010.

[44] D. J. Lewkowicz, "Perception of auditory-visual temporal synchrony in human infants," *Journal of Experimental Psychology: Human Perception and Performance*, vol. 22, no. 5, pp. 1094–1106, 1996.

[45] D. J. Lewkowicz, "Learning and discrimination of audiovisual events in human infants: the hierarchical relation between intersensory temporal synchrony and rhythmic pattern cues," *Developmental Psychology*, vol. 39, no. 5, pp. 795–804, 2003.

[46] J. Brock, C. C. Brown, J. Boucher, and G. Rippon, "The temporal binding deficit hypothesis of autism," *Development and Psychopathology*, vol. 14, no. 2, pp. 209–224, 2002.

[47] J. H. Foss-Feig, L. D. Kwakye, C. J. Cascio et al., "An extended multisensory temporal binding window in autism spectrum disorders," *Experimental Brain Research*, vol. 203, no. 2, pp. 381–389, 2010.

[48] D. J. Lewkowicz, "Infant perception of audio-visual speech synchrony," *Developmental Psychology*, vol. 46, no. 1, pp. 66–77, 2010.

[49] M. MacRoy-Higgins, R. G. Schwartz, V. L. Shafer, and K. Marton, "Influence of phonotactic probability/neighbourhood density on lexical learning in late talkers," *International Journal of Language and Communication Disorders*, vol. 48, no. 2, pp. 188–199, 2013.

[50] G. Schafer and K. Plunkett, "Rapid word learning by fifteen-month-olds under tightly controlled conditions," *Child Development*, vol. 69, no. 2, pp. 309–320, 1998.

[51] J. Fukushima, T. Hatta, and K. Fukushima, "Development of voluntary control of saccadic eye movements: I. Age- related changes in normal children," *Brain and Development*, vol. 22, no. 3, pp. 173–180, 2000.

[52] C. Chevallier, G. Kohls, V. Troiani, E. S. Brodkin, and R. T. Schultz, "The social motivation theory of autism," *Trends in Cognitive Sciences*, vol. 16, no. 4, pp. 231–238, 2012.

[53] S. R. Leekam, E. Hunnisett, and C. Moore, "Targets and cues: gaze-following in children with autism," *Journal of Child Psychology and Psychiatry*, vol. 39, no. 7, pp. 951–962, 1998.

17

The 2D : 4D Digit Ratio as a Biomarker for Autism Spectrum Disorder

M. Mackus,[1] D. de Kruijff,[1] L. S. Otten,[1] A. D. Kraneveld,[1,2] J. Garssen,[1,3] and J. C. Verster[1,2,4]

[1] *Division of Pharmacology, Utrecht University, Utrecht, Netherlands*
[2] *Institute for Risk Assessment Sciences (IRAS), Utrecht University, Utrecht, Netherlands*
[3] *Nutricia Research, Utrecht, Netherlands*
[4] *Centre for Human Psychopharmacology, Swinburne University, Melbourne, VIC, Australia*

Correspondence should be addressed to J. C. Verster; j.c.verster@uu.nl

Academic Editor: Robert F. Berman

It has been suggested that the second (2D, index finger) to fourth (4D, ring finger) digit ratio, 2D : 4D, may be a biomarker for the risk of developing autism. The aim of the current study was to determine the usefulness of the 2D : 4D digit ratio as biomarker for autistic traits. $N = 401$ healthy young volunteers participated in the study. For both hands, digit lengths were measured using digital Vernier calipers. In addition to demographics, the Autism Spectrum Quotient (AQ) questionnaire was completed, comprised of five subscales, assessing "social insights and behavior," "attention switching," "communication," "imagination," and "attention to detail." Overall, no significant correlations were observed between the AQ total score, its subscales, and the 2D : 4D digit ratio. For women, the left hand 2D : 4D digit ratio correlated significantly with the subscale score "communication" ($r = -0.142$; $p = 0.036$). For men, a significant positive correlation was found between the left 2D : 4D digit ratio and the total AQ score ($r = 0.157$; $p = 0.042$) and AQ subscale "attention switching" ($r = 0.182$; $p = 0.017$). In conclusion, gender specific associations between the 2D : 4D digit ratio and specific autism traits were observed, which were stronger in men than in women. Future studies should be conducted in patients that are formally diagnosed with autism.

1. Introduction

The second (2D, index finger) to fourth (4D, ring finger) digit ratio, 2D : 4D, has been suggested as a predictor of disease predisposition [1]. More specifically, the 2D : 4D digit ratio might be a useful predictor of fertility, differentiation pattern of the central nervous system (CNS), and the expression of particular adult-onset diseases, such as immune dysfunction, myocardial infarction, and breast cancer [1]. For example, low digit ratios are associated with increased fertility and vice versa.

Relative digit lengths are established in the 14th week of fetal development [2]. Low 2D : 4D digit ratios (2D < 4D) are associated with high levels of fetal testosterone, relative to fetal estrogen levels. In contrast, high values of digit ratios (2D > 4D) are associated with high fetal estrogen levels, relative to fetal testosterone levels [3]. This sexually dimorphic difference is most strongly expressed on the right side of the body [4]. Consequently, sexual traits can be most reliably correlated with the right digit ratio [3, 5]. This is distinguished between two ranges of digit ratios; individuals with digit ratios higher than 1.00 are defined as "dove" type, and individuals with digit ratios lower than 1.00 are defined as "hawk" type. As a consequence of varying concentrations of prenatal testosterone, digit ratios are said to be sexually dimorphic, meaning that this ratio is different in men and women. Males tend to have lower digit ratios than females [6, 7]. Digit ratios have already been suggested to correlate with various sexually dimorphic traits. The best-known association with the digit ratio is the masculinity of an individual, especially in men. Previous studies have found a direct relationship between male digit ratios and traits depending on pubertal and adult testosterone levels [8].

Interestingly, evidence is found for testosterone having a major impact on the differentiation of the CNS [9]. An important implication is the correlation of high prenatal levels of testosterone and the development of traits of autism spectrum disorder (ASD): since low digit ratios are associated with high levels of prenatal testosterone, these ratios are suggested to predict an elevated expression of autistic traits [10–12]. A meta-analysis of seven studies by Hönekopp compared the 2D : 4D digit ratio in both individuals diagnosed with ASD and unaffected controls [11]. This analysis showed that the digit ratio is on average lowered by 0.5–0.6 SD in individuals diagnosed with ASD. Measures of empathizing and systemizing did not show a relationship with the digit ratio neither in ASD-affected nor in healthy controls. This may be explained by the small fraction of individuals that received prenatal testosterone levels being considerably above the male average required to see such relevant effects in behavior. A meta-analysis by Teatero and Netley extends the results found by Hönekopp. The analysis of twenty-five studies found that ASD individuals tend to have their digit ratios lowered by 0.10–0.77 SDs, and systemizing and empathizing not to be correlated with these ratios [12].

Testosterone is suggested to inhibit the growth of certain areas of the left hemisphere and on the other hand to stimulate the growth of the same areas in the right hemisphere [9]. In addition, autism has been described as extreme manifestation of certain sexually dimorphic traits and is also defined as the consequence of an "extreme male brain" [13, 14]. This phenomenon is also called hypermasculinization and is found in autistic children. Hypermasculinization is a direct consequence of relative high testosterone levels in the fetal stage and is being linked to lower digit ratios [15]. Thus, the digit ratio could serve as a useful biomarker for the development of autistic traits.

It is important to further investigate whether the 2D : 4D digit ratio is useful as noninvasive biomarker for ASD. Diagnosis of ASD at a young age will enable early intervention, and better outcomes are proven to be a direct consequence of early diagnosis [16, 17]. Addressing the risk for developing disruptive symptoms such as communication problems at an early age may prevent or reduce their expression in later life [18]. Therefore, the aim of the present study was to examine the relationship between the presence and severity of autistic traits and the 2D : 4D digit ratio in young adults between 18 and 30 years old.

2. Methods

Students of Utrecht University, Netherlands, 18 to 30 years old, were recruited to participate in this study by completing a survey. Informed consent was obtained from all participants; no medical ethics approval was required to conduct this study [19].

In addition to demographic data, the 50-item adult Autism Spectrum Quotient (AQ) was completed as a quantitative measure of autistic traits [20]. Subjects had to rate to what extent they agree or disagree with statements on personal preferences and habits on a 4-point Likert scale (answering possibilities: "definitely agree," "slightly agree," "slightly disagree," and "definitely disagree"). The AQ has 5 subscales, assessing the domains communication, social insights and behavior, imagination, attention to detail, and attention switching. A high score on a subscale implies an increased likelihood of possessing the corresponding autistic trait.

The length of the index (2D) and ring (4D) finger on both left and right hand were measured using a digital Vernier caliper. The total length of these digits was quantified from the middle of the basal crease to the tip of the finger and was determined in millimeters, with a recording accuracy of 0.01 mm. To optimize measuring precision, participants were asked to open their hands, laying them down on a flat surface, without overstretching them. All finger length measurements were conducted by the same researcher (MM), to control for between measurement errors.

IBM SPSS statistics version 24 was used for data analysis. 2D : 4D digit ratios were correlated with the total AQ score and its subscales. AQ scores were compared between those with a ratio greater than 1.00 (dove-type personality) and those with a digit ratio smaller than 1.00 (hawk-type personality). Analyses were conducted for the whole group and for men and women separately.

3. Results

$N = 401$ subjects participated in this study, with a mean (SD) age of 20.5 (2.3) years. The mean (SD) total AQ score was 102.2 (13.2). The mean left digit ratio (SD) was 0.988 (0.036), and the mean (SD) right digit ratio was 0.992 (0.034). The total AQ score was significantly higher in men compared to women ($p = 0.000$). When compared to women, men scored significantly higher on the subscales "social insights and behavior" ($p = 0.010$), "attention switching" ($p = 0.018$), "communication" ($p = 0.000$), and "imagination" ($p = 0.000$). Demographics for the group as a whole, and according to gender, are summarized in Table 1.

Overall (men and women combined), digit ratios of both hands did not significantly correlate with the total AQ score and the separate subscales. In both dove-type and hawk-type subjects, both the left hand and right hand 2D : 4D digit ratio did not significantly correlate with the total AQ score, nor with any of the AQ subscales.

3.1. Gender Differences. The right hand 2D : 4D digit ratio was significantly higher in men than in women ($p = 0.007$); no gender differences were seen for the left hand 2D : 4D digit ratio. Cohen's d indicating that effect size equals 0.01 for the left hand digit ratio and 0.03 for the right hand digit ratio in men versus women. In women, the left hand 2D : 4D digit ratio correlated significantly negative with scores on the subscale "communication" ($p = 0.036$; $r = -0.142$). In men, the left hand 2D : 4D digit ratio significantly positively correlated with the total AQ score ($p = 0.042$; $r = 0.157$) and with the subscale "attention switching" ($p = 0.017$; $r = 0.182$). No significant correlations were found between the right hand 2D : 4D digit ratio and any of the AQ subscales.

3.2. Dove-Type versus Hawk-Type Digit Ratios according to Gender. Regarding the *left* hand 2D : 4D digit ratio, in male

Table 1: Description of participating subjects.

	Overall	Men	Women
Age	20.5 (2.3)	20.7 (2.4)	20.2 (2.1)
Total AQ score	102.2 (13.2)	105.1 (12.8)*	99.9 (13.0)
Social insights and behavior	18.7 (4.4)	19.4 (4.7)*	18.2 (4.2)
Attention switching	22.5 (3.9)	23.0 (4.0)*	22.1 (3.9)
Communication	19.8 (3.8)	20.5 (3.9)*	19.2 (3.6)
Imagination	20.2 (3.9)	21.1 (3.9)*	19.5 (3.8)
Attention to detail	21.1 (4.5)	21.2 (4.1)	21.1 (4.8)
Left digit ratio	0.988 (0.036)	0.986 (0.034)	0.990 (0.036)
Right digit ratio	0.992 (0.034)	0.987 (0.034)	0.996 (0.034)

Mean (SD) values are presented for the total group and for men and women separately. Significant differences ($p < 0.05$) are indicated by $*$.

hawk-type subjects a significant positive correlation of was found with the AQ subscale "attention to detail" ($p = 0.014$; $r = 0.221$), whereas in male dove-type subjects the left hand 2D : 4D digit ratio correlated significantly positive with both the total AQ score ($p = 0.004$; $r = 0.408$) and the subscales "attention switching" ($p = 0.005$; $r = 0.389$), "imagination" ($p = 0.020$; $r = 0.328$), and "attention switching" ($p = 0.020$; $r = 0.324$). In women, none of these correlations reached significance. Regarding the *right* hand 2D : 4D digit ratio, the only significant correlation for the right hand 2D : 4D digit ratio was found with the total AQ score in male dove-type subjects ($p = 0.043$; $r = 0.274$). All other correlations were not significant.

4. Discussion

Our findings confirm that for the population as a whole the 2D : 4D digit ratio does not significantly correlate with the total AQ score and its subscales. These correlations were also not significant when analyzing the data separately for dove-type and hawk-type subjects.

From these overall conclusions it may seem tempting to conclude that the 2D : 4D digit ratio is a poor biomarker of autistic traits in a healthy study population. However, the data do also show several interesting gender differences that should not be ignored. Whereas the left hand 2D : 4D digit ratio correlated significantly only with scores on the subscale "communication" in women, in men it significantly correlated with the total AQ score and the subscale "attention switching." Moreover, in dove-type men both the left and right hand digit ratio significantly correlated with the total AQ score. Their left hand digit ratio further correlated significantly with the AQ subscales for "attention switching," "imagination," and "attention to detail." In male hawk-type subjects, left hand digit ratios correlated significantly only with the subscale "detail oriented." In women, these correlations were not significant.

The observed gender differences may be explained by the fact that ASD must be viewed as sexually dimorphic, just as the 2D : 4D digit ratio, with males on average having lower ratios than females [3, 21]. Low digit ratios correspond to high prenatal testosterone levels and relate to the expression of autistic traits and possible development of autism [10]. The latter also corresponds to the observation that ASD is strongly sex-dependent, that is, much more common in men than in women (with a male/female ratio of 4 to 1) [22]. Supportive evidence for the role of prenatal testosterone levels in the development of ADS also comes from a study that examined the expression of autistic traits in children with congenital adrenal hyperplasia (CAH). CAH is a genetic disorder causing excess adrenal androgen production, testosterone amongst others, already beginning in the fetal stage. Girls with CAH show masculinization of mood and behavior, relative to their unaffected siblings [23, 24]. Knickmeyer and Baron-Cohen identified girls with CAH to exhibit more autistic traits, compared to their unaffected siblings, and suggested it to be the result of higher prenatal androgen exposure [25].

Although several studies have suggested an association between prenatal levels of testosterone, the 2D : 4D digit ratio, and the risk of autism, other studies could not confirm these findings [10, 26–28]. For example, by comparing digit ratios of autistic children to those of their close relatives, Manning et al. predicted that high levels of prenatal testosterone do not invariably result in an autistic phenotype and that other factors may also precipitate an autistic phenotype [10]. In addition to the results of Manning and Taylor [8], Hönekopp [11] and Barona et al. [29] suggest high prenatal testosterone levels to predispose to autism only in individuals exposed to extremely high prenatal testosterone. The majority of our study population consisted of individuals with a 2D : 4D digit ratio that is as low as the ratio described by Hönekopp and Teatero and Netley to be a risk factor in developing ASD.

The absence of significant associations may further have been caused by differences in study design, that is, comparing 2D : 4D digit ratios of people with and without a formal ASD diagnosis versus associating the 2D : 4D digit ratio with severity of ADS trait measures in the general population [30].

A limitation of the current study is that data was collected from a relative healthy and young sample. University students are highly educated individuals who usually possess a more than average level of skills that are seen impaired in ADS, such as communication and attention switching. Recruitment of participants in a clinical setting would have provided qualitatively different data and stronger associations between the 2D : 4D digit ratio and specific aspects of autism spectrum disorder [31]. Therefore, future research concerning the association between ASD and the 2D : 4D digit ratio should include a broader age range, including the nonstudent population and patients.

5. Conclusion

Although the overall association between ADS and the 2D : 4D digit ratio was not significant, significant gender specific associations between the 2D : 4D digit ratio and specific autism traits were observed, which were stronger in men than in women. Future research should focus on these gender differences.

Disclosure

Preliminary data of this study has been presented as poster at the 2016 ECNP conference in Vienna, Austria. The corresponding abstract has been published as follows: M. Mackus, D. de Kruijff, L. S. Otten, J. Garssen, and J. C. Verster. The developmental origins of autism spectrum disorder: the 2D : 4D digit ratio as biomarker? European Neuropsychopharmacology 2016, 26: S724 – S724.

References

[1] J. T. Manning and P. E. Bundred, "The ratio of 2nd to 4th digit length: A new predictor of disease predisposition?" *Medical Hypotheses*, vol. 54, no. 5, pp. 855–857, 2000.

[2] S. M. Garn, A. R. Burdi, W. J. Babler, and S. Stinson, "Early prenatal attainment of adult metacarpal-phalangeal rankings and proportions," *American Journal of Physical Anthropology*, vol. 43, no. 3, pp. 327–332, 1975.

[3] J. T. Manning, D. Scutt, J. Wilson, and D. I. Lewis-Jones, "The ratio of 2nd to 4th digit length: a predictor of sperm numbers and concentrations of testosterone, luteinizing hormone and oestrogen," *Human Reproduction*, vol. 13, no. 11, pp. 3000–3004, 1998.

[4] J. M. Tanner, *Foetus into Man: Physical Growth from Conception to Maturity*, Harvard University Press, Cambridge, MA, USA, 1990.

[5] G. Ronalds, D. I. W. Phillips, K. M. Godfrey, and J. T. Manning, "The ratio of second to fourth digit lengths: A marker of impaired fetal growth?" *Early Human Development*, vol. 68, no. 1, pp. 21–26, 2002.

[6] J. Manning, L. Kilduff, C. Cook, B. Crewther, and B. Fink, "Digit ratio (2D:4D): a biomarker for prenatal sex steroids and adult sex steroids in challenge situations," *Frontiers in Endocrinology*, vol. 5, 2014.

[7] R. George, "Human finger types," *The Anatomical Record*, vol. 46, no. 2, pp. 199–204, 1930.

[8] J. T. Manning and R. P. Taylor, "Second to fourth digit ratio and male ability in sport: Implications for sexual selection in humans," *Evolution and Human Behavior*, vol. 22, no. 1, pp. 61–69, 2001.

[9] N. Geschwind and A. M. Galaburda, "Biological mechanisms, association, and pathology: a hypothesis and a program for research," *Archives of Neurology*, vol. 43, pp. 428–654, 1985.

[10] J. T. Manning, S. Baron-Cohen, S. Wheelwright, and G. Sanders, "The 2nd to 4th digit ratio and autism," *Developmental Medicine and Child Neurology*, vol. 43, no. 3, pp. 160–164, 2001.

[11] J. Hönekopp, "Digit ratio 2D:4D in relation to autism spectrum disorders, empathizing, and systemizing: a quantitative review," *Autism Research*, vol. 5, no. 4, pp. 221–230, 2012.

[12] M. L. Teatero and C. Netley, "A critical review of the research on the extreme male brain theory and digit ratio (2D:4D)," *Journal of Autism and Developmental Disorders*, vol. 43, no. 11, pp. 2664–2676, 2013.

[13] S. Baron-Cohen, S. Wheelwright, R. Skinner, J. Martin, and E. Clubley, "The autism-spectrum quotient (AQ): evidence from Asperger syndrome/high-functioning autism, males and females, scientists and mathematicians," *Journal of Autism and Developmental Disorders*, vol. 31, no. 1, pp. 5–17, 2001.

[14] S. Baron-Cohen, "The extreme male brain theory of autism," *Trends in Cognitive Sciences*, vol. 6, no. 6, pp. 248–254, 2002.

[15] B. Auyeung, S. Baron-Cohen, E. Ashwin, R. Knickmeyer, K. Taylor, and G. Hackett, "Fetal testosterone and autistic traits," *British Journal of Psychology*, vol. 100, no. 1, pp. 1–22, 2009.

[16] B. A. Iwata, M. F. Dorsey, K. J. Slifer, K. E. Bauman, and G. S. Richman, "Toward a functional analysis of self-injury," *Journal of Applied Behavior Analysis*, vol. 27, no. 2, pp. 197–209, 1994.

[17] L. K. Koegel, R. L. Koegel, K. Ashbaugh, and J. Bradshaw, "The importance of early identification and intervention for children with or at risk for autism spectrum disorders," *International Journal of Speech-Language Pathology*, vol. 16, no. 1, pp. 50–56, 2014.

[18] R. H. Horner, E. G. Carr, P. S. Strain, A. W. Todd, and H. K. Reed, "Problem behavior interventions for young children with autism: a research synthesis," *Journal of Autism and Developmental Disorders*, vol. 32, no. 5, pp. 423–446, 2002.

[19] http://www.ccmo.nl/en/questionnaire-research.

[20] R. A. Hoekstra, M. Bartels, D. C. Cath, and D. I. Boomsma, "Factor structure, reliability and criterion validity of the autism-spectrum quotient (AQ): A study in Dutch population and patient groups," *Journal of Autism and Developmental Disorders*, vol. 38, no. 8, pp. 1555–1566, 2008.

[21] F. Baker, "Anthropological notes on the human hand," *American Anthropologist*, vol. A1, no. 1, pp. 51–76, 1888.

[22] D. M. Werling and D. H. Geschwind, "Understanding sex bias in autism spectrum disorder," *Proceedings of the National Academy of Sciences of the United States of America*, vol. 110, no. 13, pp. 4868-4869, 2013.

[23] E. Hampson, J. F. Rovet, and D. Altmann, "Spatial reasoning in children with congenital adrenal hyperplasia due to 21-hydroxylase deficiency," *Developmental Neuropsychology*, vol. 14, no. 2-3, pp. 299–320, 1998.

[24] M. Hines, B. A. Fane, V. L. Pasterski, G. A. Mathews, G. S. Conway, and C. Brook, "Spatial abilities following prenatal androgen abnormality: Targeting and mental rotations performance in individuals with congenital adrenal hyperplasia," *Psychoneuroendocrinology*, vol. 28, no. 8, pp. 1010–1026, 2003.

[25] R. C. Knickmeyer and S. Baron-Cohen, "Fetal testosterone and sex differences," *Early Human Development*, vol. 82, no. 12, pp. 755–760, 2006.

[26] S. Baron-Cohen, B. Auyeung, B. Nørgaard-Pedersen et al., "Elevated fetal steroidogenic activity in autism," *Molecular Psychiatry*, vol. 20, pp. 369–376, 2015.

[27] A. L. Guyatt, J. Heron, B. L. C. Knight, J. Golding, and D. Rai, "Digit ratio and autism spectrum disorders in the Avon Longitudinal Study of Parents and Children: A birth cohort study," *BMJ Open*, vol. 5, no. 8, article no. A21, 2015.

[28] A. D. Abbott, R. J. Colman, R. Tiefenthaler, D. A. Dumesic, and D. H. Abbott, "Early-to-mid gestation fetal testosterone increases right hand 2D:4D finger length ratio in polycystic ovary syndrome-like monkeys," *PLoS ONE*, vol. 7, no. 8, Article ID e42372, 2012.

[29] M. Barona, R. Kothari, D. Skuse, and N. Micali, "Social communication and emotion difficulties and second to fourth digit ratio in a large community-based sample," *Molecular Autism*, vol. 6, no. 1, article no. 63, 2015.

[30] T. Lilley, T. Laaksonen, O. Huitu, and S. Helle, "Maternal corticosterone but not testosterone level is associated with the ratio of second-to-fourth digit length (2D:4D) in field vole offspring (Microtus agrestis)," *Physiology and Behavior*, vol. 99, no. 4, pp. 433–437, 2010.

[31] E. I. De Bruin, F. Verheij, T. Wiegman, and R. F. Ferdinand, "Differences in finger length ratio between males with autism, pervasive developmental disorder-not otherwise specified, ADHD, and anxiety disorders," *Developmental Medicine and Child Neurology*, vol. 48, no. 12, pp. 962–965, 2006.

18

A Preliminary Investigation of a Specialized Music Therapy Model for Children with Disabilities Delivered in a Classroom Setting

Jenna Mendelson,[1] Yasmine White,[2] Laura Hans,[3] Richard Adebari,[3] Lorrie Schmid,[3] Jan Riggsbee,[4] Ali Goldsmith,[3] Burcu Ozler,[3] Kristen Buehne,[3] Sarah Jones,[3] Jennifer Shapleton,[3] and Geraldine Dawson[2]

[1] *Department of Psychology, The University of North Carolina at Greensboro, Greensboro, NC, USA*
[2] *Department of Psychiatry and Behavioral Sciences, Duke University, Durham, NC, USA*
[3] *Education and Human Development Incubator and Social Science Research Institute, Duke University, Durham, NC, USA*
[4] *Program in Education, Duke University, Durham, NC, USA*

Correspondence should be addressed to Jenna Mendelson; jennalmendelson@gmail.com

Academic Editor: Mohammad Ghaziuddin

Music therapy is gaining popularity as an intervention strategy for children with developmental disabilities, including autism spectrum disorder (ASD). This study was a pilot investigation of a classroom-based music-based intervention, *Voices Together*®, for improving communication skills in children with ASD and children with intellectual disabilities. Four local public elementary school special education classrooms, serving 5 children with a classification of autistic disorder and 32 children with intellectual disability without autism, were randomly selected to receive one of two levels of exposure to *Voices Together* music therapy: "long-term" (15 weeks beginning in January 2015 (Time 1), $n = 14$) or "short-term" (7 weeks beginning 7 weeks later in February (Time 2), $n = 17$). Using observational ratings, investigators reliably scored participants live in terms of their level of verbal responsiveness to prompts during three songs featured each week of the program. Both groups demonstrated increases in verbal responses over time; however, only the long-term group demonstrated significant within-group increases. Preliminary findings suggest that music therapy delivered in a classroom in 45-minute weekly sessions for 15 weeks can promote improvements in verbal responsiveness among individuals with autism and other developmental disabilities. Findings warrant further investigation into the efficacy of classroom-based music therapy programs.

1. Introduction

Over the last 12 years, the prevalence of developmental disabilities in US children has increased by 17.1% [1]. Students with developmental disabilities often have challenges in the areas of communication and social/emotional learning, which can lead to social isolation, problematic behaviors, and deficits in academic learning [2]. However, individuals with developmental disabilities have been found to respond well to the incorporation of music in intervention programs, in terms of both gains in communication skills and stronger social functioning [3], suggesting that music therapy may present an effective means of improving communication and social skills in this population. The American Music Therapy Association (AMTA) defines music therapy as "the clinical and evidence-based use of music interventions to accomplish individualized goals within a therapeutic relationship by a credentialed professional who has completed an approved music therapy program" [4].

Early research examining the efficacy of music therapy for improving communication and social skills for children with developmental disabilities suggested that it may be an effective approach for enhancing nonverbal and verbal communication, as well as social engagement [3]. Based on these findings, the AMTA lists improvements in communication skills as among the primary functions of music therapy interventions [4]. Music has been found to be an effective tool in the promotion of communication and social skills among children with developmental disabilities, including those with and without ASD (e.g., [5, 6]), and with varying levels of symptom severity, including nonverbal children with ASD (e.g., [7]). Moreover, incorporation of music therapy with other intervention strategies in the classroom has been found to positively impact social skills among children with a range of developmental disabilities [8].

Buday [9] conceptualized the patterns presented in musical compositions as a potential mechanism for this efficacy. Patterns in music have been theorized to help hold children's attention and promote language development [10]. Moreover, children with ASD and intellectual disability (ID) have been found to be more likely to attend to auditory than visual cues when the auditory stimulus is musical [11], supporting the hypothesis of music as an effective vehicle for intervention through its unique ability to hold children's attention. Positive affective responses that occur with music have also been hypothesized to increase participation in therapy, as well as progress toward goals (Buday, 1995). Moreover, music has been described as an inherently social activity and has been directly linked to social interaction [12].

Further supporting the potential efficacy of music-based interventions for individuals with developmental disabilities, research has demonstrated that individuals with developmental disabilities, including those with ASD, process information in unique ways, which can be manifested in relatively enhanced musical abilities [13]. For example, individuals with ASD have been found to respond emotionally to music in a way that is similar to neurotypical individuals [14]. Music abilities are not limited to individuals with ASD who demonstrate exceptional musical skills [15]. Stanutz and colleagues [13] demonstrated that even those children with ASD who had no previous musical training possessed better pitch discrimination abilities and superior long-term memory for melody, compared to IQ- and age-matched neurotypical controls. Given the centrality of communication and social deficits among children with developmental disabilities [2, 16], therapists may be able to leverage the unique ability of music to hold children's attention and increase participation in therapy while promoting positive affect and social interactions in order to help children with developmental disabilities improve their communication and social skills.

Taken together, music therapy may be an excellent fit for the therapeutic needs of individuals with developmental disabilities, especially given research indicating its impact on communication and social skills, which are among the core deficits of ASD and are also implicated in a range of other developmental disabilities [2, 16]. Perhaps for these reasons, music is already commonly incorporated into therapeutic interventions of children with ASD, featuring in some capacity in as many as 12% of classroom-based interventions [17]. However, to date, very few controlled studies exist that examine the feasibility and efficacy of music-based interventions in a classroom setting.

This project was designed to be a pilot study of a classroom-based music therapy program, *Voices Together*, on the social and communication skills of children with developmental disabilities. Pilot studies have been determined to be a key component to the research process as a precursor to randomized controlled trials (RCTs; [18]). Pilot studies can be valuable tools in determining the feasibility of participant recruitment in completion of the research protocol [19] prior to conducting a full-scale RCT. However, while pilot studies may provide some early support for research hypotheses, findings must be interpreted with caution [18].

The *Voices Together* program is a proprietary and specialized music therapy model that integrates music and multisensory experiences to teach communication and social/emotional skills to people with intellectual and developmental disabilities. Among the core methods employed in the program is VOICSS™: Vocal Interactive Communication and Social Strategies. This method uses structured music-based interactions to help participants develop their skills in domains of communication and social/emotional learning.

The first hypothesis of this study was that participation in the *Voices Together* program would lead to increases in social and communicative behavior both in terms of behavioral observations made during participation in the *Voices Together* program and in terms of general classroom participation (as measured by teacher ratings). Secondly, while increases in social behavior were expected in both groups, improvements were expected to be more robust in the long-term group. Thirdly, because all songs in the *Voices Together* program employ comparable strategies to evoke social and communicative responses, no differences in improvements to social and communicative responses were hypothesized across the three songs employed in this project.

2. Method

2.1. Participants. Four special education classrooms (two Kindergarten-2nd grade and two grades 3–5 classrooms) in the Durham Public Schools participated in this study. Thirty-three children, including 5 children with ASD and 32 with intellectual disability without ASD, participated. Diagnosis was based on the school system classification of the children. Communication skills of students, as assessed by qualitative teacher report, were also variable, ranging from minimally verbal to conversational speech. Because participants were selected directly by the school district, information pertaining to age, IQ, symptom severity, gender, and the specific classroom placements of the 5 children with ASD was not made available to the researchers.

2.2. Procedure. Within each level of classroom (Kindergarten-2nd grade versus 3rd–5th grade), classrooms were randomly selected to receive one of two levels of exposure to *Voices Together* music therapy: "long-term" (15 weeks beginning in January 2015 (Time 1), n = 14) or "short-term" (7 weeks beginning 7 weeks later in February (Time 2), n = 17).

2.2.1. Voices Together Program. *Voices Together* is a specialized music therapy model designed to encourage communication and social behavior. Technique strategies and songs are interactive by design and inherently have a high expectation of a reciprocal response by establishing a pattern of prompt-response as part of each song. These strategies and songs are geared to initiate and maintain conversation, while exploring emotional, behavioral, and conceptual areas critical to social connection. The trained and licensed music therapist uses vocal exchange, a social/emotional curriculum, and musical instruments all geared toward eliciting social and communicative responses from participants. *Voices Together* is based on the VOICSS (Vocal Interactive Communication and Social Strategies) approach, which aims to increase social and communication outcomes by using program songs aimed at encouraging social interaction and verbal responses. The basic structure of the songs within the VOICSS method, which is unique to the *Voices Together* program, follows this pattern:

(1) Brainstorming and providing written responses on a whiteboard for the group on a predetermined topic (VT curriculum) that supports the social/emotional and communication objectives
(2) Choosing a peer leader for the song who facilitates the song with support from the therapist
(3) Singing and speaking; reciprocal and simple metered patterns
(4) Listening
(5) Responding
(6) Repeating and reinforcing responses by group

Songs incorporate specific techniques to make communication more likely, including leaving requests for a response on an unresolved musical note, internal structure for turn-taking that alternates between group and individual response, and directly asking each individual questions that alternate between singing and speaking. Therapists also regularly employ a strategy known as "responsive prompting" (consisting of prompts for communication that vary in intensity based on each participant's ability level) to encourage verbal responses, both within the structure of program songs and during spontaneous group interactions. To ensure fidelity to the treatment protocol, *Voices Together* providers are observed and rated across 7 domains: (1) providing appropriate energy to engage participants, (2) facilitating peer-to-peer awareness and connection, (3) facilitating client self-awareness, (4) facilitating and adapting appropriate speech/communication goals, (5) facilitating emotional awareness, (6) modifying techniques based on participant ability, and (7) appropriate support of self-management of behaviors.

Three *Voices Together* songs were selected for the purpose of this study: the "*Hello*" song, which comprises an introduction to the session and requires participants to greet each other and each say their name as part of the song; the "*Feelings*" song, which requires participants to respond to group by describing how they are feeling that day; and the "*Topic*" song, which requires participants to respond to song lyrics by bringing up a topic of interest with the group. All three songs use VOICSS strategies to evoke social responses from participants and are designed to improve social and communication skills by encouraging participants to generate novel social and communicative responses within the structure of a familiar format.

A licensed music therapist trained in the *Voices Together* program led all therapy sessions. As per the *Voices Together* curriculum, participants sat in a horseshoe shape in the classroom, with the music therapist sitting centrally, facing the students. Students participated in a single 45-minute session of *Voices Together* once weekly for 15 weeks in the long-term group and 7 weeks in the short-term group.

2.3. Dependent Variables

2.3.1. Behavioral Observations. Four advanced level undergraduate students and three research staff rated students' behavior, focusing on communication. Raters were trained to code both student and therapist behavior during twice-weekly coding meetings led by one of the coinvestigators of this project during the month leading up to the first session. The coding procedure was designed specifically for the aims of this project, and each participant was coded individually. Coding was completed during live observations that took place in the classroom during the therapy sessions at each of the three time points. Two raters attended each coding session, coded independently of each other to calculate reliability, and then adjudicated differences through discussion at the end of the session. Although videotaped coding using a standardized coding procedure was initially planned for this project, a live-coding strategy was ultimately employed due to difficulty obtaining consent from parents of all participants to use video recordings of their children in the classroom.

Both therapist prompts and child responses were coded. Therapist prompts were reverse-scored such that the lowest level of prompting (representing the highest level of spontaneity in participant response) received the highest score. Therapists' level of prompt required to elicit a response was coded, with prompts ranked from the least directive (pause alone) to the most directive (full verbal modeling). Visual prompts were initially included among the coded prompts but dropped when it became apparent that they were used systematically in one classroom and as such were not reflective of participant ability level. Each participant was coded individually. If a participant was absent at the time of a scheduled behavioral observation, the observation was rescheduled for a time during the week when all participants could be present. There was one instance where this was not possible, and the absent participant's data was not included in statistical analyses.

Participants' levels of verbal and social responses were coded on a Likert scale of 1–8 for each domain. Responses were numerically ranked from the least social/verbal (8 = body orientation/no response) to the most social/verbal (1 = full sentence verbal response). Prompts were scored on a similar Likert rating scale ranging from 1 (pause alone) to 5 (hand-over-hand). Lower mean score prompts indicate less intrusive prompts. Scores for the prompts and requisite responses for all three songs were combined to form the composite "*All Songs*" score. Lower mean scores indicated more positive responses. These scores were then summed to provide a total overall score for social/verbal responsiveness during the observation for each participant. Thus, scores closer to 0 are indicative of *higher* levels of social and verbal interaction. Given previous research suggesting that music may be an effective mode of therapy based in part on the promotion of positive affect (Buday, 1995), participants were also coded for positive affect, defined simply as whether or not the participant smiled over the course of the observation.

Reliability was calculated by the intraclass coefficient (ICC). ICC was selected as an appropriate measure of interrater reliability for this project because it allows for calculation of overall reliability for teams of larger than three coders and incorporates into reliability calculation the magnitude of disagreement (as opposed to an all-or-nothing agreement, such as what is calculated by Cohen's kappa; [20–22]). Because a series of pilot videos were coded by multiple coders as a measure of overall reliability, the single-measure ICC is reported. Based on general guidelines delineated by Cicchetti [23], reliability is considered fair when the ICC is between .40 and .59, good when the ICC falls between .60 and .74, and excellent when it is between .75 and 1.0. An ICC of 1.0 represents perfect interrater agreement. The ICC was used to calculate overall reliability for the prompts, responses, and positive affect coding across three training videos featuring implementation of the *Voices Together* program in a classroom setting, very similar to the *in vivo* coding completed by the coding team. For the prompt coding, the ICC ranged from fair to excellent across the three training videos (the full range is reported here; $ICC_{(2,1)} = .52–.80$). Reliability for coding responses also ranged from fair to excellent across the three videos ($ICC_{(2,1)} = .52–.97$), and reliability for positive affect was slightly poorer, in the fair range across the three training videos ($ICC_{(2,1)} = .42–.54$).

2.3.2. Teacher Ratings. Teachers completed the Social Skills Improvement System-Rating Scale (SSIS-RS; [24]), an 83-item scale designed to assess the efficacy of interventions targeting social skills and to demonstrate both social and intervention validity [25]. The SSIS-RS has been found to have strong psychometric properties across both the Social Skills and Problem Behaviors subscales, including high internal consistency and test-retest reliability [26]. The SSIS-RS Teacher rating survey consists of 13 subscales encompassing social skills, problem behaviors, autism spectrum behaviors, and academic achievement. Social skills, problem behaviors, and autism spectrum behaviors were rated using a 4-point Likert scale labeled "Never," "Seldom," "Often," and "Almost Always." Additionally, the academic achievement subscale uses a 5-point Likert scale for the participant's percentile rank in the classroom from "Lowest 10%" to "Highest 10%." The scale takes 20–25 minutes to complete and is used to evaluate social skills and competing problem behaviors such as communication, self-control, bullying, hyperactivity, and autism spectrum behaviors. For the purposes of this study, main analyses focused on the Assertion, Communication, and Engagement subscales, as these were hypothesized to be most closely related to the goals of the therapy program.

Teachers completed the SSIS-RS about each participant at Time 1 (the first week of the program for the long-term group), Time 2 (7 weeks into the program, the starting point for the short-term group), and Time 3 (15 weeks into the program). Teachers were compensated with $200.00 after completing the SSIS-RS at Time 3. A new teacher was hired in one of the two short-term classrooms at Time 2 of the study. To account for possible differences in reporting due to the second teacher's new status in the classroom at Time 2, both the new teacher and the previous teacher completed the questionnaire at Time 2 and scores were averaged. The new teacher then completed questionnaires independently at Time 3. Given the necessity of organizing the classroom schedule in order to hold therapy sessions during the school day, teachers were not blind to whether participants were in the short- or long-term groups.

3. Results

To assess improvements in social and communicative behavior, data were analyzed using a series of repeated measures ANOVAs, first to assess increases in behavioral observations of responsiveness and next to assess increases in the level of prompt used (level of prompt was reverse-scored such that increased scores represent more the use of more minimal prompts). Scores from individual participants in each classroom were then averaged according to classroom to provide a single score for each participating class. The one participant who was not present for one of the behavioral observations was excluded from this average and from all subsequent analyses. Separate repeated measures ANOVAs were run for each song (*Hello*, *Feelings*, and *Topic*), as well as one for combined observations from all three songs (*All Songs*) and one to assess change in terms of positive affect. Where ANOVAs demonstrated significant differences across time points, within-group paired t-tests were run to examine more specifically whether changes occurred in both the short- and the long-term groups. Lastly, a series of paired t-tests were run to examine improvements in social skills as rated by teachers on the SSIS-RS. In cases where live-coders provided discrepant responses, results using the averaged scores from both coders are reported here.

3.1. Behavioral Observations. To assess hypothesis 1 (that both groups would demonstrate improvements in the observed level of social and communicative response over time), groups were combined and levels of prompts and responses were examined across both the short- and the long-term groups from $T2$ to $T3$. A repeated measures ANOVA examining the level of response across both groups over time indicated a significant increase in level of response to the *Feelings* song from Time 1 to Time 3 (Figure 1; *Feelings response*, $F(2, 28) = 3.32$, $p < .05$). Follow-up paired t-tests using combined scores from both groups indicate higher level responses across time points for the *Feelings* song ($t(29) = 1.77$, $p = .09$, *Hello* song, $t(29) = 1.78$, $p = .08$, and

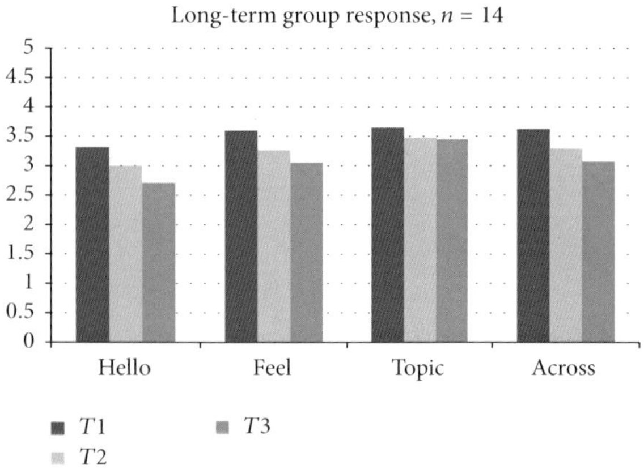

FIGURE 1: Long-term group response across time points.

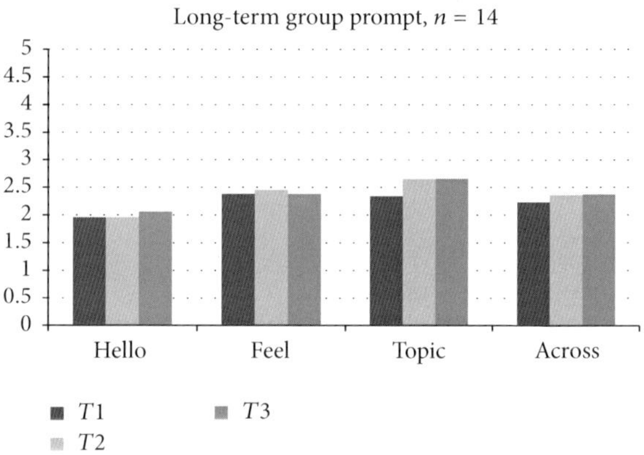

FIGURE 2: Long-term group prompt scores across time points.

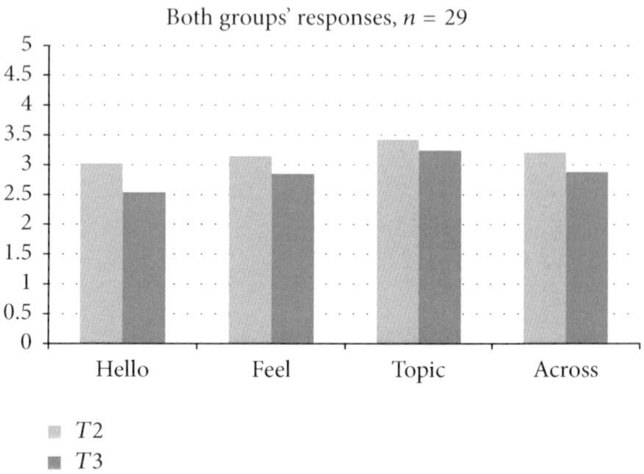

FIGURE 3: Combined responses across time points.

trending significance in *All Songs* $t(29) = 1.91$, $p = .0.07$; see Figure 3). A closer examination, however, indicates that while these improvements were a trend in the short-term group, they were only significant in the long-term group. The long-term group demonstrated significant increases in response to the *Feelings* song between Time 1 and Time 2 ($t(14) = 2.63$, $p < .05$). The long-term group also demonstrated a significant increase in average level of response across all *Voices Together* songs from Time 1 to Time 2, $t(14) = 2.47$, $p < .05$, and between Time 1 and Time 3, $t(14) = 2.46$, $p < .05$. Additionally, the long-term group demonstrated a significant increase in average level of response across all *Voices Together* songs from Time 1 to Time 2, $t(14) = 2.47$, $p < .05$, and between Time 1 and Time 3, $t(14) = 2.46$, $p < .05$. Neither group demonstrated significant improvements in terms of level of response to the *Topic* song, or in terms of the expression of positive affect during therapy sessions. Although the short-term group demonstrated increases in level of response from $T2$ to $T3$, these improvements were not statistically significant. Overall, the first hypothesis (that both groups would demonstrate significant improvements in terms of level of response) was not supported at a statistically significant level, although the short-term group did demonstrate improvements that were not statistically significant. However, hypothesis 2 (that improvements would be more robust in the long-term group) was supported in terms of the *Feelings* song, *Hello* song, and *All Songs*.

A repeated measures ANOVA across time points indicated differences in average long-term group mean scores for level of *Topic prompt* (the level of prompt required during the Topic song; $F(2, 28) = 3.32$, $p < .05$; Figure 2). Follow-up paired t-tests were conducted to determine changes in mean prompt levels across the time points for each group. Unexpectedly, paired t-tests indicated significant *increases* in level of prompt needed during the Topic song in the long-term group from Time 1 to Time 3 ($t(14) = 2.55$, $p < .05$). Classroom observations suggest that this may be due to increasing difficulty of the *Topic* song over time. Paired t-tests indicate no statistically significant differences in level of prompts used between time points Time 2 and Time 3 for the short-term control group. Overall, groups did not differ significantly for prompts at Time 2 or Time 3, or in terms of level of prompt required for any other *Voices Together* song. Thus, the hypothesis of no differences in terms of improvements in behavioral observations across songs was actually *not* supported, in that the long-term group demonstrated an unexpected increase in terms of level of prompt required for the *Topic* song.

Although information regarding individual participant age was unavailable for this project, follow-up analyses were run using grade level as a proxy for participant age. As might be expected due to developmental level, participants in grades 3–5 demonstrated a higher level of response and required fewer prompts across all time points and songs than those in grades K-2. Follow-up subsets of paired t-tests for all songs between Time 2 and Time 3 revealed comparable improvements across both grades K-2 and 3–5 in terms of prompts during the *Hello* song (K-2: $t(15) = 2.54$, $p = .023$; 3–5 $t(13) = 3.03$, $p = .01$). However, only grades 3–5 demonstrated significant improvements in terms of responses to the *Feelings* song ($t(13) = 2.55$, $p = .024$).

3.2. Teacher Questionnaires. Increases were predicted across the Assertion, Communication, and Engagement subscales of the SSIS-RS for both groups while participating in the *Voices Together* program. Paired t-tests were run on all subscales, focusing primarily on assertion, communication, and engagement for both long- and short-term groups. Contrary to the hypotheses, paired t-tests comparing scores from within each group across time points indicated no statistically significant differences between time points for either the long- or the short-term group on any of the SSIS-RS subscales. Thus, neither hypothesis 1 nor hypothesis 2 was supported by teacher ratings on the SSIS-RS.

4. Discussion

Significant improvements in terms of responses found in the long-term group, but not the short-term group, suggest that longer duration of exposure to *Voices Together* may promote a greater degree of improvement. Further research in the form of an RCT examining dosage effect of *Voices Together*, including the impact of longer or more frequent sessions, smaller versus larger groups, and time period over which the program is administered, is warranted to determine whether a greater degree of exposure to *Voices Together* promotes improvement in social and communicative behavior.

Unexpectedly, findings varied not only in terms of prompts versus responses, but also with regard to each *Voices Together* song. The *Topic* song in particular, which required participants to respond to musical prompts by bringing up a topic of interest with the group, did not appear to elicit improved responses from participants and resulted in an *increasing* level of prompts from therapists over time, counter to hypotheses. This may be due to the increasing complexity of topics expected from participants as they became familiar with the song, or to the more open-ended nature of the required response than with the *Feelings* or *Hello* song. Notably, the more structured nature of the *Feelings* and *Hello* songs may have allowed participants to rely more heavily on the musical pattern to generate a response. Overall, this finding suggests that further research as to the impact of specific song styles and musical patterns on level of communicative response from participants in music therapy programs is warranted. Also bearing consideration, songs were presented in the same order each session, suggesting that these differences may be attributable to the order of presentation rather than characteristics of the songs themselves. Counterbalancing song presentation as part of an RCT will be better able to assess the relative efficacy of each song and contribute to the understanding of mechanisms of efficacy for the *Voices Together* program.

While behavioral observations indicated significant improvement in response to *Voices Together* songs in the long-term group, these improvements were not reflected in teacher ratings on the SSIS-RS. Findings may have been obstructed by variability in rating tendencies between teachers, as well as the potential of a ceiling effect among participants who received higher scores on the SSIS-RS at baseline. Future studies may benefit from inclusion of the SSIS-RS parent report form as a means of obtaining perspectives of multiple raters for each participant as well as assessing generalization of findings outside of the school setting.

Importantly, this study was intended as a pilot study to determine the feasibility of both the research protocol and the *Voices Together* intervention itself in a public school setting. As a result, methods were subjected to significant limitations that can be used to inform methodology in future iterations of this project. Perhaps most notably, individual information about participants (including age, IQ, and diagnostic status) was not available. The lack of this information represents a major limitation of this study in terms of its ability to respond to hypotheses. Exploratory analyses using grade as proxy for age may suggest that participant age can impact the efficacy of the program, although this data should be interpreted with caution. Future RCTs of the *Voices Together* will need to ensure that demographic information for each individual participant can be made available in the selected school setting, most likely through a more lengthy and detailed consent process that was not possible as part of this project. Inclusion of relevant individual information for each participant will allow for analysis of possible moderation and mediation effects of individual characteristics, including age. Overall, however, findings from this study are promising in terms of both the feasibility and the efficacy of music-based intervention in special-needs classrooms and point to the value of a full-scale RCT to examine the impact of music-based therapy on individuals with different diagnostic classifications and individual characteristics.

Notably, again due to challenges with the consent procedure in the specific school setting, coding of behavioral observations from this project was limited to live-coding, which restricted the coding scheme to more broad-stroke observations for the sake of reliability and represents a limitation of this study. Future studies that are able to implement more detailed coding systems will allow for more nuanced and fine-tuned scoring of behavioral observations. Along these lines, video coding that allows for incorporation of more advanced behavioral coding technology may facilitate scoring of more subtle social and communicative behaviors that may not have been captured by this study.

Finally, while this study attempted to capture dosage effect by including long- and short-term treatment groups, it did not include a true control group. Future research using a randomized controlled design is warranted to examine whether the *Voices Together* program is truly effective relative to treatment-as-usual. Moreover, this project was limited to a relatively small sample size, and school selection of participants resulted in a diagnostically variable sample on whom limited demographic information is available. Thus, while these findings are promising, RCTs involving larger, better characterized samples will be key to determining whether classroom-based music therapy merits categorization as an efficacious or possibly efficacious treatment for children with developmental disabilities.

5. Conclusions

Findings from this preliminary investigation of *Voices Together* in the classroom indicate that children receiving 15 weeks of intervention show significant increases in level of communicative response from Time 1 to Time 3, whereas the short-term group receiving only 7 weeks of therapy showed improvements that were not statistically significant. These results lend tentative empirical support to the growing case for music therapy as an efficacious treatment in the promotion of social and communication skills among individuals with developmental disabilities. Notably, these increases were observed following 45 minutes weekly of classroom-based music therapy administered over 7 weeks and continued to increase over the 15 weeks of treatment, suggesting that *Voices Together* may be able to have a positive impact on communicative responses even in relatively small doses delivered in a classroom setting. However, teacher ratings of social and communicative behavior did not reveal significant improvements in overall level of social and communication skills in the broader classroom settings. Findings and limitations of this preliminary investigation can be used as a basis for further research into the efficacy of the *Voices Together* program in the promotion of social and communication skills among children with developmental disabilities.

Competing Interests

The authors declare that they have no competing interests.

Acknowledgments

This research was conducted with funding from the Education and Human Development Incubator, Social Science Research Institute, and Bass Connections, Duke University.

References

[1] C. A. Boyle, S. Boulet, L. A. Schieve et al., "Trends in the prevalence of developmental disabilities in US children, 1997–2008," *Pediatrics*, vol. 127, no. 6, pp. 1034–1042, 2011.

[2] American Psychiatric Association, *Diagnostic and Statistical Manual of Mental Disorders*, American Psychiatric Association, Arlington, Va, USA, 5th edition, 2013.

[3] C. Gold, T. Wigram, and C. Elefant, "Music therapy for autism spectrum disorder," *Cochrane Database of Systematic Reviews*, no. 2, 2010.

[4] American Music Therapy Association, 2016, http://www.musictherapy.org/.

[5] M. Braithwaite and J. Sigafoos, "Effects of social versus musical antecedents on communication responsiveness in five children with developmental disabilities," *Journal of Music Therapy*, vol. 35, no. 2, pp. 88–104, 1998.

[6] M. M. R. Perry, "Relating improvisational music therapy with severely and multiply disabled children to communication development," *Journal of Music Therapy*, vol. 40, no. 3, pp. 227–246, 2003.

[7] G. A. Sandiford, K. J. Mainess, and N. S. Daher, "A pilot study on the efficacy of melodic based communication therapy for eliciting speech in nonverbal children with autism," *Journal of Autism and Developmental Disorders*, vol. 43, no. 6, pp. 1298–1307, 2013.

[8] L. F. Gooding, "The effect of a music therapy social skills training program on improving social competence in children and adolescents with social skills deficits," *Journal of Music Therapy*, vol. 48, no. 4, pp. 440–462, 2011.

[9] E. M. Buday, "The effects of signed and spoken words taught with music on sign and speech imitation by children with autism," *Journal of Music Therapy*, vol. 32, no. 3, pp. 189–202, 1995.

[10] L. L. Morton, J. R. Kershner, and L. S. Siegel, "The potential for therapeutic applications of music on problems related to memory and attention," *Journal of Music Therapy*, vol. 27, no. 4, pp. 195–209, 1990.

[11] D. J. Kolko, L. Anderson, and M. Campbell, "Sensory preference and overselective responding in autistic children," *Journal of Autism and Developmental Disorders*, vol. 10, no. 3, pp. 259–271, 1980.

[12] D. Hargreaves, N. Marshall, and A. North, "Music education in the twenty- first century: a psychological perspective," in *Collected Work: Music Education. II: Psychology and Musical Development*, vol. 2, pp. 325–344, Routledge, New York, NY, USA, AN: 2012-24804, 2012.

[13] S. Stanutz, J. Wapnick, and J. A. Burack, "Pitch discrimination and melodic memory in children with autism spectrum disorders," *Autism*, vol. 18, no. 2, pp. 137–147, 2014.

[14] T. Ouimet, N. E. V. Foster, A. Tryfon, and K. L. Hyde, "Auditory-musical processing in autism spectrum disorders: a review of behavioral and brain imaging studies," *Annals of the New York Academy of Sciences*, vol. 1252, no. 1, pp. 325–331, 2012.

[15] R. Accordino, R. Comer, and W. B. Heller, "Searching for music's potential: a critical examination of research on music therapy with individuals with autism," *Research in Autism Spectrum Disorders*, vol. 1, no. 1, pp. 101–115, 2007.

[16] S. Mrug, B. S. G. Molina, B. Hoza et al., "Peer rejection and friendships in children with attention-deficit/hyperactivity disorder: contributions to long-term outcomes," *Journal of Abnormal Child Psychology*, vol. 40, no. 6, pp. 1013–1026, 2012.

[17] S. M. Srinivasan and A. N. Bhat, "A review of 'music and movement' therapies for children with autism: Embodied interventions for multisystem development," *Frontiers in Integrative Neuroscience*, vol. 7, no. 22, 2013.

[18] G. A. Lancaster, S. Dodd, and P. R. Williamson, "Design and analysis of pilot studies: recommendations for good practice," *Journal of Evaluation in Clinical Practice*, vol. 10, no. 2, pp. 307–312, 2004.

[19] S. Ross, A. Grant, C. Counsell, W. Gillespie, I. Russell, and R. Prescott, "Barriers to participation in randomised controlled trials: a systematic review," *Journal of Clinical Epidemiology*, vol. 52, no. 12, pp. 1143–1156, 1999.

[20] J. Cohen, "A coefficient of agreement for nominal scales," *Educational and Psychological Measurement*, vol. 20, no. 1, pp. 37–46, 1960.

[21] J. L. Fleiss and P. E. Shrout, "Intraclass correlations: uses in assessing rater reliability," *Psychological Bulletin*, vol. 86, no. 2, pp. 420–428, 1979.

[22] K. A. Hallgren, "Computing inter-rater reliability for observational data: an overview and tutorial," *Tutorials in Quantitative Methods for Psychology*, vol. 8, no. 1, pp. 23–34, 2012.

[23] D. V. Cicchetti, "Guidelines, criteria, and rules of thumb for evaluating normed and standardized assessment instruments in psychology," *Psychological Assessment*, vol. 6, no. 4, pp. 284–290, 1994.

[24] F. M. Gresham and S. N. Elliott, *Social Skills Improvement System-Rating Scales*, Pearson Assessments, Minneapolis, Minn, USA, 2008.

[25] S. N. Elliott, F. M. Gresham, J. L. Frank, and P. I. Beddow, "Intervention validity of social behavior rating scales: features of assessments that link results to treatment plans," *Assessment for Effective Intervention*, vol. 34, no. 1, pp. 15–24, 2008.

[26] F. M. Gresham, S. N. Elliott, M. J. Vance, and C. R. Cook, "Comparability of the social skills rating system to the social skills improvement system: content and psychometric comparisons across elementary and secondary age levels," *School Psychology Quarterly*, vol. 26, no. 1, pp. 27–44, 2011.

19

Illness Severity, Social and Cognitive Ability, and EEG Analysis of Ten Patients with Rett Syndrome Treated with Mecasermin (Recombinant Human IGF-1)

Giorgio Pini,[1] Laura Congiu,[1] Alberto Benincasa,[1] Pietro DiMarco,[1] Stefania Bigoni,[1] Adam H. Dyer,[2] Niall Mortimer,[3] Andrea Della-Chiesa,[4] Sean O'Leary,[2] Rachel McNamara,[2] Kevin J. Mitchell,[3] Michael Gill,[5] and Daniela Tropea[1,5,6]

[1]*Tuscany Rett Center, Ospedale Versilia, 55043 Lido di Camaiore, Italy*
[2]*School of Medicine, Trinity College Dublin, College Green, Dublin 2, Ireland*
[3]*Department of Genetics, Trinity College Dublin, College Green, Dublin 2, Ireland*
[4]*Trinity College Institute of Neuroscience, College Green, Dublin 2, Ireland*
[5]*Department of Psychiatry, Trinity College Dublin, College Green, Dublin 2, Ireland*
[6]*Neuropsychiatric Genetics, Trinity Centre for Health Sciences, St. James Hospital, Dublin 8, Ireland*

Correspondence should be addressed to Daniela Tropea; tropead@tcd.ie

Academic Editor: Robert F. Berman

Rett Syndrome (RTT) is a severe neurodevelopmental disorder characterized by an apparently normal development followed by an arrest and subsequent regression of cognitive and psychomotor abilities. At present, RTT has no definitive cure and the treatment of RTT represents a largely unmet clinical need. Following partial elucidation of the underlying neurobiology of RTT, a new treatment has been proposed, Mecasermin (recombinant human Insulin-Like Growth Factor 1), which, in addition to impressive evidence from preclinical murine models of RTT, has demonstrated safety in human studies of patients with RTT. The present clinical study examines the disease severity as assessed by clinicians (International Scoring System: ISS), social and cognitive ability assessed by two blinded, independent observers (RSS: Rett Severity Score), and changes in brain activity (EEG) parameters of ten patients with classic RTT and ten untreated patients matched for age and clinical severity. Significant improvement in both the ISS ($p = 0.0106$) and RSS ($p = 0.0274$) was found in patients treated with IGF1 in comparison to untreated patients. Analysis of the novel RSS also suggests that patients treated with IGF1 have a greater endurance to social and cognitive testing. The present clinical study adds significant preliminary evidence for the use of IGF-1 in the treatment of RTT and other disorders of the autism spectrum.

1. Introduction

Rett Syndrome (RTT) is a devastating neurodevelopmental disorder affecting approximately 1 in 10,000 females. RTT is characterized by an apparently normal period of development followed by a stagnation regression of cognitive and psychomotor abilities. Over 85% of cases are caused by mutations in the gene coding for methyl CpG-binding protein 2 (*MeCP2*) and following this discovery significant neurobiological insight has followed [1]. Moreover, a novel treatment based on such insight, IGF-1 (Insulin-Like Growth Factor 1), has shown promise in preclinical animal models [2, 3] and demonstrated safety in multiple early human studies [4–6].

Patients with RTT have no evident symptoms during the first 18 months of life. When disease becomes clinically apparent, the following symptoms appear: stagnation (cessation of growth, microcephaly, muscle loss, and hypotonia), developmental regression (deficits in social interaction, hand wringing, and clapping), decrease in BMI and musculoskeletal disorders (weight loss, osteopaenia, and scoliosis), and motor deterioration (Parkinsonian symptoms, weakness). Some authors describe the above symptoms as appearing at different stages of the disease [7]. Cardiorespiratory problems also complicate the clinical picture of RTT, contributing to the increased rates of sudden death, as does the high prevalence of epilepsy in RTT patients [8, 9].

Mutations in the *MeCP2* gene on Xq28 are responsible for RTT in the vast majority of cases [10]. The protein product of *MeCP2*, methyl-CpG-binding protein 2 (MECP2), is primarily found in the nucleus, where it binds symmetrically methylated CpG sites [11]. Also located outside the nucleus, it may act as a crucial link between synaptic activity and neuronal transcription [12, 13]. Functions of MECP2 may include transcriptional regulation and involvement in processes such as brain development, neuronal structure, and synaptic function [12]. MECP2 is critical to synaptic maturation and maintenance [14].

Importantly, *MeCP2* deletion in murine models results in a RTT-like phenotype which recapitulates many of the features of RTT in humans and is ameliorated on restoration of *MeCP2* expression. Intuitively, restoration of *MeCP2* function represents an attractive mechanism to target in the treatment of RTT [15–17]. Approaches to restore MECP2 function by gene therapy, whilst attractive, may be somewhat limited at present [18]. A more pragmatic therapeutic approach may be to target the downstream effectors of MECP2.

The best characterized downstream effector of MECP2 is Brain Derived Neurotrophic Factor (BDNF) critical in processes such as neuronal and synaptic maturation and development [19]. BDNF is downregulated in mouse models of RTT as well as in RTT patients [3, 20, 21]. Importantly, overexpression of BDNF can counteract the RTT phenotype in murine models [20]. However, the pharmacological use of BDNF is complicated by the fact that BDNF is unable to cross the Blood Brain Barrier (BBB) [22]. Another pleiotropic growth factor which has critical roles in synapse development, maturation, and maintenance is Insulin-Like Growth Factor 1 (IGF1), an activator of tyrosine kinase receptors and canonical pathways such as PI3K and MAPK signaling pathways [23, 24]. The ability of IGF-1 and its tripeptide form (GPE: Glutamate-Proline-Glycine) to cross the BBB significantly improves its potential as a therapeutic agent [11]. IGF1 pathway activation in *Mecp2* knockout mice has been shown to reverse many features of the RTT phenotype, such as anxiety levels, respiratory patterns, and irregularity in heart rate [2, 3]. The effects of IGF1 extend to increased synaptic signaling proteins, enhanced cortical excitatory transmission, and restored dendritic spine densities and amplitudes [2, 3]. Thus, IGF1 signifies a plausible therapeutic target in the treatment of RTT.

Recombinant human IGF1 (rhIGF-1, Mecasermin) is presently indicated in the pediatric population for severe growth failure and IGF1 deficiency [25]. In RTT patients, three studies to date have examined IGF-1 safety and tolerability [4–6]. The first assessed the safety of IGF1 in six RTT patients with a subsequent single case study reporting its safety in repeated cycles of IGF1 treatment [4, 5]. Further, a recent study confirmed the safety of IGF1 treatment and examined the pharmacokinetics of a multiple ascending dose and open-label extension study in 9 patients with RTT [6]. Preliminary efficacy analysis in this study noted improvements in certain cardiorespiratory measures (apnea), anxiety, and depression (indexed by reversal of frontal band alpha asymmetry on EEG).

The present clinical study investigates the changes in clinical severity (ISS) following IGF-1 treatment in ten RTT patients treated with IGF1 in comparison to untreated patients matched for clinical severity, age, and study duration. We also investigated the social and cognitive abilities of these patients in comparison to untreated patients using a novel video-based analysis, the Rett Severity Score (RSS). EEG analysis was performed following precedent in the literature for the RTT population. Although the present study is open-labeled in nature, it represents the first report in the literature on social and cognitive parameters in IGF-1 treated patients and IGF1 effects on endurance, adding significant weight to the preliminary evidence base for IGF-1 treatment in RTT patients.

2. Materials and Methods

2.1. Patient Screening and Selection. The procedures were approved by Comitato Etico Locale Sperimentazioni (CELS) Viareggio Delibera number 328 del 28/10/2009. Of twenty-five girls screened using the inclusion criteria, ten were selected for treatment with IGF1 [4]. A list of inclusion/exclusion criteria is reported in [4]. In brief: all patients had classic RTT with mutations in the *MeCP2* gene. Exclusion criteria included being aged <2 or >13 years, not in the third-stage of the disorder (according the stage-subdivision of the disease [7]), displaying nonclassical variants of RTT, presence of neoplasia, or a medical history of hypoglycaemia. Younger patients included in the study had demonstrated the regression of acquired abilities such as language and showed manual dyspraxia, all symptoms allowing an early diagnosis. Also, they demonstrated an improvement of interactive behavior, typical of a "transitory autism."

All ten treated patients (subjects 1–10; S1–10) had International Scoring System (ISS) score assessment before (T0) and after treatment (T1). Nine of the ten treated patients had social and cognitive ability assessment at T0 and T1 by two independent blinded assessors. All had adequate EEG recordings available at T0 and T1.

Ten untreated RTT patients who were selected on matching for age and disease severity (untreated subjects 1–10; U1–10) were also included. Nine of these untreated patients had ISS ascertained at comparable time periods to treated patients (24 weeks apart at T0 and T1), with all having social and cognitive ability assessed at T0 and T1 and nine having adequate EEG available at T0 and T1. Details of the individual patients can be found in Table 1.

2.2. IGF1 Administration. Families gave written consent for participation in the study prior to commencing IGF1 treatment. IGF1 (Mecasermin-Increlex*) was administered subcutaneously twice/day for 20–24 weeks to all ten patients. For the first and last week of the study, 0.05 mg/Kg was administered. For the intervening weeks, a dose of 0.1 mg/Kg was administered. The dose used is identical to that for other pediatric indications. The safety of IGF1 at this dose and similar doses in this population has been demonstrated [4–6].

TABLE 1: Patients included in the present study.

Patient	Age	Epilepsy (Y/N)	Mutation	ISS before study
IGF-1 treated subjects				
S1	4.7	Y	R270X (nonsense)	19
S2	4.8	Y	Del exons 3 and 4	21
S3	5.11	Y	R133C (missense)	18
S4	10.8	N	1155 del 12 + 1157 del 44 (frameshift)	20
S5	8.1	Y	T158M (missense)	21
S6	5.9	Y	C13ins in GCCGC in exon 1 (frameshift)	19
S7	9.49	Y	R306C	12
S8	4.46	N	T158M (missense)	14
S9	3.72	N	1096 del 89	12
S10	3.92	Y	1157 del46n	18
Untreated subjects				
U1	2.19	N	C468G (missense)	—
U2	6.74	Y	P152R (missense)	17
U3	2.41	N	753 del C (frameshift)	12
U4	4.61	Y	R294X (nonsense)	16
U5	4.7	N	R270X (nonsense)	20
U6	12.06	Y	Y141X (nonsense)	7
U7	1.92	N	R106W (missense)	15
U8	2.66	Y	1085 del 183 (frameshift)	15
U9	3.09	N	R168X (nonsense)	18
U10	4.96	Y	T158M (missense)	21

Details of ten subjects treated with IGF-1 and ten untreated subjects included for analysis in the present study. Subjects treated with IGF-1 are numbered S1–S10 and untreated subjects are named U1–10. Age is included in years. Epilepsy status at any time point in the present study is included as is the mecp2 mutation in each individual subject. The ISS (International Scoring System) before treatment is also included, except in U1 where it was not available.

2.3. Subgroup Analysis

2.3.1. Mutation Severity Status of RTT Patients. Despite its monogenic classification, there is significant genetic heterogeneity in RTT. Stratification of RTT patients by mutation severity may indicate a variability in the benefit of IGF1 which correlates with varying degrees of mutation severity. There were eight unique mutations in the IGF-1 treated group of patients, with two individuals carrying the T158M mutation. Within the untreated group all individuals had a unique mutation. This is detailed in Table 1. Mutation severity was grouped into 3 discrete groups in accordance with previous classification in the literature [26].

2.4. Outcomes/Parameters Measured

2.4.1. International Scoring System (ISS). The International Scoring System (ISS) [27, 28] was used to evaluate the severity of disease in each of the patients, with a lower score indicating a lower disease severity. ISS considers scores on 5 separate subscales: (i) Growth and Development, (ii) Muscular-Skeletal Appearance, (iii) Movement, (iv) Mental-Cortical, and (v) Brainstem-Autonomic. Each item is scored as follows: 0: no abnormality, 1: mild abnormality, and 2: severe abnormality. At baseline, ISS was compared between IGF1 treated and untreated groups to assess the similarity of the groups and hence applicability of the present study to the RTT population. Following this, the change in ISS score of the ten treated patients at T0 and T1 was compared to that of the RTT untreated patients at a comparable time interval (T0 and T1).

TABLE 2: Positive and negative features of the novel Rett Severity Score (RSS).

Rett Severity Score features	
Positive features	Negative features
Pointing	Hand wringing
Manipulating	Biting
Reaching for something	Rocking
Ability to mimic/imitate	Hitting
Indicating yes/no with head gesture	Indiscriminate moaning
Reactivity to a call	Tongue, chewing
Reactivity to an object	Vacant staring
Siming to stimulus	Bruxism
Deliberate Vocalisation	Breath holding, apnoea
Attention	Valsalva Maneuver

A full description can be found in the supplementary materials of the present paper.

2.4.2. Social and Cognitive Analysis. In order to assess social and cognitive parameters, video footage of both treated and untreated groups was analysed by two blinded, independent observers. The observers had no prior exposure or knowledge of the treatment status of the patients. 60 minutes minimum of video footage was analysed at T0 and T1. Nine of the ten treated patients had video footage of sufficient quality available and all ten untreated patients had adequate footage available. In the remaining treated patient, adequate video footage was unavailable. Three of the subjects were evaluated only by one observer.

Preliminarily footage was observed in order to design the scoring criteria design the novel tool, the Rett Severity Scale (RSS). Patients were scored on 20 features in total (Table 2): (i) 10 positive features: pointing, manipulating, reaching for something, ability to mimic/imitate, indicating yes/no with a head gesture, reactivity to a call, reactivity to an object, smiling in response to a stimulus, deliberate vocalisation, and attention, and (ii) 10 negative features: hand wringing, biting, rocking, hitting, indiscriminate moaning, tongue chewing, vacant starting, bruxism, breath-holding apnea, and Valsalva maneuver. To assure that the scale selected was appropriate and would not lead to false positive or negative results, analysis of scores was performed twice, using an initial scoring system followed by a recoded scoring system.

In the first system each of these features was rated on a scale of 1 to 5 by severity with the following system: 1: extreme impairment, 2: severe impairment, 3: moderate impairment, 4: mild impairment, and 5: absence of impairment. The second score system, based on the average of raters initial assessment, is in the range of 1 (severe impairment), 2 (medium impairment), 3 (no impairment). In order to ensure interrater reliability and validity of the novel RSS, the correlation between both rater scores was calculated for both positive and negative symptoms at T0 and T1. For this correlation, we used the scoring system 1–5 as it is the one which more stringently considers input from independent observers. The tool is included in the supplementary materials (see Supplementary Material available online at http://dx.doi.org/10.1155/2016/5073078) of this paper as is a detailed description of each severity rating for each of the 20 features.

In addition, observers rated scores for different time points during each visit (T0 and T1). This enabled comparison of scores at the beginning and end of each visit and was carried out in order to enable analysis of testing endurance in IGF1 treated and untreated patients. Importantly, all girls who had video footage recorded had it recorded in the same room, for the same period of time with the same level of external stimulation, noise, and activity. Such a methodology has clear benefits in terms of assessment standardization.

2.4.3. EEG Analysis. All ten treated patients and nine untreated patients had EEG measurements carried out using ten electrodes EEG at the same time as video footage (above) was recorded. Electrodes were positioned in accordance with the 10–20 layouts and lasted 1-2 hours. Analysis was performed for a minimum duration of 28 minutes each, sampled at a frequency of 128 kHz (samples/sec). Analysis was conducted using a custom-made script in MATLAB consisting of a Fast Fourier Transform (FFT) function which analyses the signal divided in five second bins. Peak and mean frequencies and amplitudes for the different ranges were separately averaged over the whole signal and grouped into bins to be used as comparative variables between and within groups [4]. Following precedent literature on EEG findings in RTT, mean theta and delta wave amplitude and frequencies and alpha band power were examined [4, 6, 9, 29].

2.5. Statistical Analysis. Due to the nature of data used and the small sample size in the present study, nonparametric tests were used. The Mann-Whitney U test was used for unpaired analysis and the Wilcoxon signed rank test for paired analysis. A Kruskal-Wallis test was used to mutation severity subgroups. For parametric data, paired and unpaired t-tests were used. For inferential analysis, tests used were two-tailed, with the threshold for statistical significance being set at $p < 0.05$. Statistical analysis was performed using Minitab 17 and GraphPad Prism 6.0, with the latter also being used to create figures of the relevant results.

3. Results

3.1. Significant Improvement in ISS Scores in IGF-1 Treated RTT Patients. The International Scoring System (ISS) was used to assess RTT severity as detailed above. There was no difference in ISS ratings between treated and untreated groups at baseline ($p = 0.967$, Mann-Whitney U test), reflecting the clinical similarity of the treated and untreated RTT patients.

In the treated group, six patients showed an improvement (decrease) in ISS with three patients showing no change. One of the treated patients (S2) had an ISS increased by one point at follow-up. In the untreated group, six patients showed an increase in ISS, with two patients demonstrating no change and one patient showing an improvement in ISS. The mean change (T1–T0) in ISS was significant in the treated versus untreated patients ($p = 0.0106$, Mann-Whitney U test) (Figure 1). On paired analysis of treated patients, the change in ISS as a result was just short of significance ($p = 0.052$, Wilcoxon Signed Ranks Test), possibly resulting from the small sample size and the nonparametric nature of the statistics used. In sum, the change in ISS was significantly different between treated and untreated RTT patients, with the vast majority (nine from ten) of treated RTT patients showing an improvement or stability in disease severity.

3.2. Social and Cognitive Abilities. In order to measure the ability of patients in interacting with objects and people in the environment, we introduced a new evaluation score: the Rett Severity Score (RSS), which is described in detail in the methods and supplementary sessions. Two independent observers, blinded to the patient condition and to the time point scored the footages of treated and untreated patients. To assure the reliability of this new scoring system, the outcomes were analysed according to two different scoring systems: one ranking 1–5 and the other 1–3.

3.2.1. Blinded Observers Have Correlated Evaluations' Scores. In order to assess the interrater reliability of the Rett Severity Score (RSS), the consistency between the two blinded assessors was analysed. The change in RSS ratings between each visit for each patient was calculated (T1–T0). Using a nonparametric Spearman correlation for random seven treated patients and six untreated patients, there was significant correlation between assessors ratings for positive, negative, and combined features in both treated ($p = 0.008$, $p = 0.014$, and $p < 0.005$) and untreated ($p = 0.042$, $p = 0.015$, and $p < 0.015$) groups.

3.2.2. Significant Improvement in Social and Cognitive Ability in IGF1 Treated Patients. In order to appreciate RSS changes between T0 and T1, the similarity of groups at baseline was analysed. There was no difference in the average social and cognitive ratings between treated and untreated groups for positive, negative, or combined features between treatment groups.

In order to compare RSS changes before and after treatment, the mean change in RSS (T1–T0) ratings by the two

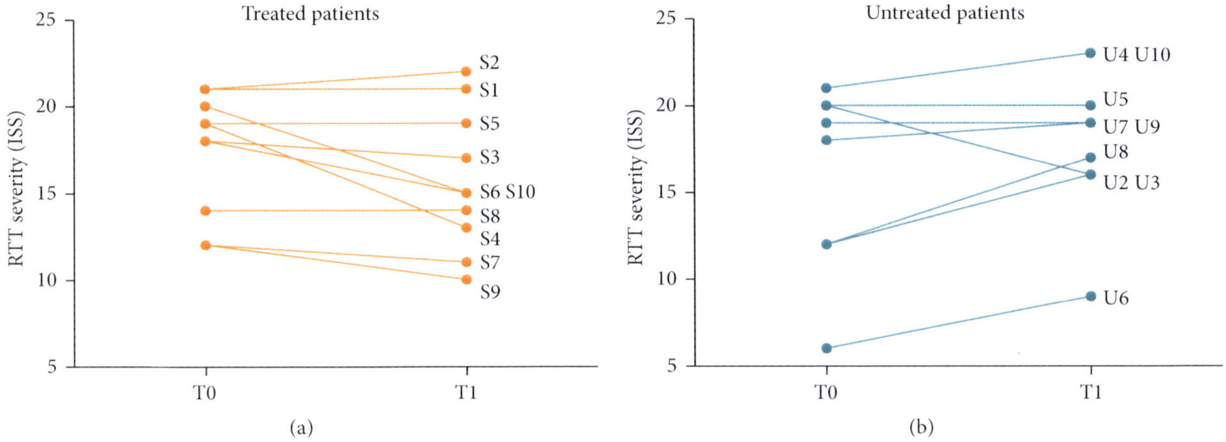

FIGURE 1: ISS before and after treatment for (a) IGF1 treated and (b) untreated patients. The Mean change in ISS in IGF1 treated versus untreated patients ($p = 0.0106$, Mann-Whitney U test, two-tailed). The change in ISS for the treated group was short of significance ($p = 0.052$, Wilcoxon Signed Ranks Test, two-tailed). ISS: International Scoring System. S1–10: treated patients 1–10; U2–10: untreated patients 1–10.

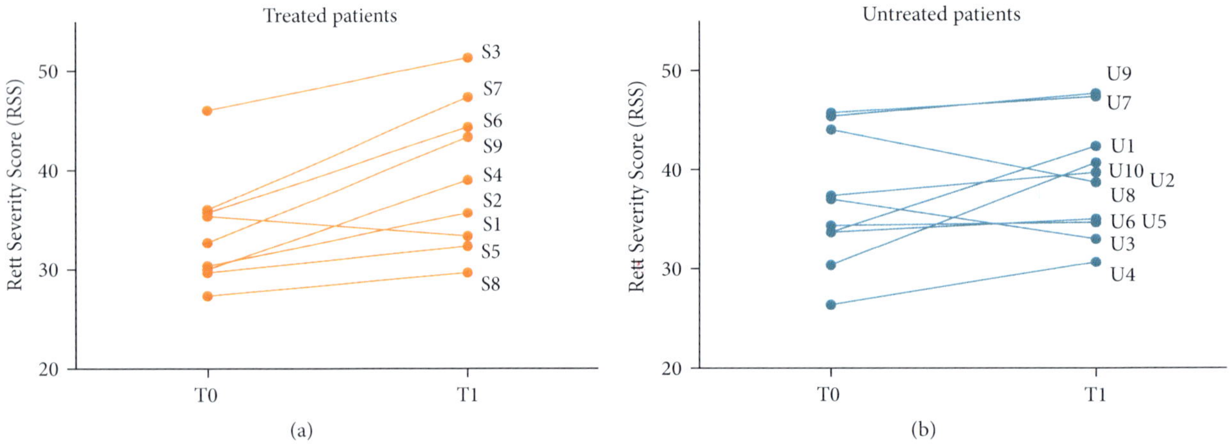

FIGURE 2: Combined features of social and cognitive scores before and after treatment for IGF1 treated patients in comparison to untreated patients. The change in Rett Severity Score (RSS) was significant for RSS 1–3 ($p = 0.0078$) as analysed by Wilcoxon Matched-Pairs Signed Ranks Test. A higher score correlates to better social/cognitive ability.

observers was taken. On paired analysis, the improvement in IGF1 treated patients from T0 to T1 was significant with both scoring systems ($p = 0.009$ (score: 1–5), $p = 0.008$ (score: 1–3), Wilcoxon Signed Ranks Test) but not for untreated RTT patients illustrating that significance cannot be fully accounted for by improvement with repeated testing. Thus, the patients treated with IGF1 demonstrated a significant improvement in social and cognitive scores between T0 and T1 in comparison to untreated patients (Figure 2).

Considering between-group analysis, there was a significant level of improvement in the total RSS of IGF1 treated patients in comparison to untreated patients measured with the 1–5 score system ($p = 0.0274$, Mann-Whitney U test). Improvement in negative features ($p = 0.0498$, Mann-Whitney U test) was significant in the treatment group in comparison to untreated patients, with positive features falling just short of significance ($p = 0.061$, Mann-Whitney U test). The same analysis with 1–3 score system just fails to reach significance ($p = 0.056$) probably for the limited number of patients in the study and the nonparametric test used for the analysis.

3.2.3. Improvement in Endurance in IGF1 Treated Patients. As detailed in the Methods section above, social and cognitive features were rated over the course of both T0 and T1. In order to examine endurance to testing in both groups, the RSS at the beginning and end of each visit was compared. In assessing both groups of patients ($n = 19$) at baseline (T0) before IGF1 treatment, all patients showed a significant decrease in cognitive and social abilities from the beginning to the end of the assessment ($p = 0.003$ (score: 1–5) $p = 0.021$ (score: 1–3), Wilcoxon Signed Ranks Test). In assessing untreated patients on the second visit (T1), there was also a significant decrease in social and cognitive abilities from the beginning to the end of testing at T1 in positive and negative features combined ($p = 0.014$ (score: 1–5), $p = 0.016$ (score: 1–3)). Thus, repeated testing did not seem to significantly alter endurance to testing in untreated patients at T1. In IGF1 treated patients, there

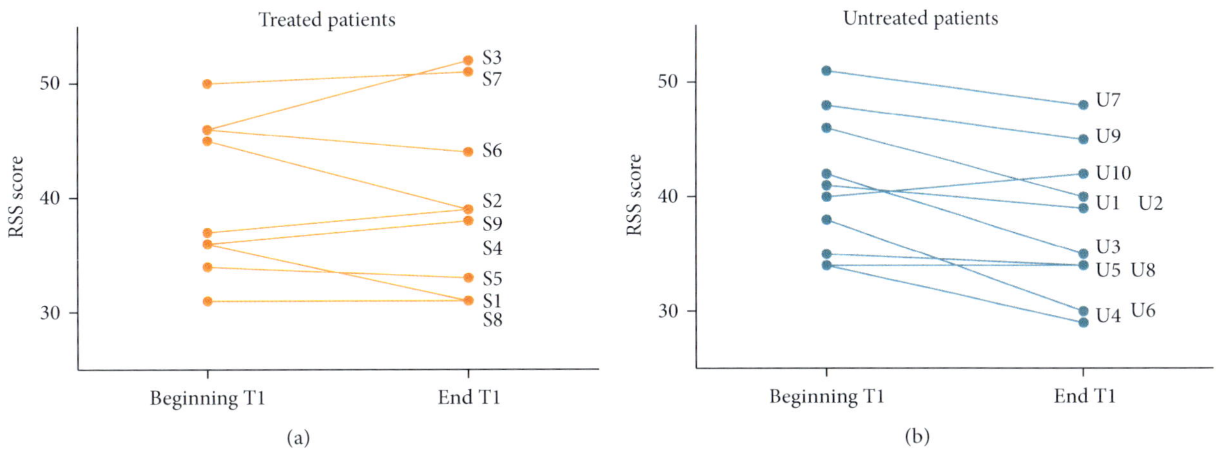

FIGURE 3: IGF1 treated patients do not show the same decrease in endurance to testing as untreated RTT patients. Endurance refers to the decrease in social/cognitive rating (RSS) from the beginning to the end of each visit (T0 and T1). In untreated patients, there is a significant decrease in scores from the start to the end of testing at T1. In treated patients, such a decrease was not seen following IGF-1 treatment. Recall that an increasing (positive on the graph above) score indicates improvement in social and cognitive ability.

was no trend of increased or decreased scoring as testing progressed for both features combined ($p = 1$) or individually for negative ($p = 0.678$) or positive ($p = 0.374$) features at T1 with both scoring ranges. Thus, IGF1 may prevent the decrease in social and cognitive testing endurance in RTT patients seen over visit duration (Figure 3).

3.3. EEG Analysis

3.3.1. Analysis of Alpha Band Desynchronisation. Following previous reports in the RTT literature changes in frontal alpha band asymmetry in the ten RTT patients treated with IGF-1 in comparison to the ten untreated patients were investigated. Left > Right ($L > R$) activation is interpreted as more anxious and Right > Left ($R > L$) as less anxious. At T0, six patients in the treatment group had $L > R$ desynchronisation index and four had a $R > L$ desynchronisation index.

Overall, the change in alpha band desynchronisation in the treated group from T0 to T1 was not significant in the ten patients treated with IGF1 in comparison to the nine untreated patients ($p = 0.8$, unpaired t-test). Similarly, the change from T0 to T1 wasn not significant when performing paired analysis ($p = 0.69$, paired t-test). However, when analysis was limited to only those patients who had a $L > R$ desynchronisation at baseline, there was a trend towards reversal on paired analysis at T0 ($p = 0.21$, paired t-test). The change was much weaker on unpaired analysis with the four patients in the untreated group with $L > R$ index at baseline ($p = 0.8196$, unpaired t-test). When the same analysis was repeated only on the first five minutes of EEG analysis at T0 and T1, the change in alpha band desynchronisation index was not significant ($p = 0.68$ and $p = 0.64$, unpaired t-test and paired t-test).

3.3.2. Delta and Theta Amplitudes and Frequencies. Delta and theta amplitude and frequencies were examined. Both paired and unpaired analyses were performed examining changes in the ten IGF1 treated RTT patients in comparison to the nine untreated RTT patients. Whilst a significant signal was seen for significant changes in the mean frequency of theta waves at C4-T4 ($p = 0.015$, paired t-test, Figure 4), as well as for the mean amplitude of delta waves at T3-O1 ($p = 0.019$, paired t-test, Figure 4), the results do not survive Bonferroni correction for multiple testing. No significant results were found on unpaired analysis.

4. Discussion

The present clinical study examined disease severity, social cognitive ability, and brain activity (EEG) measures of ten girls with classic RTT treated with Mecasermin (rh-IGF1) in comparison to ten untreated girls. Significant improvement was found when comparing disease severity and social and cognitive abilities of patients treated with IGF-1 for 6 months before (T0) and after (T1) treatment to the untreated patients at two similar time points 6 months apart (T0/T1). Analysis of brain activity (EEG) demonstrated a trend towards a reversal of alpha band desynchronisation in IGF-1 treated patients; however the result did not reach statistical significance. Importantly, the present study represents the first empirical report into the social and cognitive abilities of RTT patients treated with IGF-1 using the novel Rett Severity Score (RSS), a novel scoring tool for blinded assessors. This analysis gives some insights into the possible effects of IGF1 in RTT, in particular when considering the increased endurance to testing seen in IGF-1 treated patients. These findings add significant preliminary evidence for the use of IGF-1 in the treatment of RTT.

Notwithstanding the open-label nature of the present study, we present the development of a novel scoring tool (the RSS) in the video-based assessment of social and cognitive abilities in RTT. This analysis, based on ratings by two blinded and independent assessors, gives the first indication to date of the possible effects of IGF-1 treatment on the social and cognitive abilities of patients with RTT. In fact, it can be suggested

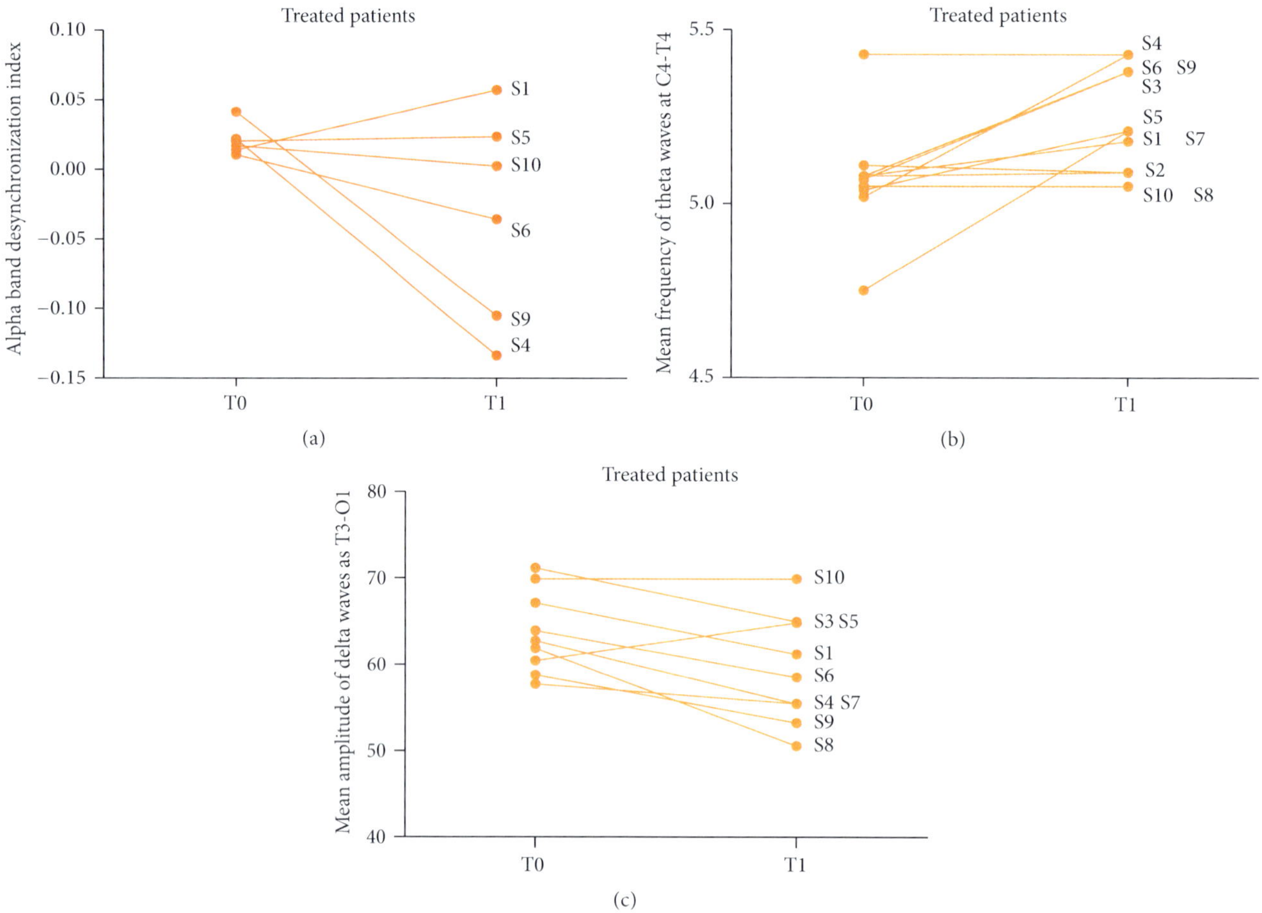

Figure 4: EEG parameters assessed before (T0) and after (T1) IGF-1 treatment. Alpha band desynchronisation is shown for those patients who were more anxious at baseline $L > R$ (a). The mean frequency of theta waves at C4-T4 (b) is also shown as is the mean amplitude of delta waves at T3-O1 (c). S1–10: treated subjects 1–10.

from the current study that part of the effect of IGF-1 may be due to an increased ability to endure assessment. Such a proposal is corroborated by anecdotal evidence from patient's clinicians and families reported with IGF-1. Although the major effect of IGF1 treatment can be appreciated only on the improvement of negative symptoms, whilst improvements of positive symptoms fail to reach significance, the number of subjects and the nonparametric nature of statistics used may have contributed to this outcome. Of note, the significant change in social and cognitive abilities as well as endurance to testing is seen using both scoring systems. This novel RSS can be considered a complementary assessment of social and cognitive ability to clinical evaluation of RTT subjects. It would be useful to examine the RSS in formal efficacy studies to confirm our preliminary results.

The International Scoring System (ISS), a clinician based assessment, is widely accepted in the assessment of disease severity in RTT. In addition to analysis of social and cognitive features, the ISS includes parameters for the assessment of movement and musculoskeletal function. All treated patients and all untreated patients except for one in the present study had their ISS assessed at T0 and T1. A note here on potential bias is prudent. Due to the open-label nature of the present study, clinicians were aware of which patients were receiving treatment with IGF-1 and which patients were not. However, notwithstanding such a limitation, all patients in the treatment group, except for one, experienced an improvement or stabilisation in ISS from T0 to T1. This is in stark contrast to the untreated group of patients, where only one patient's ISS improved from T0 to T1. The mean change in ISS from T0 to T1 was significant on both unpaired (Mann-Whitney, $p = 0.0106$) and paired (Wilcoxon, $p = 0.009$) analysis.

An important paper has reported reversal of alpha band desynchronisation on treatment with IGF-1 [6]. In the first instance, we were not able to replicate such result. However, when limited to patients with $L > R$ alpha band desynchronisation at T0 (more anxious), paired analysis demonstrated a trend to reversal in the previously reported direction ($p = 0.21$, paired t-test). Such a result may not reach statistical significance due to the small sample size of IGF-1 treated patients with $L > R$ desynchronisation at T0 ($n = 6$). Further EEG analysis in larger studies of IGF-1 treatment in RTT may help add clarity to this issue, which is complicated by the small sample sizes in the RTT population.

When analysing theta and delta waves, thought to be important in the RTT population for their role in cognition and learning, a significant change in the mean frequency of theta waves at C4-T4 ($p = 0.015$, paired t-test) and mean amplitude of delta waves at T3-O1 ($p = 0.019$, paired t-test) was demonstrated. Such results may be complex to interpret, as they do not survive testing for multiple correction and may represent false positives. The fact that the results cannot pass Bonferroni correction, as well as the fact that they cannot be seen on unpaired analysis, complicates the interpretation. It is important that future studies on IGF-1 treatment in RTT revisit such associations to enable further clarification.

A limitation of the present report is the open-label nature of the study. Whilst the ISS was not fully blinded, the RSS was assessed by blinded assessors. Notably, the strongest results in the present study are seen for the RSS. When interpreting the results of this study a key aspect is the sample size, which is a common factor of rare diseases and in this case is also affected by limited availability of IGF1; hence this study should be considered a presentation of clinical cases rather than a clinical trial. Several statistical tests fail to reach significance because of the limited sample size and the statistic test used; hence the replication of study results by additional clinical studies and trials is particularly important. In sum, the present study adds significant preliminary evidence for the use of IGF-1 in the treatment of RTT.

5. Conclusions

The present study demonstrated significant improvement in clinical severity and social and cognitive scores of patients with classical RTT before and after IGF-1 treatment in comparison to untreated patients matched for age and disease severity assessed at a similar interval. The present study is the first report in the literature to examine the social and cognitive abilities of RTT patients before and after treatment using the blinded RSS. Further, analysis by subgroups and analysis of various EEG parameters, whilst not meeting the threshold for statistical significance, provide preliminary evidence for parameters and variables that may be examined in the interpretation of formal efficacy data when it becomes available from clinical trials. In addition, this is first study showing that IGF1 improves endurance of treated patients, hence giving insights into the possible mechanisms of action of the treatment. The present report adds significant preliminary evidence for the use of IGF-1 in the treatment of Rett Syndrome and other disorders of the autism spectrum.

Acknowledgments

The authors sincerely thank all the RTT families who contributed to this study and all the personnel of the Versilia Hospital. HRB Ireland provided scholarship for Adam H. Dyer. IRC 13063 to Niall Mortimer is also acknowledged.

References

[1] C. A. Chapleau, J. Lane, J. Larimore, W. Li, L. Pozzo-Miller, and A. K. Percy, "Recent progress in Rett syndrome and MECP2 dysfunction: assessment of potential treatment options," *Future Neurology*, vol. 8, no. 1, pp. 21–28, 2013.

[2] D. Tropea, E. Giacometti, N. R. Wilson et al., "Partial reversal of Rett Syndrome-like symptoms in MeCP2 mutant mice," *Proceedings of the National Academy of Sciences of the United States of America*, vol. 106, no. 6, pp. 2029–2034, 2009.

[3] J. Castro, R. I. Garcia, S. Kwok et al., "Functional recovery with recombinant human IGF1 treatment in a mouse model of Rett Syndrome," *Proceedings of the National Academy of Sciences of the United States of America*, vol. 111, no. 27, pp. 9941–9946, 2014.

[4] G. Pini, M. F. Scusa, A. Benincasa et al., "Repeated insulin-like growth factor 1 treatment in a patient with rett syndrome: a single case study," *Frontiers in Pediatrics*, vol. 2, article 52, 2014.

[5] G. Pini, M. F. Scusa, L. Congiu et al., "IGF1 as a potential treatment for Rett Syndrome: safety assessment in six Rett patients," *Autism Research and Treatment*, vol. 2012, Article ID 679801, 14 pages, 2012.

[6] O. S. Khwaja, E. Ho, K. V. Barnes et al., "Safety, pharmacokinetics, and preliminary assessment of efficacy of mecasermin (recombinant human IGF-1) for the treatment of Rett syndrome," *Proceedings of the National Academy of Sciences of the United States of America*, vol. 111, no. 12, pp. 4596–4601, 2014.

[7] B. Hagberg, "Clinical manifestations and stages of Rett syndrome," *Mental Retardation and Developmental Disabilities Research Reviews*, vol. 8, no. 2, pp. 61–65, 2002.

[8] P. O. Julu, A. M. Kerr, F. Apartopoulos et al., "Characterisation of breathing and associated central autonomic dysfunction in the Rett disorder," *Archives of Disease in Childhood*, vol. 85, no. 1, pp. 29–37, 2001.

[9] B. Cardoza, A. Clarke, J. Wilcox et al., "Epilepsy in Rett syndrome: association between phenotype and genotype, and implications for practice," *Seizure*, vol. 20, no. 8, pp. 646–649, 2011.

[10] R. E. Amir, I. B. Van Den Veyver, M. Wan, C. Q. Tran, U. Francke, and H. Y. Zoghbi, "Rett syndrome is caused by mutations in X-linked MECP2, encoding methyl-CpG-binding protein 2," *Nature Genetics*, vol. 23, no. 2, pp. 185–188, 1999.

[11] O. S. Khwaja and M. Sahin, "Translational research: Rett syndrome and tuberous sclerosis complex," *Current Opinion in Pediatrics*, vol. 23, no. 6, pp. 633–639, 2011.

[12] W. E. Kaufmann, M. V. Johnston, and M. E. Blue, "MeCP2 expression and function during brain development: implications for Rett syndrome's pathogenesis and clinical evolution," *Brain and Development*, vol. 27, supplement 1, pp. S77–S87, 2005.

[13] M. Chahrour, Y. J. Sung, C. Shaw et al., "MeCP2, a key contributor to neurological disease, activates and represses transcription," *Science*, vol. 320, no. 5880, pp. 1224–1229, 2008.

[14] R. Z. Chen, S. Akbarian, M. Tudor, and R. Jaenisch, "Deficiency of methyl-CpG binding protein-2 in CNS neurons results in a Rett-like phenotype in mice," *Nature Genetics*, vol. 27, no. 3, pp. 327–331, 2001.

[15] J. Guy, B. Hendrich, M. Holmes, J. E. Martin, and A. Bird, "A mouse Mecp2-null mutation causes neurological symptoms that mimic rett syndrome," *Nature Genetics*, vol. 27, no. 3, pp. 322–326, 2001.

[16] M. D. Shahbazian, J. I. Young, L. A. Yuva-Paylor et al., "Mice with truncated MeCP2 recapitulate many Rett syndrome features and display hyperacetylation of histone H3," *Neuron*, vol. 35, no. 2, pp. 243–254, 2002.

[17] K. K. E. Gadalla, M. E. S. Bailey, and S. R. Cobb, "MeCP2 and Rett syndrome: reversibility and potential avenues for therapy," *Biochemical Journal*, vol. 439, no. 1, pp. 1–14, 2011.

[18] W. G. Chen, Q. Chang, Y. Lin et al., "Derepression of BDNF transcription involves calcium-dependent phosphorylation of MeCP2," *Science*, vol. 302, no. 5646, pp. 885–889, 2003.

[19] Q. Chang, G. Khare, V. Dani, S. Nelson, and R. Jaenisch, "The disease progression of Mecp2 mutant mice is affected by the level of BDNF expression," *Neuron*, vol. 49, no. 3, pp. 341–348, 2006.

[20] Z. Zhou, E. J. Hong, S. Cohen et al., "Brain-specific phosphorylation of MeCP2 regulates activity-dependent Bdnf transcription, dendritic growth, and spine maturation," *Neuron*, vol. 52, no. 2, pp. 255–269, 2006.

[21] D. Wu and W. M. Pardridge, "Neuroprotection with noninvasive neurotrophin delivery to the brain," *Proceedings of the National Academy of Sciences of the United States of America*, vol. 96, no. 1, pp. 254–259, 1999.

[22] A. M. Fernandez and I. Torres-Alemán, "The many faces of insulin-like peptide signalling in the brain," *Nature Reviews Neuroscience*, vol. 13, no. 4, pp. 225–239, 2012.

[23] C. A. Bondy and C. M. Cheng, "Signaling by insulin-like growth factor 1 in brain," *European Journal of Pharmacology*, vol. 490, no. 1–3, pp. 25–31, 2004.

[24] M. Itoh, S. Ide, S. Takashima et al., "Methyl CpG-binding protein 2 (a mutation of which causes Rett syndrome) directly regulates insulin-like growth factor binding protein 3 in mouse and human brains," *Journal of Neuropathology and Experimental Neurology*, vol. 66, no. 2, pp. 117–123, 2007.

[25] P. F. Backeljauw and S. D. Chernausek, "The insulin-like growth factors and growth disorders of childhood," *Endocrinology and Metabolism Clinics of North America*, vol. 41, no. 2, pp. 265–282, 2012.

[26] V. A. Cuddapah, R. B. Pillai, K. V. Shekar et al., "Methyl-CpG-binding protein 2 (MECP2) mutation type is associated with disease severity in Rett Syndrome," *Journal of Medical Genetics*, vol. 51, no. 3, pp. 152–158, 2014.

[27] A. M. Kerr, Y. Nomura, D. Armstrong et al., "Guidelines for reporting clinical features in cases with *MECP2* mutations," *Brain & Development*, vol. 23, no. 4, pp. 208–211, 2001.

[28] J. Kagan and N. Snidman, "Early childhood predictors of adult anxiety disorders," *Biological Psychiatry*, vol. 46, no. 11, pp. 1536–1541, 1999.

[29] R. Thibodeau, R. S. Jorgensen, and S. Kim, "Depression, anxiety, and resting frontal EEG asymmetry: a meta-analytic review," *Journal of Abnormal Psychology*, vol. 115, no. 4, pp. 715–729, 2006.

20

The Association between Adult Participation and the Engagement of Preschoolers with ASD

Ann M. Sam,[1] Stephanie S. Reszka,[2] Brian A. Boyd,[2] Yi Pan,[1] Kara Hume,[1] and Samuel L. Odom[1]

[1]*Frank Porter Graham Child Development Institute, University of North Carolina, Chapel Hill, 517 S. Greensboro Road, Carrboro, NC 27510, USA*
[2]*Department of Allied Health, University of North Carolina, Chapel Hill, NC 27599, USA*

Correspondence should be addressed to Ann M. Sam; ann.sam@unc.edu

Academic Editor: Hansen Wang

The ability for a child to engage in the classroom is associated with better academic outcomes. Yet, there is limited information on how child characteristics of autism and adult behavior impact engagement. This study examined (1) the pattern of adult participation and child engagement in preschool classrooms that serve children with ASD, (2) the associations between child engagement and adult participation, and (3) how characteristics of ASD (autism severity, language ability, and challenging behavior) moderate the relationship between adult participation and child engagement. Overall, children were less likely to be engaged when adults were actively or passively participating with them. Moderators impacted this relationship. Children with higher levels of autism severity were more likely to be engaged when adults were actively or passively participating with them. Similarly, children with lower language abilities were more likely to be engaged when adults were actively or passively participating with them. Finally, children with higher levels of challenging behaviors were less likely to be engaged when adults were actively or passively participating with them. These findings have important implications for how adults can best support the engagement of children with ASD.

1. Introduction

The National Research Council of the United States [1] recommended that young children with autism spectrum disorder (ASD) receive intensive services for 25 hours per week to promote communication, social skills, cognitive skills, and appropriate behavior. While young children with ASD are spending many hours in various programs and classrooms, there is limited information concerning the efficacy of various comprehensive treatment models or how these models are implemented in schools [2]. Even less is known about how adults are participating with children in school-based classrooms and how adult participation impacts child engagement.

Teachers and other adults in classrooms play a key role in a child's developmental process as they assist in regulating a child's activity level and interactions with peers and adults [3]. Early interactions with teachers provide a working model of teacher-child relationships and create a pattern of how children engage with other adults in the school environment [3, 4]. The relationship between teachers and children can shape and alter developmental trajectories of children with more positive relationships with teachers associated with better academic and social outcomes for young children [5–7]. On a day to day basis, these interactions may influence the quality of instruction a child receives by impacting the level of a child's engagement in the classroom environment [7].

Child engagement is defined as "the amount of time children spend interacting with the environment (with adults, children, or other materials) in a manner that is developmentally appropriate" [8, p. 60]. Higher levels of engagement are correlated with better outcomes for learners [9, 10]. For example, kindergarteners who were identified as more engaged in classroom activities had higher literacy achievement scores at the end of the year than kindergarteners with lower levels of engagement in classroom activities [10].

The amount and quality of child engagement differ between children who are typically developing and children with disabilities. Kemp and colleagues [11] found that young children with a range of disabilities in inclusive childcare settings were engaged approximately for 67% of the time in free play, group, and meal activities. Brown and colleagues [12] found that preschool-aged children with disabilities in inclusive classrooms were engaged for 54% of the time. This level of engagement did not cause concern for Brown and colleagues [12] because the active engagement category did not take into account more passive forms of engagement such as listening to peers/teachers or transitioning between activities that the coding system might not have captured.

Odom and colleagues [13] found that the engagement level for children with ASD in inclusive settings (51%) was comparable to children with other disabilities (52%) and slightly lower when compared to children who were developing typically (59%). However, Kemp and colleagues [11] found that children with ASD were engaged during free play activities only for 47.6% of the time compared to children with other disabilities who were engaged in free play activities for 84.6% of the time in inclusive settings. Wong and Kasari [14] found that preschoolers with ASD in self-contained classrooms were unengaged for a lower amount of time (37%) during classroom activities (e.g., free play, centers, circle, and self-care activities). Possible reasons for the variability of engagement across research studies include various definitions of engagement used, observation of different activities within the preschool day (e.g., free play, circle time, and routines), type of classroom (e.g., self-contained versus inclusive), and child to adult ratio.

Child engagement levels can vary based upon specific child characteristics. For example, McWilliam and Bailey Jr. [15] observed that children with disabilities with younger developmental ages were more likely to be unengaged for longer period of time than typically developing children in an inclusive childcare center. A study by de Kruif and McWilliam [16] found that children identified by both teacher report and researchers' observations to be more developmentally mature (in an inclusive childcare center) spent more time in higher level engagement activities. Negative behavior exhibited by children has been shown to reduce the level of engagement [13]. Additionally, when children are not engaged, repetitive behaviors are more likely [16].

Adults in classrooms also play a key role in fostering child engagement. Adult participation has been defined in various ways throughout the literature [17–19]. Three common categories of adult participation are (1) active adult participation (i.e., interacting directly with the focal child), (2) passive adult participation (i.e., within a close distance to the focal child but not interacting directly), and (3) no adult participation towards a focal child (i.e., the adult is not interacting directly with the focal child or within close proximity of focal child). Powell and colleagues [18] found that adults in public school early childhood classrooms were out of range or disengaged with typically developing children in play settings for about 76% of the time.

The level of adult participation influences the degree of child engagement. For example, preschool children with disabilities demonstrated higher levels of engagement in activities when activities were selected by children versus adults [13]. When adults initiated the activity, children with disabilities interacted more often with adults rather than with other children [19]. Similarly, two-year-old boys with ASD were found to have higher levels of engagement when the child selected a toy to play with versus when a teacher made the toy selection for them [20]. Furthermore, McWilliam and colleagues [17] found that teacher's interaction style impacted the engagement of the preschoolers in an inclusive childcare setting. Specifically, when a teacher elaborated on a child's activity and provided the child with information, the child was more engaged than when the teacher responded to a child, asked a question of a child, or made a request of the child.

Researchers have found that teachers and adults interact with a child differently based upon disability status, thereby influencing child engagement levels. Adults tend to provide much more support and assistance to children with disabilities compared to children developing typically [12, 13]. Hamilton [21] found that teachers in inclusive classrooms focused more upon children with disabilities engaging with materials rather than interacting with peers. Overall, teachers and other adults tend to provide more support for children with disabilities to remain engaged when compared to peers developing typically.

While researchers have explored how children with and without disabilities engage in preschool classrooms throughout the day [11–13], very little is known about how preschoolers with ASD engage in free play or center time activities. Child characteristics, such as disability, maturity, and autism severity, have been shown to influence how children engage in classroom activities [11, 15, 16]. Yet, no studies have addressed how levels of adult participation (i.e., active adult participation, passive adult participation, or no adult participation) influence the engagement of children with ASD. Further, characteristics of ASD (e.g., severity, language ability, and challenging behavior) have not been examined to determine if these characteristics moderate the relationship between child engagement and adult participation.

Given the intensive education recommendations for preschool children with ASD [1], research needs to specifically focus on the relationships and interactions between adults in these programs and preschool children with ASD. Furthermore, research needs to address how specific characteristics of ASD (i.e., severity, language ability, and challenging behavior) moderate the relationship between adult participation and child engagement. The purpose of this study is to address the research gap through the following research questions:

(i) What are the patterns of adult participation and child engagement in preschool classrooms that serve children with ASD?

(ii) What are the associations between child engagement and adult participation?

(iii) Does autism severity moderate the relationship between adult participation and child engagement?

(iv) Does language ability moderate the relationship between adult participation and child engagement?

(v) Does challenging behavior moderate the relationship between adult participation and child engagement?

2. Method

This study was part of a larger study comparing two comprehensive treatment models, high fidelity LEAP (i.e., Learning Experiences Alternative Programs for Preschoolers and Parents) and TEACCH Autism Program classrooms, to each other and a control condition (Business as Usual (BAU)). The term BAU was used instead of treatment as usual to refer to non-model-specific special education programs where children receive standard or recommended school-based services [22]. While the current study did not address how engagement of children or participation of adults varied as a function of the model, model type was used as a covariate to remove possible confounds (see [22]). Sites included four states: North Carolina, Florida, Colorado, and Minnesota. For the larger study, data were collected at three time points: pretest (start of school year), posttest (end of school year), and follow-up (6 months after posttest collected). For this study, only data from the first time point were used.

2.1. Program Settings. Established in 1972 by Schopler, the TEACCH Autism Program foundation is in behavioral principles and cognitive social learning theory. The TEACCH program stresses using the environment to enhance the learning of individuals with ASD [23]. In 1981, Strain established LEAP, a preschool program which includes children with ASD in an inclusive program. LEAP adapts early childhood curriculum and applied behavioral analysis and developmental theory [24–26]. While BAU classrooms include children with ASD, the curriculum used is not designed to specifically address characteristics of ASD. These programs use an eclectic approach to address the needs of children with ASD [27].

2.2. Participants. Classrooms met the following inclusion/exclusion criteria: (1) classrooms were within a public school system, (2) teacher was licensed to teach in respective state, (3) TEACCH and LEAP teachers attended a formal training either from personnel directly associated with the model/program or from someone formally trained (trainings varied from 3 to 5 days and occurred with no affiliation with the study), (4) teachers worked in their respective classroom type for a minimum of two years prior to the start of the study, and (5) teachers met prior-determined criteria of an "average" rating (score of 3 out 5) on four subscales of a classroom quality measure, the PDA Program Assessment [28].

To be enrolled, children met the following criteria: (1) between 3 and 5 years of age at time of enrollment; (2) previous clinical diagnosis or educational label consistent with ASD or developmental delay; (3) meeting diagnostic criteria on Autism Diagnostic Observation Schedule (ADOS) [29]; and (4) no previous exposure to the comparison treatment model (e.g., a child enrolled in a TEACCH classroom could not have prior exposure to the LEAP model). Children were excluded from the study with significant uncorrected vision or hearing impairment, uncontrolled seizure disorder, or traumatic brain injury. Lastly, in order to complete parent rating scales, families had to be proficient in English.

Table 1: Child assessments.

Assessment	Mean	SD	Range
Mullen (standard score)	64.12	18.99	49–136
CARS	33.43	7.26	15.5–55.5
PLS4	63.96	28.17	4–129
CBCL	51.23	22.92	3–107

Child participants included 187 preschool-aged children (age 3–5) diagnosed with ASD. Children were enrolled in TEACCH programs (43.16%), BAU classrooms (28.95%), and LEAP classrooms (27.89%). Child participants included 83.96% males. Child participants were white (79.86%), black (10.70%), Asian (5.35%), multiracial (3.74%), and other (0.53%). At pretest, children ranged in age from 2.9 to 5.18 years (mean 4.01 years).

Teacher participants included 69 female teachers and 1 male teacher. Teachers were white (97.14%) and black (2.86%). The mean number of years teaching was 10.37 years (range 2–29.5 years). Teachers had a master's degree (55.7%), a bachelor's degree (38.6%), education above a master's degree (4.3%), or an associate's degree (1.43%). Within classrooms, the mean child to adult ratio was 3.55 students per teacher.

2.3. Measures. Child assessments were conducted by trained research staff within a six-week period at the beginning of the school year. See Table 1 for assessment information. The Mullen Standard Score at pretest was 64.12 (SD 18.99) [30]. The Preschool Language Scale-IV (PLS-IV) assesses auditory comprehension and expressive communication to obtain a total language score [31]. The mean score for the PLS-IV was 63.96. The Childhood Autism Rating Scale (CARS) assesses the severity of autism as normal (scores below 30), mildly and moderately autistic (scores 30–36.5), and severely autistic (scores 37–60) [32]. The mean CARS score was 33.43. The Child Behavior Checklist (CBCL) provides a summary of internalizing, externalizing, and total problems [33]. The total problems raw score was used to determine challenging behavior. The mean CBCL total problem raw score was 51.23 (normative sample mean is 33.30 with a standard deviation of 18.70).

Research staff videotaped each participant for a total of 30 minutes during center time (a common feature across all classrooms where children participate in a variety of activities located in different centers such as blocks or art). During center time, children selected different activity areas (including dramatic play, large blocks, art, computer, sensory, and manipulatives). PROCODER software [34] was used to assist in coding each video using the *Code for Active Student Participation and Engagement-Revised (CASPER-III)* [35]. *CASPER-III* is an ecobehavioral assessment. Ecobehavioral assessments have been used to examine such variables as child engagement, teacher instruction/support, and peer social interactions [12, 21, 36–38]. These assessments typically examine three variables: adult behavior, classroom/environment characteristics, and student behavior [36].

TABLE 2: Interobserver agreement.

	$A/(A+D)$		Kappa	
	Mean	Range	Mean	Range
Adult Support	0.93	0.73–0.99	0.84	0.48–0.94
Arrangement	0.93	0.83–0.99	0.88	0.70–0.99
Child Behavior	0.9	0.73–0.97	0.83	0.57–0.91

The *CASPER-III* variables included Activity Area, Group Arrangement, Child Behavior, Initiator of Activity, Adult Support, and Social Behavior [35]. Momentary time sampling at 10-second intervals was used to code each video.

Videos were coded by one of our trained research assistants trained with the *CASPER-III Training Manual for Observers* [35]. Raters practiced coding until all raters reached consensus with at least 80% agreement (i.e., the number of agreements divided by the number of agreements plus disagreements) or a Kappa of at least 0.80 for each variable. Twenty percent of observations were coded by an additional rater for interobserver agreement for each variable (Group Arrangement, Adult Support, and Child Behavior). Both *Kappa* and agreement measures were used. Note that the agreement measure is based upon observed agreement. See Table 2 for the interobserver agreement.

The current study examined both adult participation in reference to an identified focal child and the focal child's engagement level. Each child participant served as a focal child. The focal child's environmental context was videotaped (i.e., the identified focal child, the center or area the focal child participated in, and other children/adults in the immediate area were filmed). The child engagement and adult participation variables were created by combining existing *CASPER* variables. Adult participation included the *CASPER* variables of Active Participation, Passive Participation, and No Participation. Table 3 presents the *CASPER* variables and definitions used to create these variables. Child engagement variables included Active Child Engagement and No Active Child Engagement by combining *CASPER* variables. Table 3 presents the *CASPER* variables and definitions used to create the child engagement variables.

2.4. Data Analysis. Descriptive statistics were used to determine the pattern of child engagement and adult participation. To address the repeated measures within children, children nested within classrooms, and both adult level and child level variables, multilevel logistic regression was used for the remaining research questions. The question regarding the associations between child engagement and active (γ_{001} adultactive$_{tij}$) and passive (γ_{002} adultpassive$_{tij}$) adult participation was addressed using multilevel logistic regression controlling for comprehensive model type (TEACCH (γ_{101} TEACCH$_j$) and LEAP (γ_{102} LEAP$_j$)), child to adult ratio (γ_{100} ratio$_j$), child ASD severity (γ_{010} severity$_{ij}$), child language ability (γ_{011} language$_{ij}$), and child challenging behavior (γ_{012} behavior$_{ij}$) (Model 1). Model 1 was

$$\begin{aligned}\text{logit } P_{tij} = {} & \gamma_{000} + \gamma_{001}\,\text{adultactive}_{tij} \\ & + \gamma_{002}\,\text{adultpassive}_{tij} + \gamma_{100}\,\text{ratio}_j \\ & + \gamma_{101}\,\text{TEACCH}_j + \gamma_{102}\,\text{LEAP}_j \\ & + \gamma_{010}\,\text{severity}_{ij} + \gamma_{011}\,\text{language}_{ij} \\ & + \gamma_{012}\,\text{behavior}_{ij} + \mu_{oij} + R_{1j}.\end{aligned} \tag{1}$$

Finally, to answer the three moderation effect questions, one interaction model was used. Covariates included comprehensive model type (TEACCH (γ_{101} TEACCH$_j$) and LEAP (γ_{102} LEAP$_j$)), child to adult ratio (γ_{100} ratio$_j$), child ASD severity (γ_{010} severity$_{ij}$), child language ability (γ_{011} language$_{ij}$), child challenging behavior (γ_{012} behavior$_{ij}$), interactions between active adult participation (γ_{001} adultactive$_{tij}$) and each of the three moderators (child ASD severity (γ_{003} adultactive$_{tij}$ $*$ severity$_{ij}$), child language ability (γ_{003} adultactive$_{tij}$ $*$ language$_{ij}$), child behavioral issue (γ_{003}adultactive$_{tij}$ $*$ behavior$_{ij}$)) and interactions between passive adult participation (γ_{002} adultpassive$_{tij}$) and each of the three moderators (child ASD severity (γ_{004} adultpassive$_{tij}$ $*$ severity$_{ij}$), child language ability (γ_{004} adultpassive$_{tij}$ $*$ language$_{ij}$), and child behavioral issue (γ_{004} adultpassive$_{tij}$ $*$ behavior$_{ij}$)) (Model 2). Model 2 was

$$\begin{aligned}\text{logit } P_{tij} = {} & \gamma_{000} + \gamma_{001}\,\text{adultactive}_{tij} \\ & + \gamma_{002}\,\text{adultpassive}_{tij} + \gamma_{003}\,\text{adultactive}_{tij} \\ & * \text{severity}_{ij} + \gamma_{004}\,\text{adultpassive}_{tij} \\ & * \text{severity}_{ij} + \gamma_{003}\,\text{adultactive}_{tij} \\ & * \text{language}_{ij} + \gamma_{004}\,\text{adultpassive}_{tij} \\ & * \text{language}_{ij} + \gamma_{003}\,\text{adultactive}_{tij} \\ & * \text{behavior}_{ij} + \gamma_{004}\,\text{adultpassive}_{tij} \\ & * \text{behavior}_{ij} + \gamma_{100}\,\text{ratio}_j + \gamma_{101}\,\text{TEACCH}_j \\ & + \gamma_{102}\,\text{LEAP}_j + \gamma_{010}\,\text{severity}_{ij} \\ & + \gamma_{011}\,\text{language}_{ij} + \gamma_{012}\,\text{behavior}_{ij} + \mu_{oij} \\ & + R_{1j}.\end{aligned} \tag{2}$$

Post hoc tests were used to examine the linear combinations of parameter estimates at crucial values (i.e., at the mean, a standard deviation above the mean, and a standard deviation below the mean) for significant associations.

3. Results

The first research question examined the pattern of child engagement and adult participation. Adults spent most of their time passively participating with focal children (36.5%), followed by actively participating with focal children (34.1%), and then no adult participation with focal children (29.4%). Children spent the majority of their time engaged in activities (72.3%) with only 27.7% of time spent not engaged.

Table 3: Operational definitions.

	CASPER variables	*CASPER* definitions
Adult participation		
Active Participation	Direction Adult Support	Adult provides instruction to focal child or assistance in performing a task or activity.
	Adult approval	Adult expresses praise, appreciation, or satisfaction (verbally or physically) with the focal child.
	Adult comment	Adult talks or gestures to focal child without providing direct support or approval.
Passive Participation	Group discussion/directions	Adult reads aloud to a group of children, sings to group, or gives direction to a group of children including focal child.
	No adult behavior to focal child and one of the following group arrangements: 1 : 1 with adult Small group with adult Large group with adult	Adult is directing no coded behavior to focal child or group of children with focal child, but adult is in close proximity to focal child.
No Participation	No adult behavior to focal child and one of the following group arrangements: Solitary Small group Large group	Adult is directing no coded behavior to focal child or a group of children with focal child, and an adult is not in close proximity to focal child.
Child engagement		
Active Child Engagement	Book	Focal child actively involved with books.
	Preacademics	Focal child engages in preacademic behavior.
	Pretend/sociodramatic play	Focal child uses objects or materials in symbolic manner or performs a role in play theme.
	Art	Focal child interacting in art activity.
	Games with rules	Focal child participating in game with rules.
	Dance/music/recitation	Focal child engaging in songs, poems, nursery rhymes, or dances.
	Self-care/self-help	Focal child involved in caring for his or her personal needs.
	Manipulating	Focal child using coordinated eye-hand movements to interact meaningfully with materials or objects.
	Large motor	Focal child using large muscle movements.
	Clean-up	Focal child is putting away toys, equipment, furniture, dishes, and so forth.
No Active Child Engagement	Not engaged	Focal child is not actively engaged in any *CASPER* child engagement category.
	Stereotypic/repetitive	Focal child involved in some type of repetitive or stereotypic behavior.

Table 4: Model one results for associations between child engagement and adult participation.

Effect	Est.	SE	t stat.	p
Intercept	1.066	0.135	7.91	<0.0001
Active adult participation	−0.108	0.043	−2.52	0.0116
Passive adult participation	−0.095	0.042	−2.25	0.0243
TEACCH	0.031	0.190	0.16	0.8693
LEAP	0.164	0.182	0.9	0.3679
PLS 4	0.371	0.051	7.27	<0.0001
CARS	−0.021	0.044	−0.49	<0.6268
CBCL	−0.225	0.037	−6.01	<0.0001
Child-adult ratio	−0.159	0.081	−1.95	0.0513

Table 5: Model 2 results for moderators of relationship between child engagement and adult participation.

Effect	Est.	SE	t stat.	p
Intercept	1.055	0.136	7.74	<0.0001
Active adult participation	−0.114	0.043	−2.63	0.0085
Passive adult participation	−0.084	0.042	−1.99	0.047
TEACCH	0.030	0.192	0.15	0.8772
LEAP	0.161	0.184	0.88	0.3809
PLS 4	0.476	0.066	7.23	<0.0001
CARS	−0.090	0.061	−1.48	0.1385
CBCL	−0.120	0.049	−2.43	0.0152
Child-adult ratio	−0.167	0.082	−2.03	0.0423
Active adult participation ∗ PLS 4	−0.143	0.059	−2.43	0.0151
Passive adult participation ∗ PLS 4	−0.137	0.057	−2.39	0.0169
Active adult participation ∗ CARS	0.128	0.057	2.27	0.0235
Passive adult participation ∗ CARS	0.034	0.056	0.6	0.5488
Active adult participation ∗ CBCL	−0.143	0.050	−2.88	0.0039
Passive adult participation ∗ CBCL	−0.154	0.049	−3.15	0.0016

Associations between child engagement and adult participation were examined in the second research questions. Model 1 results are presented in Table 4. Focal children were less likely to be engaged when adults were actively participating with a focal child ($t = -2.52$, $p = 0.012$, log OR = −0.108, and SE = 0.043). The odds ratio (OR) of focal child engagement between actively and not actively participating adults was estimated at 0.90. Focal children were also less likely to be engaged when adults were passively participating with a focal child ($t = -2.25$, $p = 0.024$, log OR = −0.095, and SE = 0.042). The estimated OR was 0.91.

The final three research questions addressed how autism severity, child language ability, and child challenging behavior moderated the relationship between adult participation and child engagement. Model 2 results are presented in Table 5. The interaction between child engagement and active adult participation was moderated by autism severity (log OR = 0.128, SE = 0.057, $t = 2.27$, and $p = 0.024$) with active adult participation supporting child engagement. Children with higher autism severity ratings (i.e., CARS scores a standard deviation above the mean) were likely to be engaged when adults were actively participating. Post hoc test examined the

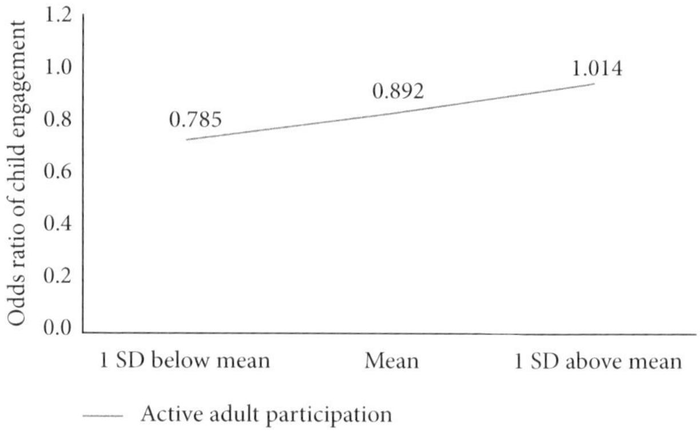

Figure 1: Interaction of active adult participation and child ASD severity on child engagement.

linear combinations of parameter estimates at crucial values (i.e., at the mean and a standard deviation above and below the mean). The estimated OR of engagement between actively and not actively participating adults for children with CARS scores at one standard deviation above the mean (+1 SD) was not statistically significantly different from 1 (log OR = 0.014, SE = 0.074, $t = 0.19$, and $p = 0.8493$); the estimated OR for children with CARS scores at the mean was 0.89 (log OR = −0.114, SE = 0.043, $t = -2.63$, and $p = 0.0085$); the estimated OR for children with CARS one standard deviation below the mean (−1 SD) was 0.78 (log OR = −0.243, SE = 0.068, $t = -3.54$, and $p = 0.0004$). Figure 1 shows the odds ratios of child engagement between active adult participation and no active adult participation for children with different levels of ASD severity measured by CARS. No evidence was found for differential associations between child engagement and passive adult participation for children with different ASD severity levels (log OR = 0.034, SE = 0.056, $t = 0.6$, and $p = 0.549$). Overall, children with higher autism severity ratings were more likely to be involved when adults were interacting with them.

As shown in Table 5, there was evidence that the association between child engagement and active adult participation was negatively moderated by child language ability (log OR = −0.143, SE = 0.059, $t = -2.43$, and $p = 0.015$). Post hoc analysis showed that estimated OR of engagement between actively and not actively participating adults for children with language scores at +1 SD was 0.77 (log OR = −0.258, SE = 0.076, $t = -3.37$, and $p = 0.0008$); the estimated OR for children with language ability at the mean was 0.89 (log OR = −0.114, SE = 0.043, $t = -2.63$, and $p = 0.0085$); the estimated OR for children with language ability at −1 SD was not statistically significantly different from 1 (log OR = 0.029, SE = 0.070, $t = 0.42$, and $p = 0.6768$). The association between passive adult participation and child engagement was also negatively moderated by child language ability (log OR = −0.137, SE = 0.057, $t = -2.39$, and $p = 0.0169$). Post hoc test showed that estimated OR of engagement between passively and not passively participating adults for children with language score at +1 SD was 0.80 (log OR = −0.221, SE = 0.074, $t = -3$, and $p = 0.0027$); the estimated OR for students

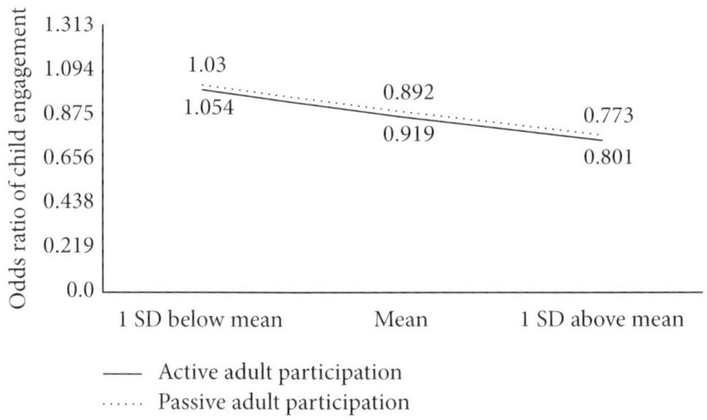

FIGURE 2: Interaction of active/passive adult participation and child language ability on child engagement.

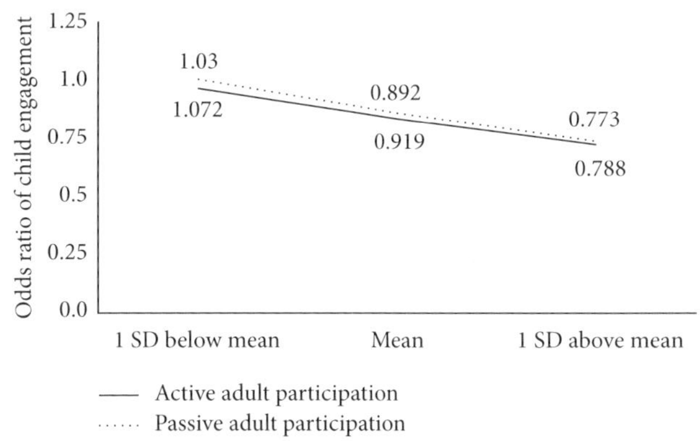

FIGURE 3: Interaction of active/passive adult participation and Child Behavior on child engagement.

with language score at the mean was 0.92 (log OR = −0.084, SE = 0.042, $t = -1.99$, and $p = 0.047$); the estimated OR for students with language score at −1 SD was not statistically significantly different from 1 (log OR = 0.053, SE = 0.069, $t = 0.76$, and $p = 0.4445$). Figure 2 shows the impact of the significant interaction between active and passive adult participation and child language ability on child engagement. Overall, children with higher language abilities were less likely to be engaged when adults were actively or passively participating with them.

Similar to the effect of language scores, the association between child engagement and active adult participation was negatively moderated by child challenging behavior (log OR = −0.143, SE = 0.050, $t = -2.88$, $p = 0.004$, and $p = 0.0039$). Post hoc analysis showed that estimated OR of engagement between actively and not actively participating adults for children with problem behavior score at +1 SD was 0.77 (log OR = −0.258, SE = 0.065, $t = -3.96$, and $p = 0.0001$); the estimated OR for children with problem behavior score at the mean was 0.89 (log OR = −0.114, SE = 0.043, $t = -2.63$, and $p = 0.0085$); the estimated OR for children with problem behavior score at −1 SD was not statistically significantly different from 1 (log OR = 0.029, SE = 0.067, $t = 0.43$, and $p = 0.6638$). Similarly, the association between passive adult participation and child engagement was negatively moderated by child challenging behavior (log OR = −0.154, SE = 0.049, $t = -3.15$, and $p = 0.002$). Post hoc test showed that estimated OR of engagement between passively and not passively participating adults for children with problem behavior score at +1 SD was 0.79 (log OR = −0.238, SE = 0.064, $t = -3.71$, and $p = 0.002$); the estimated OR for students with language score at the mean was 0.92 (log OR = −0.084, SE = 0.042, $t = -1.99$, and $p = 0.047$); the estimated OR for students with language score at −1 SD was not statistically significantly different from 1 (log OR = 0.069, SE = 0.065, $t = 1.06$, and $p = 0.2873$). Figure 3 shows the impact of the significant interactions between active and passive adult participation and child challenging behavior on child engagement. Overall, children rated with higher amounts of challenging behavior were less likely to be engaged when adults were actively or passively participating with them.

To summarize, higher levels of adult participation were associated with less child engagement. However, when children had greater autism severity or less language ability, higher levels of adult participation were associated with higher levels of child engagement. For children with more challenging behaviors, higher adult participation was associated with less engagement.

4. Discussion

This study provides information on how adult participation is associated with child engagement in preschool classrooms that serve children with ASD. This is the first study that explored how specific characteristics (i.e., autism severity, child language ability, and challenging behavior) moderate this relationship.

During center time activities, preschoolers with ASD were engaged in classroom activities for 72.3% of the time. The percentage of time engaged was higher in this study than previous research which found that children with ASD were engaged approximately half the time (47.6% and 51%) [11, 13]. Brown and colleagues [12] observed preschoolers with disabilities in inclusive settings across multiple activities and settings resulting in numerous transitions where students might not be "engaged." In contrast, this study focused on center time and included both inclusive and separate/self-contained settings. While preschoolers could transition between activities, the transitions were minimal and relatively short in duration. The inclusion of high quality classrooms in the current study is another possible explanation for the higher rates of child engagement. Previous studies have linked classroom quality to child engagement levels in preschool, kindergarten, and third grade classrooms [9, 10, 15]. While the models used for analysis controlled for covariates of model type (LEAP an inclusive setting and TEACCH a self-contained setting) and adult to child ratios, the teachers in these classrooms had received formal trainings on models and classrooms met quality measures (see [23]).

Adults divided their time with focal children fairly evenly spending 36.5% of the time passively participating with the identified focal child, 34.1% of the time actively participating, and 29.4% of the time not participating with the focal child. Adults in this study spent more time actively and passively participating with focal children than what is found in a previous study for preschoolers without disabilities in urban public preschool classrooms [18]. The current studies definition of adult participation and inclusion of high quality classrooms could account for these differences. The inclusion of high quality classrooms possibly resulted in preselecting adults who were more likely to regularly interact with children.

The current study found that children were less likely to be engaged when an adult was actively or passively participating with them. To explore this relationship further, this study examined the possible impact of several potential moderators on child engagement. First, autism severity positively moderated the relationship between adult participation and child engagement with children rated with more severe forms of autism more likely to be engaged when adults were actively participating with them. Previous research found that adults are more likely to interact with children who are involved in more solitary activities or passive forms of play in childcare centers and inclusive preschools [39, 40]. Given this, adults might seek out children with more severe forms of ASD who are isolated and need more support and guidance in the preschool classroom. Second, the association between child engagement and adult participation was negatively moderated by child language ability with children with lower language abilities more likely to be engaged when adults were actively or passively participating with them. Similar to children with more severe forms of autism, children with lower language abilities may have required more assistance from adults in the classroom to engage in classroom activities successfully. Finally, challenging behavior was negatively associated with adult participation and child engagement. Children with higher amounts of challenging behavior engaged less frequently when adults were actively or passively participating with them. This finding is supported by previous research that found that children with more challenging behavior are less likely to be engaged in activities in inclusive classrooms [13]. Children with more challenging behavior might require additional support from adults in the classroom. For example, when a child is exhibiting challenging behavior (such as throwing toys, hitting, and kicking) an adult is more likely to support the child to ensure the safety of the child and other peers in the class. However, the behavior of the child during this period would be coded as not engaged.

Several limitations should be noted for this study. First, the analysis only included data collected at pretest during the beginning of the year. Adults might alter their behavior towards children throughout the year as children gain more independence. Next, the quality of the video impacted the ability to code behaviors. For example, the context of the video was not always captured. If an adult or child was off screen the time point, coding was not possible during the affected time point. Third, the definition of child engagement was based upon an ecobehavioral assessment and differs from other engagement literatures [12]. A more precise coding of child engagement using hierarchical engagement codes might have resulted in different findings. The cooccurrence of adult participation and child engagement was examined which prevented the ability to determine how adult participation predicts child engagement. Finally, past research regarding child engagement levels has focused on inclusive settings [11, 13] or self-contained, separate settings [14]. This study included both self-contained and inclusive classroom settings. While treatment model (i.e., TEACCH and LEAP) was controlled for in the analysis, the results were not interpreted by inclusive or separate settings.

5. Conclusion

The present study provides information on the association of adult behavior and the engagement of preschoolers with ASD. Given that children were more engaged when adults were not present or interacting with the focal child, arranging the environment to promote the active engagement of children is critical. Arranging the environment to promote learning has been emphasized as best practice for young children [41] and as helpful for children with ASD [24]. The arrangement of the environment might be particularly important for children who display more challenging behaviors as these children were less likely to be engaged when adults were actively participating with them. Children with more severe forms of autism and less language ability were more likely to be actively engaged when adults were actively participating with them. These children might need more support from adults to engage with materials or the environment. The current study examined the association between child engagement and adult participation based upon the selected characteristics as moderators. However, these moderators are not independent of one another. For example, a child with ASD might display challenging behavior, low language ability, and more severe forms of ASD. This child might benefit from a more structured environment and support from an adult when needed to actively engage with the environment.

Future research is needed to determine how potential characteristics of adults (e.g., education level, experience, training, and burnout) moderate child outcomes. Additionally, future research should focus on exploring the causal relationship between adult behavior and child engagement. Engagement is critical to enhance positive outcomes for children. Based upon this study, child moderators have the potential to impact how teachers and other adults can best support the engagement of children.

Disclaimer

The opinions expressed represent those of the authors and do not represent views of the Institute or the US Department of Education.

Acknowledgment

The research reported here was supported by the Institute of Education Sciences, US Department of Education, through Grant R324B070219 awarded to UNC-Chapel Hill.

References

[1] National Research Council, *Educating Children with Autism*, National Academy Press, Washington, DC, USA, 2001.

[2] S. L. Odom, B. A. Boyd, L. J. Hall, and K. Hume, "Evaluation of comprehensive treatment models for individuals with autism spectrum disorders," *Journal of Autism and Developmental Disorders*, vol. 40, no. 4, pp. 425–436, 2010.

[3] R. C. Pianta, *Enhancing Relationships between Children and Teachers*, American Psychological Association, Washington, DC, USA, 1999.

[4] C. Howes, L. C. Phillipsen, and E. Peisner-Feinberg, "The consistency of perceived teacher–child relationships between preschool and kindergarten," *Journal of School Psychology*, vol. 38, no. 2, pp. 113–132, 2000.

[5] M. R. Burchinal, E. Peisner-Feinberg, R. Pianta, and C. Howes, "Development of academic skills from preschool through second grade: family and classroom predictors of developmental trajectories," *Journal of School Psychology*, vol. 40, no. 5, pp. 415–436, 2002.

[6] A. J. Mashburn, R. C. Pianta, B. K. Hamre et al., "Measures of classroom quality in prekindergarten and children's development of academic, language, and social skills," *Child Development*, vol. 79, no. 3, pp. 732–749, 2008.

[7] B. K. Hamre and R. C. Pianta, "Early teacher-child relationships and the trajectory of children's school outcomes through eighth grade," *Child Development*, vol. 72, no. 2, pp. 625–638, 2001.

[8] R. A. McWilliam, C. M. Trivette, and C. J. Dunst, "Behavior engagement as a measure of the efficacy of early intervention," *Analysis and Intervention in Developmental Disabilities*, vol. 5, no. 1-2, pp. 59–71, 1985.

[9] J. T. Downer, S. E. Rimm-Kaufman, and R. C. Pianta, "How do classroom conditions and children's risk for school problems contribute to children's behavioral engagement in learning?" *School Psychology Review*, vol. 36, no. 3, pp. 413–432, 2007.

[10] C. C. Ponitz, S. E. Rimm-Kaufman, K. J. Grimm, and T. W. Curby, "Kindergarten classroom quality, behavioral engagement, and reading achievement," *School Psychology Review*, vol. 38, no. 1, pp. 102–120, 2009.

[11] C. Kemp, Y. Kishida, M. Carter, and N. Sweller, "The effect of activity type on the engagement and interaction of young children with disabilities in inclusive childcare settings," *Early Childhood Research Quarterly*, vol. 28, no. 1, pp. 134–143, 2013.

[12] W. H. Brown, S. L. Odom, S. Li, and C. Zercher, "Ecobehavioral assessment in early childhood programs: a portrait of preschool inclusion," *Journal of Special Education*, vol. 33, no. 3, pp. 138–153, 1999.

[13] S. L. Odom, W. H. Brown, I. S. Schwartz, C. Zercher, and S. R. Sandall, "Classroom ecology and child participation," in *Widening the Circle*, pp. 25–45, Teachers College Press, New York, NY, USA, 2002.

[14] C. Wong and C. Kasari, "Play and joint attention of children with autism in the preschool special education classroom," *Journal of Autism and Developmental Disorders*, vol. 42, no. 10, pp. 2152–2161, 2012.

[15] R. A. McWilliam and D. B. Bailey Jr., "Effects of classroom social structure and disability on engagement," *Topics in Early Childhood Special Education*, vol. 15, no. 2, pp. 123–147, 1995.

[16] R. E. L. de Kruif and R. A. McWilliam, "Multivariate relationships among developmental age, global engagement, and observed child engagement," *Early Childhood Research Quarterly*, vol. 14, no. 4, pp. 515–536, 1999.

[17] R. A. McWilliam, A. A. Scarborough, and H. Kim, "Adult interactions and child engagement," *Early Education & Development*, vol. 14, no. 1, pp. 7–28, 2003.

[18] D. R. Powell, M. R. Burchinal, N. File, and S. Kontos, "An eco-behavioral analysis of children's engagement in urban public school preschool classrooms," *Early Childhood Research Quarterly*, vol. 23, no. 1, pp. 108–123, 2008.

[19] L. L. Tsao, S. L. Odom, V. Buysse, M. Skinner, T. West, and J. Vitztum-Komanecki, "Social participation of children with disabilities in inclusive preschool programs: program typology and ecological features," *Exceptionality*, vol. 16, no. 3, pp. 125–140, 2008.

[20] D. B. Reinhartsen, A. N. Garfinkle, and M. Wolery, "Engagement with toys in two-year-old children with autism: teacher selection versus child choice," *Research & Practice for Persons with Severe Disabilities*, vol. 27, no. 3, pp. 175–187, 2002.

[21] D. Hamilton, "An ecobehavioural analysis of interactive engagement of children with developmental disabilities with their peers in inclusive preschools," *International Journal of Disability, Development and Education*, vol. 52, no. 2, pp. 121–137, 2005.

[22] B. A. Boyd, K. Hume, M. T. McBee et al., "Comparative efficacy of LEAP, TEACCH and non-model-specific special education programs for preschoolers with autism spectrum disorders," *Journal of Autism and Developmental Disorders*, vol. 44, no. 2, pp. 366–380, 2014.

[23] G. B. Mesibov, V. Shea, and E. Schopler, *The TEACCH Approach to Autism Spectrum Disorders*, Kluwer Academic Publishers, Plenum Publishers, New York, NY, USA, 2005.

[24] P. S. Strain and E. H. Bovey, "Randomized, controlled trial of the leap model of early intervention for young children with autism spectrum disorders," *Topics in Early Childhood Special Education*, vol. 31, no. 3, pp. 133–154, 2011.

[25] P. Strain and L. Cordisco, "LEAP preschool," in *Preschool Education Programs for Children with Autism*, S. H. J. Handleman, Ed., pp. 225–244, PRO-ED, Austin, Tex, USA, 1994.

[26] P. S. Strain and M. Hoyson, "The need for longitudinal, intensive social skill intervention: LEAP follow-up outcomes for children with autism," *Topics in Early Childhood Special Education*, vol. 20, no. 2, pp. 116–122, 2000.

[27] J. S. Howard, C. R. Sparkman, H. G. Cohen, G. Green, and H. Stanislaw, "A comparison of intensive behavior analytic and eclectic treatments for young children with autism," *Research in Developmental Disabilities*, vol. 26, no. 4, pp. 359–383, 2005.

[28] Professional Development in Autism Center, *PDA Program Assessment*, PDA Center at University of Washington, Seattle, Wash, USA, 2008.

[29] C. Lord, M. Rutter, P. C. DiLavore, and S. Risi, *The Autism Diagnostic Observation Schedule (ADOS)*, Western Psychological Corporation, Los Angeles, Calif, USA, 1999.

[30] E. M. Mullen, *Mullen Scales of Early Learning (AGS Edition)*, Western Psychological, Los Angeles, Calif, USA, 1995.

[31] I. Zimmerman, V. Steiner, and R. Pond, *Preschool Language Scale-IV*, Psychological Corporation, San Antonio, Tex, USA, 2003.

[32] E. Schopler, R. J. Reichler, and B. R. Renner, *The Childhood Autism Rating Scale*, Western Psychological Services, Los Angeles, Calif, USA, 1988.

[33] T. M. Achenbach and L. A. Rescorla, *Manual for the ASEBA Preschool Forms and Profiles*, University of Vermont, Research Center for Children, Youth, and Families, Burlington, Vt, USA, 2000.

[34] J. Tapp and T. A. Walden, "PROCODER: a system for collection and analysis of observational data from videotape," in *Behavioral Observation: Technology and Applications in Developmental Disabilities*, T. Thompson, D. Felece, and F. J. Symons, Eds., pp. 61–70, Paul H. Brookes, Baltimore, Md, USA, 2000.

[35] L. Tsao, S. L. Odom, and W. B. Brown, *Code for Active Student Participation and Engagement—Revised (CASPER III): A Training Manual for Observers*, Indiana University, Bloomington, Ind, USA, 2001.

[36] K. R. Logan, R. Bakeman, and E. B. Keefe, "Effects of instructional variables on engaged behavior of students with disabilities in general education classrooms," *Exceptional Children*, vol. 63, no. 4, pp. 481–497, 1997.

[37] D. M. Kamps, B. R. Leonard, E. P. Dugan, B. Boland, and C. R. Greenwood, "The use of ecobehavioral assessment to identify naturally occurring effective procedures in classrooms serving students with autism and other developmental disabilities," *Journal of Behavioral Education*, vol. 1, no. 4, pp. 367–397, 1991.

[38] S. L. Odom and C. Peterson, "Ecobehavioral analysis of early education/specialized classroom settings and peer social interaction," *Education and Treatment of Children*, vol. 13, no. 4, pp. 316–330, 1990.

[39] R. J. Coplan and K. Prakash, "Spending time with teacher: characteristics of preschoolers who frequently elicit versus initiate interactions with teachers," *Early Childhood Research Quarterly*, vol. 18, no. 1, pp. 143–158, 2003.

[40] L. V. Harper and K. S. McCluskey, "Teacher-child and child-child interactions in inclusive preschool settings: do adults inhibit peer interactions?" *Early Childhood Research Quarterly*, vol. 18, no. 2, pp. 163–184, 2003.

[41] Division for Early Childhood, *DEC Recommended Practices in Early Intervention/Early Childhood Special Education 2014*, Division for Early Childhood, 2014, http://www.dec-sped.org/recommendedpractices.

21

Theory of Mind Indexes the Broader Autism Phenotype in Siblings of Children with Autism at School Age

Tawny Tsang,[1] Kristen Gillespie-Lynch,[2] and Ted Hutman[3]

[1]*Department of Psychology, University of California, Los Angeles, CA 90024, USA*
[2]*Department of Psychology, College of Staten Island and The Graduate Center, CUNY, New York, NY 10314, USA*
[3]*Department of Psychiatry & Bio-Behavioral Sciences, David Geffen School of Medicine at UCLA, University of California, Los Angeles, CA 90024, USA*

Correspondence should be addressed to Tawny Tsang; tsangtt89@ucla.edu

Academic Editor: Klaus-Peter Ossenkopp

Subclinical variants of the social-communicative challenges and rigidity that define autism spectrum disorder (ASD) are known as the broader autism phenotype (BAP). The BAP has been conceptualized categorically (as specific to a subset of relatives of individuals with ASD) and dimensionally (as continuously distributed within the general population). The current study examined the compatibility of these two approaches by assessing associations among autism symptoms and social-communicative skills in young school-age children with ASD, children who have a sibling with ASD, and children without a sibling with ASD. Autism symptoms were associated with reduced Theory of Mind (ToM), adaptive skills, cognitive empathy, and language skills across the full sample. Reduced ToM was a core aspect of the BAP in the current sample regardless of whether the BAP was defined categorically (in terms of siblings of children with ASD who exhibited atypical developmental) or dimensionally (in terms of associations with autism symptoms across the entire sample). Early language skills predicted school-age ToM. Findings support the compatibility of categorical and dimensional approaches to the BAP, highlight reduced ToM as a core aspect of the school-age BAP, and suggest that narrative-based approaches to promoting ToM may be beneficial for siblings of children with ASD.

1. Introduction

Subclinical characteristics associated with autism, such as difficulties with social communication and rigidity, are continuously distributed in the general population and are particularly common among relatives of people with autism [1–5]. Collectively, these traits are referred to as the "broader autism phenotype" (BAP). Investigations of the BAP range from operationalizing it as a categorical entity restricted to a subgroup of relatives of people with autism who show elevated social-communicative impairments and/or restricted behaviors [3, 6–9] to exploring it as a dimensional phenomenon associated with a range of mental health issues and personality-related characteristics in the general population [10–13].

These different conceptualizations of the BAP often use distinct measures and sampling techniques (e.g., [14, 15]). Few studies have attempted to bridge categorical and dimensional perspectives of the BAP by determining whether specific challenges present among individuals with autism are also present among some relatives of individuals with autism, and if such challenges are continuously associated with autistic-like traits across a general population sample (see [16] for a rare example of a study that melded both approaches). Studies that include both categorical and dimensional approaches to the BAP are essential for demonstrating that they represent a common construct. The current study examines the compatibility of these two approaches by assessing autistic-like traits and social-communicative skills among young children with autism, children who have a sibling with autism, and children without a sibling with autism. This study is grounded in the idea that the BAP is akin to the "'duality' of light, a phenomenon with both wave- and particle-like properties" [17, p. 529].

1.1. Relations between the BAP and Autism. Autistic-like social-communicative atypicalities and rigid behaviors may share common genetic underpinnings with autism spectrum disorder (ASD; [2]). Heightened levels of autistic-like traits are more likely to be present in parents [13, 18] and siblings of children with ASD [3, 6, 7, 19–22] than in individuals with no family history of ASD. The incidence of subclinical autistic-like traits is also greater for families with multiple instances of ASD relative to simplex families [18, 23–27]. The BAP may reflect an intermediate expression of genetic susceptibility to ASD, similar to the proposed intermediate phenotypes associated with other highly heritable psychiatric conditions, like schizophrenia and bipolar disorder (e.g., [28, 29]). Better characterization of the BAP may help identify mechanisms underlying ASD.

Variations in the nature and magnitude of phenotypic expression of the BAP observed across studies suggest heterogeneity in the aggregation of autistic-like characteristics (for review, see [4]). Although this heterogeneity may partially reflect differences in how the BAP is conceptualized, heterogeneity remains as much of a challenge for the BAP as it is for ASD itself. While the BAP is defined by milder variants of the behavioral challenges associated with ASD, it does not necessarily entail functional impairment [30] and may even be associated with giftedness (e.g., [31]). Furthermore, there is currently no agreed upon gold standard measure like the Autism Diagnostic Observation Scale [32] to quantify the extent to which an individual manifests BAP features. Instead, several instruments have been adapted or developed to characterize the BAP in family members (for a review, see [15]) and/or the general population (e.g., [14]).

1.2. Characterization of the BAP. An emerging body of research examines the BAP dimensionally by administering self-report measures to "general population" samples (commonly consisting of convenience samples of college students). These studies have revealed associations between heightened autistic-like traits and reduced ToM and enhanced perceptual skills [33], difficulty interpreting emotions [12, 13, 16, 34], and social challenges [11, 35].

These dimensional approaches to characterizing the BAP are believed to build upon earlier research evaluating the BAP categorically among relatives of individuals with ASD. In the first study to provide clear evidence of the BAP, Folstein and Rutter [36] found that monozygotic twins of individuals with ASD who did not themselves have ASD exhibited cognitive, linguistic, and/or social challenges. Subsequent researchers have evaluated the BAP categorically by comparing relatives of individuals with ASD more generally to those without a relative on the spectrum. For example, comparisons of parents who did or did not have a child with ASD revealed that decreased Theory of Mind (ToM; [37]) and enhanced perceptual skills may be characteristics of the BAP [38]. Other researchers have used cut-off scores on structured interviews, surveys, and/or observational measures to identify subgroups of relatives of individuals with ASD who exhibit heightened autistic-like traits [3, 6, 7, 39, 40]. A subset of parents of children with ASD who were classified as aloof based on interviews exhibited difficulties with ToM and emotion recognition relative to those who were not classified as aloof and control parents [8, 39].

In addition to subclinical levels of core autistic-like traits, studies of relatives have also revealed that developmental language atypicalities (including spelling and reading difficulties; [6]), anxiety and mood disorders, difficulties with executive functioning, and cognitive challenges are present in a subset of relatives of individuals with ASD (reviewed in [41]). However, a number of other studies have revealed no evidence that cognitive and/or language difficulties are elevated among relatives of individuals with ASD (reviewed in [42]).

1.3. The BAP at School Age. Among younger siblings of children with ASD who have reached school-age (the focus of this report), the BAP has been characterized broadly based on risk group [43–46] or more narrowly by focusing on a subset of siblings who exhibit heightened autistic-like symptoms and/or atypicalities in language, cognition, and academic skills [42, 47, 48]. Indeed, there is no consensus in the field regarding inclusionary criteria for BAP classification among younger siblings of children with ASD (reviewed by [49]).

The small body of emerging research focusing on the school-age outcomes of younger siblings has revealed limited evidence of the BAP at school-age. For instance, Warren and colleagues [46] compared 39 younger siblings of children with ASD (sibs-ASD) to 22 younger siblings of typically developing children (sibs-TD) at 5 years of age and found no significant differences in IQ, language, social symptoms, or behavior problems. However, reduced executive functioning and heightened levels of restricted interests/behaviors were observed among sibs-ASD. Given that sibs-ASD had exhibited reduced joint attention relative to sibs-TD as toddlers [50], the researchers surmised that sibs-ASD may have demonstrated developmental resilience by overcoming initial challenges.

Evidence suggestive of resilience was also obtained by Gamliel and colleagues [42] when they compared 37 sibs-ASD to 47 sibs-TD at multiple time points between 4 months and 7 years of age. They found that almost a third of the sibs-ASD exhibited linguistic and cognitive impairments on standardized measures at some point in development. However, most of the sibs-ASD had caught up to their peers—often without intervention—by 54 months of age, although some of them still exhibited language difficulties. Notably, the proportion of sibs-ASD who exhibited the BAP at 7 years was substantially higher than it had been between 4 and 54 months of age. Cognitive, language, and/or academic difficulties reemerged at 7 years of age and were apparent in 40% of the sibs-ASD (relative to 16% of the sibs-TD) according to parent reports and/or direct tests. The authors suggested that BAP related issues may (re)emerge as children are faced with increasingly challenging academic and social environments.

In contrast, a different research group found no evidence of impairments in expressive/receptive language, pragmatic language, or reading among a slightly older sample (8–11 years old) of 18 sibs-ASD relative to national norms [43]. Similarly, comparisons of 31 sibs-ASD and 23 sibs-TD at approximately 7.5 years of age (including some of the participants who will be described in this report) revealed no evidence of pragmatic or structural language impairments associated with the BAP [44].

However, group-level comparisons of sibs-ASD to sibs-TD may obscure atypicalities among a subset of relatives. Indeed, a recent cross-institutional study (including some of the participants described in this report) compared a subset of sibs-ASD, who were not diagnosed with ASD but who were identified as clinically concerning, to typically developing children at early school age [51]. Clinical concerns included elevated autistic-like symptoms, ADHD symptoms, speech-language challenges, anxiety/mood problems, and learning difficulties. Clinically concerning sibs-ASD had higher parent-reported autism symptoms and psychopathology and lower language skills than typically developing sibs-ASD and sibs-TD, who did not differ from one another.

In the current report, we define the BAP categorically as clinical concerns in individuals who do not meet criteria for ASD. This operational definition is consistent with prior school-age research wherein the BAP was defined in terms of a range of concerns rather than by focusing only on participants with elevated autistic-like symptoms (e.g., [42]). Miller and colleagues viewed the BAP as specific to the subset of clinically concerning children who exhibited heightened autism symptoms. However, they acknowledged that mood, language, learning, and attention difficulties are common among relatives of individuals with ASD and stated that research is needed to determine how to define the BAP among younger siblings. A primary aim of this report is to determine whether clinically concerning non-ASD outcomes are an appropriate definition of the BAP by evaluating if difficulties that are elevated among clinically concerning participants are dimensionally associated with autistic-like symptoms across the entire sample.

1.4. Is ToM an Aspect of the BAP at School Age? Given that the majority of studies examining the BAP at school age have focused on linguistic, cognitive, and academic outcomes, we examine potential social-cognitive contributors to the BAP at school age. The school-age time point is a developmentally appropriate period to assess explicit ToM reasoning because evidence of rudimentary ToM (i.e., passing false-belief tasks) emerges by 4 years of age among typically developing children and becomes more sophisticated over time [52]. A subset of the children in the studies conducted by Gamliel and colleagues (24 sibs-ASD and 24 sibs-TD) participated in ToM tasks (the false belief and strange stories tasks) at 54 months of age [45]. After observing no differences in ToM between sibs-ASD and sibs-TD, the researchers concluded that sibs-ASD show resilience in terms of ToM abilities. However, this finding contrasts with research demonstrating reduced ToM among three-year-old siblings of children with ASD [53], slightly older sibs-ASD [54], and parents of children with ASD [37, 38]. Impaired ToM was also apparent among a subset of parents of children with ASD who were classified as socially aloof (e.g., [8, 39]).

Nevertheless, Shaked and colleagues' lack of evidence that reduced ToM is an aspect of the BAP at school age is consistent with null effects obtained in a study comparing 18 siblings of children with ASD (between 8 and 18 years of age) to 18 siblings of children with a learning disability [55], although the authors of the latter study concluded that their study was insufficiently powered to detect an effect if one were present. Similarly, dimensional associations between autistic-like traits and challenges with mentalizing have been demonstrated in the general population [33], but such associations are not always observed (e.g., [56]).

Contradictory evidence concerning whether ToM is an aspect of the BAP may reflect an often unexamined factor in the aforementioned studies, that is, variation in language skills. Language is concurrently associated with performance on ToM tasks for people with and without ASD (e.g., [57–59]). Language ability also predicts subsequent ToM development among children with and without ASD [60–62]. Therefore, a secondary aim of the current study is to examine associations between language (at 3 years of age and school age) and school-age ToM.

In the current study, we utilize both a behavioral measure of ToM and a parent-report measure of cognitive empathy (i.e., understanding of others' perspectives) and affective empathy (i.e., emotional responsiveness to others' emotions). Although ToM and cognitive empathy are often described as synonymous (e.g., [63]), a behavioral measure of ToM (the Eyes Test) was unrelated to cognitive and affective empathy among adults in the general population [64]. In contrast, behavioral ToM was associated with *both* cognitive and affective empathy among individuals with ASD and parents of children with ASD, who exhibited reduced cognitive and affective empathy and ToM relative to controls. Given variable associations between behavioral ToM and cognitive empathy, we evaluate both in the current study. We also include a behavioral proxy (attention to an examiner in distress) and a parent-report measure of affective empathy. However, we do not expect affective empathy to be an aspect of the BAP based on theoretical work suggesting that affective empathy may be unimpaired or enhanced in ASD [65].

1.5. Study Aims. A primary aim of the current study is to evaluate the compatibility of findings derived from a categorical and a dimensional approach to defining the BAP at school age. Given the broad range of variables that have been associated with the BAP in prior research, we examine categorical and dimensional associations between the BAP and a range of social-cognitive and social-affective characteristics. Study measures include observational and parent-report measures of autistic-like traits (assessed by severity scores on the ADOS), ToM, language, nonverbal IQ, affective and cognitive empathy, responses to others' distress, and adaptive behaviors. We first evaluate the extent to which these skills differ across groups to identify atypicalities apparent among younger siblings identified as clinically concerning (a categorical analysis) and then examined dimensional interrelationships between autistic-like symptoms and social-communicative variables. We then examine whether language development (at 3 years and at school age) is associated with school-age social-cognitive challenges.

TABLE 1: Participant characteristics by group.

	HR-ASD (n = 11)	HR-Other (n = 12)	HR-Typical (n = 24)	LR-Typical (n = 22)	p^1
Male, %	63.64	50.00	37.50	59.09	0.39
Caucasian, %	36	31	58	84	0.001
High SES^2, %	60	50	24	52	0.25
Age at testing in years, M (SD)	5.46 (0.46)	6.04 (1.29)	5.52 (0.45)	5.89 (0.41)	0.01

Note. Some families did not provide complete demographic data. Percentages are relative to all responses received.
[1] p value = significance level for Kruskal-Wallis test of overall group differences.
[2] High SES = annual family income ≥ USD $125,000.

Participants took part in a larger longitudinal study employing an infant-sibling design and thus the data reflect a wide range of social (dis)ability. The study seeks to determine whether a high level of shared variance among measures reflects a common underlying social-communicative deficit in the BAP, or whether individual measures uniquely account for heterogeneity in the BAP. Given the scope of skills examined, this study also examines the utility of converging measurement tools in clinical settings. The current investigation is not exhaustive but focuses on behavioral impairments in the social-affective and social-cognitive domain. In sum, the current study uses categorical and dimensional approaches to identify social characteristics associated with the BAP among young school-age children and to determine if early language predicts social challenges at school age.

2. Methods

2.1. Participants. Enrollment criteria, recruitment strategy, and a large proportion of the sample itself have been described elsewhere [44]. Infant siblings of children with autism (HR group) and low-risk (LR) controls were seen at 5 time points from infancy to toddlerhood (6, 12, 18, 24, and 36 months) and at school-age (M = 5.74 years, SD = 0.69 years). This study focuses on the latest time point in the longitudinal study and includes the subset of children who were seen at the school-age visit (n = 69).

Clinical psychologists observed participants at the school-age visit to determine whether they met diagnostic criteria for an ASD upon reviewing reports provided by the ADOS, the ADI-R, and the *Social Communication Questionnaire* (SCQ; [66]). Participants were classified into 4 groups for statistical comparisons (see Table 1 for sample characterization): (a) "ASD": HR participants who met DSM-IV criteria for ASD (n = 9) and LR participants who received an ASD diagnosis (n = 2); (b) "HR-Other": HR participants who showed other developmental concerns (e.g., heightened autistic traits, language, learning and/or cognitive delays, attention deficits, and anxiety/mood difficulties; see [51]) based on clinical judgment but did not meet clinical criteria for ASD (n = 12); (c) "HR-Typical": HR participants who exhibited typical development according to the ADOS, DAS-II, CELF-4, and VABS-II (HR-TD; n = 24); (d) "LR-Typical": LR participants who exhibited typical development using the aforementioned criteria (LR-TD; n = 22). Two additional LR participants were judged to exhibit developmental concerns and were excluded from analyses.

2.2. Measures

2.2.1. Autism Diagnostic Observation Schedule (ADOS, [32]). The ADOS is a semistructured play-based observational measure that is designed to elicit autism symptomatology. The appropriate ADOS module (2 or 3) was administered based on participant's age and language abilities as prescribed by the authors of the measure. Symptom severity was compared across modules using the ADOS Calibrated Severity Score (ADOS-CSS; [67]), where higher scores denote more severe social disability and/or restricted interests and repetitive behaviors. ADOS severity scores exhibit more stability over time than raw scores and have therefore been recommended as a more valid measure of the severity of autistic traits [68].

2.2.2. Differential Ability Scales, 2nd Edition (DAS; [69]). The DAS is a cognitive assessment measuring verbal, nonverbal, and spatial abilities. Here we focus on nonverbal cognitive ability (NVIQ), which was derived from the Nonverbal Reasoning and Spatial Abilities Standard Score.

2.2.3. Clinical Evaluation of Language Fundamentals-4 (CELF-4; [70]). The CELF-4 is a standardized behavioral assessment of general language abilities in children 5 to 21 years of age. The Core Language Standard Score (CLS) is calculated based on performance on four subtests measuring receptive and expressive language skills fundamental to effective communication (e.g., semantics, syntax, morphology, auditory memory, and phonological awareness).

2.2.4. Mullen Scales of Early Learning [71]. The Mullen is a standardized play-based assessment that measures nonverbal and verbal cognitive skills. This assessment was administered at the 36-month visit. Here we focus on the age-normed verbal score, which is computed from the expressive and receptive subscales.

2.2.5. Griffith Empathy Measure (GEM; [72]). The GEM is a parent-report measure used to quantify individual differences in cognitive and affective empathy. Cognitive empathy refers to the ability to take another person's perspective by decoding emotions and situational cues. The affective component of empathy refers to showing appropriate or congruent affective responses to other person's situation. Cognitive and affective empathy scores are derived from parent ratings of 23 questions on a 9-point Likert scale (−4 to 4).

Table 2: Descriptive statistics by group.

	ASD	HR-Other	HR-TD	LR-TD	F	p	η^2
ADOS CSS	7.18[a] (0.98)	5.00[b] (2.63)	1.75 (0.94)	1.59 (1.18)	50.66	<0.001	0.70
ToM scaled score	6.67[c] (3.17)	9.09[d] (3.65)	11.13 (3.72)	12.36 (2.85)	7.84	<0.001	0.27
CELF-4 Core Language SS	90.00[c] (22.23)	93.17[d] (18.82)	108.04 (11.95)	109.73 (10.65)	7.76	<0.001	0.27
Griffith cognitive empathy	0.63[c] (5.73)	6.25 (8.61)	9.55 (7.39)	8.84 (6.29)	4.23	0.009	0.19
VABS ABC	86.82 (15.17)	93.63 (18.95)	102.09 (25.62)	105.87 (12.41)	2.41	0.08	0.12
DAS NVIQ	105.27 (12.91)	104.92 (16.67)	107.71 (13.43)	104.32 (9.66)	0.17	0.92	0.08
Social reference to examiner (%time)	76.63 (31.81)	79.10 (30.31)	69.75 (32.77)	72.00 (25.18)	0.69	0.56	0.03
Griffith affective empathy	6.13 (9.30)	9.67 (8.18)	9.64 (7.56)	6.42 (11.29)	0.612	0.61	0.03

Note. Standard deviations appear in parentheses below means. Analyses of variance were covaried by age.
[a]ASD > LR-TD; [b]HR-Other > LR-TD; [c]ASD < LR-TD; [d]HR-Other < LR-TD.

2.2.6. Observational Empathy Task. This study included an observational measure of attentional and affective response to an examiner's display of distress during a play interaction. The measure has also been employed in previous research in our lab (e.g., [73, 74]). An examiner and the child took turns playing with a toy xylophone while the parent sat near the child. After the examiner determined that the child was focused on the play interaction, the examiner feigned injury by pretending to hit her hand with the toy mallet. At that point, the examiner withdrew from the play interaction and focused on her "hurt" hand for 15 seconds before reengaging the child and assuring the child that she felt fine. The child and examiner were filmed and the child's responses to the examiner's distress were coded offline (see [73] for additional details). Looking time at the examiner or parent is considered a proxy for attentiveness to the examiner's distress.

2.2.7. Theory of Mind Task (ToM). ToM indexes the understanding of others' mental states and represents a critical social cognitive skill for social adaptation. The task presented here is derived from Wellman and Liu [52] and assesses multiple milestones in social cognitive development. This approach has been validated in a group of children with ASD [75]. Participants were verbally presented with four brief scenarios and asked questions about each scenario that tapped into increasingly sophisticated aspects of understanding other people's mental states. Control questions were also posed to confirm comprehension of the scenario. The aspects of ToM that were evaluated proceeded in the following order: recognizing diverse desires, taking different perspectives (knowledge access), making judgments about explicit false beliefs, and making judgments about differences between real and apparent emotions (i.e., people can feel a different emotion from the one they display). Correct responses were scaled by question difficulty (i.e., 1 point for the diverse desire question, 2 points for each of the two knowledge access questions, 3 points for each of the two false-belief questions, and 4 points for the real-apparent emotion question). A ToM score was calculated by summing correct responses for each question type such that a maximum score of fifteen could be achieved.

2.2.8. Vineland Adaptive Behaviors Scales-II (VABS-II; [76]). The VABS is a semistructured parent questionnaire gauging adaptive functioning in daily living, socialization, communication, and motor skill domains. The adaptive behavior composite (ABC) is a standardized measure of adaptive behavior across the four domains.

2.3. Statistical Analyses. All participants provided data for at least 5 of the 7 measures. Descriptive statistics by outcome group (i.e., ASD, HR-Other, HR-TD, and LR-TD) for ADOS CSS, cognitive and affective empathy, VABS ABC, CELF CLS, ToM, observational empathy, and DAS NVIQ are reported in Table 2. The mean age of the ASD group was significantly younger than the mean ages of the other outcome groups at the time of the school-age visit (see Table 1). Therefore, age was included as a covariate in the reported analyses (ANCOVAs). Planned simple contrasts comparing ASD, HR-Other, and HR-TD to LR-TD evaluated differences among groups. ToM scores were negatively skewed and were inverse-log transformed to normalize the distribution. Subsequent tests were conducted with the transformed scores; however, to facilitate interpretation, scores reported in tables reflect original values.

In addition to examining group differences (a categorical approach), we conducted zero-order correlations among constructs related to social cognition and social communication across the entire sample (a dimensional approach). This aspect of the study aimed to quantify convergence and divergence among measures via Spearman correlations. Spearman correlations were used because some of our measures are bounded and it is a more conservative measure than Pearson correlations. Missing data were excluded pairwise to make use of all available data.

To evaluate the extent to which social-communicative, cognitive, and adaptive skills account for variability in macrolevel autism symptom severity, measures that were significantly correlated were included as predictors in a regression model using ADOS CSS as the criterion. Lastly, separate regressions (due to collinearity of the language variables) were run to evaluate whether 3-year and concurrent language skills were associated with school-age ToM. Analyses were conducted using IBM SPSS version 22 (IBM, 2013).

Table 3: Behavioral intercorrelations.

	Variable	1	2	3	4	5	6	7
1	DAS NVIQ							
2	CELF-4 Core Language SS	0.28[a]						
3	ADOS CSS	−0.02	−0.42[b]					
4	Griffith affective empathy	0.01	−0.08	−0.14				
5	Griffith cognitive empathy	−0.04	0.30[a]	−0.24	0.11			
6	Social reference %	0.30[a]	−0.15	0.03	0.14	−0.001		
7	ToM scaled score	0.09	0.40[b]	−0.46[b]	−0.17	0.25[a]	0.07	
8	VABS ABC	0.21	0.55[b]	−0.35[a]	−0.13	0.51[b]	−0.08	0.44[b]

Note. [a] $p < 0.05$; [b] $p < 0.01$.

Table 4: Behavioral intercorrelations, excluding ASD participants.

	Variable	1	2	3	4	5	6	7
1	DAS NVIQ							
2	CELF-4 Core Language SS	0.38[b]						
3	ADOS CSS	−0.04	−0.32[a]					
4	Griffith affective empathy	0.02	−0.05	−0.13				
5	Griffith cognitive empathy	0.02	0.26	−0.09	0.04			
6	Social reference %	0.23	−0.08	0.02	0.17	0.05		
7	ToM scaled score	0.07	0.33[b]	−0.30[a]	−0.23	0.15	0.09	
8	VABS ABC	0.35[a]	0.34[a]	−0.11	−0.12	0.42[b]	0.07	0.33[a]

Note. [a] $p < 0.05$; [b] $p < 0.01$.

3. Results

3.1. Categorical Evaluations of the BAP. ANCOVAs (see Table 2) revealed group differences in ADOS CSS, ToM, core language standard score (CLS), and cognitive empathy. Group differences were not observed for the adaptive behavior composite (VABS ABC) scores, nonverbal cognitive scores (NVIQ), affective empathy, and attention to the examiner feigning distress. Planned simple contrasts indicated that both ASD and HR-Other groups had significantly higher ADOS CSS scores, and lower ToM and CLS scores than the LR-TD group. Individuals with ASD on average had significantly lower cognitive empathy scores than those in the LR-TD group. The HR-TD group did not differ significantly from the LR-TD group on any measure.

3.2. Dimensional Evaluations of the BAP. Spearman correlations among measures are summarized in Table 3. Nonverbal scores were only correlated with CLS and social referencing. CLS, ADOS CSS, cognitive empathy, ToM, and VABS ABC scores were intercorrelated (all p's < 0.05). Cognitive empathy was not related to affective empathy. This pattern of zero-order correlations was not strongly influenced by scores from ASD participants. Associations between ADOS CSS, CLS, ToM, VABS ABC, and cognitive empathy were similar even when participants with ASD were excluded from analyses (see Table 4). Inter-related measures in the correlation matrix were entered into a regression model with ADOS CSS as the criterion. Regression diagnostics indicated that the regression model was not influenced by any outliers or influential cases [77]. ToM, VABS ABC, CLS, and cognitive empathy accounted for 27.7% of the variance in ADOS CSS scores over and above the effects of chronological age ($F(4,46) = 4.28$, $p = 0.005$). With all predictors included in the model, only ToM uniquely accounted for a significant portion of the variance in symptom severity (ToM $\beta = -0.37$, $t = -2.53$, $p = 0.02$, partial correlation = −0.36; VABS ABC $\beta = -0.02$, $t = 0.11$, and $p = 0.91$; cognitive empathy $\beta = -0.13$, $t = 0.85$, $p = 0.40$, CLS $\beta = -0.21$, $t = -1.20$, and $p = 0.23$). This finding was followed up using a holdout cross-validation method [78] to confirm the predictive validity of the regression model.

3.3. Predictive and Concurrent Associations between Language and ToM. Early (36-month) and school-age language scores were highly correlated with each other ($r = 0.71$, $p < 0.001$). Given excessive collinearity between the two variables, separate regressions were run to evaluate their effects on ToM, controlling for age and diagnostic classification at the school-age visit. 36-month Mullen Verbal T scores significantly predicted school-age ToM ($\beta = 0.24$, $t = 2.21$, $p = 0.03$; partial correlation = 0.27); however, school-age language (CLS) was not concurrently associated with ToM ($\beta = 0.16$, $t = 1.41$, $p = 0.16$; partial correlation = 0.17). The partial correlation coefficient provides an estimate of the effect size.

3.4. Is Early Language or Concurrent ToM More Predictive of the School-Age BAP? When 36-month Mullen Verbal T-Scores were entered into the regression model predicting school-age ADOS CSS scores from all concurrent variables that were significantly associated with CSS scores (except concurrent language due to excessive collinearity with

36-month language), the model was significant ($F(4,44) = 3.48$, $p = 0.01$). Again, only ToM uniquely accounted for a significant portion of the variance in symptom severity at school age (ToM $\beta = -0.368$, $t = -2.35$, $p = 0.02$, and partial correlation $= -0.33$; VABS ABC $\beta = -0.008$, $t = 0.05$, and $p = 0.96$; cognitive empathy $\beta = -0.23$, $t = -1.51$, and $p = 0.14$; 36-month Mullen Verbal $\beta = -0.09$, $t = -0.59$, and $p = 0.55$). Thus, concurrent ToM was a better index of school-age BAP than early language skills.

4. Discussion

Converging findings from categorical and dimensional approaches to the BAP in the current study suggest that researchers should consider defining the BAP among siblings of children with ASD in terms of a range of characteristics (including atypicalities of attention, language, and mood) and possibly perceptual strengths (e.g., [38, 79]) rather than by focusing only on siblings who exhibit elevated autistic-like symptoms. This recommendation is consistent with a large body of prior work demonstrating that family members of people with ASD are more likely than others to exhibit attentional, cognitive, linguistic, mood, and personality-related atypicalities (reviewed in [41]).

4.1. ToM and the BAP. Reduced ToM was a characteristic of the BAP among school-aged participants in the current study when assessed categorically (i.e., ToM was a challenge for children with ASD and siblings of children with ASD who were developing atypically) and dimensionally (when related to ADOS severity scores across a combined sample of high-risk and low-risk children). In fact, associations between severity scores and a number of intercorrelated measures (i.e., ToM, adaptive skills, and language) across the full sample were driven by individual differences in ToM. This finding provides support for the compatibility of categorical and dimensional approaches to the BAP while highlighting a key social-cognitive skill that contributes to the BAP at school age. The current study extends prior evidence that ToM is an aspect of the BAP among younger [53] and older individuals [8, 33, 37–39, 54] by suggesting that ToM may be a core aspect of the BAP underlying associations between autistic-like traits and other individual differences among young children who are just beginning elementary school.

Nevertheless, the current findings are inconsistent with the only other study to examine ToM among young school age siblings of children with ASD [45] as well as other studies that did not document reduced ToM among somewhat older siblings of children with ASD [55, 80]. Studies that did not observe reduced ToM among sibs-ASD used a broadly defined high-risk versus low-risk approach to characterizing the BAP. That analytic approach may have attenuated effects as only a subset of relatives of individuals with ASD exhibit categorically distinctive aspects of the BAP (e.g., [22, 39, 81]). Similarly, the contributions of ToM to the BAP that were observed in the current study may sometimes [33] but not always [56] be observed in general population samples. Therefore, replication of the current findings is needed. Nevertheless, the current study suggests that a developmentally oriented measure of ToM, which assesses the ability to achieve different mentalizing milestones, combined with analytic approaches that focus specifically on siblings of children with ASD who are developing atypically and/or that use more dimensional analytic techniques (which are more powerful than categorical approaches; [17]) may be needed to detect ToM-related atypicalities associated with the BAP.

Indeed, a reduced capacity to understand others' mental states (at least at certain points in development and when assessed with certain tests) may be integral to the BAP and compromise the quality of interpersonal relationships. Delayed development of ToM among school-aged children with ASD is believed to underlie social immaturity and atypical peer relations [75]. These difficulties with social cognition associated with the BAP may continue to create social challenges across the lifespan [8, 82].

Future research should examine mechanisms underlying atypical social cognition associated with the BAP. Given that difficulty with emotion reading is a commonly observed characteristic of the BAP when assessed categorically among relatives of individuals with ASD (reviewed by [4]) and dimensionally among college students [12, 34, 82], difficulty interpreting emotions may contribute to atypical development of ToM in the BAP. Indeed, the Reading the Mind in the Eyes Task (one of the most widely used measures of ToM) is essentially a test of complex emotion reading. However, attention to the examiner's distress and parent-reported affective empathy were not associated with either the BAP or ToM performance in the current study. This absence of associations between aspects of affective empathy and the BAP is consistent with Smith's [65] hypothesis that affective empathy is *not* impaired in ASD. Together, these findings suggest that difficulty *deciphering* others' perspectives is an aspect of the BAP at school-age while difficulty *sharing* emotions with others is not. Difficulty deciphering one's own and others' emotions may contribute to reduced ToM at school-age. Indeed, findings from the aforementioned study that employed a combined categorical and dimensional approach to exploring the BAP suggest that difficulty reading one's own emotions (alexithymia) may be a core characteristic of the BAP that should be explored in future research [16]. Alexithymia may contribute to BAP-related difficulties with ToM as challenges reading one's own emotions likely contribute to obstacles interpreting others' emotions as well.

Future research should also examine if the family environment contributes to atypical ToM development among a subset of siblings of children with ASD. For example, the presence of an older child with ASD in the household may reduce attention (and associated opportunities to practice understanding others' minds through conversation) directed towards younger siblings. Younger siblings may also mimic behaviors indicative of atypical ToM exhibited by older siblings with ASD. Alternatively, having an older sibling whose behavior is atypical (particularly if the older child cannot explain his or her behaviors) may encourage younger siblings to work at understanding their older sibling's perspective and thus support ToM development. Prior research has demonstrated that having an older sibling *without* ASD is associated with *decreased* ToM for children with ASD, presumably because the older child may compensate for the younger child's difficulties [83]. Although complicated to assess, investigations of how sibling and parental behaviors impact the ToM development of younger siblings with and without ASD are needed.

4.2. Language, ToM, and the BAP. As in the broader sample of which the current participants are a subset [51], younger siblings of children with ASD who were developing atypically exhibited language difficulties relative to typically developing high-risk and low-risk children. Language was also associated dimensionally with the BAP in the current study. Consistent with a large body of research demonstrating that language is associated with ToM in typical and atypical development [59, 61], baseline correlations revealed associations between school-age structural language and parent-reported cognitive (but not affective) empathy and behavioral ToM. Nevertheless, ToM uniquely contributed to the BAP at school-age; language was no longer associated with the BAP once ToM was accounted for. In addition, concurrent language was *not* associated with ToM after controlling for age and outcome group. Therefore, difficulties deciphering other minds may be a core characteristic of the BAP at school age irrespective of concurrent language ability.

In contrast to the lack of strong associations between concurrent language and ToM at school-age, language at 36 months of age *was* predictive of subsequent ToM. This finding extends prior research demonstrating that early language skills support the development of explicit ToM reasoning among typically developing children [61] and children with autism [59, 62] by suggesting that early variations in language ability among children with and without a sibling with ASD contribute to later ToM. Longitudinal associations between early language and later ToM mirror evidence that the manifestation of core symptoms of ASD varies with age (reviewed in [84]) by suggesting that skills affected by the BAP also change with time.

While 36-month language contributed to school-age ToM, school-age ToM remained uniquely associated with school-age autistic-like symptoms even after 36-month language was accounted for in analyses. This finding supports a nonlinear interpretation of development wherein early language development gives rise to a variety of social-cognitive skills which may be used to ameliorate potential autistic-like symptoms. Future research is needed to determine whether specific difficulties (re)emerge as the children grow and encounter more challenging social environments, as suggested by Gamliel and colleagues [42].

4.3. Developmental Profiles of HR and LR School-Age Children. Despite our observation of significant group differences in performance on a number of measures, it is worth noting that mean scores in cognitive empathy, adaptive behaviors, and language for the HR-Other group fell well within 2 standard deviations of normed mean scores. Similarly, children in the ASD group achieved verbal and nonverbal intelligence scores that are considered "average." Several other groups using the sibling-risk design have also reported normative cognitive skills among HR participants (e.g., [22, 85]), including a similar rate of cognitive development between HR and LR children from infancy to school age [42]. Furthermore, a recent population-based study found a positive association between common genetic risk variants for ASD and general cognitive ability [86]. Our results converge with those from other samples to suggest that familial autism may represent a particular form of ASD with high nonverbal intelligence and relatively spared adaptive and language skills (see also [87–93]). A dissociation between intelligence and social skills is commonly observed in "high-functioning" individuals with ASD (e.g., [94]) and this uneven profile may be a manifestation of BAP. Further investigation of these findings is advisable before conclusions can be drawn regarding the population of later-born siblings of children with ASD.

Participants in the current sample were at the beginning of their school years when assessed. Social and academic stressors of the school environment may have progressively disruptive effects on social-communicative and social cognitive development, especially in children with social vulnerabilities (e.g., [42, 55, 95, 96]). Increased vulnerability for social-communicative difficulties during school years may also arise from genetic factors exerting a greater influence on the phenotypic expression of highly heritable traits in later childhood (e.g., [97]). Peer relations during childhood and adolescence play a pivotal role in social affective development, including social competency and emotional understanding (for review see [98]). Adults exhibiting the BAP report reduced quality and quantity of friendships [40], alluding to a history of diminished or atypical peer relations and social networks not unlike that in ASD [99]. Poor quality of social interactions may have cascading effects on the development of ToM (e.g., [100]) and other social skills. In other words, BAP features may accrue over time due to environmental and genetic factors coupled with reduced opportunities for healthy peer interactions, presenting the possibility that high-risk children may appear more impaired than low-risk children in later years than they do at the beginning of elementary school. However, substantial evidence for resilience among the siblings of children with ASD suggests that many of those who encounter such challenges will overcome them.

Data presented in this study includes both parent interviews (VABS, Griffith Empathy) and observational assessments (ToM, CELF, DAS, ADOS, and response to distress). Our results suggest that both types of information contribute to a comprehensive profile of social cognitive and communicative behaviors associated with the BAP among school-age children. We found that ToM, cognitive empathy, adaptive functioning, and language ability collectively reflected level of autism symptom severity. Furthermore, relations across a broad range of measures of social ability were apparent when evaluated via correlations, suggesting that performance on measures of ToM, cognitive empathy, adaptive functioning, and language ability may be driven by a common underlying mechanism.

Relations among social skills, social cognition, and the BAP are also apparent in adults (e.g., [8, 13]), providing some indication of developmental stability in the observed correlations. Our pattern of results corroborates previous studies demonstrating associations between language and social cognition [57, 101–103] and adaptive social functioning and social impairments [104] in ASD. The null association between affective and cognitive components of empathy also corroborates prior work [72]. Limited evidence was obtained that behavioral ToM and cognitive empathy are indeed the same construct (as stated by [63]), as associations between ToM and parent-reported cognitive empathy were relatively weak and were no longer apparent once participants with ASD were excluded from analyses.

4.4. Limitations. Our manner of defining what constituted the categorical operationalization of the BAP in the current study may have impacted findings. Children in our "BAP group" were judged to have a broad range of developmental concerns including social, language, and cognitive delays, as well as disruptive attention deficits and anxiety. This heterogeneity in developmental concerns is not surprising given genetic liability: autism risk genes have been associated with social anxiety [105, 106], language impairments [30], attention-deficit/hyperactivity disorder [51], bipolar disorder, major depressive disorder, and schizophrenia [107]. Differential expression, number of risk alleles, and environmental factors may give rise to a wide range of phenotypic expression among high-risk individuals without ASD (e.g., [108, 109]). Therefore, the etiologies underlying the different developmental atypicalities in the HR-Other group were likely diverse, which coupled with small sample size limits power to detect effects.

A second limitation lies in uncertainty regarding the extent to which our high-risk sample is truly at high risk for ASD. Genetic research indicates that the presence of *de novo* copy number variants (CNVs) is greater in simplex families (those with only one child with ASD) than in multiplex families (for review see [110]). If *de novo* mutations caused ASD in some probands in the current study, younger siblings may be at lower risk for ASD than in cases where mutations or other genetic risk markers were inherited. In other words, some high-risk participants in this sample may have an older sibling with sporadic as opposed to familial autism and risk for the BAP may be reduced in cases of sporadic ASD. Efforts to examine the BAP to characterize behavioral profiles and the genetic basis of ASD would benefit from studying unaffected individuals in multiplex families. The field of genetics in ASD is progressing at a rapid rate to include repositories of genetic information from families in multiple sites (e.g., Autism Genetic Resource Exchange, MSSNG, Simons Simplex Collection). Comparable behavioral databases will also move the field forward.

The small number of high- and low-risk participants with ASD and "other outcomes" in the current sample did not permit us to examine whether categorical differences between groups and dimensional associations among variables within each group index convergent aspects of the BAP. Attrition is inevitable in longitudinal research and this was a limiting factor in this study. Future research following high- and low-risk participants through and beyond toddlerhood would benefit from multisite collaboration. This would both increase power to detect effects and improve generalizability of results.

5. Conclusions and Future Directions

The current study provides support for the compatibility of categorical and dimensional approaches to the BAP and suggests that ToM may be a key aspect of the BAP among children with a sibling with ASD who are just starting out in school. Therefore, supports for siblings of children with ASD who are preparing to enter school should focus proactively on helping them develop ToM skills. Reading has been associated with ToM development among children [111]. Narrative-based approaches to promoting ToM, such as reading groups where children practice reflecting on and telling stories, may be beneficial for preschool and school-age siblings of children with ASD. Literacy-based ToM supports may also help to avoid the potential exacerbation of language difficulties among younger siblings as they develop and encounter more challenging environments.

Greater understanding of potential precursors to ToM may yield insights into the development of social functioning and the emergence of the BAP. One theoretical precursor to ToM is joint attention (e.g., [112]). Joint attention is believed to be crucial for social cognitive development, language acquisition, and social competence (for a review, see [113]). Furthermore, difficulties with joint attention are often (but not always) an aspect of the BAP in infancy [114–117]. Empirically evaluating a relation between early joint attention skills and subsequent ToM reasoning among high- and low-risk toddlers would be a promising future endeavor.

Authors' Contribution

The first author contributed to the conceptual framing of the study, analytic approach, and writing of the paper. The second author played a guiding role in developing the conceptual framework and analytic approach for this study and contributed very substantially to the literature review and writing of the paper. The third author supervised clinical aspects of the study and contributed to the research design, data analysis, and writing of the paper.

Acknowledgments

The authors wish to thank the families who generously shared their time to participate in this longitudinal research program. The following research assistants administered assessments that are the cornerstone of this research: Stephany Cox, James Earhart, Lovella Gomez, Brigid McCarthy, Jenna Mendelson, Joanna Mussey, Nuri Reyes, Mithi del Rosario, and Stephanie Sharma. The authors wish to express deepest gratitude to their mentor, Marian Sigman, who launched this study and the larger domain of infant-sibling research. This research was funded by United States National Institutes of Health, Grants U54-MH-68172 (Sigman), P50-HD-55784 (Bookheimer), and K01-MH-96961 (Hutman).

References

[1] J. N. Constantino and R. D. Todd, "Autistic traits in the general population: a twin study," *Archives of General Psychiatry*, vol. 60, no. 5, pp. 524–530, 2003.

[2] S. Lundström, Z. Chang, M. Råstam et al., "Autism spectrum disorders and autisticlike traits: similar etiology in the extreme end and the normal variation," *Archives of General Psychiatry*, vol. 69, no. 1, pp. 46–52, 2012.

[3] A. Pickles, E. Starr, P. Bolton et al., "Variable expression of the autism broader phenotype: findings from extended pedigrees," *Journal of Child Psychology and Psychiatry*, vol. 41, no. 4, pp. 491–502, 2000.

[4] E. Sucksmith, I. Roth, and R. A. Hoekstra, "Autistic traits below the clinical threshold: re-examining the broader autism phenotype in the 21st century," *Neuropsychology Review*, vol. 21, no. 4, pp. 360–389, 2011.

[5] J. Gerdts and R. Bernier, "The broader autism phenotype and its implications on the etiology and treatment of autism spectrum disorders," *Autism Research and Treatment*, vol. 2011, Article ID 545901, 19 pages, 2011.

[6] A. Bailey, S. Palferman, L. Heavey, and A. Le Couteur, "Autism: the phenotype in relatives," *Journal of Autism and Developmental Disorders*, vol. 28, no. 5, pp. 369–392, 1998.

[7] P. Bolton, H. Macdonald, A. Pickles et al., "A case-control family history study of autism," *Journal of Child Psychology and Psychiatry*, vol. 35, no. 5, pp. 877–900, 1994.

[8] M. Losh and J. Piven, "Social-cognition and the broad autism phenotype: identifying genetically meaningful phenotypes," *Journal of Child Psychology and Psychiatry*, vol. 48, no. 1, pp. 105–112, 2007.

[9] S. Ozonoff, G. S. Young, A. Belding et al., "The broader autism phenotype in infancy: when does it emerge?" *Journal of the American Academy of Child & Adolescent Psychiatry*, vol. 53, no. 4, pp. 398.e2–407.e2, 2014.

[10] E. J. Austin, "Personality correlates of the broader autism phenotype as assessed by the Autism Spectrum Quotient (AQ)," *Personality and Individual Differences*, vol. 38, no. 2, pp. 451–460, 2005.

[11] L. E. Jobe and S. W. White, "Loneliness, social relationships, and a broader autism phenotype in college students," *Personality and Individual Differences*, vol. 42, no. 8, pp. 1479–1489, 2007.

[12] E. Poljac, E. Poljac, and J. Wagemans, "Reduced accuracy and sensitivity in the perception of emotional facial expressions in individuals with high autism spectrum traits," *Autism*, vol. 17, no. 6, pp. 668–680, 2013.

[13] N. J. Sasson, K. S. L. Lam, D. Childress, M. Parlier, J. L. Daniels, and J. Piven, "The broad autism phenotype questionnaire: prevalence and diagnostic classification," *Autism Research*, vol. 6, no. 2, pp. 134–143, 2013.

[14] B. Ingersoll, C. J. Hopwood, A. Wainer, and M. B. Donnellan, "A comparison of three self-report measures of the broader autism phenotype in a non-clinical sample," *Journal of Autism and Developmental Disorders*, vol. 41, no. 12, pp. 1646–1657, 2011.

[15] M. Losh, R. Adolphs, and J. Piven, "The broad autism phenotype," in *Autism Spectrum Disorders*, pp. 457–476, Oxford University Press, Oxford, UK, 2011.

[16] S. Berthoz, C. Lalanne, L. Crane, and E. L. Hill, "Investigating emotional impairments in adults with autism spectrum disorders and the broader autism phenotype," *Psychiatry Research*, vol. 208, no. 3, pp. 257–264, 2013.

[17] A. Pickles and A. Angold, "Natural categories or fundamental dimensions: on carving nature at the joints and the rearticulation of psychopathology," *Development and Psychopathology*, vol. 15, no. 3, pp. 529–551, 2003.

[18] C. R. Maxwell, J. Parish-Morris, O. Hsin, J. C. Bush, and R. T. Schultz, "The broad autism phenotype predicts child functioning in autism spectrum disorders," *Journal of Neurodevelopmental Disorders*, vol. 5, no. 1, article 25, 2013.

[19] M. Rutter, "Genetic studies of autism: from the 1970s into the millennium," *Journal of Abnormal Child Psychology*, vol. 28, no. 1, pp. 3–14, 2000.

[20] R. Paul, Y. Fuerst, G. Ramsay, K. Chawarska, and A. Klin, "Out of the mouths of babes: vocal production in infant siblings of children with ASD," *Journal of Child Psychology and Psychiatry*, vol. 52, no. 5, pp. 588–598, 2011.

[21] K. Chawarska, F. Shic, S. Macari et al., "18-month predictors of later outcomes in Younger siblings of children with autism spectrum disorder: a baby siblings research consortium study," *Journal of the American Academy of Child and Adolescent Psychiatry*, vol. 53, no. 12, pp. 1317–1327.e1, 2014.

[22] S. Georgiades, P. Szatmari, L. Zwaigenbaum et al., "A prospective study of autistic-like traits in unaffected siblings of probands with autism spectrum disorder," *JAMA Psychiatry*, vol. 70, no. 1, pp. 42–48, 2013.

[23] J. N. Constantino, C. Lajonchere, M. Lutz et al., "Autistic social impairment in the siblings of children with pervasive developmental disorders," *American Journal of Psychiatry*, vol. 163, no. 2, pp. 294–296, 2006.

[24] J. A. Gerdts, R. Bernier, G. Dawson, and A. Estes, "The broader autism phenotype in simplex and multiplex families," *Journal of Autism and Developmental Disorders*, vol. 43, no. 7, pp. 1597–1605, 2013.

[25] M. Losh, D. Childress, K. Lam, and J. Piven, "Defining key features of the broad autism phenotype: a comparison across parents of multiple- and single-incidence autism families," *American Journal of Medical Genetics Part B: Neuropsychiatric Genetics*, vol. 147, no. 4, pp. 424–433, 2008.

[26] A. J. Schwichtenberg, G. S. Young, M. Sigman, T. Hutman, and S. Ozonoff, "Can family affectedness inform infant sibling outcomes of autism spectrum disorders?" *Journal of Child Psychology and Psychiatry*, vol. 51, no. 9, pp. 1021–1030, 2010.

[27] R. Bernier, J. Gerdts, J. Munson, G. Dawson, and A. Estes, "Evidence for broader autism phenotype characteristics in parents from multiple-incidence autism families," *Autism Research*, vol. 5, no. 1, pp. 13–20, 2012.

[28] A. Meyer-Lindenberg and D. R. Weinberger, "Intermediate phenotypes and genetic mechanisms of psychiatric disorders," *Nature Reviews Neuroscience*, vol. 7, no. 10, pp. 818–827, 2006.

[29] Q. Zhang, Q. Shen, Z. Xu et al., "The effects of *CACNA1C* gene polymorphism on spatial working memory in both healthy controls and patients with schizophrenia or bipolar disorder," *Neuropsychopharmacology*, vol. 37, no. 3, pp. 677–684, 2012.

[30] J. Piven, "The broad autism phenotype: a complementary strategy for molecular genetic studies of autism," *American Journal of Medical Genetics*, vol. 105, no. 1, pp. 34–35, 2001.

[31] P. M. Vital, A. Ronald, G. L. Wallace, and F. Happé, "Relationship between special abilities and autistic-like traits in a

large population-based sample of 8-year-olds," *Journal of Child Psychology and Psychiatry and Allied Disciplines*, vol. 50, no. 9, pp. 1093–1101, 2009.

[32] C. Lord, M. Rutter, P. C. DiLavore, and S. Risi, *Autism Diagnostic Observation Schedule: ADOS*, Western Psychological Services, Los Angeles, Calif, USA, 2002.

[33] C. S. Best, V. J. Moffat, M. J. Power, D. G. C. Owens, and E. C. Johnstone, "The boundaries of the cognitive phenotype of autism: theory of mind, central coherence and ambiguous figure perception in young people with autistic traits," *Journal of Autism and Developmental Disorders*, vol. 38, no. 5, pp. 840–847, 2008.

[34] R. Kothari, D. Skuse, J. Wakefield, and N. Micali, "Gender differences in the relationship between social communication and emotion recognition," *Journal of the American Academy of Child and Adolescent Psychiatry*, vol. 52, no. 11, pp. 1148–1157, 2013.

[35] S. W. White, B. C. Bray, and T. H. Ollendick, "Examining shared and unique aspects of social anxiety disorder and autism spectrum disorder using factor analysis," *Journal of Autism and Developmental Disorders*, vol. 42, no. 5, pp. 874–884, 2012.

[36] S. Folstein and M. Rutter, "Infantile autism: a genetic study of 21 twin pairs," *Journal of Child Psychology and Psychiatry*, vol. 18, no. 4, pp. 297–321, 1977.

[37] S. Gokcen, E. Bora, S. Erermis, H. Kesikci, and C. Aydin, "Theory of mind and verbal working memory deficits in parents of autistic children," *Psychiatry Research*, vol. 166, no. 1, pp. 46–53, 2009.

[38] S. Baron-Cohen and J. Hammer, "Parents of children with Asperger syndrome: what is the cognitive phenotype?" *Journal of Cognitive Neuroscience*, vol. 9, no. 4, pp. 548–554, 1997.

[39] M. Losh, R. Adolphs, M. D. Poe et al., "Neuropsychological profile of autism and the broad autism phenotype," *Archives of General Psychiatry*, vol. 66, no. 5, pp. 518–526, 2009.

[40] J. Piven, P. Palmer, D. Jacobi, D. Childress, and S. Arndt, "Broader autism phenotype: evidence from a family history study of multiple-incidence autism families," *The American Journal of Psychiatry*, vol. 154, no. 2, pp. 185–190, 1997.

[41] N. Garon, S. E. Bryson, L. Zwaigenbaum et al., "Temperament and its relationship to autistic symptoms in a high-risk infant sib cohort," *Journal of Abnormal Child Psychology*, vol. 37, no. 1, pp. 59–78, 2009.

[42] I. Gamliel, N. Yirmiya, D. H. Jaffe, O. Manor, and M. Sigman, "Developmental trajectories in siblings of children with autism: cognition and language from 4 months to 7 years," *Journal of Autism and Developmental Disorders*, vol. 39, no. 8, pp. 1131–1144, 2009.

[43] E. Drumm, S. Bryson, L. Zwaigenbaum, and J. Brian, "Language-related abilities in 'unaffected' school-aged siblings of children with ASD," *Research in Autism Spectrum Disorders*, vol. 18, pp. 83–96, 2015.

[44] K. Gillespie-Lynch, A. Khalulyan, M. del Rosario et al., "Is early joint attention associated with school-age pragmatic language?" *Autism*, vol. 19, no. 2, pp. 168–177, 2015.

[45] M. Shaked, I. Gamliel, and N. Yirmiya, "Theory of mind abilities in young siblings of children with autism," *Autism*, vol. 10, no. 2, pp. 173–187, 2006.

[46] Z. E. Warren, J. H. Foss-Feig, E. E. Malesa et al., "Neurocognitive and behavioral outcomes of younger siblings of children with autism spectrum disorder at age five," *Journal of Autism and Developmental Disorders*, vol. 42, no. 3, pp. 409–418, 2012.

[47] N. Ben-Yizhak, N. Yirmiya, I. Seidman, R. Alon, C. Lord, and M. Sigman, "Pragmatic language and school related linguistic abilities in siblings of children with autism," *Journal of Autism and Developmental Disorders*, vol. 41, no. 6, pp. 750–760, 2011.

[48] I. Gamliel, N. Yirmiya, and M. Sigman, "The development of young siblings of children with autism from 4 to 54 months," *Journal of Autism and Developmental Disorders*, vol. 37, no. 1, pp. 171–183, 2007.

[49] E. J. H. Jones, T. Gliga, R. Bedford, T. Charman, and M. H. Johnson, "Developmental pathways to autism: a review of prospective studies of infants at risk," *Neuroscience & Biobehavioral Reviews*, vol. 39, pp. 1–33, 2014.

[50] E. Malesa, J. Foss-Feig, P. Yoder, Z. Warren, T. Walden, and W. L. Stone, "Predicting language and social outcomes at age 5 for later-born siblings of children with autism spectrum disorders," *Autism*, vol. 17, no. 5, pp. 558–570, 2013.

[51] M. Miller, A.-M. Iosif, G. S. Young et al., "School-age outcomes of infants at risk for autism spectrum disorder," *Autism Research*, 2015.

[52] H. M. Wellman and D. Liu, "Scaling of theory-of-mind tasks," *Child Development*, vol. 75, no. 2, pp. 523–541, 2004.

[53] T. Gliga, A. Senju, M. Pettinato, T. Charman, and M. H. Johnson, "Spontaneous belief attribution in younger siblings of children on the autism spectrum," *Developmental Psychology*, vol. 50, no. 3, pp. 903–913, 2014.

[54] L. Dorris, C. A. E. Espie, F. Knott, and J. Salt, "Mind-reading difficulties in the siblings of people with Asperger's syndrome: evidence for a genetic influence in the abnormal development of a specific cognitive domain," *Journal of Child Psychology and Psychiatry and Allied Disciplines*, vol. 45, no. 2, pp. 412–418, 2004.

[55] S. Ozonoff, S. J. Rogers, J. M. Farnham, and B. F. Pennington, "Can standard measures identify subclinical markers of autism?" *Journal of Autism and Developmental Disorders*, vol. 23, no. 3, pp. 429–441, 1993.

[56] Y. Kunihira, A. Senju, H. Dairoku, A. Wakabayashi, and T. Hasegawa, "'Autistic' traits in non-autistic Japanese populations: relationships with personality traits and cognitive ability," *Journal of Autism and Developmental Disorders*, vol. 36, no. 4, pp. 553–566, 2006.

[57] F. G. Happé, "The role of age and verbal ability in the theory of mind task performance of subjects with autism," *Child Development*, vol. 66, no. 3, pp. 843–855, 1995.

[58] E. Peterson and S. F. Miller, "The eyes test as a measure of individual differences: how much of the variance reflects verbal IQ?" *Frontiers in Psychology*, vol. 3, article 220, 2012.

[59] H. Tager-Flusberg, "Evaluating the theory-of-mind hypothesis of autism," *Current Directions in Psychological Science*, vol. 16, no. 6, pp. 311–315, 2007.

[60] J. W. Astington and J. M. Jenkins, "A longitudinal study of the relation between language and theory-of-mind development," *Developmental Psychology*, vol. 35, no. 5, pp. 1311–1320, 1999.

[61] K. Milligan, J. W. Astington, and L. A. Dack, "Language and theory of mind: meta-analysis of the relation between language ability and false-belief understanding," *Child Development*, vol. 78, no. 2, pp. 622–646, 2007.

[62] S. Steele, R. M. Joseph, and H. Tager-Flusberg, "Brief report: developmental change in theory of mind abilities in children with autism," *Journal of Autism and Developmental Disorders*, vol. 33, no. 4, pp. 461–467, 2003.

[63] S. Baron-Cohen and S. Wheelwright, "The empathy quotient: an investigation of adults with Asperger syndrome or high functioning autism, and normal sex differences," *Journal of Autism and Developmental Disorders*, vol. 34, no. 2, pp. 163–175, 2004.

[64] R. Grove, A. Baillie, C. Allison, S. Baron-Cohen, and R. A. Hoekstra, "The latent structure of cognitive and emotional empathy in individuals with autism, first-degree relatives and typical individuals," *Molecular Autism*, vol. 5, no. 1, article 42, 2014.

[65] A. Smith, "The empathy imbalance hypothesis of autism: a theoretical approach to cognitive and emotional empathy in autistic development," *The Psychological Record*, vol. 59, no. 3, pp. 489–510, 2009.

[66] M. Rutter, A. Bailey, C. Lord, C. Cianchetti, and G. S. Fancello, *SCQ: Social Communication Questionnaire: Manuale*, Giunti OS, Firenze, Italy, 2007.

[67] K. Gotham, A. Pickles, and C. Lord, "Standardizing ADOS scores for a measure of severity in autism spectrum disorders," *Journal of Autism and Developmental Disorders*, vol. 39, no. 5, pp. 693–705, 2009.

[68] S. Shumway, C. Farmer, A. Thurm, L. Joseph, D. Black, and C. Golden, "The ADOS calibrated severity score: relationship to phenotypic variables and stability over time," *Autism Research*, vol. 5, no. 4, pp. 267–276, 2012.

[69] C. D. Elliott, *Differential Ability Scales: Administration and Scoring Manual*, Psychological Corporation, 1990.

[70] E. Semel, E. H. Wiig, and W. A. Secord, *Clinical Evaluation of Language Fundamentals (CELF-4)*, The Psychological Corporation, San Antonio, Tex, USA, 2003.

[71] E. M. Mullen, *Mullen Scales of Early Learning*, AGS, Circle Pines, Minn, USA, 1995.

[72] M. R. Dadds, K. Hunter, D. J. Hawes et al., "A measure of cognitive and affective empathy in children using parent ratings," *Child Psychiatry and Human Development*, vol. 39, no. 2, pp. 111–122, 2008.

[73] T. Hutman, A. Rozga, A. D. Delaurentis, J. M. Barnwell, C. A. Sugar, and M. Sigman, "Response to distress in infants at risk for autism: a prospective longitudinal study," *Journal of Child Psychology and Psychiatry*, vol. 51, no. 9, pp. 1010–1020, 2010.

[74] T. Hutman, M. K. Chela, K. Gillespie-Lynch, and M. Sigman, "Selective visual attention at twelve months: signs of autism in early social interactions," *Journal of Autism and Developmental Disorders*, vol. 42, no. 4, pp. 487–498, 2012.

[75] C. C. Peterson, H. M. Wellman, and V. Slaughter, "The mind behind the message: advancing theory-of-mind scales for typically developing children, and those with deafness, autism, or Asperger syndrome," *Child Development*, vol. 83, no. 2, pp. 469–485, 2012.

[76] S. S. Sparrow, D. V. Cicchetti, and D. A. Balla, *Vineland Adaptive Behavior Scales: (Vineland II), Survey Interview Form/Caregiver Rating Form*, Pearson Assessments, Livonia Township, Minn, USA, 2005.

[77] X. Chen, P. Ender, M. Mitchell, and C. Wells, "Regression with SPSS," 2003, http://www.ats.ucla.edu/stat/spss/webbooks/reg/default.htm.

[78] T. Hastie, R. Tibshirani, and J. Friedman, *The Elements of Statistical Learning*, Springer, New York, NY, USA, 2009.

[79] J. P. McCleery, E. Allman, L. J. Carver, and K. R. Dobkins, "Abnormal magnocellular pathway visual processing in infants at risk for autism," *Biological Psychiatry*, vol. 62, no. 9, pp. 1007–1014, 2007.

[80] R. J. Holt, L. R. Chura, M.-C. Lai et al., "'Reading the Mind in the Eyes': an fMRI study of adolescents with autism and their siblings," *Psychological Medicine*, vol. 44, no. 15, pp. 3215–3227, 2014.

[81] D. Messinger, G. S. Young, S. Ozonoff et al., "Beyond autism: a baby siblings research consortium study of high-risk children at three years of age," *Journal of the American Academy of Child and Adolescent Psychiatry*, vol. 52, no. 3, pp. 300–308, 2013.

[82] N. J. Sasson, R. B. Nowlin, and A. E. Pinkham, "Social cognition, social skill, and the broad autism phenotype," *Autism*, vol. 17, no. 6, pp. 655–667, 2013.

[83] K. O'Brien, V. Slaughter, and C. C. Peterson, "Sibling influences on theory of mind development for children with ASD," *Journal of Child Psychology and Psychiatry and Allied Disciplines*, vol. 52, no. 6, pp. 713–719, 2011.

[84] C. Lord and R. M. Jones, "Annual research review: re-thinking the classification of autism spectrum disorders," *Journal of Child Psychology and Psychiatry*, vol. 53, no. 5, pp. 490–509, 2012.

[85] K. Hudry, S. Chandler, R. Bedford et al., "Early language profiles in infants at high-risk for autism spectrum disorders," *Journal of Autism and Developmental Disorders*, vol. 44, no. 1, pp. 154–167, 2014.

[86] T.-K. Clarke, M. K. Lupton, A. M. Fernandez-Pujals et al., "Common polygenic risk for autism spectrum disorder (ASD) is associated with cognitive ability in the general population," *Molecular Psychiatry*, 2015.

[87] T. Pilowsky, N. Yirmiya, R. S. Shalev, and V. Gross-Tsur, "Language abilities of siblings of children with autism," *Journal of Child Psychology and Psychiatry*, vol. 44, no. 6, pp. 914–925, 2003.

[88] M. Dawson, I. Soulières, M. A. Gernsbacher, and L. Mottron, "The level and nature of autistic intelligence," *Psychological Science*, vol. 18, no. 8, pp. 657–662, 2007.

[89] M. McGonigle-Chalmers and M. McSweeney, "The role of timing in testing nonverbal iq in children with ASD," *Journal of Autism and Developmental Disorders*, vol. 43, no. 1, pp. 80–90, 2013.

[90] A.-M. Nader, V. Courchesne, M. Dawson, and I. Soulières, "Does WISC-IV underestimate the intelligence of autistic children?" *Journal of Autism and Developmental Disorders*, pp. 1–8, 2014.

[91] I. Soulières, M. Dawson, M. A. Gernsbacher, and L. Mottron, "The level and nature of autistic intelligence II: what about Asperger syndrome?" *PLoS ONE*, vol. 6, no. 9, Article ID e25372, 2011.

[92] M. G. Edelson, "Are the majority of children with autism mentally retarded? A systematic evaluation of the data," *Focus on Autism and Other Developmental Disabilities*, vol. 21, no. 2, pp. 66–83, 2006.

[93] B. J. Freeman and M. Van Dyke, "Are the majority of children with autism mentally retarded?" *Focus on Autism and Other Developmental Disabilities*, vol. 21, no. 2, pp. 86–88, 2006.

[94] S. Baron-Cohen, *Mindblindness: An Essay on Autism and Theory of Mind*, MIT Press, 1997.

[95] P. Boutin, M. Maziade, C. Mérette, M. Mondor, C. Bédard, and J. Thivierge, "Family history of cognitive disabilities in first-degree relatives of autistic and mentally retarded children," *Journal of Autism and Developmental Disorders*, vol. 27, no. 2, pp. 165–176, 1997.

[96] J. Piven, J. Gayle, G. A. Chase et al., "A family history study of neuropsychiatric disorders in the adult siblings of autistic

individuals," *Journal of the American Academy of Child and Adolescent Psychiatry*, vol. 29, no. 2, pp. 177–183, 1990.

[97] E. M. Tucker-Drob, D. A. Briley, and K. P. Harden, "Genetic and environmental influences on cognition across development and context," *Current Directions in Psychological Science*, vol. 22, no. 5, pp. 349–355, 2013.

[98] G. W. Ladd, "Peer relationships and social competence during early and middle childhood," *Annual Review of Psychology*, vol. 50, no. 1, pp. 333–359, 1999.

[99] B. Chamberlain, C. Kasari, and E. Rotheram-Fuller, "Involvement or isolation? The social networks of children with autism in regular classrooms," *Journal of Autism and Developmental Disorders*, vol. 37, no. 2, pp. 230–242, 2007.

[100] J. W. Astington, "Sometimes necessary, never sufficient: false-belief understanding and social competence," in *Individual Differences in Theory of Mind: Implications for Typical and Atypical Development*, B. Repacholi and V. Slaughter, Eds., pp. 13–38, Psychology Press, New York, NY, USA, 2003.

[101] W. P. Hresko, D. K. Reid, and D. D. Hammill, *The Test of Early Language Development*, Pro-Ed, Austin, Tex, USA, 1981.

[102] A. L. Cutting and J. Dunn, "Theory of mind, emotion understanding, language, and family background: individual differences and interrelations," *Child Development*, vol. 70, no. 4, pp. 853–865, 1999.

[103] H. Tager-Flusberg, "Language and understanding minds: connections in autism," in *Understanding Other Minds: Perspectives from Developmental Cognitive Neuroscience*, vol. 2, pp. 124–149, Oxford University Press, Oxon, UK, 2000.

[104] A. Klin, C. A. Saulnier, S. S. Sparrow, D. V. Cicchetti, F. R. Volkmar, and C. Lord, "Social and communication abilities and disabilities in higher functioning individuals with autism spectrum disorders: the Vineland and the ADOS," *Journal of Autism and Developmental Disorders*, vol. 37, no. 4, pp. 748–759, 2007.

[105] M. B. Stein, B.-Z. Yang, D. A. Chavira et al., "A common genetic variant in the neurexin superfamily member cntnap2 is associated with increased risk for selective mutism and social anxiety-related traits," *Biological Psychiatry*, vol. 69, no. 9, pp. 825–831, 2011.

[106] C. M. Freitag, "The genetics of autistic disorders and its clinical relevance: a review of the literature," *Molecular Psychiatry*, vol. 12, no. 1, pp. 2–22, 2007.

[107] J. W. Smoller, "Cross Disorder Group of the Psychiatric Genomics Consortium. Identification of risk loci with shared effects on five major psychiatric disorders: a genome-wide analysis (vol 381, pg 1371, 2013)," *The Lancet*, vol. 381, no. 9875, p. 1360, 2013.

[108] D. H. Geschwind, "Genetics of autism spectrum disorders," *Trends in Cognitive Sciences*, vol. 15, no. 9, pp. 409–416, 2011.

[109] S. S. Jeste and D. H. Geschwind, "Disentangling the heterogeneity of autism spectrum disorder through genetic findings," *Nature Reviews Neurology*, vol. 10, no. 2, pp. 74–81, 2014.

[110] M. W. State and P. Levitt, "The conundrums of understanding genetic risks for autism spectrum disorders," *Nature Neuroscience*, vol. 14, no. 12, pp. 1499–1506, 2011.

[111] R. A. Mar, J. L. Tackett, and C. Moore, "Exposure to media and theory-of-mind development in preschoolers," *Cognitive Development*, vol. 25, no. 1, pp. 69–78, 2010.

[112] T. Charman, S. Baron-Cohen, J. Swettenham, G. Baird, A. Cox, and A. Drew, "Testing joint attention, imitation, and play as infancy precursors to language and theory of mind," *Cognitive Development*, vol. 15, no. 4, pp. 481–498, 2000.

[113] P. Mundy and L. Newell, "Attention, joint attention, and social cognition," *Current Directions in Psychological Science*, vol. 16, no. 5, pp. 269–274, 2007.

[114] T. D. Cassel, D. S. Messinger, L. V. Ibanez, J. D. Haltigan, S. I. Acosta, and A. C. Buchman, "Early social and emotional communication in the infant siblings of children with autism spectrum disorders: an examination of the broad phenotype," *Journal of Autism and Developmental Disorders*, vol. 37, no. 1, pp. 122–132, 2007.

[115] W. A. Goldberg, K. L. Jarvis, K. Osann et al., "Brief report: early social communication behaviors in the younger siblings of children with autism," *Journal of Autism and Developmental Disorders*, vol. 35, no. 5, pp. 657–664, 2005.

[116] A. G. Presmanes, T. A. Walden, W. L. Stone, and P. J. Yoder, "Effects of different attentional cues on responding to joint attention in younger siblings of children with autism spectrum disorders," *Journal of Autism and Developmental Disorders*, vol. 37, no. 1, pp. 133–144, 2007.

[117] M. Sullivan, J. Finelli, A. Marvin, E. Garrett-Mayer, M. Bauman, and R. Landa, "Response to joint attention in toddlers at risk for autism spectrum disorder: a prospective study," *Journal of Autism and Developmental Disorders*, vol. 37, no. 1, pp. 37–48, 2007.

22

Investigating the Evidence of Behavioral, Cognitive, and Psychiatric Endophenotypes in Autism

Kavita Ruparelia,[1,2] Karim Manji,[2] Amina Abubakar,[3] and Charles R. Newton[4]

[1] *Open University, Milton Keynes, UK*
[2] *Department of Pediatrics and Child Health, Muhimbili University of Health and Allied Sciences, Dar es Salaam, Tanzania*
[3] *KEMRI-Wellcome Trust Research Programme, Centre for Geographic Medicine Research (Coast), Kilifi, Kenya*
[4] *Department of Psychiatry, University of Oxford, Oxford, UK*

Correspondence should be addressed to Kavita Ruparelia; ruparelia.kavita@gmail.com

Academic Editor: Roberto Canitano

Substantial evidence indicates that parents of autistic individuals often display milder forms of autistic traits referred to as the broader autism phenotype (BAP). To determine if discrete endophenotypes of autism can be identified, we reviewed the literature to assess the evidence of behavioral, cognitive, and psychiatric profiles of the BAP. A systematic review was conducted using EMBASE, MEDLINE, PsycINFO, PsycEXTRA, and Global Health. Sixty papers met our inclusion criteria and results are discussed according to the proportion of studies that yield significant deficits per domain. The behavioral, cognitive, and psychiatric endophenotypes in parents of autistic probands are still not clarified; however, evidence suggests mild social/communication deficits, rigid/aloof personality traits, and pragmatic language difficulties as the most useful sociobehavioral candidate endophenotype traits. The existence of deficits in the cognitive domain does suggest familial vulnerability for autism. Furthermore, increased depressed mood and anxiety can also be useful markers; however, findings should be interpreted with caution because of the small number of studies in such heterogeneously broad domains and several methodological limitations.

1. Introduction

Autism is a life-long complex neurodevelopmental disorder which has heterogeneous clinical manifestations and multifactorial aetiology. It is characterized by impairments in social interaction and communication and restricted patterns of behavior, interests, and activities, occurring within the first 3 years of life [1].

The heritability of autism is estimated to be from 70% to 90% [2, 3]. Research suggests the risk of developing autism in siblings of individuals with autism is between 10 and 20%, considerably higher than when compared to about 1% for siblings of typically developing children [4, 5]. These data suggest a strong genetic basis, despite the clinical heterogeneity. Since numerous studies using linkage or candidate gene approaches have not discovered a single genetic locus of major effect, it is thought that the definition of the endophenotypes may provide insights into the biological basis of this condition.

Studies have provided substantial evidence indicating that first-degree relatives of autistic individuals often display milder forms of autistic traits referred to as the broader autism phenotype (BAP) [6]. This milder expression includes a set of behavioral and cognitive characteristics that reflect the phenotypic expression that is qualitatively similar in unaffected relatives of autistic individuals. For instance, mild challenges in social cognition in using facial cues and other features to determine mental states have been noted in parents of children with autism [7]. Additional studies report similar differences in emotion processing abilities, particularly emotion identification [8, 9] and phonological processing [10]. Research that includes such quantitative measures of autistic traits and underlying mechanisms responsible for such features in first-degree relatives is fundamental in studying the genetic basis of autism as it can help to identify which characteristics aggregate in family members and are thus likely to be potential endophenotypes for autism at the neurocognitive level.

Endophenotypes are heritable markers associated with a given condition and can provide insight into its etiology. Gottesman and Gould [11] offered a set of criteria for identification of useful endophenotypes suggesting that deficits must be (a) associated with illness in the population; (b) heritable; (c) state-independent (manifesting in an individual whether or not illness is active); (d) cosegregated with the condition within families; and (e) also found in unaffected relatives at a higher prevalence than in the general population. The study of endophenotypes is particularly useful in understanding developmental disorders such as autism that are diagnosed on clinical features but are of neurobiological origin and can aid to better identify and characterize the nature of the genetic contributions to this complex disorder.

Several researchers have reviewed the BAP traits in first-degree relatives of autistic probands [12–14]. Some reviews include studies that have examined the BAP in parents and siblings of autistic probands. Although features of the autism phenotype have been found in the "at risk" infant sibling studies, no clear distinction can be made to determine whether they are the characteristics of the BAP or whether the infant siblings may later receive an autism diagnosis. Thus, we limited this review process to parents only by employing a systematic approach to focus on the sociobehavioral, cognitive and psychiatric profiles of the broader autism phenotype to determine candidate endophenotypic traits for autism.

We conducted a systematic review of the literature to assess the evidence of behavioral, cognitive, and psychiatric endophenotypes of autism in parents. The aim of this review was to ascertain whether parents of probands with autism have higher prevalence of various components of the BAP and more specifically of behavioral, cognitive, and other psychiatric conditions. The questions addressed were as follows:

(1) What are the behavioral, cognitive, and other psychiatric (focusing primarily on depression and anxiety) endophenotypes of autism as manifested through the broader autism phenotype in biological parents of autistic probands?

(2) What are the tools used to measure these endophenotypes and the magnitude of effect?

(3) Do patterns evident in endophenotypes of autism provide insight into cultural and geographical differences?

2. Review Methods

2.1. Data Sources and Search Strategy. A comprehensive literature search was performed to collate evidence of behavioral, cognitive, and psychiatric endophenotypes in autism. Literature searches for published and grey literature were subsequently carried out using 5 databases, EMBASE, MEDLINE, PsycINFO, PsycEXTRA, and Global Health, from inception to August 2014 without language restriction. The strategy was developed by breaking down the review questions into elemental facets according to the recommendations of the National Health Service Centre for Reviews and Disseminations [15]. These facets included exposure, outcome, population, publication language, and keywords (Table 1). The initial search strategy used the words "autis* AND endophenotyp* OR phenotyp*". These searches were further refined by the addition of the outcome terms and population ("parent* OR relative OR famil*"). The bibliographies of key references were later hand-searched to identify articles missed in the database search. Figure 1 illustrates our literature search strategy.

2.2. Data Selection Criteria. The titles and abstracts of papers identified were reviewed and the full versions of potential papers were read to decide on final selection. The inclusion criteria were

(1) original studies that employed a quantitative methodological approach to investigate behavioral, cognitive, and psychiatric (depression and anxiety) endophenotypes in biological parents,

(2) the fact that autistic proband (other conditions on the spectrum such as Asperger Syndrome, Pervasive Developmental Disorder, and Pervasive Developmental Disorder Not Otherwise Specified were also included) must have a clinically established diagnosis of autism (minimum DSM III) and no concomitant medical conditions associated with autistic symptomatology and visual, auditory, and motor impairment such as Fragile X or Tuberous Sclerosis.

(3) Studies that carried out a comparison of endophenotypes between parents of individuals diagnosed with autism and unaffected adults, a normative parental control group, and/or a clinical parental control group.

We excluded any studies investigating the BAP in the general population, studies on genetics and autism, and studies examining the neuroanatomical and neurofunctional dimensions of the BAP. All single case studies, case series, book chapters, theoretical papers, review papers, unpublished dissertations/theses, and studies not published in English were excluded.

The final set of papers was restricted to those that quantitatively evaluated behavioral, cognitive, and psychiatric endophenotypes in biological parents of autistic probands.

2.3. Data Extraction. The author (KR) examined the titles, abstracts, and studies with study selection criteria. Data were organized into broad domains for each of the three categories: sociobehavioral, that is, direct assessment of BAP expression, other measures of personality and friendships, social interaction, repetitive/restrictive interests, and social and narrative language; cognitive, that is, intellectual functioning, structural language, social cognition, executive function, local visual processing (central coherence), and visual perception; other psychiatric conditions, specifically depression and anxiety.

Table 1: Description of search strategy.

Search element	EMBASE	MEDLINE	PsycINFO	PsycEXTRA	Global Health
Exposure	Thesaurus terms explored: Autis*				
Keywords	Endophenotyp* OR Phenotyp*				
Outcome	*Thesaurus terms explored* Behavior Language Social interaction Repetitive Restrictive Cognitive Executive function Central coherence Theory of mind Social cognition Visual Attention Depression anxiety	*Thesaurus terms explored* Behavior Language Social interaction Repetitive Restrictive Cognitive Executive function Central coherence Theory of mind Social cognition Visual Attention Depression anxiety	*Thesaurus terms explored* Behavior Language Social interaction Repetitive Restrictive Cognitive Executive function Central coherence Theory of mind Social cognition Visual Attention Depression anxiety	*Thesaurus terms explored* Behavior Language Social interaction Repetitive Restrictive Cognitive Executive function Central coherence Theory of mind Social cognition Visual Attention Depression anxiety	*Thesaurus terms explored* Behavior Language Social interaction Repetitive Restrictive Cognitive Executive function Central coherence Theory of mind Social cognition Visual Attention Depression anxiety
Population	Parent* OR Relative* OR Famil*				
Language	Any				

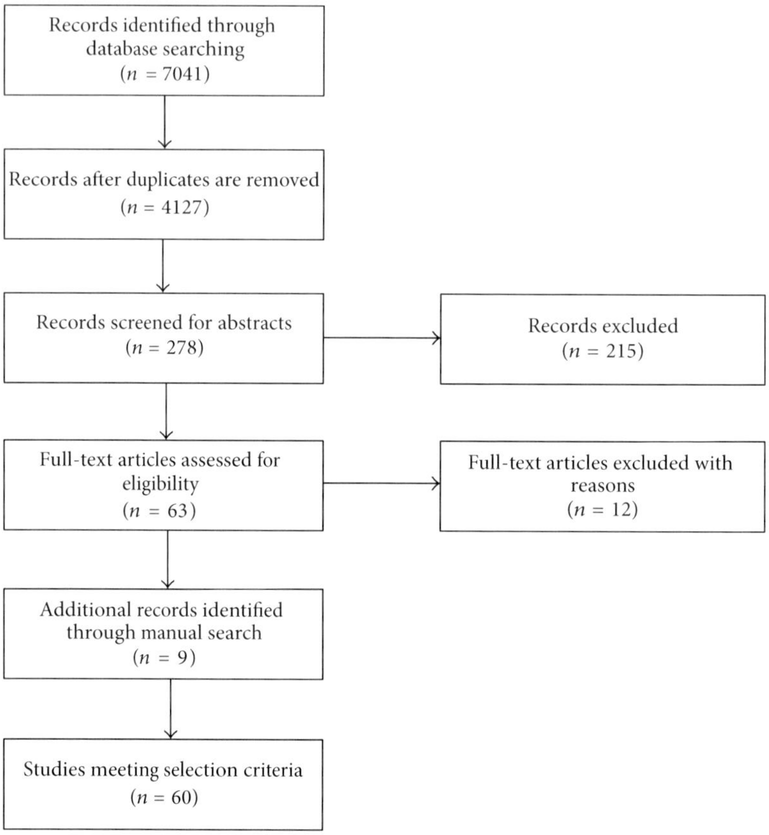

Figure 1: Flow chart of study selection.

2.4. Effect Sizes. The data extracted was based on heterogeneous measures and outcomes, so pooling the data in a meta-analysis was inappropriate. To compare the robustness of the measures used, for each behavioral, cognitive, and psychiatric variable of interest an effect size (ES) was computed from the data reported in each study. Cohen's effect size statistic (d) was calculated as the difference between the means of both groups divided by the pooled standard deviation. The following criteria were used to assess the magnitude of effect: $d < 0.2$ (small), $d > 0.5$ (medium), and $d > 0.8$ (large) [16].

3. Results

3.1. Search Results. The initial electronic search identified 7,041 records, of which 4,127 records remained after duplicates were removed. 278 articles were eligible for full review after examination of titles and abstracts (Figure 1). After full text review, we excluded 12 articles for the following reasons: in 9 studies it was not possible to distinguish parent and sibling data when results were reported for combined first-degree relatives, and, in 3 studies, proband diagnosis was established using criteria prior to DSM III. The search criteria, additional articles identified through manual search, and total numbers of articles meeting selection criteria are shown in Figure 1.

3.2. Results of Literature Extraction. Twenty-five of the 60 studies that fulfilled the inclusion criteria directly evaluated the BAP expression (including personality, social behavior, and pragmatic language features of the BAP). An additional 7 studies assessed other aspects within the sociobehavioral domain. Thirty-seven reports assessed the broad domain of cognitive functioning and seven studies investigated other psychiatric conditions. Twenty-seven of the studies were conducted in North America, 24 in Western Europe, 4 in the Middle East, and 3 in Western Pacific and 1 was conducted in South America and 1 used combined samples from North America, Western Europe, and Western Pacific. However, no studies were conducted in Asia or Africa. Index families included a total of 4,833 mothers and 3,065 fathers that took part across all studies reviewed (few studies did not specify sex breakdown). Studies varied greatly in their choice of comparison control group, with 26 studies using a nonclinical comparison group, 21 studies using a normative control sample, and 13 studies using a combined sample of clinical and nonclinical control groups. Thirteen studies evaluated the gradation of expression across family types using families with multiple incidence autism (MPX) and single incidence autism (SPX).

We summarized the results of the literature search according to different sociobehavioral, cognitive and psychiatric domains. For each domain we present the measures used within that domain and any significant differences found between index parents and parental controls, and so results are described in relation to proband diagnosis. All background measures used to establish BAP status without using a comparison group as well as control tasks are not reported under the specific criteria in this review.

3.3. Sociobehavioral Domain (Supplementary Table 1). This domain includes studies that evaluated the BAP expression using measures designed specifically to assess social abilities, communication skills, and personality traits characteristic of the BAP, as well as measures of reciprocal interaction, restrictive, and repetitive interest and social and narrative language.

3.3.1. BAP Expression through Direct Clinical Assessment. Studies explored the BAP using a variety of measures and research designs with some studies utilizing conservative selection criteria, dividing parents of autistic probands into "BAP present" (BAP+) and "BAP absent" (BAP−) groups. As shown in Supplementary Table 1 in Supplementary Material available online at https://doi.org/10.1155/2017/6346912, from eight of the measures specifically designed to assess the BAP, four are more recent questionnaires aiming to assess the BAP quantitatively, and four use interviews and direct behavioral observations. Of the four questionnaires, one is a self-report measure (Autism Spectrum Quotient (AQ)), two are informant report measures (Communication Checklist-Adult (CCA); and Social Responsiveness Scale (SRS)), and one is a self-report and informant report questionnaire (Broader Autism Phenotype Questionnaire (BAPQ)). Of the four remaining measures, two are semistructured interviews (Family History Interview (FHI)/Family History Schedule (FHS) and Modified Personality Assessment Schedule (MPAS)/Modified Personality Assessment Schedule-Revised (MPAS-R)) and two assess BAP via interviews and direct clinical observation/assessment (Broader Phenotype Autism Symptom Scale (BPASS) and Pragmatic Rating Scale (PRS)).

Autism Spectrum Quotient (AQ). A total of ten reports measured the BAP using the self-report AQ (ES range: 0.01–1.34). Three studies used adaptations of the AQ: one in Italian [17], one in Turkish [18], and one in French [19]. Within the "social skills" factor, five studies found significantly higher deficits in social skills compared to parents of typically developing children [17, 18, 20–22]. Two studies reported significantly higher prevalence of "Attention Switching" deficits between the index parents and parents of typically developing children [22] and parents of children with specific language impairment [23]. One study evaluating the "Attention to Detail" subscale reported mothers of typically developing children scoring significantly higher than index mothers [24]. Within the "Communication" subscale, five out of eight studies reported significantly higher communication deficits between index parents and parents of typically developing children [17, 18, 20, 22] and parents of children with a specific language impairment [23]. However, only Wheelwright et al.'s (2010) [22] study reported a significant trend for index parents to have more deficits in "Imagination" subscale compared to a sample of parents of typically developing children. For the total AQ score, four studies reported higher combined total scores among index parents when compared to parents of typically developing children [17, 18, 22] and parents of children with specific language impairment [23].

Ingersoll et al. (2011) [25] combined the social skill and communication factors and revealed index mothers to score significantly higher than normative mothers on the AQ.

Furthermore, in a more recent study, using a validated French Autism Quotient (FAQ), Robel et al. (2014) [19] distributed AQ scores between two main factors, F1 corresponding to socialization and communication and F2 corresponding to imagination and rigidity. They reported index parents to have more symptomatic scores in the F1 domain compared to parents of typically developing children. No significant differences were found for the F2 domain; however, the global score (F1 and F2 combined) remained significant with index parents scoring higher.

Broader Autism Phenotype Questionnaire (BAPQ). Two studies evaluated the BAP using the BAPQ (ES range: 0.26–1.49). Hurley et al. (2007) [26] used the method of preestablishing parents of autistic probands into "BAP present" (BAP+) and "BAP absent" (BAP–) groups by direct assessment on MPAS-R and PRS, reporting consistently higher scores for "BAP+" group compared to "BAP–" group and community control parents on all subscales: aloof, rigid, pragmatic language, and the total score. More recently, Sasson et al. (2013) [27] reported similar results for all BAPQ subscales and total score, with index fathers scoring significantly higher than normative fathers, and the same trend was significant for mothers of both groups.

Broader Phenotype Autism Symptom Scale (BPASS). Bernier et al. (2012) [28] used the BPASS to assess the BAP in MPX parents compared to parents of SPX families, parents of developmentally delayed children, and parents of typically developing children (ES range 0.75–1.28). Differences among groups were found in the "Social Motivation" subscale where MPX parents showed significantly more deficits than the SPX parents, parents of developmentally delayed children, and parents of typically developing children. In both "Expressiveness" and "Restricted Interests" subscales a significant difference was found only between the MPX parents scoring higher than parents of typically developing children. No group differences were found within the "Communication" subscale and, interestingly, SPX parents did not differ from parents of children with developmental delay or typical development.

Communication Checklist-Adult Version (CC-A). Whitehouse et al. (2010) [29] assessed the BAP using the CC-A (ES range: 0.04–0.43), and found only the "Social Engagement" subscale had statistically significant differences between the index parents and a normative sample, suggesting a more passive communication style for the index parents. No group differences were found in the "Language Structure" and "Pragmatic Language" subscales; however, analysis of the total score of the two groups (1 standard deviation below mean) was found to be significant.

Family History Interview/Family History Schedule (FHI/FHS). Three studies evaluated the BAP using the FHI/FHS semistructured interview method (no ES available). Folstein et al. (1999) [30] analyzed four items (language delays, reading difficulties, spelling difficulties, and articulation) on the "Communication" subscale. Accordingly, "early language-related cognitive difficulties" (ELRCD) were scored and a "definite" or "probable" rating was applied. Significantly higher rates of definite and probable ELRCD were found in index parents compared to parents of children with Down's Syndrome. However, two other studies found index parents to perform equally to comparison groups on the "Communication" subscale [6, 31]. Within the "social" factor, Piven et al. (1997) [6] found parents from MPX families had significantly higher prevalence of social deficits than parents of Down's Syndrome children, particularly in index fathers. Similarly, Pickles et al. (2013) [31] reported significantly increased social deficits in index parents compared to parents of children with a specific language impairment. Interestingly, no group differences were found between index parents and parents of children with a combined diagnosis of specific language impairment and autism. Only Piven et al. (1997) [6] assessed the "Stereotyped Behaviors" subscale and reported MPX parents to have significantly more repetitive stereotyped behaviors compared to parents of Down's Syndrome children.

Modified Personality Assessment Schedule (MPAS/MPAS-R). One study used the MPAS to evaluate the BAP (Piven et al., 1994) [32] and three subsequent studies have used a modified version (MPAS-R) [33–35] (ES not available). Three out of the four studies assessing the "Aloof" subscale found significantly higher rates of aloofness in index parents compared to parents of Down's Syndrome children [32, 33], with one study reporting MPX parents to score significantly higher than SPX parents who in turn scored significantly higher than parents of children with Down's Syndrome [35]. Similarly, the same trend for the "Anxious," "Hypersensitive," "Rigid," and "Untactful" personality traits was reported [35]. Piven et al. (1997) [33] reported significantly higher rates of anxiousness, hypersensitiveness, and rigidity in MPX parents in comparison to parents of Down's Syndrome; however, they found no significant differences between the two groups in the "Untactful," "Undemonstrative," and "Unresponsive" traits. Piven et al. (1994) [32], however, did find significantly higher rates of untactfulness and undemonstrativeness in index parents compared to parents of children with Down's Syndrome. In a more recent study, Losh et al. (2012) [35] failed to find a significant difference for the "Overly Conscientious" subscale, but they did find a significant difference in the "Rigidity" subscale.

Pragmatic Rating Scale (PRS/PRS-M). A total of five studies assessed the BAP using the PRS (ES range: 0–1.14). Landa et al. (1992) [36] combined blind and nonblind ratings and reported higher total scores for the index parents compared to their control sample of parents of Down's Syndrome and typical development. Losh et al. (2012) [35] found in their sample of mothers only that index mothers had similar pragmatic language violations to mothers of children with Fragile X Syndrome, and both these groups had higher frequency of violations than mothers of typically developing children. Piven et al. (1997) [33] reported higher frequency of pragmatic language violations and speech errors in MPX parents compared to parents of Down's Syndrome children. Additionally, Losh et al. (2008) [34] found a linear trend for both pragmatic language violations and speech errors, reporting MPX parents to score significantly higher than SPX parents who in turn scored significantly higher than parents of children with Down's Syndrome. Ruser et al. (2007) [37] used a modified version of the PRS (PRS-M) and reported index parents to have significantly higher deficits in subscales of emotional expressiveness and awareness of the other, overtalkativeness, and language in comparison to parents of children with Down's Syndrome. Group differences in the communicative factor were not found to be significant; however, index fathers showed significantly increased communication deficits than index mothers. The total PRS-M score revealed significant group differences between index parents and Down's Syndrome parents, with index fathers scoring higher than index mothers.

Social Responsiveness Scale (SRS). The SRS was used as a measure to assess the BAP by two studies in our review (ES range: 0.02–0.90). De la Marche et al. (2012) [38] reported all index fathers (MPX and SPX combined) having a significantly higher total score compared to unaffected adult males; however no statistical differences were found between MPX fathers and SPX fathers and SPX fathers and male controls. In contrast, Schwichtenberg et al. (2010) [39] found that both the MPX and SPX fathers in their sample scored significantly higher than fathers of typically developing children. No differences between mothers in both groups were found.

3.3.2. Other Measures of Personality and Friendships. Another personality measure used in studies of the BAP is the NEO Personality Inventory (NEO-PI). Two studies show a trend for parents from MPX families scoring significantly higher on the neuroticism subscale in comparison to parents of children from SPX families [34] and parents of DS probands [33, 34] (ES 0.79, $n = 1$). Furthermore, the same two studies assessed quality of friendships using the Friendship Interview (FI), indicating significantly fewer friendships in parents from MPX families in comparison to parents of children from SPX families [34] and parents of Down's Syndrome children [33, 34]. Interestingly, Losh et al. (2008) [34] also found sex differences in the quality of friendships within ASD parents, with fathers from MPX families and SPX families having significantly fewer friendships than mothers from MPX families and SPX families (ES 1.14, $n = 1$).

3.3.3. Reciprocal Social Interaction. Two studies assessed alexithymia (i.e., inability to identify and describe emotions in oneself) as part of the BAP. Szatmari et al. (2008) [9] used the Toronto Alexithymia Scale (TAS-20) as a measure of alexithymia and, despite its three factors (difficulty identifying feelings, difficulty describing feelings, and externally oriented thinking) not reaching significance, the total score confirmed higher frequency of alexithymia in index parents compared to parents of children with Prader Willi syndrome. Using the same scale, however, Berthoz et al. (2013) [40] failed to find a statistically significant difference between index parents and unaffected adults (ES range: 0.14–0.25). Another measure of alexithymia used by Berthoz et al. (2013) [40] was the Bermond-Vorst Alexithymia Questionnaire-B (BVAQ-B); however no significant differences were found between the samples (ES range: 0.02–0.19).

Berthoz et al. (2013) [40] further assessed social anhedonia (i.e., inability to experience pleasure from activities usually found enjoyable), using the revised version of the Social Anhedonia Scale (SAS) (ES 0.25) and found no significant differences between the index parents and unaffected adults. However, Berthoz et al. (2013) [40] found index parents to score significantly higher than unaffected adults on physical anhedonia as measured by the Physical Anhedonia Scale (PAS) (ES 0.33).

3.3.4. Social and Narrative Language. In addition to the PRS, which was specifically designed to assess the deficits in social language as a BAP expression, two other measures have assessed social and narrative language. Di Michele et al. (2007) [8] used Grice's Conversational Maxims task to assess pragmatic conversations and found the index parents performed significantly worse when compared to parents of typically developing children and parents of children with Down Syndrome (ES not available). Landa et al. (1991) [41] used "spontaneous narrative discourse performance" to assess narrative discourse deficits. They reported control adults producing significantly more complete episodes and stories with multiple episodes, and the mean overall quality for the index parents was significantly less than that for the comparison adults (ES range: 0.35–0.73).

3.3.5. Repetitive/Restrictive Behaviors and Interests. Repetitive and restrictive behaviors are a core symptom of autism. The majority of findings in parents of autistic probands corresponding to this domain are covered in the studies that assess the BAP in terms of rigid and perfectionistic personalities. Only one study used an experimental questionnaire designed to examine real-life, nonsocial skills and preferences such as insistence on routines and circumscribed hobbies. Briskman et al. (2001) [42] reported index parents to score significantly higher than parents of boys with dyslexia and typical development (ES range: 0.37–1.11).

3.4. Cognitive Domain (Supplementary Table 2). Most forms of neuropsychological tests involve multiple cognitive functions suggesting that cognitive domains can be related to each other. We have organized the measures for this broad domain under different categories based on the cognitive function which they predominantly assess; however, an overlap may exist. References for the different measures can be found in the studies included in this review and in more specialized text book resources [43].

3.4.1. Intellectual Functioning. Intelligence Quotient (IQ) was measured with different versions of the Wechsler Scales in the studies. Thirteen studies assessed total Verbal IQ (VIQ) (ES range: 0.05–1.28, $n = 12$), with scores for index parents similar to comparison groups in all but one study [44] with higher scores for index parents when compared to parents of Down's Syndrome children. Several VIQ subtests were also independently tested. Three studies used the digit span subtest (some modified it to assess short term memory)

(ES range: 0.04–0.67), of which two found better performance in index parents compared to parents with children with Down's Syndrome [44] and parents of children with specific language impairment [23]. Only one study used the Arithmetic subscale and found no significant differences between index parents compared to parents with children with Down's Syndrome [44] (ES: 0.25). Four studies used the vocabulary subtest (ES range: 0.04–0.96) and results were mixed, with one study indicating higher scores for index parents compared to parents of children with Down's Syndrome [44], another indicating a reverse trend with index parents scoring significantly lower than parents of typically developing children [45], and two revealing no significant differences between groups. Four studies assessed the comprehension subtest (ES range: 0.31–0.74), with only one indicating a significant difference with index parents scoring significantly higher than parents of children with Down's Syndrome [44]. Additionally, two studies used the similarities subtest (ES range: 0.13–0.35) with only one reporting a significant difference [44].

Thirteen studies also assessed total Performance IQ (PIQ) (ES range: 0–1.16, $n = 12$), with three studies reporting a significant difference, with index parents performing poorer than parents of children with Down's Syndrome [30, 46] and unaffected adults [10]. One study, however, reported an opposite trend with index fathers performing significantly better than fathers with a child with specific language impairment [47]. Several PIQ subtests were also independently tested. Four studies used the picture completion subtest (ES range: 0.07–0.65); however only two reported significant lower scores for index parents compared to parents of children with Down's Syndrome [30, 46]. Moreover, Folstein et al. (1999) [30] also reported lower scores on the picture arrangement subtest with the same trend of significance (ES range: 0.03–0.26, $n = 2$). Two studies assessed the object assembly subtest (ES range: 0.12–0.62); however only one reported a significant difference with MPX parents scoring lower than parents of Down's Syndrome children [46]. Furthermore, Schmidt et al. (2008) [10] found significantly lower scores on the matrix reasoning subtest in index parents compared to unaffected adults (ES 0.67). Interestingly, none of the five studies assessing the block design subtest (ES range: 0.04–0.43) and one study assessing the digit symbol subtest found significant differences between groups (ES range: 0.17–0.19).

Full Scale IQ (FSIQ) (ES range: 0.05–1.88, $n = 13$) was assessed in fourteen studies in our review with three studies reporting a significant poorer performance in index parents when compared to parents of children with Down's Syndrome [30, 34] and a combined clinical group of parents of children with Down's Syndrome and typical development [48].

Additionally, four studies used Raven's Progressive Matrices to report Nonverbal IQ (NVIQ), with no significant differences found between groups [49–52] (ES range: 0.05–0.57).

3.4.2. Structural Language Abilities. A number of studies assessed structural language abilities using a variety of different measures. Results are divided into specific domains. Receptive language skills were assessed by three studies using two measures. The Peabody Picture Vocabulary Test (PPVT-III) (ES range: 0.33–1.58) was used by two studies with only one study reporting index mothers as having significantly more deficits than mothers of children with autism and language impairment who in turn had more deficits compared to mothers of children with a specific language impairment [47]. Whitehouse et al. (2007) [23] used the Test for Reception of Grammar-2 (TROG-2) to evaluate receptive grammar and reported no differences between groups (ES not available). Schmidt et al. (2008) [10] assessed expressive language using the Expressive Vocabulary Test (EVT) (ES 0.10) and the verbal fluency subtest of the Delis Kaplan Executive Function System (DK-EFS) (ES: 0.16–0.39) reporting no significant differences between index parents and unaffected adults. Additionally, they assessed figurative language using the figurative language subtest from the Test of Language Competence-Expanded Edition (TOLC-E) reporting no significant differences between the two groups (ES: 0.28).

Phonological processing was assessed in five reports using five different tests. Lindgren et al. (2009) [47] used the Comprehensive Test of Phonological Processing (CTOPP) (ES range: 0.02–1.42, $n = 2$), revealing significantly better performance in phonological awareness and the nonword repetition subtests in the index mothers compared to mothers of children with a specific language impairment. In contrast, however, Schmidt et al. (2008) [10] found index parents to perform significantly lower than unaffected adults in the same nonword subtest. Bishop et al. (2004) [53] used a different Nonword Memory Test (ES range: 0.02–0.04) and a Nonsense Passage Reading test (ES range: 0.04–0.42) to assess phonological processing, none indicating significant differences between index parents and parents of typically developing children. However, Whitehouse et al. (2007) [23] did find index parents to perform significantly better than parents of children with specific language impairment in the nonsense words subtest of the NEPSY (a Developmental Neuropsychological Assessment Test Battery) (ES range: 0.04–0.88). In contrast, Plumet et al. (1995) [54] found no significant differences in composite verbal scores when comparing index parents to parents of children with Down's Syndrome using a battery of verbal tasks with an emphasis on orthographic and phonological abilities (ES: 0.22).

Reading skills were assessed by eight studies using seven different measures. Piven and Palmer (1997) [46] used the Rapid Automized Naming (RAN) task and found no differences in the number and letter categories; however, they found significant differences with MPX parents taking longer to complete the task on the color and object categories (ES range: 0.17–0.58). Similarly, Losh et al. (2010) [55] combined the color and object categories and reported index parents taking longer to complete the task when compared with parents of typically developing children (ES not available). The Woodcock-Johnson Psychoeducational Battery-Revised (WJ-R) has several subtests, and no significant differences were found in the broad reading (ES range: 0.48–2.11) and reading skill composite scores [47] (ES range: 0.40–1.84), the word attack subtest [46, 47] (ES range: 0.09–1.35), and letter word subtest [46]. However, Folstein et al. (1999) [30]

found a significantly lower reading age and reading grade using the nonsense word reading subtest in index parents compared to parents of children with Down's Syndrome (ES: 0.40). Mothers of children with autism performed better in the dictation (ES range: 0.17–0.99, $n = 2$) and passage comprehension subtests (ES range: 0.45–1.54, $n = 2$) compared to mothers of children with specific language impairment [47]. In contrast, Piven and Palmer (1997) [46] found MPX parents had more difficulties in the passage comprehension subtest when compared with parents of children with Down's Syndrome. Interestingly, no differences were noted in comprehension (ES range: 0.12–0.36) and passage reading subtests (ES range: 0.21–0.36) using the Gray Oral Reading Test (GORT) [30, 44] and the Edinburgh Reading Test (ERT) [44]. Fombonne et al. (1997) [44] also used the National Adult Reading Test (NART) (ES range: 0.20–0.44, $n = 2$) reporting index parents scoring significantly lower than parents of children with Down's Syndrome. However, Baron-Cohen and Hammer (1997) [7] found no significant differences in error scores between index parents and parents of typically developing children. Whitehouse et al. (2007) [23] used the Test of Word Reading Efficiency (ES range: 0.03–0.62) and found index parents performed better than parents of children with specific language impairment on the phonemic decoding efficiency subtest (nonsense words). Finally, Schmidt et al. (2008) [10] found no significant differences in reading difficulties using the Reading History Questionnaire (RHQ) between index parents and unaffected adults (ES: 0.34).

Three studies assessed spelling abilities using two different measures. Whitehouse et al. (2007) [23] found no group differences using a Speeded Dictation task (ES not available). Furthermore, Fombonne et al. (1997) [44] found a superior performance by index parents on the Schonell Spelling Test (SST) (ES range: 0.02–0.13, $n = 2$). Only one study assessed oromotor functioning using the oromotor sequencing subtest of the NEPSY Test Battery (ES range: 0.43–0.54) reporting index families performing better than parents of children with specific language impairment [23].

3.4.3. Social Cognition. In this domain measures assess the ability to process information relating to other people's mental states. Five reports assessed the "Theory of Mind" using different versions of Reading the Mind in the Eyes Test (ES range: 0.03–1.51, $n = 4$). Three studies reported deficits between index parents and comparison groups [7, 48, 56]. In contrast, Gocken et al. (2009) [57] and Tajmirriyahi et al. (2013) [58] found no significant group differences in mental state decoding in the eyes test. Furthermore, Gocken et al. (2009) [57] explored mental state decoding using a faces test and reported no significant differences between index parents and a normative sample (ES: 0.23). Tajmirriyahi et al. (2013) [58], however, used a novel method of Reading the Mind in the Voice Test to reveal significantly higher deficits in mental state decoding in index parents when compared to parents of children with Down's Syndrome and typical development (ES range: 0.63–0.98). Additionally, Di Michele et al. (2007) [8] used False Belief tasks (smarties task, Sally-Anne task, and unexpected transfer test) and found index parents passed fewer false belief tests in comparison to parents of children with Down's Syndrome and typical development (ES not available). Similarly, Gocken et al. (2009) [57] reported poorer performance in index parents compared to a normative sample using the Unexpected Outcomes Test (UOT) (ES: 0.58); however, they did not find a significant difference using the Hinting task (ES: 0.36).

Remarkably, only one study assessed empathy using the Empathy Quotient (EQ) reporting significant impairments in empathy in index fathers compared to unaffected males [52] (ES: 0.11–0.40).

Affect perception was assessed in eight studies using twelve different tests of emotion recognition and labeling. Using the "Bubbles" method with pictures of facial affect, Adolphs et al. (2008) [59] showed no difference in accuracy and reaction time; however, the "BAP+" group used significantly different facial information (eye region and mouth region) in comparison to the "BAP−" group and parents of typically developing children (ES not available). Using the Penn Emotion Recognition Test (ER40), das Neves et al. (2011) [60] reported significantly longer time for correct responses in index parents compared to unaffected adults (ES range: 0.54–1.09). They also reported less accurate responses, identification of female and male faces, and mild and extreme emotions. Bölte and Poustka (2003) [49] showed no significant differences in groups using the Facial Affect Recognition Test (pictures by Ekman and Friesen) (ES range: 0.32–2.06). Similarly, Sucksmith et al. (2013) [52] found no significant differences in accuracy and adjusted response time in index parents compared to unaffected adults using the Karolinska Directed Emotional Faces task (KDEF) (ES range: 0.08–0.30). Kadak et al. (2014) [21] used the Emotion Recognition Test (using photos of facial affect from Ekman and Friesen) and found index parents had impaired recognition of happy, surprised, and neutral faces compared to parents of typically developing children (ES range: 0.05–0.50).

Two studies assessed emotional labeling and matching of facial patterns using three different measures. Using Schematic Line Drawings (ES not available), Palermo et al. (2006) [61] showed impaired labeling for sad, disgust, and overall recognition of facial patterns in index parents compared to parents of typically developing children. In contrast, using the Emotion Matching task (ES: 0.06) and the Emotion Labeling task (ES: 0.19), Smalley and Asarnow (1990) [45] found no significant impairments.

3.4.4. Executive Function. Executive function encompasses abilities that underlie goal directed behavior. This broad domain was split into specific subdomains. Cognitive flexibility was assessed by four studies evaluating set-shifting tasks. Two studies using the intradimensional/extradimensional set-shifting task (IDED) revealed significantly higher rates of learned irrelevance [62] (ES: 0.52), trials to criterion [63] (ES range: 0.69–0.83), and errors to criterion [63] (ES range: 0.64–0.70) in index parents compared to control samples in the extradimensional stage only. However, Bölte and Poustka (2006) [50] used the Wisconsin Card Sorting Test (WCST) (ES range: 0.06–0.18) and the Trail Making Test (TMT, Parts A and B) (ES range: 0.13–0.38) and found no impaired cognitive control between groups. Similarly, Losh et al. (2009) [56] also showed no significant difference in the total time to complete the TMT task between groups.

Five reports assessed planning abilities using two measures. Using the Tower of London (ToL) (ES range: 0.07–0.93, $n = 2$), Hughes et al. (1997) [63] found index parents requiring a significantly increased number of extra moves to complete the task compared to unaffected adults. In contrast, Wong et al. (2006) [62] found no significant group differences in the number of extra moves and rule violations. Three studies used the Tower of Hanoi version (ToH) revealing no significant differences in the total time to complete variable (ES range: 0.01–0.45 $n = 1$) between index parents and a matched clinical sample [50] and nonclinical sample [56], and one study reported significant differences in planning efficiency between index parents and parents of children with Down's Syndrome [46].

One study assessed generativity using the Pattern Meanings test which measures ideational fluency, indicating a significantly impaired overall response generativity in index parents compared to a mixed sample of clinical and nonclinical comparison group [62] (ES: 0.51).

Spatial working memory was assessed by one study using a Visual Search Test, indicating index parents scoring significantly higher between search errors when compared to unaffected adults [63] (ES range: 0.27–0.95). In contrast, however, using the Response to Inhibition and Load (RIL) test, Wong et al. (2006) [62] tested inhibition and its interaction with working memory and found unimpaired reaction times and number of errors in index parents (ES range: 0.04–0.28).

Verbal working memory was assessed using three measures by one study. Using the Stroop Interference Test (ES: 0.2) and a Verbal Fluency Test (letters KAS in Turkish) (ES: 0.26), Gocken et al. (2009) [57] revealed no significant differences between groups. However, they did show impaired accuracy in index parents using the Auditory Consonant Trigrams (ACT) (ES: 0.55).

3.4.5. Local Visual Processing (Central Coherence). Central coherence is a specific perceptual-cognitive style leading to a local visual processing bias. Five studies assessed disembedding performance using two tests. All five studies used the Embedded Figures Test (EFT) with mixed results. Three out of the five studies found significantly longer response times for index parents [7, 50] and more specifically in index fathers, when compared to control fathers [64] (ES range: 0.01–1.60, $n = 5$). No significant results were reported within the accuracy variable [56, 64] (ES range: 0.11–0.77, $n = 2$); however, De Jonge et al. (2006) [65] reported significantly fewer incorrect responses in index parents when compared to parents of children with Down's Syndrome (ES range: 0.18–0.52). Furthermore, Happé et al. (2001) [64] revealed a similar trend with index parents making fewer errors using the Titchener Circles Illusion test (ES not available).

Mental segmentation ability was assessed with an Unsegmented/Segmented Block Design task (adaptation from the Weschler subtest) in two studies. Happé et al. (2001) [64] found faster response times in index parents in the unsegmented task (ES range: 0.24–0.84, $n = 1$), and, in contrast, Losh et al. (2009) [56] found significantly faster reaction times in the segmented task only (ES range: 0.04–0.63, $n = 1$). Furthermore, De Jonge et al. (2009) [66] showed no group differences in mean number of errors using a Block Design Reconstruction task (patterns by Akshoomoff and Stiles) (ES range: 0.10–0.16).

The sentence completion task was used by two studies to assess global sentence completions revealing significantly increased number of errors in index parents [56, 64] and longer response times in index parents [56].

3.4.6. Visual Processing. Interestingly only one study assessed visual processing using four different measures. Contrast sensitivity was measured using the Vistech Contrast Sensitivity Charts and no significant differences were found between index parents and parents of children with Down's Syndrome [67] (ES: 0.55). Similarly, tasks of motion discrimination (Motion Coherence task (ES: 0.25) and Moving Shape task (ES: 0.17)) and form discrimination (Form Discrimination (Shape) task) (ES: 0.05) revealed no significant differences between the same groups [67].

3.5. Other Psychiatric Conditions Domain (Supplementary Table 3). This domain was assessed in seven reports using nine different measures. Piven et al. (1991) [68] used the Schedule for Affective Disorders and Schizophrenia-Lifetime Version (SADS-L) and found significantly higher scores in the "anxiety" factor when compared to parents of children with Down's Syndrome, and no statistical significance was found for the "major depressive disorder" subscale between the two groups (ES not available). However, using a modified version of the Schedule for Affective Disorders and Schizophrenia-Lifetime Version Modified for the Study of Anxiety Disorders, Revised (SADS-LA-R), Piven and Palmer (1999) [69] did find significantly higher frequency of "major depressive disorder" in index parents in addition to the "social phobia" factor.

Micali et al. (2004) [70] devised a parental questionnaire and validated their results from consented medical records from GPs and found a significant trend towards higher prevalence of "depression" and "anxiety" in index parents. Using the Symptom Checklist-90-Revised (SCL-90-R), Bölte et al. (2007) [51] found significantly increased frequency in index parents in four of the nine subscales (depression, hostility, phobic anxiety, and paranoid ideation) (ES range: 0–1.33). Additionally, Bölte et al. (2007) [51] also assessed personality style and disorder using the Personality Style and Disorder Inventory (PSSI) and reported significantly higher rates in index parents in five out of fourteen factors (reserved/schizoid, self-critical/insecure, critical/negativistic, spontaneous/borderline, and quiet/depressive) (ES range: 0.02–1.18).

Gocken et al. (2009) [57] assessed depression and anxiety factors using the Brief Psychiatric Rating Scale (BPRS) between index parents and a normative comparison group and only found a statistically significant difference in the depression factor with index parents scoring higher (ES range: 0.29–0.44). Similarly, Ingersoll et al. (2011) [25] assessed depressed mood using the Centre for Epidemiological

Studies-Depression Scales (CESD) and showed index mothers as having increased rates of depression when compared to a normative sample of mothers (ES: 0.35). Interestingly, Berthoz et al. (2013) [40] reported no significant differences in levels of depressive mood using the Beck Depression Inventory (BDI) (ES: 0.50) and no significant differences were found in anxiety levels using the state (ES: 0.19) and trait portions (ES: 1.24) of State-Trait Anxiety Inventory Form Y (STAI-Y) [40].

4. Discussion

This systematic review aimed to assess the evidence of behavioral, cognitive, and psychiatric profiles of the BAP in unaffected biological parents of autistic probands by synthesizing the evidence from 60 studies meeting a priori search criteria. Results are discussed according to the following criteria: (i) the number of studies that indicate significant impairments in each domain and subdomain; (ii) quantitative criteria using effect sizes; and (iii) the possible emerging themes across studies. Table 2 represents a summary of all measures used by studies meeting our search criteria.

4.1. Summary of Findings. Findings emerging from this review are discussed according to each domain. Within the sociobehavioral domain, eight measures that directly assess the BAP expression in unaffected parents showed substantial deficits in the domain of social and communication skills (AQ, 7/10 studies; BPASS, 1 study; CC-A, 1 study; FHI/FHS, 2/2 studies; SRS, 2/2 studies), rigid and perfectionistic (BAPQ, 2/2 studies; MPAS-R, 3/3 studies) and aloof (BAPQ, 2/2; MPAS-R, 3/4 studies) personality traits, and pragmatic language difficulties (BAPQ, 2/2 studies; PRS, 4/4 studies) related to the core deficit in autism and are reported consistently across most studies. Moreover, additional deficits in social and narrative language have been highlighted using measures of spontaneous narrative discourse [36] and Grice's Conversational Maxims task [8]. Available evidence also points to index parents establishing fewer friendships (FI, 2/2 studies) and an elevated frequency of neuroticism (NEO-PI, 2/2 studies). Despite being a core domain of a clinical diagnosis for autism, the majority of findings in parents of autistic probands corresponding to restricted and repetitive behaviors and interests are covered in the studies that assess the BAP in terms of rigid and perfectionistic personality styles. Only one study used an experimental questionnaire designed to examine real-life nonsocial skills and preferences such as insistence on routines and circumscribed hobbies [42].

Within the sociobehavioral domain, reciprocal social interaction is probably the least studied subdomain in parents of autistic probands. As such, findings from alexithymia (TAS-20, 1/2 studies; BVAQ-B, 1 study with no significance found) and physical (PAS, 1/1 study) and social anhedonia (SAS, 1 study with no significance found) are modest and require further studies to explore these traits. Thus, we agree with previous reviews [12–14] indicating that mild social/communication deficits, rigid/aloof personality traits, and pragmatic language difficulties may be the most useful social behavioral candidate endophenotype traits as they meet all the established criteria [11]; however, effect sizes throughout this domain varied considerably.

At the cognitive level, a remarkable finding is the discrepancies found in intellectual functioning of parents of autistic probands compared to parents of children with and without a clinical diagnosis. One of thirteen studies revealed significantly higher VIQ scores when compared to a clinical sample of parents of a child with Down's Syndrome [44]. Three of thirteen studies assessing PIQ reached a similar significant trend when compared to parents with a Down's Syndrome child [30, 46] and unaffected adults [10]. Total PIQ scores were significantly higher in index parents when compared to parents with a child with specific language impairment [47]. Only two of twelve reports reached a significant deficit in FSIQ when index parents were compared to parents of children with Down's Syndrome [30] and when compared to a combined sample of parents of a child with Down's Syndrome and of typical development. However, it is noteworthy that scores for all parents were well within the average range in all studies. Thus there is limited evidence for the role of intellectual functioning as an endophenotype for autism with no clear clinical significance.

Several measures were used to assess the structural language abilities within the cognitive domain. Interestingly, no significant differences were found in the expressive language (TROG-2, 1 study with no significance found; EVT, 1 study with no significance found; DK-EFS verbal fluency subtest, 1 study with no significance found) and figurative language categories (TOLCE-E figurative language subtest, 1 study with no significance found). Lindgren et al. (2009) [47] found index parents to perform better than parents with a child with a specific language impairment on measures assessing receptive language (PPVT-III, 1/2 studies; TROG-2, 1 study with no significance found) refuting the hypothesis that families with autism and specific language impairment do not share similar genetic loading for language.

In phonological awareness, findings are mixed with studies only reporting few deficits in nonsense word/passage reading tests (2/3 studies) with index parents performing better than parents with a specific language impairment child [23] and parents of children with Down's Syndrome [30]. Using the RAN measure for reading skills, two studies reported faster times to complete the color and object only tasks in index parents when compared to parents of children with Down's Syndrome [46] and parents of typically developing children [55]. This may have relevance with regard to perceptual load in autism. However, no significant differences were found in the rapid naming subtest of the CTOPP [47].

Findings from the social cognition domain including mental state decoding, affect perception, emotion recognition, and labeling in the BAP also report mixed and conflicting results. Remarkably only one studied assessed empathy warranting further research in this subdomain.

Evidence from the broad domain of executive function in the BAP is also inconsistent but the few studies that have found impairments did not appropriately match experimental and control groups for IQ are worth noting (e.g., [63]).

Similarly, findings from studies assessing performance on tests where local visual processing is an advantage (central

Table 2: Summary of the frequency of all measures used by studies meeting our search criteria and effect size ranges for each domain.

	Frequency
Sociobehavioral category	
BAP expression (ES range: 0.01–1.49)	
Autism Spectrum Quotient (AQ)	10
Broader Autism Phenotype Questionnaire (BAPQ)	2
Broader Phenotype Autism Spectrum Scale (BPASS)	1
Communication Checklist-Adult (CC-A)	1
Family History Interview/Family History Schedule (FHI/FHS)	3
Modified Personality Assessment Schedule-Revised (MPAS-R)	4
Pragmatic Rating Scale (PRS)	4
Social Responsiveness Scale (SRS)	2
Other measures of personality and friendships (ES range: 0.79–1.14)	
The Friendship Interview (FI)	2
The Neo Personality Interview (NEO-PI)	2
Reciprocal social interaction (ES: 0.33)	
Alexithymia	
Toronto Alexithymia Scale (TAS-20)	2
Bermond-Vorst Alexithymia Questionnaire-B (BVAQ-B)	1
Anhedonia	
Revised Social Anhedonia Scale (SAS)	1
Physical Anhedonia Scale (PAS)	1
Social and narrative language (ES: 0.50–0.73)	
Grice's Conversational Maxims task	1
Spontaneous Narrative Language	1
Repetitive, restrictive behaviors & interests (ES: 0.37–1.11)	
Everyday Preferences & Abilities	
Real Life Skills & Preferences	1
Cognitive category	
General intellectual functioning (ES range: 0.14–1.16)	
Wechsler Scales	19
Raven's Progressive Matrices (RPM)	4
Structural language abilities (ES range: 0.04–1.65)	
Receptive language	
Peabody Picture Vocabulary Test (PPVT-III)	2
Test for Reception of Grammar-2 (TROG-2)	1
Expressive language	
Expressive Vocabulary Test (EVT)	1
Verbal Fluency Subtest-Delis Kaplan Executive Function System (DK-EFS)	1
Figurative language	
Figurative Language Subtest-Test of Language Competence-Expanded (TOLC-E)	1
Phonological awareness	
Comprehensive Test of Phonological Processing (CTOPP)	2
Nonword Memory Test	1
Nonsense Passage Reading Test	1
Nonsense Words Subtest-NEPSY Test Battery	1
Battery of Verbal tasks (including orthographic & phonological abilities)	1

TABLE 2: Continued.

	Frequency
Reading abilities	
Rapid Automized Naming (RAN)	2
Woodcock-Johnson Psychoeducational Battery-Revised (WJ-R)	3
Gray Oral Reading Test (GORT)	2
Edinburgh Reading Test (ERT)	1
National Adult Reading Test (NART)	2
Test of Word Reading Efficiency	1
Reading History Questionnaire (RHQ)	1
Spelling abilities	
Schonell Spelling Test (SST)	1
Speeded Dictation task	2
Oromotor functioning	
Oromotor Sequencing Subtest-NEPSY Test Battery	1
Social cognition (ES range: 0.05–1.51)	
Theory of Mind	
Reading the Mind in the Eyes Test (different versions)	5
The Faces Test	1
Reading the Mind in the Voice Test	1
False Belief tasks (Smarties task; Sally-Anne task; unexpected transfer test)	1
Unexpected Outcomes Test (UOT)	1
The Hinting task	1
Empathy	
Empathy Quotient (EQ)	1
Affect perception/emotion recognition	
Pictures of facial affect, "Bubbles" method	1
Penn Emotion Recognition Test (ER40)	1
Facial Affect Recognition Test	1
Emotion Recognition Test	1
Karolinska Directed Emotional Faces task (KDEF)	1
Point Light Basic Emotions task	1
Trustworthiness of Faces task	1
The Morphed Faces task	1
The Movie Still task	1
Schematic Line Drawings task	1
Emotion Matching task	1
Emotion Labeling task	1
Executive function (ES range: 0.27–1.27)	
Set-shifting	
intradimensional-extradimensional Set-Shifting task (IDED)	2
Wisconsin Card Sorting Test (WCST)	1
Trail Making Test (A & B)	2
Planning	
Tower of London (ToL)	2
Tower of Hanoi (ToH)	3
Generativity/ideational fluency	
Pattern Meanings	1

Table 2: Continued.

	Frequency
Spatial working memory/inhibition	
Visual Search Test	1
The Delayed Oculomotor task	1
Response Inhibition & Load (RIL)	1
Verbal working memory	
Auditory Consonant Trigrams (ACT)	1
Verbal Fluency Test	1
Stroop Interference Test	1
Central coherence (local visual processing) (ES range: 0.18–1.60)	
Disembedding performance	
Embedded Figures Test (EFT)	5
Titchener Circles Illusion	1
Mental segmentation ability	
Unsegmented Block Design task (adapted from Wechsler Scales)	2
Segmented Block Design task (adapted from Wechsler Scales)	2
Block Design task (Wechsler scales)	2
Block Design Reconstruction task	1
Attentional engagement	
Detection task	1
Global sentence completions	
Sentence completion task	2
Visual processing (ES not available)	
Contrast sensitivity	
Vistech Contrast Sensitivity Charts	1
Motion discrimination	
Motion Coherence task	1
Moving Shape task	1
Form discrimination	
Form Discrimination (Shape) task	1
Other psychiatric conditions category (depression and anxiety) (ES range: 0–1.33)	
Brief Psychiatric Rating Scale (BPRS)	1
Personality Style & Disorder Inventory (PSSI)	1
Symptom Checklist 90-Revised (SCL-90-R)	1
Schedule for Affective Disorders and Schizophrenia-Lifetime Version (SADS-L)	1
Schedule for Affective Disorders and Schizophrenia-Lifetime Version Modified for the Study of Anxiety Disorders-Revised (SADS-LA-R)	1
Parental questionnaire	1
The Centre for Epidemiological Studies-Depression Scales (CESD)	1
Beck Depression Inventory	1
State-Trait Anxiety Inventory Form Y (STAI-Y)	1

coherence) were mixed in studies of the BAP. Conflicting results in the disembedding performance were noted (EFT, 4/8 studies; Titchener Circles Illusion, 1 study) as well as mental segmentation abilities (Unsegmented Block Design task, 1/2 studies; Segmented Block Design task, 1/2 studies; Block Design Reconstruction task, 1 study with no significance found). Two studies, however, indicate higher frequency of errors and response times in index parents during a global

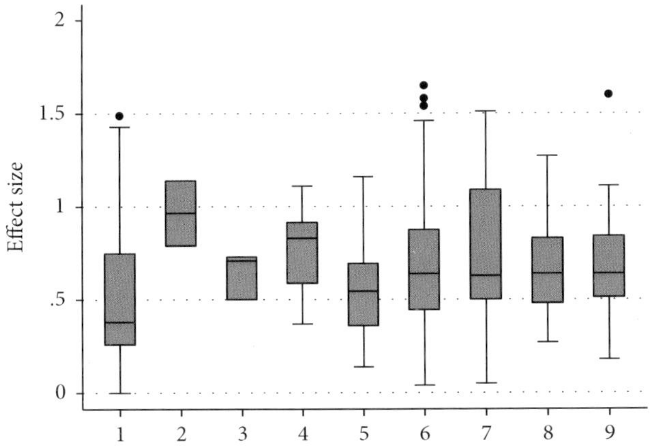

FIGURE 2: Boxplot reflecting effect size ranges for the sociobehavioral and cognitive domains. 1 = BAP expression. 2 = other measures of personality and friendships. 3 = social and narrative language. 4 = repetitive, restrictive behaviors, and interests. 5 = general intellectual functioning. 6 = structural language abilities. 7 = social cognition. 8 = executive function. 9 = local visual processing (central coherence).

sentence completion task (sentence completion task, 2/2 studies). Nonetheless, this area of cognition in the BAP also warrants further research.

Lastly, a number of studies have documented higher rates of depression (in 5/7 measures), anxiety (in 2/6 measures), and social phobia/social phobic anxiety (in 4/6 measures) in parents of children with autism compared to normative samples (e.g., [57]) and a clinical sample (e.g., [51]). We also note depression and anxiety to be more prevalent (2/6 studies) in mothers of children with autism. Ingersoll et al. (2011) [25] reported increased depressed mood in index mothers when compared to mothers of typically developing children, with similar findings from Micali et al. (2004) [70]. Although one can assume that having a child with a disability can affect mood and anxiety levels, many studies indicate an onset of these conditions before the birth of the child with autism, suggesting that the stress of caring for a child with a disability did not cause the symptoms. Findings from our review revealed moderate to high magnitude of effect; thus, depression and anxiety may have a genetic link with autism, supporting findings from a previous meta-analysis of psychiatric disorders in parents of children with autism [71].

Figure 2 displays the boxplots reflecting effect size ranges for the sociobehavioral and cognitive domains and subdomains. It was not possible to include effect size ranges for the domain of other psychiatric conditions as depression and anxiety could not be divided into separate subdomains due to the measures used in the studies. The reciprocal social interaction subdomain was omitted as there was only one effect size available for one significant finding. Similarly, the visual processing subdomain was also omitted as findings were not significant.

4.2. Emerging Themes. A number of studies reviewed suggest that subclinical autistic traits aggregate in MPX families and occur less frequently in SPX families [28, 34]. For instance decreased number and intensity of BAP traits observed in parents of SPX in comparison to MPX provide behavioral evidence consistent with findings of increased de novo, noninherited genetic events in SPX families (e.g., [72]). Losh et al. (2008) [34] suggest that the BAP gradation expression across family types is consistent with increasing genetic liability to autism.

A male bias is a well-documented feature in autism [73]. Findings from our review also indicate few sex differences, indicating this male bias [37–39]. However, despite this and the clear sex bias in autism, many studies do not suggest sex differences for most BAP features (e.g., [74]).

Furthermore, our findings indicate that the majority of the studies reviewed were conducted in Western countries. There were too few studies from non-Western countries to make any meaningful comparisons. Further cross-cultural research is required to understand the endophenotypes of autism within different cultural and geographical settings in order to tackle this geographical distribution bias.

4.3. Measure Quality. It is clear from this review that a large number of measures have been utilized to assess the BAP in relation to different domains and the constructs analyzed are heterogeneous. However it should be noted that the current review does not assess in depth whether the BAP measures are valid or reliable in measuring BAP. Domain wise, in many cases the same measures have been used by other studies. We discuss whether results for each measure in the same domain show the same magnitude and are in the same direction.

For instance, Davidson et al. (2014) [75] reported that frequency of BAP traits varies significantly depending upon the measure utilized, highlighting the need for a different approach that utilizes multiple informants and relies on the assessment of distinct BAP traits.

4.4. Methodological Limitations of Studies. Any discordant findings in the studies reviewed may be partly explained by methodological differences between studies. Sample size and choice of comparison group play an important role in the outcome of results. Six studies enrolled 30 or less index parents. Thus, relatively small sample sizes may lead to false negative results and/or limit the power to detect the BAP in the three domains.

Studies vary in their choice of a comparison group with some relying on the convenience of clinic-based samples where selection biases may lead to distorted results and others emphasizing the use of population based samples. For example, parents of children with Down Syndrome were frequently used, but these parents are likely to be older and possibly of different socioeconomic status. Few studies matched index parents to control groups on intellectual functioning, age, and socioeconomic basis, thus making it difficult to assimilate if differences on specific cognitive tasks represent a specific impairment in functioning or are attributable to differences in demographic data.

4.5. Limitations and Future Directions. In addition to the limitation outlined above, there are other limitations. Given that nine additional studies were found through a manual search after the initial search, it is possible that other studies were not ascertained by our search terms. To address this limitation, future research may also consider additional search terms beyond those used here.

This review aimed to identify endophenotypes in behavioral, cognitive, and psychiatric domains independently, and as such we did not assess associations between the BAP features across different domains. Losh et al. (2009) [56] suggest that it is likely that specific BAP traits cosegregate with performance in other domains. For instance, parents displaying rigid/perfectionistic personality traits could perform differently on tasks requiring cognitive flexibility. Additionally, most studies meeting our search criteria assessed only one or two domains, rendering it difficult to establish whether an endophenotypic overlap, if any, exists.

Future reviews should also include studies that examine neuroanatomical and neurofunctional correlates of the BAP. These are essential in furthering our understanding of the neural correlates of the behavioral, cognitive, and psychiatric aspects of autism.

More sophisticated research of the endophenotypes of parents of children with autism may help develop better measures of evaluation of the BAP. Future studies should use a more comprehensive and quantitative framework using more robust measures to detect subtle subclinical autistic traits in the BAP in cross-cultural settings. To the best of our knowledge, no study assessing the endophenotypic profile of autism in Africa has been published yet. Such research by our team is underway.

4.6. Conclusions. In summary, the current review increases our understanding of the BAP and extends the findings of previous reviews [13, 14]. It also supplements a systematic review [12] and a meta-analysis [71] with a broader scope. However, findings should be interpreted with caution because of the small number of studies in such heterogeneously broad domains and methodological limitations.

The assessment of the BAP profile in parents of autistic probands allows us to have a better insight into the varying underlying genetic mechanisms in autism. The behavioral, cognitive, and psychiatric endophenotypes in parents of autistic probands are still not clarified; however, evidence points towards mild social/communication deficits, rigid/aloof personality traits, and pragmatic language difficulties as the most useful social behavioral candidate endophenotype traits. The existence of some deficits in the cognitive domain does suggest familial vulnerability for autism; however, more research is required to elucidate these findings within this domain. Furthermore, increased depressed mood and anxiety can also be useful markers of vulnerability.

Acknowledgments

The authors would like to thank Catherine McGowan for help with database searches.

References

[1] American Psychiatric Association, *Diagnostic and Statistical Manual of Mental Disorders (DSM-5)*, American Psychiatric Publishing, Arlington, VA, USA, 5th edition, 2013.

[2] A. Bailey, A. Le Couteur, I. Gottesman et al. et al., "Autism as a strongly genetic disorder: Evidence from a British twin study," *Psychological Medicine*, vol. 25, pp. 63–77, 1995.

[3] J. Hallmayer, S. Cleveland, A. Torres et al., "Genetic heritability and shared environmental factors among twin pairs with autism," *Archives of General Psychiatry*, vol. 68, no. 11, pp. 1095–1102, 2011.

[4] S. Ozonoff, G. S. Young, A. Carter et al., "Recurrence risk for autism spectrum disorders: a baby siblings research consortium study," *Pediatrics*, vol. 128, pp. 488–495, 2011.

[5] J. N. Constantino, Y. Zhang, T. Frazier, A. M. Abbacchi, and P. Law, "Sibling recurrence and the genetic epidemiology of autism," *The American Journal of Psychiatry*, vol. 167, no. 11, pp. 1349–1356, 2010.

[6] J. Piven, P. Palmer, D. Jacobi, D. Childress, and S. Arndt, "Broader autism phenotype: evidence from a family history study of multiple-incidence autism families," *The American Journal of Psychiatry*, vol. 154, no. 2, pp. 185–190, 1997.

[7] S. Baron-Cohen and J. Hammer, "Parents of children with Asperger syndrome: what is the cognitive phenotype?" *Journal of Cognitive Neuroscience*, vol. 9, no. 4, pp. 548–554, 1997.

[8] V. Di Michele, M. Mazza, R. Cerbo, R. Roncone, and M. Casacchia, "Deficits in pragmatic conversation as manifestation of genetic liability in autism," *Clinical Neuropsychiatry*, vol. 4, pp. 144–151, 2007.

[9] P. Szatmari, S. Georgiades, E. Duku, L. Zwaigenbaum, J. Goldberg, and T. Bennett, "Alexithymia in parents of children with autism spectrum disorder," *Journal of Autism and Developmental Disorders*, vol. 38, pp. 1859–1865, 2008.

[10] G. L. Schmidt, L. K. Kimel, E. Winterrowd, B. F. Pennington, S. L. Hepburn, D. C. Rojas et al., "Impairments in phonological processing and nonverbal intellectual function in parents of children with autism," *Journal of Clinical and Experimental Neuropsychology*, vol. 30, no. 5, pp. 557–567, 2008.

[11] I. I. Gottesman and T. D. Gould, "The endophenotype concept in psychiatry: etymology and strategic intentions," *The American Journal of Psychiatry*, vol. 160, no. 4, pp. 636–645, 2003.

[12] L. D. L. P. Cruz, W. Camargos-Júnior, and F. L. Rocha, "The broad autism phenotype in parents of individuals with autism: A systematic review of the literature," *Trends in Psychiatry and Psychotherapy*, vol. 35, no. 4, pp. 252–263, 2013.

[13] J. Gerdts and R. Bernier, "The broader autism phenotype and its implications on the etiology and treatment of autism spectrum disorders," *Autism Research and Treatment*, Article ID 545901, 2011.

[14] E. Sucksmith, I. Roth, and R. A. Hoekstra, "Autistic traits below the clinical threshold: re-examining the broader autism phenotype in the 21st century," *Neuropsychology Review*, vol. 21, no. 4, pp. 360–389, 2011.

[15] K. S. Khan, G. Ter Riet, J. Glanville, A. J. Sowden, and J. Kleijnen, *Undertaking Systematic Reviews of Research on Effectiveness: CRD Guidelines for Those Carrying Out or Commissioning Reviews*, York Publishing Services, York, UK, 2nd edition, 2001.

[16] J. Cohen, *Statistical Power Analysis for the Behavioural Science*, Lawrence Erlbaum Associates, Hillsdale, NJ, USA, 2nd edition, 1988.

[17] L. Ruta, D. Mazzone, L. Mazzone, S. Wheelwright, and S. Baron-Cohen, "The Autism-Spectrum Quotient- Italian Version: A Cross-Cultural Confirmation of the Broader Autism Phenotype," *Journal of Autism and Developmental Disorders*, vol. 42, pp. 625–633, 2012.

[18] S. Kose, E. Bora, S. Erermiş, B. Özbaran, T. Bildik, and C. Aydin, "Broader autistic phenotype in parents of children with autism: Autism Spectrum Quotient-Turkish version," *Psychiatry and Clinical Neurosciences*, vol. 67, no. 1, pp. 20–27, 2013.

[19] L. Robel, B. Rousselot-Pailley, C. Fortin, M. Levy-Rueff, B. Golse, and B. Falissard, "Subthreshold traits of the broad autistic spectrum are distributed across different subgroups in parents, but not siblings, of probands with autism," *European Child and Adolescent Psychiatry*, vol. 23, no. 4, pp. 225–233, 2014.

[20] D. V. M. Bishop, M. Maybery, A. Maley, D. Wong, W. Hill, and J. Hallmayer, "Using self-report to identify the broad phenotype in parents of children with autistic spectrum disorders: a study using the autism-spectrum quotient," *Journal of Child Psychology and Psychiatry and Allied Disciplines*, vol. 45, no. 8, pp. 1431–1436, 2004.

[21] M. T. Kadak, Ö. F. Demirel, M. Yavuz, and T. Demir, "Recognition of emotional facial expressions and broad autism phenotype in parents of children diagnosed with autistic spectrum disorder," *Comprehensive Psychiatry*, vol. 55, no. 5, pp. 1146–1151, 2014.

[22] S. Wheelwright, B. Auyeung, C. Allison, and S. Baron-Cohen, "Defining the broader, medium and narrow autism phenotype among parents using the Autism Spectrum Quotient (AQ)," *Molecular Autism*, pp. 1–10, 2010.

[23] A. J. O. Whitehouse, J. G. Barry, and D. V. M. Bishop, "The broader Language Phenotype of Autism: a comparison with specific language impairment," *Journal of Child Psychology and Psychiatry*, vol. 48, no. 8, pp. 822–830, 2007.

[24] A. M. Scheeren and J. E. A. Stauder, "Broader Autism Phenotype in Parents of Autistic Children: Reality or Myth?" *Journal of Autism and Developmental Disorders*, vol. 28, pp. 276–287, 2008.

[25] B. Ingersoll, K. Meyer, and M. W. Becker, "Increased rates of depressed mood in mothers of children with ASD associated with the presence of the broader autism phenotype," *Autism Research*, vol. 4, no. 2, pp. 143–148, 2011.

[26] R. S. E. Hurley, M. Losh, M. Parlier, J. S. Reznick, and J. Piven, "The broad autism phenotype questionnaire," *Journal of Autism and Developmental Disorders*, vol. 37, pp. 1679–1690, 2007.

[27] N. J. Sasson, K. S. L. Lam, M. Parlier, J. L. Daniels, and J. Piven, "Autism and the broad autism phenotype: Familial patterns and intergenerational transmission," *Journal of Neurodevelopmental Disorders*, vol. 5, no. 1, pp. 1–7, 2013.

[28] R. Bernier, J. Gerdts, J. Munson, G. Dawson, and A. Estes, "Evidence for broader autism phenotype characteristics in parents from multiple-incidence autism families," *Autism Research*, vol. 5, no. 1, pp. 13–20, 2012.

[29] A. J. O. Whitehouse, H. Coon, J. Miller, B. Salisbury, and D. V. M. Bishop, "Narrowing the broader autism phenotype: a study using the Communication Checklist -Adult version (CC-A)," *Autism*, vol. 14, no. 6, pp. 559–574, 2010.

[30] S. E. Folstein, S. L. Santangelo, S. E. Gilman et al., "Predictors of cognitive test patterns in autism families," *Journal of Child Psychology and Psychiatry and Allied Disciplines*, vol. 40, no. 7, pp. 1117–1128, 1999.

[31] A. Pickles, M. C. St Clair, and G. Conti-Ramsden, "Communication and social deficits in relatives of individuals with sli and relatives of individuals with Asd," *Journal of Autism and Developmental Disorders*, vol. 43, no. 1, pp. 156–167, 2013.

[32] J. Piven, R. Landa, J. Lainhart, P. Bolton, and G. A. Chase, "Personality characteristics of the parents of autistic individuals," *Psychological Medicine*, vol. 24, no. 3, pp. 783–795, 1994.

[33] J. Piven, P. Palmer, R. Landa, S. Santangelo, D. Jacobi, and D. Childress, "Personality and language characteristics in parents from multiple-incidence autism families," *American Journal of Medical Genetics Part B (Neuropsychiatric Genetics)*, vol. 74, pp. 398–411, 1997.

[34] M. Losh, D. Childress, K. Lam, and J. Piven, "Defining key features of the broad autism phenotype: a comparison across parents of multiple- and single-incidence autism families," *American Journal of Medical Genetics Part B (Neuropsychiatric Genetics)*, vol. 147B, pp. 424–433, 2008.

[35] M. Losh, J. Klusek, G. E. Martin, J. Sideris, M. Parlier, and J. Piven, "Defining genetically meaningful language and personality traits in relatives of individuals with fragile X syndrome and relatives of individuals with autism," *American Journal of Medical Genetics, Part B: Neuropsychiatric Genetics*, vol. 159, no. 6, pp. 660–668, 2012.

[36] R. Landa, J. Piven, M. M. Wzorek, J. O. Gayles, G. A. Chase, and S. E. Folstein, "Social language use in parents of autistic individuals," *Psychological Medicine*, vol. 22, pp. 245–254, 1992.

[37] T. F. Ruser, D. Arin, M. Dowd et al., "Communicative competence in parents of children with autism and parents of children with specific language impairment," *Journal of Autism and Developmental Disorders*, vol. 37, no. 7, pp. 1323–1336, 2007.

[38] W. De la Marche, I. Noens, J. Luts, E. Scholte, S. Van Huffel, and J. Steyaert, "Quantitative autism traits in first degree relatives: evidence for the broader autism phenotype in fathers, but not in mothers and siblings," *Autism*, vol. 16, no. 3, pp. 247–260, 2012.

[39] A. J. Schwichtenberg, G. S. Young, M. Sigman, T. Hutman, and S. Ozonoff, "Can family affectedness inform infant sibling outcomes of autism spectrum disorders?" *Journal of Child Psychology and Psychiatry*, vol. 51, no. 9, pp. 1021–1030, 2010.

[40] S. Berthoz, C. Lalanne, L. Crane, and E. L. Hill, "Investigating emotional impairments in adults with autism spectrum disorders and the broader autism phenotype," *Psychiatry Research*, vol. 208, no. 3, pp. 257–264, 2013.

[41] R. Landa, S. E. Folstein, and C. Isaacs, "Spontaneous narrative-discourse performance of parents of autistic individuals," *Journal of Speech and Hearing Research*, vol. 34, pp. 1339–1345, 1991.

[42] J. Briskman, F. Happé, and U. Frith, "Exploring the cognitive phenotype of autism: Weak "central coherence" in parents and siblings of children with autism: II. Real-life skills and preferences," *Journal of Child Psychology and Psychiatry*, vol. 42, no. 3, pp. 309–316, 2001.

[43] M. D. Lezak, D. B. Howieson, E. D. Bigler, and D. Tranel, *Neuropsychological Assessment*, Oxford University Press, New York, 5th edition, 2012.

[44] E. Fombonne, P. Bolton, J. Prior, H. Jordan, and M. Rutter, "A family study of autism: cognitive patterns and levels in parents and siblings," *Journal of Child Psychology and Psychiatry*, vol. 38, no. 6, pp. 667–683, 1997.

[45] S. L. Smalley and R. F. Asarnow, "Cognitive subclinical markers in autism," *Journal of Autism and Developmental Disorders*, vol. 20, no. 2, pp. 271–278, 1990.

[46] J. Piven and P. Palmer, "Cognitive deficits in parents from multiple-incidence autism families," *Journal of Child Psychology and Psychiatry*, vol. 38, no. 8, pp. 1011–1021, 1997.

[47] K. A. Lindgren, S. E. Folstein, J. B. Tomblin, and H. Tager-Flusberg, "Language and reading abilities of children with autism spectrum disorders and specific language impairment and their first-degree relatives," *Autism Research*, vol. 2, pp. 22–38, 2009.

[48] M. Losh and J. Piven, "Social-cognition and the broad autism phenotype: identifying genetically meaningful phenotypes," *Journal of Child Psychology and Psychiatry*, vol. 48, no. 1, pp. 105–112, 2007.

[49] S. Bölte and F. Poustka, "The recognition of facial affect in autistic and schizophrenic subjects and their first-degree relatives," *Psychological Medicine*, vol. 33, pp. 907–915, 2003.

[50] S. Bölte and F. Poustka, "The broader cognitive phenotype of autism in parents: how specific is the tendency for local processing and executive dysfunction?" *Journal of Child Psychology and Psychiatry*, vol. 47, no. 6, pp. 639–645, 2006.

[51] S. Bölte, S. Knecht, and F. Poustka, "A case-control study of personality style and psychopathology in parents of subjects with autism," *Journal of Autism and Developmental Disorders*, vol. 37, pp. 243–250, 2007.

[52] E. Sucksmith, C. Allison, S. Baron-Cohen, B. Chakrabarti, and R. A. Hoekstra, "Empathy and emotion recognition in people with autism, first-degree relatives, and controls," *Neuropsychologia*, vol. 51, no. 1, pp. 98–105, 2013.

[53] D. V. M. Bishop, M. Maybery, D. Wong, A. Maley, W. Hill, and J. Hallmayer, "Are phonological processing deficits part of the broad autism phenotype?" *American Journal of Medical Genetics Part B (Neuropsychiatric Genetics)*, vol. 128, no. B, pp. 54–60, 2004.

[54] M.-H. Plumet, M.-C. Goldblum, and M. Leboyer, "Verbal skills in relatives of autistic females," *Cortex*, vol. 31, no. 4, pp. 723–733, 1995.

[55] M. Losh, D. Esserman, and J. Piven, "Rapid automatized naming as an index of genetic liability to autism," *Journal of Neurodevelopmental Disorders*, vol. 2, no. 2, pp. 109–116, 2010.

[56] M. Losh, R. Adolphs, M. D. Poe et al., "Neuropsychological profile of autism and the broad autism phenotype," *Archives of General Psychiatry*, vol. 66, no. 5, pp. 518–526, 2009.

[57] S. Gokcen, E. Bora, S. Erermis, H. Kesikci, and C. Aydin, "Theory of mind and verbal working memory deficits in parents of autistic children," *Psychiatry Research*, vol. 166, pp. 46–53, 2009.

[58] M. Tajmirriyahi, V. Nejati, H. Pouretemad, and R. M. Sepehr, "Reading the mind in the face and voice in parents of children with Autism Spectrum Disorders," *Research in Autism Spectrum Disorders*, vol. 7, no. 12, pp. 1543–1550, 2013.

[59] R. Adolphs, M. L. Spezio, M. Parlier, and J. Piven, "Distinct face-processing strategies in parents of autistic children," *Current Biology*, vol. 18, pp. 1090–1093, 2008.

[60] M. D. C. L. das Neves, F. Tremeau, R. Nicolato, H. Lauar, M. A. Romano-Silva, and H. Correa, "Facial emotion recognition deficits in relatives of children with autism are not associated with 5HTTLPR," *Revista Brasileira de Psiquiatria*, vol. 33, no. 3, pp. 261–267, 2011.

[61] M. T. Palermo, P. Pasqualetti, G. Barbati, F. Intelligente, and P. M. Rossini, "Recognition of schematic facial displays of emotion in parents of children with autism," *Autism*, vol. 10, no. 4, pp. 353–364, 2006.

[62] D. Wong, M. Maybery, D. V. M. Bishop, A. Maley, and J. Hallmayer, "Profiles of executive function in parents and siblings of individuals with autism spectrum disorders," *Genes, Brain and Behavior*, vol. 5, pp. 561–576, 2006.

[63] C. Hughes, M. Leboyer, and M. Bouvard, "Executive function in parents of children with autism," *Psychological Medicine*, vol. 27, pp. 209–220, 1997.

[64] F. Happé, J. Briskman, and U. Frith, "Exploring the cognitive phenotype of autism: weak "central coherence" in parents and siblings of children with autism: I. Experimental Tests," *Journal of Child Psychology and Psychiatry*, vol. 42, pp. 299–307, 2001.

[65] M. V. De Jonge, C. Kemner, and H. Van Engeland, "Superior disembedding performance of high-functioning individuals with autism spectrum disorders and their parents: The need for subtle measures," *Journal of Autism and Developmental Disorders*, vol. 36, no. 5, pp. 677–683, 2006.

[66] M. De Jonge, C. Kemner, F. Naber, and H. Van Engeland, "Block design reconstruction skills: Not a good candidate for an endophenotypic marker in autism research," *European Child and Adolescent Psychiatry*, vol. 18, no. 4, pp. 197–205, 2009.

[67] M. V. de Jonge, C. Kemner, E. H. de Haan, J. E. Coppens, T. J. van den Berg, H. van Engeland et al., "Visual information processing in high-functioning individuals with autism spectrum disorders and their parents," *Neuropsychology*, vol. 21, pp. 65–73, 2007.

[68] J. Piven, G. A. Chase, R. Landa, M. Wzorek, J. Gayle, D. Cloud et al., "Psychiatric disorders in the parents of autistic individuals," *Journal of the American Academy of Child and Adolescent Psychiatry*, vol. 30, no. 3, pp. 471–478, 1991.

[69] J. Piven and P. Palmer, "Psychiatric disorder and the broad autism phenotype: evidence from a family study of multiple-incidence autism families," *American Journal of Psychiatry*, vol. 156, no. 4, pp. 557–563, 1999.

[70] N. Micali, S. Chakrabarti, and E. Fombonne, "The broad autism phenotype: findings from an epidemiological survey," *Autism*, vol. 8, no. 1, pp. 21–37, 2004.

[71] N. Yirmiya and M. Shaked, "Psychiatric disorders in parents of children with autism: A meta-analysis," *Journal of Child Psychology and Psychiatry and Allied Disciplines*, vol. 46, no. 1, pp. 69–83, 2005.

[72] J. Sebat, B. Lakshmi, D. Malhotra et al., "Strong association of de novo copy number mutations with autism," *Science*, vol. 316, no. 5823, pp. 445–449, 2007.

[73] Werling & Geschwind, "Sex differences in autism spectrum disorders," *Current Opinion in Neurology*, vol. 26, no. 2, pp. 146–153, 2013.

[74] J. Klusek, M. Losh, and G. E. Martin, "Sex differences and within-family associations in the broad autism phenotype," *Autism*, vol. 18, no. 2, pp. 106–116, 2014.

[75] J. Davidson, R. P. Goin-Kochel, L. A. Green-Snyder, R. J. Hundley, Z. Warren, and S. U. Peters, "Expression of the broad autism phenotype in simplex autism families from the simons simplex collection," *Journal of Autism and Developmental Disorders*, vol. 44, no. 10, pp. 2392–2399, 2014.

23

Calcium and Vitamin D Supplement Prescribing Practices among Providers Caring for Children with Autism Spectrum Disorders: Are We Addressing Bone Health?

Shylaja Srinivasan,[1] Julia O'Rourke,[2] Sara Bersche Golas,[2,3] Ann Neumeyer,[2,3] and Madhusmita Misra[1]

[1] *Pediatric Endocrinology, Massachusetts General Hospital and Harvard Medical School, Boston, MA, USA*
[2] *Lurie Center for Autism, Massachusetts General Hospital for Children, Boston, MA, USA*
[3] *Pediatric Neurology, Massachusetts General Hospital and Harvard Medical School, Boston, MA, USA*

Correspondence should be addressed to Shylaja Srinivasan; ssrinivasan5@mgh.harvard.edu and Madhusmita Misra; mmisra@mgh.harvard.edu

Academic Editor: Roberto Canitano

Children with autism spectrum disorders (ASD) have several risk factors for low bone mineral density. The gluten-free, casein-free (GFCF) diet is a complementary therapy sometimes used in ASD that raises concerns for the adequacy of calcium and vitamin D intake. This study evaluated the prescribing practices of calcium and vitamin D supplements and the practice of checking 25-hydroxy vitamin D (25(OH)D) levels by providers in 100 children with ASD, 50 of whom were on the GFCF diet. Fifty-two percent and 46% of children on the GFCF diet were on some form of vitamin D and calcium supplements, respectively, compared to 18% and 14% of those not on this diet. Twenty-four percent of children in the GFCF group had a documented 25(OH)D level compared to none in the non-GFCF group. The data highlight a gap in calcium and vitamin D supplement prescribing practices among providers caring for children with ASD as well as a gap in the practice of checking 25(OH)D levels.

1. Introduction

Autism spectrum disorder (ASD) is a developmental disorder with various degrees of severity that can cause significant social, communication, and behavioral challenges. Data from the Center for Disease Control's Autism and Developmental Disabilities Monitoring (ADDM) Network show that the estimated number of children identified with ASD continues to rise in the United States with 1 in 68 children estimated to have an ASD in 2014 [1]. Peak bone mass, an important determinant of future bone health, is achieved by early adulthood, and the childhood and adolescent years are a critical period for bone accrual. Factors that affect bone accrual in childhood include genetics, nutritional status, calcium and vitamin D intake, weight bearing activity, hormonal alterations, and the use of certain medications [2]. Children with ASD have several risk factors that could potentially contribute to low bone mineral density (BMD), including decreased exercise, restricted diets, and use of medications that are deleterious to bone health. Nutritional status is a potentially modifiable factor and is very relevant to bone accrual in children. In the absence of curative options for the management of ASD, many parents turn towards alternative therapies and the gluten-free, casein-free (GFCF) diet is one such dietary therapy. A systematic review of studies published from 1970 to 2014 related to the GFCF diet in ASD patients showed that the evidence on this topic is currently limited and weak [3]. However, this diet continues to be used by children with ASD, largely based on anecdotal evidence for improvement.

In the US, most of one's dietary intake of calcium comes from dairy products while the dietary intake of vitamin D is derived from fortified foods such as milk and milk products with vitamin D [4]. In addition, children derive vitamin D through sun exposure. A diet limited in dairy products such as the GFCF diet raises concerns for the adequacy of calcium and vitamin D intake in the absence of supplementation. Additionally, outdoor physical activity and sun exposure may be limited in children with ASD compared to their typical peers limiting their endogenous vitamin D production, which is already limited in the northern latitudes. A low serum phosphorus level could be one of the initial signs of mild vitamin D deficiency that occurs even before serum calcium level falls [5].

Other risk factors for low BMD in children with ASD include reduced weight bearing activity and high rates of comorbid neurologic and psychiatric illnesses, including epilepsy and mood disorders. The latter may contribute to low BMD by increasing cortisol levels [6, 7]. Medications used to treat these conditions, including antiepileptics, antidepressants, and antipsychotic medications, also have influences on bone indices and vitamin D metabolism [7–12]. Finally, children with ASD are often on proton pump inhibitors, which may influence bone health by impairing insoluble calcium absorption.

We have previously examined the relationship between ASD and BMD in peripubertal boys [13]. In this study, boys with ASD had lower BMD at the hip, femoral neck, and lumbar spine compared to typically developing controls. BMD was even lower in boys with ASD on a GFCF diet. In a subsequent study that examined the prevalence of fractures in children and adults with and without ASD using a national database of emergency room visits, we found a higher odds ratio for hip fractures in children and young adults (3–22 years) as well as older adults (23–50 years) with ASD than those without ASD and a higher odds ratio for forearm and spine fractures in women aged 23–50 years with ASD [14].

With the knowledge that children with ASD have multiple risk factors for low BMD and with increasing evidence to show that individuals with ASD may have low BMD and increased risk of fractures, there is a compelling need to determine how physicians are addressing the issue of bone health in these children. Little is known about the prescribing practice of vitamin D and calcium supplements in this population or the practice of checking vitamin D levels in this group, particularly in children on the GFCF diet, who may be at higher risk. The primary objective of our study was to review the calcium and vitamin D supplement prescribing practices of physicians caring for children with ASD on a GFCF diet. Our secondary objectives were to review the practice of checking 25(OH)D and phosphorus levels in this group and to describe the use of medications in these children that may affect bone health.

2. Methods

2.1. Study Design and Subject Selection. This was a retrospective study of patients who presented to the Lurie Center for Autism at the Massachusetts General Hospital for routine clinic visits. The Lurie Center is a multidisciplinary clinical and research center dedicated to the care of individuals with autism spectrum disorders and other developmental disorders. The Lurie Center Data Repository (LCDR) obtains patient data via batched data transfer from the Partners Research Patient Data Registry (RPDR) into a secure, relational database, which is organized and queried using the Structured Query Language (SQL) Server Management Studio. Data available from the RPDR include patient demographics, encounter billing data, diagnosis billing data, outpatient clinical notes, and prescribed medications.

The patient population was identified by searching the database for individuals who had encounters at MGH with a billed diagnosis of ASD ("299" ICD-9 codes) when they were between 3 and 25 years of age and had been seen at the Lurie Center between 2004 and 2014, with a total of 2814 subjects identified. All subjects met Diagnostic and Statistical Manual of Mental Disorders (either IV or V) criteria for diagnosis of an ASD. Clinical notes in the longitudinal medical record for these patients were then reviewed for language referring to the patient being on a gluten and/or casein-free diet (e.g., "gluten-free," "casein-free," "dairy-free," and "gluten and casein"). To do this, an SQL code was written that would extract portions of note text surrounding occurrences of the word "diet" which also contained the GFCF terms, excluding notes with terms such as "not on a gluten-free" or "not on a strict casein or gluten-free" diet. These clinical note extracts were then reviewed by study staff to determine which patients were on a dedicated GFCF diet. Using this strategy, a total of 837 subjects were identified to be on a GFCF diet. We excluded subjects who had a condition known to influence bone health such as celiac disease, inflammatory bowel disease, or renal disease. We then randomly selected 100 subjects for our study of whom 50 were on the GFCF diet and 50 were not. According to the Endocrine Society's Clinical Practice guidelines, we defined vitamin D deficiency as a 25(OH)D level below 20 ng/mL and vitamin D insufficiency as a 25(OH)D level of 21–29 ng/mL [15].

This protocol was approved by the Partners Health Care Institutional Review Board, and procedures used for data collection were in compliance with the Health Insurance Portability and Accountability Act (HIPAA). Due to the retrospective nature of the study, and in accordance with the guidelines of our Institutional Review Board, informed consent and assent were not obtained.

2.2. Data Collection. We collected the following demographic data: age, sex, race, and self-reported ethnicity. The clinical data that were collected included information regarding vitamin D and calcium supplementation, 25(OH)D and phosphorus levels, and use of antiepileptic, antipsychotic, and antidepressant medications and proton pump inhibitors. Information regarding Tanner stage of subjects was not available because the clinical information was collected at specialized neurodevelopmental visits. Similarly, subjects did not have parathyroid hormone (PTH) levels measured.

To determine vitamin D and calcium supplementation status, medication data was queried in the LCDR to find who in the study population had been prescribed vitamin D or calcium by their provider. Additionally, active and inactive medication lists were reviewed in the electronic medical record. Clinical notes were also queried using the same text extraction method described above for notes containing references to patients supplementing their diet with vitamin

D or calcium, with or without a prescription from their provider. These note extracts were then reviewed by study staff to confirm that subjects were on supplements. For the purpose of our study, we counted the use of multivitamins towards supplementation of both vitamin D and calcium. When we surveyed some of the commonly used brands of children's multivitamins, we found that in general most brands tend to have around 600 IU of vitamin D and around 100 mg of elemental calcium. To determine vitamin D and phosphorus levels, the laboratory results section of the subject's electronic medical record was reviewed. Also, clinical note text extraction was performed for notes containing references to 25(OH)D and phosphorus level laboratory results with subsequent confirmation done by study staff. The same methods were used to determine the use of antiepileptic, antipsychotic, and antidepressant medications, or proton pump inhibitors in the study population.

2.3. Data Analysis. Data analysis was performed using JMP® statistical software version 11 (SAS Institute, Cary, NC). Analyses were performed using Student's t-test for continuous variables and Pearson's χ^2 test for categorical variables. A p value of less than 0.05 was considered to be significant.

3. Results

The clinical characteristics of children with ASD on a GFCF diet versus those not on a GFCF diet are summarized in Table 1. The groups did not differ for demographic characteristics, including age, sex, and self-reported ethnicity.

3.1. Vitamin D and Calcium Supplementation. Fifty-two percent of the children on the GFCF diet were taking vitamin D supplementation in comparison to 18% of those in the non-GFCF group. Forty-six percent of subjects who were on the GFCF diet were taking or prescribed calcium supplementation in comparison with 14% in the non-GFCF group (Figure 1). Compared to children on a non-GFCF diet, children on the GFCF diet were more likely to be taking vitamin D [OR 4.94, 95% CI (1.99–12.26), and $p = 0.0006$] and calcium supplements [OR 5.23, 95% CI (2.63–10.41), and $p < 0.0001$].

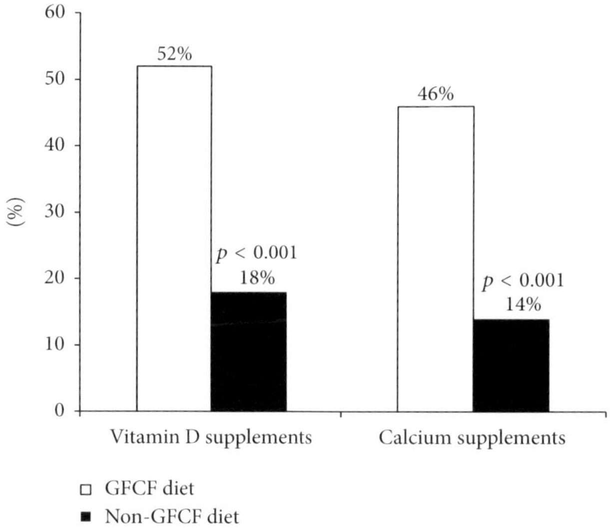

FIGURE 1: Percentage of children on the GFCF diet versus the non-GFCF diet taking vitamin D and calcium supplements.

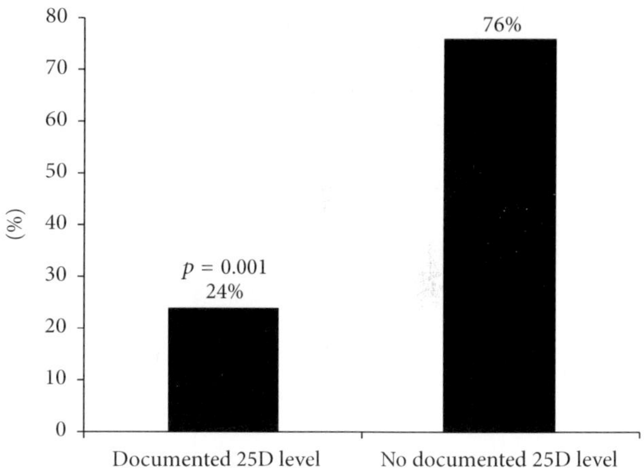

FIGURE 2: Percentage of subjects on the GFCF diet who had a documented 25(OH)D level.

3.2. 25(OH) Vitamin D Levels and Phosphorus Levels. Twenty-four percent of children in the GFCF group had a documented 25(OH)D level compared to none in the non-GFCF group (Figure 2). The mean 25(OH)D level in children on the GFCF diet was 41.4 ng/mL (SD 11.4). Of subjects on the GFCF diet who had a 25(OH)D level checked, 92% had a level greater than 30 ng/mL, the lower limit for sufficiency as suggested by the Endocrine Society's Clinical Practice guidelines. Of the 24% of subjects on the GFCF diet with a documented 25(OH)D level, 83% were taking a vitamin D supplement (Figure 3). We further looked at the season in which the 25(OH)D levels were measured and it is worthy to note that the only two insufficient values were measured in the winter months. We were unable to make a statistical inference regarding seasonality because of our limited sample size. The mean vitamin D level was higher in the GFCF group that received supplementation (mean 42.8 ng/dL, SD 11.72) than in the group that did not (mean 32.5 ng/dL, SD 3.54). Sixteen percent of children on the GFCF diet had a documented phosphorus level in comparison to 2% on the non-GFCF diet. The mean phosphorus level when checked was 5.4 mg/dL (SD 1.0) in the GFCF group and 3.05 mg/dL (SD 0.5) in the non-GFCF group.

3.3. Medication Use. The use of antiepileptic, antipsychotic, and antidepressant medication was similar between the two groups. Some of the more commonly prescribed antiepileptic medications were topiramate, valproic acid, lamotrigine, and levetiracetam. The most commonly prescribed antipsychotic medications included risperidone, quetiapine, and aripiprazole. Fluoxetine, sertraline, and citalopram were the most commonly prescribed antidepressant medications. Children in the GFCF group were more likely to be on a proton pump inhibitor ($p = 0.02$).

TABLE 1: Clinical characteristics of children on the GFCF diet versus those not on a GFCF diet.

	Gluten-free, casein-free (GFCF) diet	Non-GFCF diet	*p* value
Mean age in years (SD)	9.62 (4.66)	11.7 (4.66)	0.069
Sex (% male)	74	78	0.644
Self-reported ethnicity (%)	Non-Hispanic White: 66 Hispanic: 2 African American: 4 Asian: 16 Other: 12	Non-Hispanic White: 62 Hispanic: 10 African American: 4 Asian: 4 Other: 20	0.378
% on vitamin D supplements	52	18	*<0.001*
% on calcium supplements	46	14	*<0.001*
% with documented 25(OH)D level	24	0	*0.001*
Mean 25(OH)D level in ng/mL (SD)	41.4 (11.4)	N/A	N/A
% with documented phosphorus level	16	2	*0.013*
Mean phosphorus level in mg/dL (SD)	5.4 (1.0)	3.05 (0.5)	0.062
% on antiepileptic drugs	14	22	0.303
% on antipsychotics	14	28	0.087
% on antidepressants	18	32	0.108
% on proton pump inhibitors	30	8	*0.002*

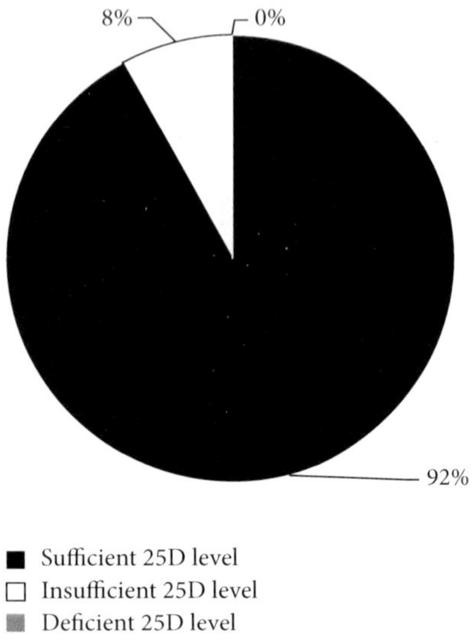

FIGURE 3: Proportion of subjects on the GFCF diet with documented 25(OH)D levels, with sufficient levels. In accordance with the Endocrine Society Practice guidelines [15], a sufficient level was considered to be ≥30 ng/mL, an insufficient level was considered to be between 21 and 29 ng/mL, and a deficient level was considered to be ≤20 ng/dL.

4. Discussion

Our results suggest that, in both groups, a large proportion of subjects were not supplemented with calcium or vitamin D. Children who were on the GFCF diet were more likely to be supplemented with calcium and vitamin D than those not on the diet. However, even in the GFCF group, approximately 50% of the subjects did not receive supplementation with either nutrient. As stated earlier, for the purpose of this study, we counted the use of multivitamins towards both vitamin D and calcium supplementation as most children's multivitamins contain vitamin D and many contain calcium. Therefore, our results may even be an overestimate of the actual proportion of children with ASD receiving supplements.

Our results also indicate that only a small proportion of children on the GFCF diet and none on the non-GFCF diet had vitamin D levels checked, even when on multiple medications that could potentially affect vitamin D metabolism and bone health. Of note, a large proportion of the vitamin D levels that were checked were above 30 ng/mL, the recommended lower limit for sufficient levels according to the Clinical Practice guidelines of the Endocrine Society [15]. This suggests that those providers who were checking levels were also supplementing their patients with vitamin D, leading to sufficient levels in these children. Of note, serum phosphate levels may decrease slightly following an oral glucose load [16], a phenomenon that is thought to be mediated through insulin. However, we do not believe that this would significantly confound the serum phosphate results and clinically do not require patients to be fasting when measuring serum phosphorus levels.

Regarding medication usage, both groups of subjects were on multiple medications that could potentially affect bone health. Antiepileptic drugs such as phenytoin, primidone, carbamazepine, oxcarbazepine, ethosuximide, and phenobarbital induce the cytochrome p450 enzyme system. This induction leads to increased catabolism of vitamin D to inactive metabolites and a subsequent rise in parathyroid hormone (PTH) levels. The rise in PTH increases mobilization of calcium from bone and thereby modifies bone turnover [8]. In contrast, sodium valproate inhibits the cytochrome p450 system, and its use is also associated with abnormal biochemical indices of bone and mineral metabolism, bone loss, and higher fracture rates in adults and children [7, 9]. Few studies have examined the newer antiepileptic medications in relation to vitamin D and bone metabolism and fracture risk. The use of lamotrigine, increasingly common in children, is associated with lower BMD and higher markers of bone turnover compared to children not receiving antiepileptic medications [10]. Furthermore, atypical antipsychotics may impact bone by increasing prolactin secretion and causing hypogonadism [11]. Both tricyclic antidepressants and selective serotonin reuptake inhibitors are associated with an increased risk of fragility fractures in observational studies in adults [12]. Whether the effects of these medications on fractures are from direct effects of these drugs on bone or from indirect effects related to sedation and falls needs further investigation. A longitudinal study of 96 boys between the ages of 7 and 17 years showed that chronic SSRI treatment in children was associated with reduced but stable bone mass for age, while chronic risperidone treatment was associated with failure to accrue bone mass [17]. Drugs such as proton pump inhibitors (PPIs) that reduce gastric acid secretion may decrease calcium absorption because insoluble calcium such as in calcium carbonate requires an acidic environment for absorption. Whether PPI use is associated with increased fracture risk is yet to be definitively established.

To our knowledge, this is one of the first studies evaluating the prescribing practices of calcium and vitamin D by providers caring for children with ASD and the practice of checking vitamin D levels in these children. Stewart et al. in 2015 reported the results of a cross-sectional study in 288 children with ASD that examined dietary supplement use and micronutrient intake. A GFCF diet was consumed by 12% of participants. Their results showed that even after supplementation, about 50% of children with ASD had inadequate intake of calcium, and about 30% had inadequate intake of vitamin D. Similar to our results, their study showed that children on the GFCF diet were more likely to be on supplements [18].

One of the strengths of our study is that it was conducted in a specialized tertiary care outpatient center with access to a large number of patients with ASD on the GFCF diet. The use of the electronic medical record and SQL code to extract text for keywords ensured that a thorough chart review was completed. This study also has limitations that are inherent to a retrospective chart review. One such limitation is that we were unable to quantify the duration of exposure of subjects to the GFCF diet. However, because we looked at whether subjects were ever on vitamin D and calcium supplementation at our center, we likely also covered the period that they were on the GFCF diet. Another limitation is that parents may not have reported medication use, especially over the counter vitamins and supplements, and providers may not have accurately documented medications especially when considering drugs such as multivitamins or supplements.

5. Conclusions

This study highlights a significant gap in the practice of prescribing vitamin D and calcium supplements in children with ASD and the practice of checking vitamin D and phosphorus levels in this group. Children with ASD have several risk factors that may affect BMD that providers caring for these children need to be aware of. Given that the childhood years are critical for bone accrual, we believe that children with ASD should be screened for vitamin D status with 25(OH)D levels and serum phosphorus levels and assessed for vitamin D and calcium intake. Supplementation should be implemented based on clinical judgment after evaluation of risk factors. This is particularly necessary in children on restrictive diets such as the GFCF diet and those on medications that can have adverse effects on bone. Prospective studies are needed to examine the effects of the GFCF diet on bone health and incidence of fractures in individuals with ASD and the impact of supplementation on these endpoints.

Abbreviations

ASD: Autism spectrum disorders
GFCF: Gluten-free, casein-free
BMD: Bone mineral density
AED: Antiepileptic medication
AP: Antipsychotic medication
AD: Antidepressant medication
PPI: Proton pump inhibitor
SQL: Structured Query Language
HIPAA: Health Insurance Portability and Accountability Act
LCDR: Lurie Center Data Repository
RPDR: Research Patient Data Registry
PTH: Parathyroid hormone.

Acknowledgments

The results of this study were presented as a poster presentation at the Pediatric Academic Societies and Pediatric Endocrine Society meeting in San Diego, California, on April 26th, 2015. This work was partly supported by NIH Grant K24 HD071843. Shylaja Srinivasan contributed to the concept of the study, data analysis and interpretation, and the writing of the paper. Julia O'Rourke contributed to data extraction and analysis and provided input regarding the final version of the paper. Sara Bersche Golas contributed to data interpretation and provided input regarding the final version of the paper. Ann Neumeyer contributed to study concept and data interpretation and provided input regarding the final version of the paper. Madhusmita Misra contributed to the concept of the study and data interpretation and provided input regarding the final version of the paper. All authors approved the final version of the paper.

References

[1] Centers for Disease Control and Prevention, "Prevalence of autism spectrum disorder among children aged 8 years—autism and developmental disabilities monitoring network, 11 sites, United States, 2010," *Morbidity and Mortality Weekly Report Surveillance summaries*, vol. 63, no. 2, pp. 1–21, 2014.

[2] J. H. Davies, B. A. J. Evans, and J. W. Gregory, "Bone mass acquisition in healthy children," *Archives of Disease in Childhood*, vol. 90, no. 4, pp. 373–378, 2005.

[3] S. Marí-Bauset, I. Zazpe, A. Mari-Sanchis, A. Llopis-González, and M. Morales-Suárez-Varela, "Food selectivity in autism spectrum disorders: a systematic review," *Journal of Child Neurology*, vol. 29, no. 11, pp. 1554–1561, 2014.

[4] M. Misra, D. Pacaud, A. Petryk, P. F. Collett-Solberg, and M. Kappy, "Vitamin D deficiency in children and its management: review of current knowledge and recommendations," *Pediatrics*, vol. 122, no. 2, pp. 398–417, 2008.

[5] M. A. Levine, C. Zapalowski, and M. S. Kappy, "Disorders of calcium, phosphate, parathyroid hormone, and vitamin D," in *Principles and Practice of Pediatric Endocrinology*, M. S. Kappy, D. B. Allen, and M. E. Geffner, Eds., Charles C Thomas, Springfield, Ill, USA, 2005.

[6] N. L. Lopez-Duran, M. Kovacs, and C. J. George, "Hypothalamic-pituitary-adrenal axis dysregulation in depressed children and adolescents: a meta-analysis," *Psychoneuroendocrinology*, vol. 34, no. 9, pp. 1272–1283, 2009.

[7] R. D. Sheth, C. A. Wesolowski, J. C. Jacob et al., "Effect of carbamazepine and valproate on bone mineral density," *The Journal of Pediatrics*, vol. 127, no. 2, pp. 256–262, 1995.

[8] A. M. Pack, M. J. Morrell, R. Marcus et al., "Bone mass and turnover in women with epilepsy on antiepileptic drug monotherapy," *Annals of Neurology*, vol. 57, no. 2, pp. 252–257, 2005.

[9] Y. Sato, I. Kondo, S. Ishida et al., "Decreased bone mass and increased bone turnover with valproate therapy in adults with epilepsy," *Neurology*, vol. 57, no. 3, pp. 445–449, 2001.

[10] C.-Y. Guo, G. M. Ronen, and S. A. Atkinson, "Long-term valproate and lamotrigine treatment may be a marker for reduced growth and bone mass in children with epilepsy," *Epilepsia*, vol. 42, no. 9, pp. 1141–1147, 2001.

[11] J. R. Bostwick, S. K. Guthrie, and V. L. Ellingrod, "Antipsychotic-induced hyperprolactinemia," *Pharmacotherapy*, vol. 29, no. 1, pp. 64–73, 2009.

[12] B. Liu, G. Anderson, N. Mittmann, T. To, T. Axcell, and N. Shear, "Use of selective serotonin-reuptake inhibitors or tricyclic antidepressants and risk of hip fractures in elderly people," *The Lancet*, vol. 351, no. 9112, pp. 1303–1307, 1998.

[13] A. M. Neumeyer, A. Gates, C. Ferrone, H. Lee, and M. Misra, "Bone density in peripubertal boys with autism spectrum disorders," *Journal of Autism and Developmental Disorders*, vol. 43, no. 7, pp. 1623–1629, 2013.

[14] A. M. Neumeyer, J. A. O'Rourke, A. Massa et al., "Brief report: bone fractures in children and adults with autism spectrum disorders," *Journal of Autism and Developmental Disorders*, vol. 45, no. 3, pp. 881–887, 2015.

[15] M. F. Holick, N. C. Binkley, H. A. Bischoff-Ferrari et al., "Evaluation, treatment, and prevention of vitamin D deficiency: an endocrine society clinical practice guideline," *The Journal of Clinical Endocrinology and Metabolism*, vol. 96, no. 7, pp. 1911–1930, 2011.

[16] M. Haap, E. Heller, C. Thamer, O. Tschritter, N. Stefan, and A. Fritsche, "Association of serum phosphate levels with glucose tolerance, insulin sensitivity and insulin secretion in non-diabetic subjects," *European Journal of Clinical Nutrition*, vol. 60, no. 6, pp. 734–739, 2006.

[17] C. A. Calarge, T. L. Burns, J. A. Schlechte, and B. S. Zemel, "Longitudinal examination of the skeletal effects of selective serotonin reuptake inhibitors and risperidone in boys," *The Journal of Clinical Psychiatry*, vol. 76, no. 5, pp. 607–613, 2015.

[18] P. A. Stewart, S. L. Hyman, B. L. Schmidt et al., "Dietary supplementation in children with autism spectrum disorders: common, insufficient, and excessive," *Journal of the Academy of Nutrition and Dietetics*, vol. 115, no. 8, pp. 1237–1248, 2015.

24

Potential Role of Selenoenzymes and Antioxidant Metabolism in relation to Autism Etiology and Pathology

Laura J. Raymond,[1] Richard C. Deth,[2] and Nicholas V. C. Ralston[1]

[1] *Energy & Environmental Research Center, University of North Dakota, 15 North 23rd Street, Stop 9018, Grand Forks, ND 58202, USA*
[2] *Department of Pharmaceutical Sciences, Northeastern University, Boston, MA 02115, USA*

Correspondence should be addressed to Laura J. Raymond; lraymond@undeerc.org

Academic Editor: Klaus-Peter Ossenkopp

Autism and autism spectrum disorders (ASDs) are behaviorally defined, but the biochemical pathogenesis of the underlying disease process remains uncharacterized. Studies indicate that antioxidant status is diminished in autistic subjects, suggesting its pathology is associated with augmented production of oxidative species and/or compromised antioxidant metabolism. This suggests ASD may result from defects in the metabolism of cellular antioxidants which maintain intracellular redox status by quenching reactive oxygen species (ROS). Selenium-dependent enzymes (selenoenzymes) are important in maintaining intercellular reducing conditions, particularly in the brain. Selenoenzymes are a family of ~25 genetically unique proteins, several of which have roles in preventing and reversing oxidative damage in brain and endocrine tissues. Since the brain's high rate of oxygen consumption is accompanied by high ROS production, selenoenzyme activities are particularly important in this tissue. Because selenoenzymes can be irreversibly inhibited by many electrophiles, exposure to these organic and inorganic agents can diminish selenoenzyme-dependent antioxidant functions. This can impair brain development, particularly via the adverse influence of oxidative stress on epigenetic regulation. Here we review the physiological roles of selenoproteins in relation to potential biochemical mechanisms of ASD etiology and pathology.

1. Introduction

The causes of autism and autism spectrum disorder (collectively, ASD) remain unknown, in part because of complex behavioral phenotypes and the likelihood that multiple genetic and environmental factors contribute to its etiology [1–3]. In the absence of biochemical tests for ASD, the diagnosis is based solely on clinical assessment of behavioral criteria that define deficits in social interaction, impairments in verbal and nonverbal receptive/expression, speech, and hyperfocused repetitive behaviors. The pathophysiology of ASD is primarily expressed in the neurologic, immunologic, and gastrointestinal (GI) systems and affects four times as many boys as girls [4–6]. Regression, with loss of previously acquired skills, can also interrupt apparently normal development. Children with severe autism can exhibit mental retardation, and autistic children have an elevated rate of seizure disorders [7].

Although ASD was previously thought to be rare, the number of persons receiving treatment for ASD has increased substantially during the past several decades and continues to increase. A recent US government report estimated the prevalence of ASD increased by 78% from 2002 to 2008 [8]. In 2011-2012, a prevalence of 20 per 1000 was reported for school aged children [9]. However, a portion of ASD's increasing incidence may reflect changes in diagnostic practice and the broadening of diagnostic criteria [10]. Other studies indicate a diagnostic shift or substitution may also have contributed to the rise in diagnosis, whereby the increase in autism diagnoses corresponds with declines in the usage of other diagnostic categories [11, 12]. Based on a meta-analysis of ASD studies, McDonald and Paul [13] concluded that it does not seem possible to assess whether or how much of the observed increases in cumulative incidence are real, although the number of individuals identified as having ASD has increased dramatically.

TABLE 1: Glutathione and oxidative stress in autism.

Authors (Reference)	Control n	Autistic n	GSH status	Additional related findings
James et al. [14]	33	20	46%↓	↓GSH/GSSG, ↓SAM/SAH, ↓cysteine
James et al. [15]	73	80	32%↓	↓GSH/GSSG, ↓SAM/SAH, ↓cysteine
D. A. Geier and M. R. Geier [16]	Lab-based normal values	10	36%↓	↓Cysteine
Adams et al. [17]	55	43	21%↓	↓SAM, ↓cysteine, ↓vitamin E, ↑FIGLU
Paşca et al. [18]	13	15	33%↓	↓Cysteine
Pastural et al. [19]	12	15	35%↓	↓Cysteine
Al-Gadani et al. [20]	30	30	27%↓	↑Lipid peroxides, ↓vitamin E, ↓SOD, ↓GPx
Melnyk et al. [21]	40	40	29%↓	↓GSH/GSSG, ↓SAM/SAH, ↓cysteine, ↓DNA methylation
James et al. [22]	42	40	28%↓	↓GSH/GSSG, ↓SAM/SAH, ↓cysteine
Geier et al. [23]	120	28	24%↓	↓Cysteine
Geier et al. [24]	Lab-based normal values	28	24%↓	↑GSSG, ↓cysteine, ↓taurine, ↓sulfate

Until reliably accurate differential diagnoses are achieved, it is difficult to attain the goal of defining the biochemical and physiological lesions that initiate and/or perpetuate the dysfunctions of autism. However, one pathological mechanism present in many children with ASD involves defects in the control of oxidative damage. Distinctions in the nature of these perturbations in redox control may provide insight for identifying biochemically defined patient subgroups that may respond to specific therapeutic interventions. This paper focuses on potential associations between genetic and acquired defects in control of oxidative damage, particularly those that impinge upon selenium- (Se-)dependent enzymes (selenoenzymes). Se physiology is a vital process in the brain and neuroendocrine system, [25, 26] and, because of the high reactivity and low abundance of Se in these tissues, its vulnerability to inhibition by a variety of toxicants is markedly enhanced. However, its potential role in the pathophysiology of ASD remains largely unexplored.

2. Oxidative Stress in ASD

Chemically reactive oxygen-derived products like peroxide radicals ($^{\bullet}O_2^{2-}$), hydrogen peroxide (H_2O_2), superoxide-anion (O_2^-), singlet oxygen ($^1O_2$), and hydroxyl radicals ($^{\bullet}OH$), are products of ongoing aerobic metabolism via mitochondrial oxidative phosphorylation [27]. If not intercepted and detoxified, reactive oxygen species (ROS) are capable of chemically damaging all forms of cellular macromolecules. To avoid these consequences, numerous ROS-detoxifying reactions enable cells to maintain redox equilibrium and metabolic homeostasis. Thus, oxidative stress is a condition where the level of ROS production exceeds antioxidant capacity.

Increased oxidative stress has been observed in children with ASD [28–30]. Blood collected from autistic children shows low concentrations of membrane polyunsaturated lipids, higher phospholipase A_2, and loss of the normal asymmetry of membrane lipoproteins, which may indicate increased oxidative damage [13, 31]. Levels of endogenous and exogenous antioxidant capacity are commonly reduced in ASD. Glutathione (GSH) is the primary intracellular antioxidant, and the ratio of its reduced (GSH) and oxidized (GSSG) forms (GSH/GSSG) provides a useful index of redox status. As shown in Table 1, numerous studies have reported significantly lower plasma levels of GSH and, in some cases, lower GSH/GSSG levels. Low GSH levels are associated with oxidative stress, increased inflammation, impaired immune response, and a decreased ability to detoxify environmental contaminants. Autistic children have been reported to be increasingly susceptible to recurrent infections, neuroinflammation, gastroinflammation, and impaired antioxidant and detoxification capacity. Diminished glutathione peroxidase (GPx), superoxide dismutase, and catalase enzyme activities have been associated with ASD, as well as low cysteine, Se, zinc (Zn), and Vitamins C, E, and A [32], although these associations are not consistently observed.

Accumulation of oxidized glutathione (GS-SG) in plasma is a strong indication of intracellular oxidative stress, as cells export the GS-SG to maintain redox equilibrium. James and coworkers [14] were first to report that plasma levels of cysteine, GSH, and the GSH/GS-SG ratio were significantly decreased in autistic children. In that study, total GSH levels were decreased, and GS-SG was increased, resulting in a threefold reduction in the redox ratio of GSH/GS-SG. Cysteine, the rate-limiting amino acid for GSH synthesis, was significantly decreased relative to controls in over 65% of the autistic children tested. The finding of lower-plasma GSH has since been replicated by other research groups [17–20, 33], suggesting this is a prevalent feature of ASD. A recent meta-analysis finds that children with ASD have decreased blood GSH (27%), GPx activity (18%), and methionine (13%) and increased concentrations of GS-SG (45%) relative to nonautistic children [34]. In addition, levels of NADPH and NADH, which reflect redox status and help maintain GSH in its reduced state, were found to be significantly lower in autistic children [32]. Several studies have reported a decrease in the level of GSH in postmortem brain samples from ASD subjects, associated with a decrease in the GSH/GS-SG ratio and increased levels of oxidative stress biomarkers [35, 36].

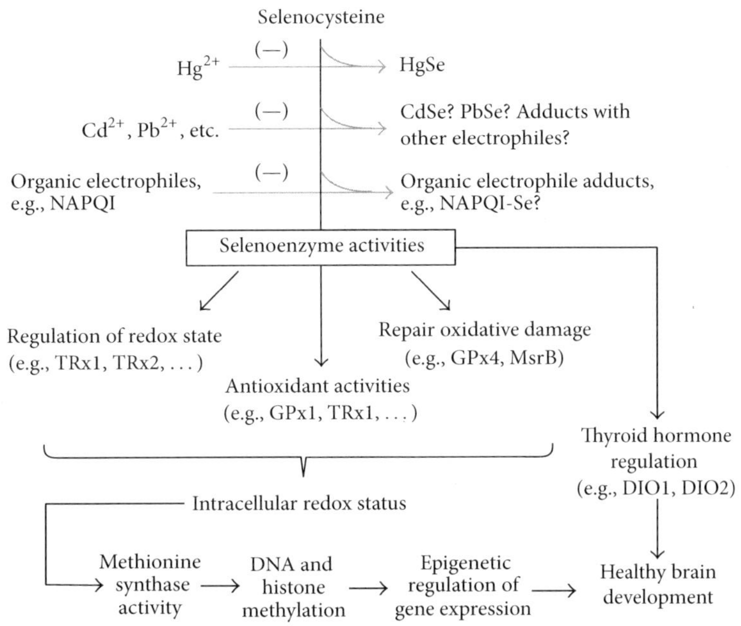

FIGURE 1: Selenoprotein synthesis and activities are sensitive to elemental and organic electrophiles. High exposures to soft electrophiles may additively impair redox regulation and thyroid hormone production, disrupting epigenetic regulation and normal brain development.

In addition, activities of several GSH-related enzymes, including the selenoenzyme GPx, were lower in cerebellums of ASD subjects [37].

The folate and Vitamin B_{12}-dependent enzyme methionine synthase (MS) is inhibited under oxidative stress conditions, resulting in a decrease in all methylation reactions, including DNA methylation [38]. The basis for MS inhibition is oxidation of its Vitamin B_{12} (cobalamin) cofactor, which is considered the most readily oxidized biomolecule, making it an ideal sensor of cellular redox status [39, 40]. Lower MS activity inhibits methylation by lowering the ratio of the methyl donor S-adenosylmethionine (SAM) to the methylation inhibitor S-adenosylhomocysteine (SAH), exerting a global dampening effect on >200 methylation reactions. Arguably, the most important among these are methylation of DNA and histones, which combine to exert epigenetic regulation over gene expression. As noted above, a decrease in SAM/SAH has been documented in plasma of ASD subjects in association with a decrease in GSH/GSSG, reflecting the reciprocal relationship between oxidative stress and methylation. In neuronal cells methionine synthase activity is stimulated by growth factors and dopamine but inhibited by neurodevelopmental toxins, including mercury (Hg) [41]. Methionine synthase mRNA levels are significantly decreased in postmortem brains of autistic subjects, indicative of a deficit in methylation capacity secondary to oxidative stress [42].

Elevated urinary levels of 8-isoprostane-$F_{2\alpha}$ (8-iso-$PGF_{2\alpha}$) and malondialdehyde (MDA), oxidative stress biomarkers, have also been noted in children with autism [28, 30]. A bimodal distribution of 8-iso-$PGF_{2\alpha}$ was reported, with the majority of autistic subjects showing moderate increases in isoprostane levels, while a smaller group of autistic children showed dramatic increases. Levels of urinary 8-hydroxy-2-deoxyguanosine (8-OHdG), a major product of DNA oxidation, were also measured but did not reach statistical significance, although they indicated a trend toward increasing concentrations in children with autism [30]. No significant correlations were noted between the levels of these biomarkers and vitamin intake, dietary supplements, medicine, medical disorders, or history of regression. Therefore, these results suggest that lipid peroxidation is increased in autistic children and that certain autistic children have much greater oxidative stress than others.

3. Selenium-Dependent Antioxidant Metabolism and ASD

Selenoproteins are essential for brain development, redox control, and preventing and reversing oxidative damage in the brain and neuroendocrine tissues (Figure 1, Table 2). Therefore, control of intracellular oxidative tone and findings of increased oxidative damage in children with ASD may be indicative of disruptions of selenoenzyme activities. The molecular forms of Se most common in foods are the amino acids selenocysteine (Sec) and selenomethionine (SeMet), although traces of water-soluble inorganic forms (e.g., selenate and selenite) can also be present in food and drinking water. For both the organic and inorganic Se forms, biochemical utilization in selenoenzymes is initiated through the common intermediate hydrogen selenide (H_2Se). Therefore, all ingested (and endogenous) forms of Se must be degraded to inorganic selenide before Se can be used for synthesis of Sec, the physiological active form of Se. Although proteins

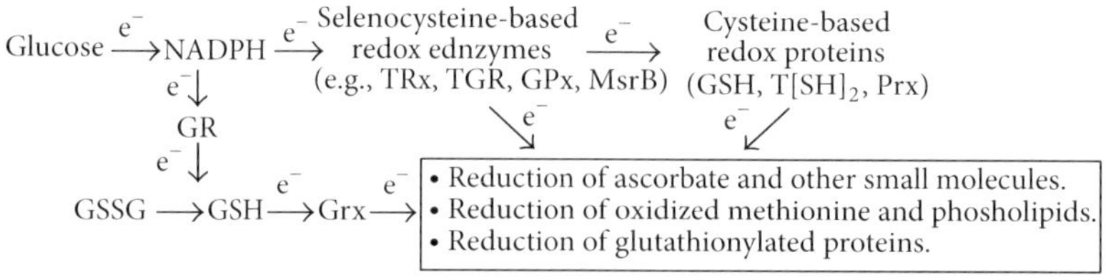

FIGURE 2: Selenoenzymes are central to providing antioxidant electrons to accomplish reduction of molecules in a number of biochemical processes. NADPH = nicotinamide adenine dinucleotide phosphate; GR = glutathione reductase; T(SH)$_2$ = reduced thioredoxin; GSH = reduced glutathione; TRx = thioredoxin reductase; GSSG = oxidized glutathione; TGR = thioredoxin-glutathione reductase; GPx = glutathione peroxidase; MsrB = methionine sulfoxide reductase; Prx = peroxiredoxin; Grx = glutaredoxin; e$^-$ = electron. Levels of plasma GSH, erythrocyte NADH, and NADPH are notably reduced ($P < 0.001$) in children with autism [16, 32].

with SeMet contain Se, they are not considered selenoproteins because SeMet is nonspecifically incorporated into proteins as if it were Met. The nonspecific insertion of SeMet or Met is directed by AUG codons and no significant distinctions in the biochemical functions have been observed. This is in contrast to Sec, which is the catalytically active primary amino acid present in all selenoproteins [43] and is responsible for the principal functions of these enzymes (Table 2). In contrast to other amino acids, Sec is not recycled for reincorporation into new proteins but is, instead, degraded to release inorganic Se which can be utilized for resynthesis of Sec.

While Cys, the analogous sulfur amino acid, is inserted at UGU/UGC codons, the insertion of Sec is in response to UGA which is otherwise the "opal" stop codon for other proteins [44–46]. The selenoprotein mRNAs include a distinct Sec insertion sequence (SECIS) stem-loop structure in their untranslated 3′ region of the mRNA. This is recognized by specific SECIS binding proteins which function together with several transacting factors as well as a unique tRNA with an anticodon complementary to UGA to initiate de novo Sec synthesis. The tRNA is aminoacylated with serine prior to biosynthesis of Sec which is inserted into the protein's primary structure. In mRNA of most selenoproteins, the UGA of the Sec insertion codon is followed by a second or terminal UGA, which is then read as the stop codon.

Since the discovery of these genetically unique proteins, their enzyme activities have become increasingly well defined. Associations between compromised Se and ASD have been reported including low Se levels in red blood cells [47]. Since blood Se is less prone to contamination and more indicative of tissue selenoenzyme activities, it is considered to be a more reliable index than hair. Indeed, hair Se is variously reported as being increased [48], decreased [49], or unchanged [50] in subjects with ASD.

When considering the developmental roles of selenoproteins, as well as their involvement in redox control and protection from oxidative stress, the potential for selenoenzyme dysregulation in relation to the pathologies associated with ASD appears worthy of investigation. The three main families of characterized selenoproteins—iodothyronine deiodinases (DIO), thioredoxin reductases (TRx), and GPx—have critical roles in thyroid function, fetal development, hormone metabolism, and oxidative stress detoxification, particularly in endocrine and brain tissues. Although ~25 selenoproteins are known, only members of the major selenoenzyme/selenoprotein families with potential relevance to autism etiology and pathology are discussed below.

3.1. Roles of Selenoenzymes in Thyroid Hormone Regulation. Selenoenzymes regulate thyroid synthesis and metabolic functions contributing to thyroid hormone biosynthesis, antioxidant defense, redox control of thyrocytes, and thyroid hormone metabolism. Thyroid hormones have important roles in regulating many key biochemical reactions, especially protein synthesis and enzymatic activity, accompanied by an increase in basal metabolic rate. Thyroid hormone regulates several processes that are associated with brain differentiation, including dendrite and axon growth, synaptogenesis, neuronal migration, and myelination [51]. Disruption of thyroid hormone production during early child development leads to permanent deficiency in intelligence and sensorimotor functions [52], and it is hypothesized that Se deficiency may be responsible for the initiation of autoimmune thyroid disorders [53]. Interestingly, thyroid hormone increases plasma Se levels, as well as the levels of selenoenzymes such as DIO [54]. This relationship is logical, since increased metabolic activity places a higher demand on antioxidant resources.

The central nervous system is very sensitive to thyroid hormone supply during growth and development. The selenoprotein family of DIOs (DIO1, 2, and 3) is involved in the formation and regulation of the active thyroid hormone, triiodothyronine (T_3). More than 80% of T_3 in the brain is derived from intracellular deiodination of T_4 by DIO2 [55, 56]. Since circulating T_3 does not readily gain access to intracellular nuclear receptors [57], DIO2 provides an important regulatory function in the brain and central nervous system (CNS). During early childhood, T_3 bound to nuclear receptors is entirely dependent on its local production from T_4 via this selenoprotein.

3.2. Roles of TRx in Redox Regulation. The three distinct forms of TRx—TRx1, TRx2, and TRx3 (collectively, TRx)—are important in controlling redox state within major compartments of the cell. While TRx1 (cytosolic) and TRx2 (mitochondrial) restore oxidized thioredoxin (T[S-S]) to its reduced (T[SH]$_2$) form and are responsible for reducing a

Table 2

Selenoprotein	Functions	References
GPx1	Detoxifies peroxides in aqueous compartment of cellular cytosol	[58]
GPx2	Expressed in cytosol of liver and tissues of the digestive system	[59]
GPx3	Synthesized primarily by kidney; secreted into plasma for transport to other tissues	[60]
GPx4	Prevents and reverses oxidative damage to lipids in brain and other tissues	[61]
TRx1	Reduces $T(SH)_2$, vitamin C, polyphenols, and other substrates to regulate intercellular redox state	[62–64]
TRx2	Located in mitochondria and controls and regulates redox state	[63, 64]
TRx3	Reduces mitochondrial glutathione disulfide, abundant in testes	[63, 64]
MsrB1	Restores oxidatively damaged methionine (R-sulfoxides) to native configuration	[64]
DIO1	Converts T_4 (thyroxine) prohormone into T_3 (active thyroid hormone)	[65]
DIO2	Regulates thyroid hormone status, activating as well as inactivating T_3	[65]
DIO3	Activates thyroid hormone in brain, placenta, important in fetal development	[65]
SPS2	Creates the Se-phosphate precursor required for synthesis of all selenoproteins	[64]
SelM	Notably high expression levels in the brain, possible thiol-disulfide oxidoreductase	[64, 66]
SelN	Interacts with ryanodine receptor, mutations result in congenital muscular dystrophy	[64]
SelP	Transports Se in plasma (10 Sec/molecule) and delivers Se to brain and endocrine tissues	[64]
SelW	Expressed in a variety of tissues and may regulate redox state of 14-3-3 proteins	[64, 66, 67]
Sel15	Oxidoreductase that may assist in disulfide formation and protein folding	[64]

variety of other essential antioxidant molecules [63] including Vitamin C [62]. Thioredoxin is a ubiquitous 12 kDa protein that employs vicinal cysteines (CXXC motif) and becomes oxidized to intramolecular disulfides T(S-S) during reduction of other molecules (Figure 2). Its action is essential for countering oxidative damage in the cytosol of aerobic organisms from bacteria to humans [68]. Since $T(SH)_2$ is a central regulator of cellular redox status that is required for the redox-regulated function of transcription factors and hormonally regulated nuclear receptors, it is critical in DNA production, gene expression, cell survival, and embryogenesis. Thus TRx maintains $T(SH)_2$ levels to enable basic processes and regulate multiple metabolic events. The antioxidant functions of TRx occur because they directly facilitate reduction of oxidized proteins through cysteine-thiol-disulfide exchange, forming an oxidized disulfide T(S-S) in the process. TRx is also directly involved in prevention and repair of damage caused by H_2O_2-based oxidative stress. Because intracellular reduction of selenite is required for de novo synthesis of Sec selenoproteins, TRx clearly has a central role in all Se physiology. It is assumed that Se's pivotal role in TRx explains why targeted disruption of the TRx1 [69] and $T(SH)_2$ [70] genes are embryonically lethal.

Additionally, investigations have shown that TRx1 synthesized without its penultimate Sec is an apoptosis initiator (GRIM-12) [71]. The only difference between the truncated GRIM-12 and full-length TRx1 is the absence of the final two amino acids, Sec and glycine. Truncation occurs when the codon UGA is interpreted as a stop codon instead of a signal for Sec insertion during times of Se deficiency or when its Sec is selectively derivatized. The Sec-deficient form of TRx1, GRIM-12, is a notably powerful apoptosis initiator that rapidly induces cell death [71].

3.3. Roles of GPx in Redox Regulation. GPx (five genetically distinct forms, GPx1–4 and GPx6) are selenoenzymes involved in antioxidant defense and redox regulation and modulation. GPx provide protection against oxidative damage and aid in the maintenance of membrane integrity by using GSH as a cofactor to catalyze reduction of hydrogen peroxide, forming oxidized glutathione (GS-SG) in the process. Thyroid hormone synthesis requires a continuous production of high concentrations of H_2O_2, which appears to be its rate-limiting step [72–74]. Therefore, since the thyrocyte is continually exposed to potentially toxic concentrations of H_2O_2 and lipid hydroperoxides, appropriate antioxidant defense systems are essential to control excess oxidative stress. Three of the five GPx are expressed in thyrocytes and thyroid tissue [75–77]. Studies indicate a distinct regulation of expression, secretion, and function of these selenoproteins for controlling thyrocyte growth, differentiation, and function [76–83]. When Se intake is adequate, the intracellular GPx and TRx systems protect the thyrocyte from peroxides; however, in Se deficiency, the thyrocyte's apoptotic response to H_2O_2 is increased [84]. Furthermore, in iodine deficiency, where hyperstimulation of the thyroid-stimulating hormone (TSH) receptor signals increased H_2O_2 production, GPx production is also stimulated, thus upregulating antioxidant protection. By virtue of its ability to increase basal metabolism, thyroid hormone increases oxygen utilization, thereby increasing the demand for antioxidant.

GPx4 reduces hydroperoxides of membrane phospholipid fatty acids and has particular relevance for autism. Along with TRx1, TRx2, DIO2, DIO3, and selenoprotein P (SelP), GPx4 is considered an essential selenoprotein whose levels are preserved in brain and endocrine tissues during Se deficiency. Suppression of neuronal GPx4 expression resulted in a selective loss of parvalbumin-expressing GABAergic interneurons [85] that are essential for dopamine-dependent regulation during attention [86] and has been linked to attention deficit hyperactivity disorder (ADHD) [87, 88]. Earlier studies also showed that expression of these interneurons was inhibited when glutathione synthesis was impaired, indicating a critical role for redox status in establishing the capacity for attention [89, 90].

3.4. Selenoenzyme Metabolism and Physiology. In addition to the TRx and GPx selenoenzyme families, further selenoproteins have recently been implicated in processes known to be involved in neurodegenerative diseases, including protein folding, degradation of misfolded membrane proteins, and control of cellular calcium homoeostasis [91]. Cerebral Se deficiency is associated with neurological disorders such as seizures and ataxia [92, 93], consistent with a restriction in the development of inhibitory interneurons. Knockout of selenoprotein synthesis in neurons specifically interfered with development of parvalbumin-expressing GABAergic interneurons, and knockout of GPx4 produced a similar deficit, indicating that these neurons have a particular requirement for Se [85]. Thus impaired selenoprotein synthesis or loss of their activities could contribute to the neurocognitive dysfunction and seizure activity in ASD.

The cerebral cortex, hippocampus, cerebellum, and olfactory bulb express the highest numbers of selenoproteins [94]. The brain and endocrine tissues are preferentially supplied with Se, predominantly through directed distribution and cellular uptake of SelP. Although other selenoproteins uniformly incorporate only a single Sec per molecule, SelP uniquely contains 10 Sec per molecule. Studies with SelP-deficient mice indicate that moderate reductions of brain Se content will impair brain function [95, 96].

Not only is SelP important for Sec transport, but it also appears to have a vital role in neurogenesis. A study of its brain distribution found a remarkably higher concentration in ependymal cells, which are found at the ventricle surface [97]. Ependymal cells are a source of neural stem cells which are produced upon asymmetric cell division and give rise to neuronal, astrocyte and oligodendrocyte lineages in the subependymal region [98]. Neurotrophic growth factors stimulate mitosis of these precursor cells [99] and provide an important source of postnatal neurons. SelP is taken up by neurons via apolipoprotein E receptor 2 (ApoER2), which is localized to synapses, and ApoER2 knockout mice show a decrease in synapse density as well as a decrease in the number of dendritic spines [100, 101].

All brain selenoenzymes are affected by loss of Se in the absence of SelP, but the DIOs, TRxs, and GPxs are the selenoproteins considered to have the most critical roles in the brain and endocrine system. Therefore, loss or compromise of their functions [96] would have dramatic effects on maturation of the neuroendocrine system. The unusual capacity of the brain and endocrine tissues (e.g., pituitary, testes) to retain their selenoenzyme activities during prolonged or even multigenerational deficiency states [43] indicates that their redox regulation effects are important in these tissues. The low GSH level of neurons (~0.2 mM) provides a unique opportunity for redox signaling as a mechanism for epigenetic control. Neurotrophic factors stimulate cysteine uptake and increase both GSH/GS-SG and SAM/SAH in association with a significant increase in DNA methylation [102]. However, Se-dependent redox regulation is more vulnerable to soft electrophiles, positively charged chemical species which bind to selenoproteins with exceptionally high affinity, as discussed below.

4. Genetic Influences and Metabolic Disturbances in ASD

Observations from family studies suggest that ASD has a strong genetic component [103–105], although the failure to identify genetic factors affecting more than a small proportion of ASD cases suggests that multiple etiologies may be responsible for the pathologies and neurobehavioral features of the disorder [106–117]. Moreover, genetic factors may increase the probability of oxidative damage and diminish the body's ability to detoxify ROS and free radicals. Interactions between genetic and environmental factors may potentiate increased oxidative stress in autistic children.

Genetic risk of autism may be related to a differential sensitivity to environmental factors. Using a strict definition of autism, a recent study found a 58% concordance rate for monozygotic male twins and 60% for females and 21% and 27% for male and female dizygotic twins, respectively [118]. Using the broader definition of ASD, monozygotic concordance increased to 77% and 50% for males and females, while dizygotic concordance was 31% and 36%, respectively. These rates are substantially lower than earlier estimates, and the authors concluded that environmental factors are more important than genetic factors, although genetic factors clearly play an important role. Moreover, no individual genetic cause of autism has been identified to account for more than 1%-2% of cases and, with the exception of Rett syndrome, there is no current evidence that ASD is linked to any specific genetic or nongenetic disorder. However, there is evidence suggesting that epigenetic factors and exposures to environmental modifiers may contribute to variable expression of autism-related traits [42]. Variants of major effect genes and numerous common variants with smaller effect genes have been identified in individuals with ASD and related conditions. These genetic variances are providing insights to common pathways and metabolic disturbances affected in ASD, particularly genes involved in oxidative stress and detoxification pathways [15, 119, 120].

Polymorphisms of genes involved in glutathione metabolism, including genes for GPx and glutathione S-transferase (GST), have been reportedly associated with ASD. GPx1 is the predominant and most abundant isoenzyme of GPx and plays an integral role in reducing oxidative stress by catalyzing the reduction of potentially harmful peroxides. Ming et al. [121] found significant disequilibrium in the overall transmission of a sequence polymorphism of GPx1 in ASD. Williams et al. [122] showed that the GSTP1-313A allele may be acting as a teratogenic allele, contributing to the phenotype of the affected child. GST proteins conjugate and detoxify products of oxidative stress and conjugate toxins that produce oxidative stress. By assessing genotypes of mothers and maternal grandparents, it was shown that the GSTP1A haplotype was significantly more frequently transmitted to mothers of individuals with ASD, suggesting that it may be acting in mothers during pregnancy to contribute to the phenotype of autism during fetal development [122].

James et al. [15] examined the frequency of several single nucleotide polymorphisms (SNPs) capable of affecting redox and methylation pathways in autistic subjects. They found significant differences in allele frequencies for the reduced folate carrier (RFC 80G>A), transcobalamin II (TCN2 776 G>C), methylenetetrahydrofolate reductase (MTHFR) 677 C>T and 1298 (A>C), catechol-O-methyltransferase (COMT 472 G>A), and GST M1 between autistic and control cohorts. These differences were associated with abnormal metabolite levels, suggesting that individuals with genetic vulnerability affecting redox and methylation capacity may be linked to a higher risk for autism. Any deficit in the function of selenoproteins could synergize with these genetic risk factors.

DNA copy number variants (CNVs) represent a major category of genetic risk for ASD and are implicated in approximately 10% of cases [123, 124]. Several of the genes likely affected by homozygous deletions are regulated by neuronal activity, and the expression of these genes can change in response to neuronal stimulation. Synapses mature partially as a function of experience-dependent neuronal activity, so disruption of those genes by mutation or copy number variation may alter the process of synaptic development. DNA methylation status is associated with the occurrence of CNVs [125], raising the possibility that impaired methylation capacity could contribute to increased CNVs in ASD.

5. Epigenetic Disturbances in ASD

Epigenetic regulation utilizes covalent modifications such as DNA methylation and the addition/removal of various chemical moieties to histone tails (collectively known as epigenetic marks) to provide stable, transgenerational changes in gene expression without alteration of the underlying nucleotide sequence [126, 127]. Epigenetic marks are dynamic and highly sensitive to cellular changes [128]. Thus, normal physiologic changes in the cellular environment, such as levels of growth factors, hormones, and neurotransmitters, as well as xenobiotic exposure, can translate into modifications in gene expression mediated by epigenetic regulation. Xenobiotic exposures affecting epigenetic status can, therefore, not only produce lifelong consequences, but their effects can be transmitted through germline cells to affect multiple succeeding generations [126, 128].

As noted above, MS exerts powerful control over all methylation reactions via its influence over the SAM/SAH ratio, and MS inhibition by oxidative stress will cause both a decrease in SAM and an increase in SAH, while reducing conditions will have the opposite effect. A twofold increase in MS activity induced by IGF-1 is associated with a twofold increase in global DNA methylation, while inhibition of MS activity by ethanol is associated with a large decrease [41]. Thus, xenobiotics affecting redox status can exert an epigenetic influence.

Beyond its direct epigenetic regulation of gene transcription, DNA methylation also regulates the activity of repetitive transposable elements dispersed throughout the human genome. Transposable elements comprise about 45% of the genome, and their earlier description as "junk DNA" has recently been revised in recognition of their ability to modulate gene transcription, mRNA splicing, microRNA formation, and other processes [129]. Reflecting their viral origin, retrotransposons such as the LINE-1 (long interspersed nuclear element-1) family are suppressed by methylation but can replicate and transpose to new locations, especially during early development and especially when methylation is suppressed. Based upon its impressive quantitative contribution to the genome, methylation of LINE-1 has been used as a surrogate for global DNA methylation [130], and factors regulating MS activity affect LINE-1 methylation [131]. LINE-1 retrotransposition is reported to occur at a higher rate in brain than to other tissues [132], and a higher rate was observed in Rett syndrome subjects carrying mutations in the methylated DNA binding protein MeCP2 [130]. Although more studies are needed to clarify their specific contribution, transposable elements such as LINE-1 are poised to provide a global genomic influence during development, so agents affecting their methylation state are likely to disrupt this process.

Oxidative stress and decreased methylation capacity are common in autism and abnormal epigenetic regulation may link the metabolic abnormalities to disruptions in brain development. Other comorbid features of autism, such as autoimmunity and gastrointestinal (GI) dysfunction [133, 134], may reflect similar manifestations of abnormal epigenetic regulation. A genome-wide comparison of DNA methylation in monozygotic twins discordant for autism found numerous differentially methylated regions associated with ASD, and the extent of these differences were correlated with severity of autistic trait scores [135].

From conception to maturation, human development is a highly orchestrated expression of epigenetic regulation, so it is not surprising that genetic and environmental factors adversely affecting oxidative tone and methylation status can contribute to developmental disorders. The exceptionally dynamic redox-dependent epigenetic regulation in the brain increases its vulnerability to neurodevelopmental disorders. Autism is a prominent feature of Rett, Angelman, Prader-Willi, and Fragile-X syndromes, each of which has been linked to interruption of methylation-dependent regulation [136–138]. Therefore, environmental exposures affecting redox and methylation status could reasonably result in neurodevelopment disorders such as ASD.

6. ASD in relation to Exposures to Potentially Neurotoxic Agents

Certain soft electrophiles are known to be neurotoxic at high exposures, presumably due to their effects on sulfur metabolism. Although these electrophilic species are highly interactive with cellular nucleophiles such as thiols, the Se of Sec is by far the strongest intracellular nucleophile. Therefore, selenoproteins are very vulnerable to enzyme inhibition by binding to neurotoxic electrophiles. Their toxic concentrations are generally miniscule in relation to sulfur, toxic levels generally equal or exceed the normal tissue concentrations of Se. Therefore, because of their high reactivity and low molar abundance, selenoenzymes are highly vulnerable to selective inhibition by high concentrations of electrophiles such as Hg. Soft electrophiles such as Hg have larger ionic radii and a more dispersed surface charge, making them more reactive with soft nucleophiles such as the Se of Sec at the active sites of enzymes.

Only certain electrophiles are notably neurotoxic. Those that bind and potentially sequester Se would cooperatively diminish the biological availability of Se for performance of its necessary physiological roles (Figure 1). For example, a multitude of electrophilic agents are naturally present in food in small amounts and the Se-sequestering effects of each would usually be minor. However, their additive effects on selenoenzyme synthesis and function could be detrimental in individuals with compromised Se status or metabolism.

Likewise, additional exposures to electrophiles are encountered in the form of environmental contaminants, such as toxic metals, pesticides, herbicides, and others. In addition, soft electrophiles are present as the active ingredients in many pharmaceuticals and food preservatives, while still others are produced during the degradation of these products. Therefore, instead of examining relationships between ASD incidence and exposures to individual agents, it may be more informative to examine ASD incidence in relation to aggregate exposures to these soft electrophiles and/or their effect on selenoenzyme activity in vulnerable individuals.

6.1. Thio-/Selenoreactive Elements. High exposures to soft electrophiles have the potential to incapacitate various sulfur- and Se-dependent metabolic processes, thus disrupting many redox regulatory mechanisms that are required for healthy cell growth and function, particularly in brain and endocrine tissues. Increased selenium status is known to counteract the adverse effects of elevated exposures to neurotoxic electrophiles such as Hg, cadmium (Cd), lead (Pb), and vanadium (V) [139]. These electrophilic elements may all be capable of selective, irreversible inhibition of selenoenzyme activities similar to the mechanism of Hg toxicity [140, 141]. However, relationships between Se status and the neurotoxic effects of these other elements have not been adequately examined, and additional mechanisms of toxicity have been recognized for some of these elements [142]. Because it is rich in cysteine, hair has often been used to provide a reflection of circulating amounts of thio-reactive electrophiles present in exposed individuals. The concentrations of Hg, As, Cd, or Pb in hair do not indicate consistent relationships with ASD incidence; however, some studies report unusually low concentrations in hair samples and suggest that individuals with ASD have diminished abilities to eliminate toxic metals [143, 144]. This is consistent with the finding that lower Hg concentrations are present in the hair of young (<6 y) children with ASD [144–146] although Majewska et al. [146] found older ASD children have higher hair Hg. Although serum was studied instead of RBC's or whole blood, a large study of Hg in relation to autism [147] reported finding no significant differences between nonautistic and ASD children. This is supported by the finding that no distinctions in expression levels of four genes that are known to respond to metal exposures were noted between ASD and typical children [148]. However, Stamova et al. [149] found a distinctive correlation between gene expression and blood Hg levels in boys with autism suggesting it is associated with a different pattern of gene transcription in response to Hg exposure. The ability of both Hg and Se to exert epigenetic effects was recently demonstrated in embryonic stem cells [150]. Several studies have reported potent toxic effects of methylmercury on neural stem cell differentiation and survival [151, 152], indicating its potential capacity for altering gene expression during development.

To prevent bacterial contamination in multiple-dose vials, thimerosal, the ethylmercury derivative of thiosalicylic acid, has been used as a preservative in various medical products, including vaccines. As autism rates increased, Bernard et al. [153] suggested that vaccine-derived Hg might be a contributing cause, a highly controversial proposal [154–156]. As a result, thimerosal was removed from all pediatric vaccines, except for some influenza vaccines, in the United States starting in 2001, but the incidence of autism continued to rise [157], furthering the doubts that vaccine-derived Hg exposures contributes to autism incidence. While a number of epidemiological studies do not indicate an association between thimerosal exposure and ASD [158, 159], possible associations between developmental disorders with Hg-containing vaccines [157] and delayed or even transgenerational influence of epigenetic changes have been suggested [160]. Such genetic or epigenetic defects of the antioxidant enzyme system could cooperatively interact with other environmental electrophiles and make vulnerable individuals more sensitive to exposure levels that would otherwise be harmless. Since deficits in selenoenzyme synthesis or function can increase the potential for oxidative stress and epigenetic dysregulation, sensitivity to neurotoxins, such as Hg and similar soft electrophiles, may differ among individuals. In this regard, there have been several reports of decreased GPx activity in autism [161, 162] and selective transmission of GPx-1 allelic variants [121]. Interestingly, Paşca et al. [120] found an inverse correlation between homocysteine and GPx activity in autistic subjects, indicating an association between low GPx activity and impaired methylation. Therefore, Castañeda et al. suggested that the removal of thimerosal from vaccines might not be immediately reflected as a reversal of epigenetic effects, especially if they involved effects on germline cells [163]. Notably, lower levels of DNA methylation increase novel insertions of transposable elements and increase the frequency of CNVs in germline cells [164–166], which are also elevated in autism. Therefore, the effects of elemental electrophiles on selenometabolism may be a contributing

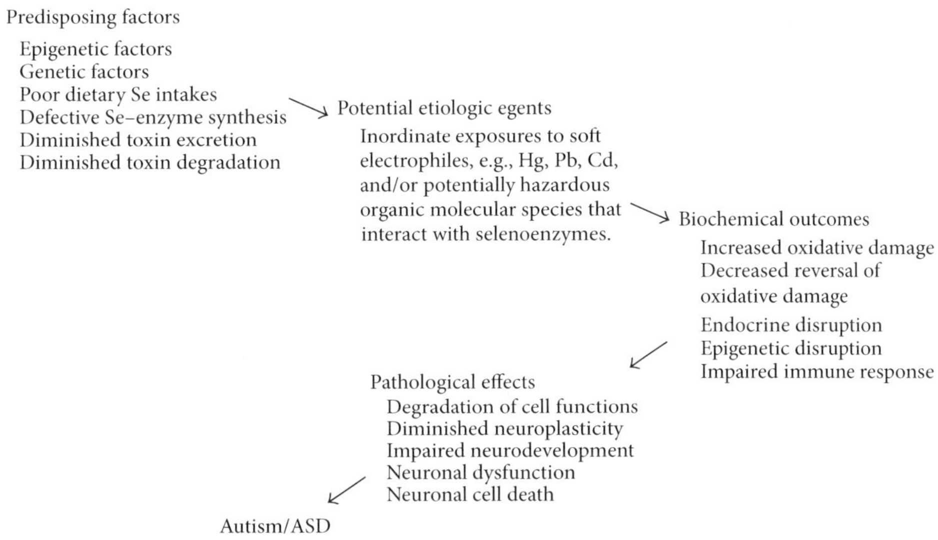

FIGURE 3: Depiction of potential etiologic contributors to disruptions of selenoenzyme physiology that may lead to disruptions of redox control and pathological consequences of autism and ASD. The factors and agents depicted are not all necessarily involved, but increases in predisposing factors along with additive contributions of increased exposures to thio- and selenoreactive electrophiles would be expected to increase the likelihood of progression to pathology.

factor to ASD etiology and/or progression in vulnerable individuals.

6.2. Thio-/Selenoreactive Organic Electrophiles. Organic molecules such as acrylamide, acrolein, and diethyldithiocarbamate are structurally diverse, but these electrophilic species all share the potential to chemically react with strong nucleophiles [167]. Just as for inorganic electrophiles, the most likely target will be the most nucleophilic moieties of enzymes, such as Sec or thiols of Cys residues. Acetaminophen, the most commonly used analgesic and antipyretic drug in much of the world, is associated with toxic effects at high exposures. Excessive intake leads to impaired sulfur metabolism and life-threatening hepatotoxicity, involving depletion of GSH [168]. A survey of parents reported a higher frequency of acetaminophen use after the MMR (measles-mumps-rubella) vaccine for autistic children than for unaffected children [169], leading to the suggestion that use of acetaminophen might be causally linked to an increase in autism rates [170].

Interestingly, the major acetaminophen-binding protein in the liver is Se binding protein-2 (SeBP2) [171, 172]. Both SeBP1 and SeBP2 bind Se, but not in the Sec form characteristic of the genetically encoded selenoproteins. Increased expression of SeBP2 is associated with increased susceptibility to acetaminophen cytotoxicity [173]. In view of the male predominance of autism, it is interesting to note that SeBP2 levels are higher in males [174] and their vulnerability to acetaminophen hepatotoxicity is also greater. Males also display a decreased capacity to restore their GSH levels to normal [175] following high acetaminophen exposures.

N-acetylcysteine protects against acetaminophen-induced hepatotoxicity by maintaining or restoring hepatic concentrations of GSH [176]. Glutathione is required to inactivate *N*-acetyl-*p*-benzoquinone imine (NAPQI), a metabolic product of acetaminophen breakdown that is thought to be the proximal cause of hepatotoxicity following acetaminophen overdoses. When excessive quantities of NAPQI are formed, the primary metabolic (glucuronide and sulfate conjugation) pathways apparently become saturated. N-acetylcysteine is thought to counteract toxicity by either reducing NAPQI to the parent compound or providing sulfhydryl for conjugation of this metabolite [176]. If supplementation with a sulfhydryl-containing compound such as N-acetylcysteine can directly inactivate NAPQI, supplementation with Se to restore selenoenzyme status may be an important adjunct therapy to restore healthy redox status in the affected tissues. The significance of the liver in providing Se for delivery to the brain suggests that compromised Se availability in the liver temporarily induced by exposures to NAPQI and/or other electrophiles could diminish the amount of Se the brain receives. Exposures to agents which could cause either prolonged or excessive diminishments in the supply of Se to neuroendocrine tissues may therefore be important factors to consider in relation to ASD.

7. Summary and Conclusions

The nosology of ASD is complicated by the difficulties to differentiate the syndrome into subsets with similar symptoms and distinct etiologies. Children that share the diagnosis of ASD represent more than one distinct pathophysiological condition. Recognizing and distinguishing between groups with separate etiologies require identification of objective laboratory indices that clinicians can use for diagnosis and to monitor progression and treatment effects. The objective of this review is to discuss metabolic defects that may contribute to the onset and pathology of ASD, particularly in relation to Se physiology.

Existing evidence indicates children with ASD have disruptions in GSH metabolism, and that impaired selenoenzyme and thiol metabolic pathways may be involved. These disruptions could occur as the result of multiple exposures to elemental and organic electrophiles (Figure 3) with exacerbations related to congenital vulnerabilities. Therefore, genetic predisposing factors for ASD may be exacerbated secondary to high aggregate exposures to electrophiles acquired through environmental, pharmaceutical, or foodborne routes. Currently, no specific causal agents or conditions have been recognized in ASD and not all children with potentially predisposing congenital defects or environmental exposures acquire ASD. This may indicate that the contributing effects of causal agents have low potency or that more than one predisposing factor is required. Therefore, a confluence of determinants of individual vulnerabilities and sufficiently high exposures to potential causal agents may be required to result in pathological effects. Likewise, the mechanisms of action may additively or synergistically accentuate risks to individuals with underlying genetic, epigenetic, or nutritional susceptibilities.

Based upon the mechanisms outlined above, interventions designed to diminish oxidative damage and support methylation capacity could improve the health of individuals afflicted with ASD, particularly those with inadequate antioxidant defenses. In such individuals, dietary interventions may offer low-risk approaches with potential for significant improvements in neurodevelopmental outcomes. Although the etiology and pathology of ASD remain poorly resolved, research suggests that afflicted children may benefit from treatments designed to improve their antioxidant capacity.

Acknowledgment

Preparation of this paper was supported by funding from the Autism Research Institute. The sponsors had no influence on the contents of this work or the decision to submit this paper for publication.

References

[1] A. M. Persico and T. Bourgeron, "Searching for ways out of the autism maze: genetic, epigenetic and environmental clues," *Trends in Neurosciences*, vol. 29, no. 7, pp. 349–358, 2006.

[2] F. R. Zahir and C. J. Brown, "Epigenetic impacts on neurodevelopment: pathophysiological mechanisms and genetic modes of action," *Pediatric Research*, vol. 69, no. 5, pp. 92R–100R, 2011.

[3] M. R. Herbert, "SHANK3, the synapse, and autism," *The New England Journal of Medicine*, vol. 365, no. 2, pp. 173–175, 2011.

[4] E. Fombonne, "Epidemiology of autistic disorder and other pervasive developmental disorders," *The Journal of Clinical Psychiatry*, vol. 66, supplement 10, pp. 3–8, 2005.

[5] I. N. Pessah, R. F. Seegal, P. J. Lein et al., "Immunologic and neurodevelopmental susceptibilities of autism," *NeuroToxicology*, vol. 29, no. 3, pp. 532–545, 2008.

[6] M. L. Bauman, "Medical comorbidities in autism: challenges to diagnosis and treatment," *Neurotherapeutics*, vol. 7, no. 3, pp. 320–327, 2010.

[7] S. J. Spence and M. T. Schneider, "The role of epilepsy and epileptiform EEGs in autism spectrum disorders," *Pediatric Research*, vol. 65, no. 6, pp. 599–606, 2009.

[8] Autism and Developmental Disabilities Monitoring Network Surveillance Year 2008 Principal Investigators and Centers for Disease Control and Prevention, "Prevalence of autism spectrum disorders—autism and developmental disabilities monitoring network, 14 sites, United States, 2008," *Morbidity and Mortality Weekly Report: Surveillance Summaries*, vol. 61, no. 3, pp. 1–19, 2012.

[9] S. J. Blumberg, M. D. Bramlett, M. D. Kogan, L. A. Schieve, J. R. Jones, and M. C. Lu, "Changes in prevalence of parent-reported autism spectrum disorder in school-aged U.S. children: 2007 to 2011-2012," *National Health Statistics Reports*, no. 65, pp. 1–7, 2013.

[10] B. Taylor, "Vaccines and the changing epidemiology of autism," *Child*, vol. 32, no. 5, pp. 511–519, 2006.

[11] P. T. Shattuck, "The contribution of diagnostic substitution to the growing administrative prevalence of autism in US special education," *Pediatrics*, vol. 117, no. 4, pp. 1028–1037, 2006.

[12] H. Jick and J. A. Kaye, "Epidemiology and possible causes of autism," *Pharmacotherapy*, vol. 23, no. 12, pp. 1524–1530, 2003.

[13] M. E. McDonald and J. F. Paul, "Timing of increased autistic disorder cumulative incidence," *Environmental Science and Technology*, vol. 44, no. 6, pp. 2112–2118, 2010.

[14] S. J. James, P. Cutler, S. Melnyk et al., "Metabolic biomarkers of increased oxidative stress and impaired methylation capacity in children with autism," *The American Journal of Clinical Nutrition*, vol. 80, no. 6, pp. 1611–1617, 2004.

[15] S. J. James, S. Melnyk, S. Jernigan et al., "Metabolic endophenotype and related genotypes are associated with oxidative stress in children with autism," *The American Journal of Medical Genetics B*, vol. 141, no. 8, pp. 947–956, 2006.

[16] D. A. Geier and M. R. Geier, "A clinical and laboratory evaluation of methionine cycle-transsulfuration and androgen pathway markers in children with autistic disorders," *Hormone Research*, vol. 66, no. 4, pp. 182–188, 2006.

[17] J. B. Adams, M. Baral, E. Geis et al., "The severity of autism is associated with toxic metal body burden and red blood cell glutathione levels," *Journal of Toxicology*, vol. 2009, Article ID 532640, 7 pages, 2009.

[18] S. P. Paşca, E. Dronca, T. Kaucsár et al., "One carbon metabolism disturbances and the C677T MTHFR gene polymorphism in children with autism spectrum disorders," *Journal of Cellular and Molecular Medicine*, vol. 13, no. 10, pp. 4229–4238, 2009.

[19] É. Pastural, S. Ritchie, Y. Lu et al., "Novel plasma phospholipid biomarkers of autism: mitochondrial dysfunction as a putative causative mechanism," *Prostaglandins Leukotrienes and Essential Fatty Acids*, vol. 81, no. 4, pp. 253–264, 2009.

[20] Y. Al-Gadani, A. El-Ansary, O. Attas, and L. Al-Ayadhi, "Metabolic biomarkers related to oxidative stress and antioxidant status in Saudi autistic children," *Clinical Biochemistry*, vol. 42, no. 10-11, pp. 1032–1040, 2009.

[21] S. Melnyk, G. J. Fuchs, E. Schulz et al., "Metabolic imbalance associated with methylation dysregulation and oxidative damage in children with autism," *Journal of Autism and Developmental Disorders*, vol. 42, no. 3, pp. 367–377, 2012.

[22] S. J. James, S. Melnyk, G. Fuchs et al., "Efficacy of methylcobalamin and folinic acid treatment on glutathione redox status in children with autism," *The American Journal of Clinical Nutrition*, vol. 89, no. 1, pp. 425–430, 2009.

[23] D. A. Geier, J. K. Kern, C. R. Garver et al., "Biomarkers of environmental toxicity and susceptibility in autism," *Journal of the Neurological Sciences*, vol. 280, no. 1, pp. 101–108, 2009.

[24] D. A. Geier, J. K. Kern, C. R. Garver, J. B. Adams, T. Audhya, and M. R. Geier, "A prospective study of transsulfuration biomarkers in autistic disorders," *Neurochemical Research*, vol. 34, no. 2, pp. 386–393, 2009.

[25] J. Chen and M. J. Berry, "Selenium and selenoproteins in the brain and brain diseases," *Journal of Neurochemistry*, vol. 86, no. 1, pp. 1–12, 2003.

[26] U. Schweizer, A. U. Bräuer, J. Köhrle, R. Nitsch, and N. E. Savaskan, "Selenium and brain function: a poorly recognized liaison," *Brain Research Reviews*, vol. 45, no. 3, pp. 164–178, 2004.

[27] M. L. Circu and T. Y. Aw, "Reactive oxygen species, cellular redox systems, and apoptosis," *Free Radical Biology and Medicine*, vol. 48, no. 6, pp. 749–762, 2010.

[28] A. Chauhan, V. Chauhan, W. T. Brown, and I. Cohen, "Oxidative stress in autism: increased lipid peroxidation and reduced serum levels of ceruloplasmin and transferrin—the antioxidant proteins," *Life Sciences*, vol. 75, no. 21, pp. 2539–2549, 2004.

[29] S. S. Zoroglu, F. Armutcu, S. Ozen et al., "Increased oxidative stress and altered activities of erythrocyte free radical scavenging enzymes in autism," *European Archives of Psychiatry and Clinical Neuroscience*, vol. 254, no. 3, pp. 143–147, 2004.

[30] X. Ming, T. P. Stein, M. Brimacombe, W. G. Johnson, G. H. Lambert, and G. C. Wagner, "Increased excretion of a lipid peroxidation biomarker in autism," *Prostaglandins Leukotrienes and Essential Fatty Acids*, vol. 73, no. 5, pp. 379–384, 2005.

[31] R. Sacco, P. Curatolo, B. Manzi et al., "Principal pathogenetic components and biological endophenotypes in autism spectrum disorders," *Autism Research*, vol. 3, no. 5, pp. 237–252, 2010.

[32] J. B. Adams, T. Audhya, S. McDonough-Means et al., "Nutritional and metabolic status of children with autism vs. neurotypical children, and the association with autism severity," *Nutrition and Metabolism*, vol. 8, article 34, 2011.

[33] D. A. Geier and M. R. Geier, "A case series of children with apparent mercury toxic encephalopathies manifesting with clinical symptoms of regressive autistic disorders," *Journal of Toxicology and Environmental Health A*, vol. 70, no. 10, pp. 837–851, 2007.

[34] A. Frustaci, M. Neri, A. Cesario et al., "Oxidative stress-related biomarkers in autism: systematic review and meta-analyses," *Free Radical Biology and Medicine*, vol. 52, no. 10, pp. 2128–2141, 2012.

[35] A. Chauhan, T. Audhya, and V. Chauhan, "Brain region-specific glutathione redox imbalance in autism," *Neurochemical Research*, vol. 37, no. 8, pp. 1681–1689, 2012.

[36] S. Rose, S. Melnyk, O. Pavliv et al., "Evidence of oxidative damage and inflammation associated with low glutathione redox status in the autism brain," *Translational Psychiatry*, vol. 2, article e134, 2012.

[37] F. Gu, V. Chauhan, and A. Chauhan, "Impaired synthesis and antioxidant defense of glutathione in the cerebellum of autistic subjects: alterations in the activities and protein expression of glutathione-related enzymes," *Free Radical Biology and Medicine*, vol. 65, pp. 488–496, 2013.

[38] R. Deth, C. Muratore, J. Benzecry, V.-A. Power-Charnitsky, and M. Waly, "How environmental and genetic factors combine to cause autism: a redox/methylation hypothesis," *NeuroToxicology*, vol. 29, no. 1, pp. 190–201, 2008.

[39] E. Mosharov, M. R. Cranford, and R. Banerjee, "The quantitatively important relationship between homocysteine metabolism and glutathione synthesis by the transsulfuration pathway and its regulation by redox changes," *Biochemistry*, vol. 39, no. 42, pp. 13005–13011, 2000.

[40] V. Bandarian, M. L. Ludwig, and R. G. Matthews, "Factors modulating conformational equilibria in large modular proteins: a case study with cobalamin-dependent methionine synthase," *Proceedings of the National Academy of Sciences of the United States of America*, vol. 100, no. 14, pp. 8156–8163, 2003.

[41] M. Waly, H. Olteanu, R. Banerjee et al., "Activation of methionine synthase by insulin-like growth factor-1 and dopamine: a target for neurodevelopmental toxins and thimerosal," *Molecular Psychiatry*, vol. 9, no. 4, pp. 358–370, 2004.

[42] C. R. Muratore, N. W. Hodgson, M. S. Trivedi et al., "Age-dependent decrease and alternative splicing of methionine synthase mRNA in human cerebral cortex and an accelerated decrease in autism," *PLoS ONE*, vol. 8, no. 2, Article ID e56927, 2013.

[43] A. Kyriakopoulos and D. Behne, "Selenium-containing proteins in mammals and other forms of life," *Reviews of Physiology Biochemistry and Pharmacology*, vol. 145, pp. 1–46, 2002.

[44] V. N. Gladyshev, F. J. Martin-Romero, X.-M. Xu et al., "Molecular biology of selenium and its role in cancer, AIDS and other human diseases," *Recent Research Developments in Biochemistry*, vol. 1, pp. 145–167, 1999.

[45] S. C. Low and M. J. Berry, "Knowing when not to stop: selenocysteine incorporation in eukaryotes," *Trends in Biochemical Sciences*, vol. 21, no. 6, pp. 203–208, 1996.

[46] S. Gromer, J. K. Eubel, B. L. Lee, and J. Jacob, "Human selenoproteins at a glance," *Cellular and Molecular Life Sciences*, vol. 62, no. 21, pp. 2414–2437, 2005.

[47] J. Jory and W. R. McGinnis, "Red-cell trace minerals in children with autism," *The American Journal of Biochemistry and Biotechnology*, vol. 4, no. 2, pp. 101–104, 2008.

[48] A. Lubkowska and W. Sobieraj, "Concentrations of magnesium, calcium, iron, selenium, zinc and copper in the hair of autistic children," *Trace Elements and Electrolytes*, vol. 26, no. 2, pp. 72–77, 2009.

[49] M. D. L. Priya and A. Geetha, "Level of trace elements (copper, zinc, magnesium and selenium) and toxic elements (lead and mercury) in the hair and nail of children with autism," *Biological Trace Element Research*, vol. 142, no. 2, pp. 148–158, 2011.

[50] G. de Palma, S. Catalani, A. Franco, M. Brighenti, and P. Apostoli, "Lack of correlation between metallic elements analyzed in hair by ICP-MS and autism," *Journal of Autism and Developmental Disorders*, vol. 42, no. 3, pp. 342–353, 2012.

[51] J. Bernal, "Thyroid hormone receptors in brain development and function," *Nature Reviews Endocrinology*, vol. 3, no. 3, pp. 249–259, 2007.

[52] I. B. Amara, H. Fetoui, F. Guermazi, and N. Zeghal, "Dietary selenium addition improves cerebrum and cerebellum impairments induced by methimazole in suckling rats," *International Journal of Developmental Neuroscience*, vol. 27, no. 7, pp. 719–726, 2009.

[53] J. Kohrle and R. Gartner, "Selenium and thyroid," *Best Practice & Research Clinical Endocrinology & Metabolism*, vol. 23, no. 6, pp. 815–827, 2009.

[54] J. Mittag, T. Behrends, C. S. Hoefig, B. Vennström, and L. Schomburg, "Thyroid hormones regulate selenoprotein expression and selenium status in mice," *PLoS ONE*, vol. 5, no. 9, Article ID e12931, 2010.

[55] F. R. Crantz, J. E. Silva, and P. R. Larsen, "An analysis of the sources and quantity of 3,5,3′-triiodothyronine specifically bound to nuclear receptors in rat cerebral cortex and cerebellum," *Endocrinology*, vol. 110, no. 2, pp. 367–375, 1982.

[56] F. Courtin, F. Chantoux, and J. Francon, "Thyroid hormone metabolism by glial cells in primary culture," *Molecular and Cellular Endocrinology*, vol. 48, no. 2-3, pp. 167–178, 1986.

[57] M. Safran, A. P. Farwell, and J. L. Leonard, "Evidence that type II 5′-deiodinase is not a selenoprotein," *The Journal of Biological Chemistry*, vol. 266, no. 21, pp. 13477–13480, 1991.

[58] X. G. Lei, W.-H. Cheng, and J. P. McClung, "Metabolic regulation and function of glutathione peroxidase-1," *Annual Review of Nutrition*, vol. 27, pp. 41–61, 2007.

[59] K. Wingler, M. Böcher, L. Flohé, H. Kollmus, and R. Brigelius-Flohé, "mRNA stability and selenocysteine insertion sequence efficiency rank gastrointestinal glutathione peroxidase high in the hierarchy of selenoproteins," *European Journal of Biochemistry*, vol. 259, no. 1-2, pp. 149–157, 1999.

[60] Y. S. Lee, A. Y. Kim, J. W. Choi et al., "Dysregulation of adipose glutathione peroxidase 3 in obesity contributes to local and systemic oxidative stress," *Molecular Endocrinology*, vol. 22, no. 9, pp. 2176–2189, 2008.

[61] M. Conrad, M. Schneider, A. Seiler, and G. W. Bornkamm, "Physiological role of phospholipid hydroperoxide glutathione peroxidase in mammals," *Biological Chemistry*, vol. 388, no. 10, pp. 1019–1025, 2007.

[62] C. L. Linster and E. van Schaftingen, "Vitamin C: biosynthesis, recycling and degradation in mammals," *The FEBS Journal*, vol. 274, no. 1, pp. 1–22, 2007.

[63] E. S. J. Arnér, "Focus on mammalian thioredoxin reductases—important selenoproteins with versatile functions," *Biochimica et Biophysica Acta*, vol. 1790, no. 6, pp. 495–526, 2009.

[64] M. A. Reeves and P. R. Hoffmann, "The human selenoproteome: recent insights into functions and regulation," *Cellular and Molecular Life Sciences*, vol. 66, no. 15, pp. 2457–2478, 2009.

[65] A. C. Bianco, D. Salvatore, B. Gereben, M. J. Berry, and P. R. Larsen, "Biochemistry, cellular and molecular biology, and physiological roles of the iodothyronine selenodeiodinases," *Endocrine Reviews*, vol. 23, no. 1, pp. 38–89, 2002.

[66] M. A. Reeves, F. P. Bellinger, and M. J. Berry, "The neuroprotective functions of selenoprotein M and its role in cytosolic calcium regulation," *Antioxidants and Redox Signaling*, vol. 12, no. 7, pp. 809–818, 2010.

[67] A. Dikiy, S. V. Novoselov, D. E. Fomenko et al., "SelT, SelW, SelH, and Rdx 12: genomics and molecular insights into the functions of selenoproteins of a novel thioredoxin-like family," *Biochemistry*, vol. 46, no. 23, pp. 6871–6882, 2007.

[68] J. Nordberg and E. S. J. Arnér, "Reactive oxygen species, antioxidants, and the mammalian thioredoxin system," *Free Radical Biology and Medicine*, vol. 31, no. 11, pp. 1287–1312, 2001.

[69] C. Jakupoglu, G. K. H. Przemeck, M. Schneider et al., "Cytoplasmic thioredoxin reductase is essential for embryogenesis but dispensable for cardiac development," *Molecular and Cellular Biology*, vol. 25, no. 5, pp. 1980–1988, 2005.

[70] M. Matsui, M. Oshima, H. Oshima et al., "Early embryonic lethality caused by targeted disruption of the mouse thioredoxin gene," *Developmental Biology*, vol. 178, no. 1, pp. 179–185, 1996.

[71] K. Anestål and E. S. J. Arnér, "Rapid induction of cell death by selenium-compromised thioredoxin reductase 1 but not by the fully active enzyme containing selenocysteine," *The Journal of Biological Chemistry*, vol. 278, no. 18, pp. 15966–15972, 2003.

[72] B. Corvilain, J. van Sande, E. Laurent, and J. E. Dumont, "The H_2O_2-generating system modulates protein iodination and the activity of the pentose phosphate pathway in dog thyroid," *Endocrinology*, vol. 128, no. 2, pp. 779–785, 1991.

[73] B. Corvilain, E. Laurent, M. Lecomte, J. van sande, and J. E. Dumont, "Role of the cyclic adenosine 3′,5′-monophosphate and the phosphatidylinositol-Ca_2^+ cascades in mediating the effects of thyrotropin and iodide on hormone synthesis and secretion in human thyroid slices," *The Journal of Clinical Endocrinology and Metabolism*, vol. 79, no. 1, pp. 152–159, 1994.

[74] U. Björkman and R. Ekholm, "Generation of H_2O_2 in isolated porcine thyroid follicles," *Endocrinology*, vol. 115, no. 1, pp. 392–398, 1984.

[75] S. Villette, G. Bermano, J. R. Arthur, and J. E. Hesketh, "Thyroid stimulating hormone and selenium supply interact to regulate selenoenzyme gene expression in thyroid cells (FRTL-5) in culture," *FEBS Letters*, vol. 438, no. 1-2, pp. 81–84, 1998.

[76] P. Zagrodzki, F. Nicol, M. A. McCoy et al., "Iodine deficiency in cattle: compensatory changes in thyroidal selenoenzymes," *Research in Veterinary Science*, vol. 64, no. 3, pp. 209–211, 1998.

[77] A. F. Howie, S. W. Walker, B. Akesson, J. R. Arthur, and G. J. Beckett, "Thyroidal extracellular glutathione peroxidase: a potential regulator of thyroid-hormone synthesis," *Biochemical Journal*, vol. 308, no. 3, pp. 713–717, 1995.

[78] A. F. Howie, J. R. Arthur, F. Nicol, S. W. Walker, S. G. Beech, and G. J. Beckett, "Identification of a 57-kilodalton selenoprotein in human thyrocytes as thioredoxin reductase and evidence that its expression is regulated through the calcium-phosphoinositol signaling pathway," *The Journal of Clinical Endocrinology and Metabolism*, vol. 83, no. 6, pp. 2052–2058, 1998.

[79] M. Oertel, R. O. Hesch, and J. Kohrle, "Expression of iodothyronine deiodinase in cultured thyroid cells," *Experimental and Clinical Endocrinology*, vol. 97, no. 2-3, pp. 182–186, 1991.

[80] R. Schreck, F. Schnieders, C. Schmutzler, and J. Kohrle, "Retinoids stimulate type I iodothyronine 5′-deiodinase activity in human follicular thyroid carcinoma cell lines," *The Journal of Clinical Endocrinology and Metabolism*, vol. 79, no. 3, pp. 791–798, 1994.

[81] S. G. Beech, S. W. Walker, A. M. Dorrance et al., "The role of thyroidal type-I iodothyronine deiodinase in tri-iodothyronine production by human and sheep thyrocytes in primary culture," *The Journal of Endocrinology*, vol. 136, no. 3, pp. 361–370, 1993.

[82] S. G. Beech, S. W. Walker, G. J. Beckett, J. R. Arthur, F. Nicol, and D. Lee, "Effect of selenium depletion on thyroidal type-I iodothyronine deiodinase activity in isolated human thyrocytes and rat thyroid and liver," *Analyst*, vol. 120, no. 3, pp. 827–831, 1995.

[83] G. Bermano, F. Nicol, J. A. Dyer et al., "Tissue-specific regulation of selenoenzyme gene expression during selenium deficiency in rats," *Biochemical Journal*, vol. 311, no. 2, pp. 425–430, 1995.

[84] A. Demelash, J.-O. Karlsson, M. Nilsson, and U. Björkman, "Selenium has a protective role in caspase-3-dependent apoptosis induced by H_2O_2 in primary cultured pig thyrocytes,"

European Journal of Endocrinology, vol. 150, no. 6, pp. 841–849, 2004.

[85] E. K. Wirth, M. Conrad, J. Winterer et al., "Neuronal selenoprotein expression is required for interneuron development and prevents seizures and neurodegeneration," *The FASEB Journal*, vol. 24, no. 3, pp. 844–852, 2010.

[86] M. Bartos, I. Vida, and P. Jonas, "Synaptic mechanisms of synchronized gamma oscillations in inhibitory interneuron networks," *Nature Reviews Neuroscience*, vol. 8, no. 1, pp. 45–56, 2007.

[87] J. de Almeida and G. Mengod, "D2 and D4 dopamine receptor mRNA distribution in pyramidal neurons and GABAergic subpopulations in monkey prefrontal cortex: implications for schizophrenia treatment," *Neuroscience*, vol. 170, no. 4, pp. 1133–1139, 2010.

[88] J. M. Swanson, M. Kinsbourne, J. Nigg et al., "Etiologic subtypes of attention-deficit/hyperactivity disorder: brain imaging, molecular genetic and environmental factors and the dopamine hypothesis," *Neuropsychology Review*, vol. 17, no. 1, pp. 39–59, 2007.

[89] J.-H. Cabungcal, D. Nicolas, R. Kraftsik, M. Cuénod, K. Q. Do, and J.-P. Hornung, "Glutathione deficit during development induces anomalies in the rat anterior cingulate GABAergic neurons: relevance to schizophrenia," *Neurobiology of Disease*, vol. 22, no. 3, pp. 624–637, 2006.

[90] P. Steullet, J.-H. Cabungcal, A. Kulak et al., "Redox dysregulation affects the ventral but not dorsal hippocampus: impairment of parvalbumin neurons, gamma oscillations, and related behaviors," *The Journal of Neuroscience*, vol. 30, no. 7, pp. 2547–2558, 2010.

[91] V. A. Shchedrina, Y. Zhang, V. M. Labunskyy, D. L. Hatfield, and V. N. Gladyshev, "Structure—function relations, physiological roles, and evolution of mammalian ER-resident selenoproteins," *Antioxidants and Redox Signaling*, vol. 12, no. 7, pp. 839–849, 2010.

[92] L. Schomburg, U. Schweizer, B. Holtmann, L. Flohé, M. Sendtner, and J. Köhrle, "Gene disruption discloses role of selenoprotein P in selenium delivery to target tissues," *Biochemical Journal*, vol. 370, no. 2, pp. 397–402, 2003.

[93] K. E. Hill, J. Zhou, W. J. McMahan et al., "Deletion of selenoprotein P alters distribution of selenium in the mouse," *The Journal of Biological Chemistry*, vol. 278, no. 16, pp. 13640–13646, 2003.

[94] Y. Zhang, Y. Zhou, U. Schweizer et al., "Comparative analysis of selenocysteine machinery and selenoproteome gene expression in mouse brain identifies neurons as key functional sites of selenium in mammals," *The Journal of Biological Chemistry*, vol. 283, no. 4, pp. 2427–2438, 2008.

[95] K. E. Hill, J. Zhou, W. J. McMahan, A. K. Motley, and R. F. Burk, "Neurological dysfunction occurs in mice with targeted deletion of the selenoprotein P gene," *The Journal of Nutrition*, vol. 134, no. 1, pp. 157–161, 2004.

[96] R. A. Sunde, A. M. Raines, K. M. Barnes, and J. K. Evenson, "Selenium status highly regulates selenoprotein mRNA levels for only a subset of the selenoproteins in the selenoproteome," *Bioscience Reports*, vol. 29, no. 5, pp. 329–338, 2009.

[97] M. Scharpf, U. Schweizer, T. Arzberger, W. Roggendorf, L. Schomburg, and J. Köhrle, "Neuronal and ependymal expression of selenoprotein P in the human brain," *Journal of Neural Transmission*, vol. 114, no. 7, pp. 877–884, 2007.

[98] I. Kazanis and C. Ffrench-Constant, "The number of stem cells in the subependymal zone of the adult rodent brain is correlated with the number of ependymal cells and not with the volume of the niche," *Stem Cells and Development*, vol. 21, no. 7, pp. 1090–1096, 2012.

[99] M. Pérez-Martín, M. Cifuentes, J. M. Grondona et al., "IGF-I stimulates neurogenesis in the hypothalamus of adult rats," *European Journal of Neuroscience*, vol. 31, no. 9, pp. 1533–1548, 2010.

[100] G. E. Olson, V. P. Winfrey, S. K. NagDas, K. E. Hill, and R. F. Burk, "Apolipoprotein E receptor-2 (ApoER2) mediates selenium uptake from selenoprotein P by the mouse testis," *The Journal of Biological Chemistry*, vol. 282, no. 16, pp. 12290–12297, 2007.

[101] R. F. Burk, K. E. Hill, G. E. Olson et al., "Deletion of apolipoprotein E receptor-2 in mice lowers brain selenium and causes severe neurological dysfunction and death when a low-selenium diet is fed," *The Journal of Neuroscience*, vol. 27, no. 23, pp. 6207–6211, 2007.

[102] N. Hodgson, M. Trivedi, C. Muratore, S. Li, and R. Deth, "Soluble oligomers of amyloid-β cause changes in redox state, DNA methylation, and gene transcription by inhibiting EAAT3 mediated cysteine uptake," *Journal of Alzheimer's Disease*, vol. 36, pp. 197–209, 2013.

[103] A. Bailey, A. Le Couteur, I. Gottesman et al., "Autism as a strongly genetic disorder: evidence from a British twin study," *Psychological Medicine*, vol. 25, no. 1, pp. 63–77, 1995.

[104] R. S. E. Hurley, M. Losh, M. Parlier, J. S. Reznick, and J. Piven, "The broad autism phenotype questionnaire," *Journal of Autism and Developmental Disorders*, vol. 37, no. 9, pp. 1679–1690, 2007.

[105] J. N. Constantino and R. D. Todd, "Intergenerational transmission of subthreshold autistic traits in the general population," *Biological Psychiatry*, vol. 57, no. 6, pp. 655–660, 2005.

[106] S. Jamain, H. Quach, C. Betancur et al., "Mutations of the X-linked genes encoding neuroligins NLGN3 and NLGN4 are associated with autism," *Nature Genetics*, vol. 34, no. 1, pp. 27–29, 2003.

[107] C. M. Durand, C. Betancur, T. M. Boeckers et al., "Mutations in the gene encoding the synaptic scaffolding protein SHANK3 are associated with autism spectrum disorders," *Nature Genetics*, vol. 39, no. 1, pp. 25–27, 2007.

[108] J. Sebat, B. Lakshmi, D. Malhotra et al., "Strong association of de novo copy number mutations with autism," *Science*, vol. 316, no. 5823, pp. 445–449, 2007.

[109] C. R. Marshall, A. Noor, J. B. Vincent et al., "Structural variation of chromosomes in autism spectrum disorder," *The American Journal of Human Genetics*, vol. 82, no. 2, pp. 477–488, 2008.

[110] L. A. Weiss, D. E. Arking, Gene Discovery Project of Johns Hopkins & the Autism Consortium, M. J. Daly, and A. Chakravarti, "A genome-wide linkage and association scan reveals novel loci for autism," *Nature*, vol. 461, no. 7265, pp. 802–808, 2009.

[111] L. A. Weiss, Y. Shen, J. M. Korn et al., "Association between microdeletion and microduplication at 16p11.2 and autism," *The New England Journal of Medicine*, vol. 358, no. 7, pp. 667–675, 2008.

[112] R. A. Kumar, S. Karamohamed, J. Sudi et al., "Recurrent 16p11.2 microdeletions in autism," *Human Molecular Genetics*, vol. 17, no. 4, pp. 628–638, 2008.

[113] K. Wang, H. Zhang, D. Ma et al., "Common genetic variants on 5p14.1 associate with autism spectrum disorders," *Nature*, vol. 459, no. 7246, pp. 528–533, 2009.

[114] B. A. Fernandez, W. Roberts, B. Chung et al., "Phenotypic spectrum associated with de novo and inherited deletions and

duplications at 16p11.2 in individuals ascertained for diagnosis of autism spectrum disorder," *Journal of Medical Genetics*, vol. 47, no. 3, pp. 195–203, 2010.

[115] J. T. Glessner, K. Wang, G. Cai et al., "Autism genome-wide copy number variation reveals ubiquitin and neuronal genes," *Nature*, vol. 459, no. 7246, pp. 569–572, 2009.

[116] D. Pinto, A. T. Pagnamenta, L. Klei, R. Anney, D. Merico, R. Regan et al., "Functional impact of global rare copy number variation in autism," *Nature*, vol. 466, no. 7304, pp. 368–372, 2010.

[117] B. Devlin, N. Melhem, and K. Roeder, "Do common variants play a role in risk for autism? Evidence and theoretical musings," *Brain Research*, vol. 1380, pp. 78–84, 2011.

[118] J. Hallmayer, S. Cleveland, A. Torres et al., "Genetic heritability and shared environmental factors among twin pairs with autism," *Archives of General Psychiatry*, vol. 68, no. 11, pp. 1095–1102, 2011.

[119] F. J. Serajee, R. Nabi, H. Zhong, and A. H. M. M. Huq, "Polymorphisms in xenobiotic metabolism genes and autism," *Journal of Child Neurology*, vol. 19, no. 6, pp. 413–417, 2004.

[120] S. P. Paşca, B. Nemeş, L. Vlase et al., "High levels of homocysteine and low serum paraoxonase 1 arylesterase activity in children with autism," *Life Sciences*, vol. 78, no. 19, pp. 2244–2248, 2006.

[121] X. Ming, W. G. Johnson, E. S. Stenroos, A. Mars, G. H. Lambert, and S. Buyske, "Genetic variant of glutathione peroxidase 1 in autism," *Brain and Development*, vol. 32, no. 2, pp. 105–109, 2010.

[122] T. A. Williams, A. E. Mars, S. G. Buyske et al., "Risk of autistic disorder in affected offspring of mothers with a glutathione S-transferase P1 haplotype," *Archives of Pediatrics and Adolescent Medicine*, vol. 161, no. 4, pp. 356–361, 2007.

[123] A. K. Merikangas, A. P. Corvin, and L. Gallagher, "Copy-number variants in neurodevelopmental disorders: promises and challenges," *Trends in Genetics*, vol. 25, no. 12, pp. 536–544, 2009.

[124] C. Guerrero-Bosagna, M. Settles, B. Lucker, and M. K. Skinner, "Epigenetic transgenerational actions of vinclozolin on promoter regions of the sperm epigenome," *PLoS ONE*, vol. 5, no. 9, Article ID e13100, 2010.

[125] J. Andrews, W. Kennette, J. Pilon et al., "Multi-platform whole-genome microarray analyses refine the epigenetic signature of breast cancer metastasis with gene expression and copy number," *PLoS ONE*, vol. 5, no. 1, Article ID e8665, 2010.

[126] J. R. McCarrey, "The epigenome as a target for heritable environmental disruptions of cellular function," *Molecular and Cellular Endocrinology*, vol. 354, no. 1-2, pp. 9–15, 2012.

[127] C. Murgatroyd and D. Spengler, "Epigenetics of early child development," *Frontiers in Psychiatry*, vol. 2, article 16, 2011.

[128] M. K. Skinner, M. Manikkam, and C. Guerrero-Bosagna, "Epigenetic transgenerational actions of endocrine disruptors," *Reproductive Toxicology*, vol. 31, no. 3, pp. 337–343, 2011.

[129] C. R. Beck, J. L. Garcia-Perez, R. M. Badge, and J. V. Moran, "LINE-1 elements in structural variation and disease," *Annual Review of Genomics and Human Genetics*, vol. 12, pp. 187–215, 2011.

[130] A. R. Muotri, M. C. N. Marchetto, N. G. Coufal et al., "L1 retrotransposition in neurons is modulated by MeCP2," *Nature*, vol. 468, no. 7322, pp. 443–446, 2010.

[131] S. M. Wernimont, A. G. Clark, P. J. Stover et al., "Folate network genetic variation, plasma homocysteine, and global genomic methylation content: a genetic association study," *BMC Medical Genetics*, vol. 12, article 150, 2011.

[132] T. Singer, M. J. McConnell, M. C. N. Marchetto, N. G. Coufal, and F. H. Gage, "LINE-1 retrotransposons: mediators of somatic variation in neuronal genomes?" *Trends in Neurosciences*, vol. 33, no. 8, pp. 345–354, 2010.

[133] T. Buie, D. B. Campbell, G. J. Fuchs III et al., "Evaluation, diagnosis, and treatment of gastrointestinal disorders in individuals with ASDs: a consensus report," *Pediatrics*, vol. 125, no. 1, supplement, pp. S1–S18, 2010.

[134] D. A. Rossignol and R. E. Frye, "A review of research trends in physiological abnormalities in autism spectrum disorders: immune dysregulation, inflammation, oxidative stress, mitochondrial dysfunction and environmental toxicant exposures," *Molecular Psychiatry*, vol. 17, no. 4, pp. 389–401, 2012.

[135] C. C. Y. Wong, E. L. Meaburn, A. Ronald et al., "Methylomic analysis of monozygotic twins discordant for autism spectrum disorder and related behavioural traits," *Molecular Psychiatry*, 2013.

[136] Y.-H. Jiang, T.-F. Tsai, J. Bressler, and A. L. Beaudet, "Imprinting in Angelman and Prader-Willi syndromes," *Current Opinion in Genetics and Development*, vol. 8, no. 3, pp. 334–342, 1998.

[137] T. Bienvenu and J. Chelly, "Molecular genetics of Rett syndrome: when DNA methylation goes unrecognized," *Nature Reviews Genetics*, vol. 7, no. 6, pp. 415–426, 2006.

[138] N. Dolzhanskaya, G. Merz, J. M. Aletta, and R. B. Denman, "Methylation regulates the intracellular protein-protein and protein-RNA interactions of FMRP," *Journal of Cell Science*, vol. 119, no. 9, pp. 1933–1946, 2006.

[139] P. D. Whanger, "Selenium and the brain: a review," *Nutritional Neuroscience*, vol. 4, no. 2, pp. 81–97, 2001.

[140] N. V. C. Ralston and L. J. Raymond, "Dietary selenium's protective effects against methylmercury toxicity," *Toxicology*, vol. 278, no. 1, pp. 112–123, 2010.

[141] C. M. L. Carvalho, E.-H. Chew, S. I. Hashemy, J. Lu, and A. Holmgren, "Inhibition of the human thioredoxin system: a molecular mechanism of mercury toxicity," *The Journal of Biological Chemistry*, vol. 283, no. 18, pp. 11913–11923, 2008.

[142] A. P. Neal and T. R. Guilarte, "Mechanisms of lead and manganese neurotoxicity," *Toxicology Research*, no. 2, pp. 99–114, 2013.

[143] J. K. Kern, B. D. Grannemann, M. H. Trivedi, and J. B. Adams, "Sulfhydryl-reactive metals in autism," *Journal of Toxicology and Environmental Health A*, vol. 70, no. 8, pp. 715–721, 2007.

[144] M. E. Obrenovich, R. J. Shamberger, and D. Lonsdale, "Altered heavy metals and transketolase found in autistic spectrum disorder," *Biological Trace Element Research*, vol. 144, no. 1–3, pp. 475–486, 2011.

[145] A. S. Holmes, M. F. Blaxill, and B. E. Haley, "Reduced levels of mercury in first baby haircuts of autistic children," *International Journal of Toxicology*, vol. 22, no. 4, pp. 277–285, 2003.

[146] M. D. Majewska, E. Urbanowicz, P. Rok-Bujko, I. Namysłowska, and P. Mierzejewski, "Age-dependent lower or higher levels of hair mercury in autistic children than in healthy controls," *Acta Neurobiologiae Experimentalis*, vol. 70, no. 2, pp. 196–208, 2010.

[147] I. Hertz-Picciotto, P. G. Green, L. Delwiche, R. Hansen, C. Walker, and I. N. Pessah, "Blood mercury concentrations in CHARGE study children with and without autism," *Environmental Health Perspectives*, vol. 118, no. 1, pp. 161–166, 2010.

[148] S. E. Owens, M. L. Summar, K. K. Ryckman et al., "Lack of association between autism and four heavy metal regulatory genes," *NeuroToxicology*, vol. 32, no. 6, pp. 769–775, 2011.

[149] B. Stamova, P. G. Green, Y. Tian et al., "Correlations between gene expression and mercury levels in blood of boys with and without autism," *Neurotoxicity Research*, vol. 19, no. 1, pp. 31–48, 2011.

[150] Y. Arai, J. Ohgane, S. Yagi et al., "Epigenetic assessment of environmental chemicals detected in maternal peripheral and cord blood samples," *The Journal of Reproduction and Development*, vol. 57, no. 4, pp. 507–517, 2011.

[151] T. C. Stummann, L. Hareng, and S. Bremer, "Hazard assessment of methylmercury toxicity to neuronal induction in embryogenesis using human embryonic stem cells," *Toxicology*, vol. 257, no. 3, pp. 117–126, 2009.

[152] C. Tamm, J. Duckworth, O. Hermanson, and S. Ceccatelli, "High susceptibility of neural stem cells to methylmercury toxicity: effects on cell survival and neuronal differentiation," *Journal of Neurochemistry*, vol. 97, no. 1, pp. 69–78, 2006.

[153] S. Bernard, A. Enayati, L. Redwood, H. Roger, and T. Binstock, "Autism: a novel form of mercury poisoning," *Medical Hypotheses*, vol. 56, no. 4, pp. 462–471, 2001.

[154] J. G. Dórea, "Making sense of epidemiological studies of young children exposed to thimerosal in vaccines," *Clinica Chimica Acta*, vol. 411, no. 21-22, pp. 1580–1586, 2010.

[155] D. A. Geier, B. S. Hooker, J. K. Kern, P. G. King, L. K. Sykes, and M. R. Geier, "A two-phase study evaluating the relationship between Thimerosal-containing vaccine administration and the risk for an autism spectrum disorder diagnosis in the United States," *Translational Neurodegeneration*, vol. 2, no. 1, article 25, 2013.

[156] C. M. Gallagher and M. S. Goodman, "Hepatitis B vaccination of male neonates and autism diagnosis, NHIS 1997–2002," *Journal of Toxicology and Environmental Health A*, vol. 73, no. 24, pp. 1665–1677, 2010.

[157] R. Schechter and J. K. Grether, "Continuing increases in autism reported to California's developmental services system: mercury in retrograde," *Archives of General Psychiatry*, vol. 65, no. 1, pp. 19–24, 2008.

[158] S. T. Schultz, H. S. Klonoff-Cohen, D. L. Wingard, N. A. Akshoomoff, C. A. Macera, and J. Ming, "Acetaminophen (paracetamol) use, measles-mumps-rubella vaccination, and autistic disorder: the results of a parent survey," *Autism*, vol. 12, no. 3, pp. 293–307, 2008.

[159] C. S. Price, W. W. Thompson, B. Goodson et al., "Prenatal and infant exposure to thimerosal from vaccines and immunoglobulins and risk of autism," *Pediatrics*, vol. 126, no. 4, pp. 656–664, 2010.

[160] D. M. Walker and A. C. Gore, "Transgenerational neuroendocrine disruption of reproduction," *Nature Reviews Endocrinology*, vol. 7, no. 4, pp. 197–207, 2011.

[161] O. Yorbik, A. Sayal, C. Akay, D. I. Akbiyik, and T. Sohmen, "Investigation of antioxidant enzymes in children with autistic disorder," *Prostaglandins Leukotrienes and Essential Fatty Acids*, vol. 67, no. 5, pp. 341–343, 2002.

[162] N. A. Meguid, A. A. Dardir, E. R. Abdel-Raouf, and A. Hashish, "Evaluation of oxidative stress in autism: defective antioxidant enzymes and increased lipid peroxidation," *Biological Trace Element Research*, vol. 143, no. 1, pp. 58–65, 2011.

[163] J. Castañeda, P. Genzor, and A. Bortvin, "PiRNAs, transposon silencing, and germline genome integrity," *Mutation Research*, vol. 714, no. 1-2, pp. 95–104, 2011.

[164] O. Gokcumen, P. L. Babb, R. C. Iskow et al., "Refinement of primate copy number variation hotspots identifies candidate genomic regions evolving under positive selection," *Genome Biology*, vol. 12, no. 5, article R52, 2011.

[165] J. Li, R. A. Harris, S. W. Cheung et al., "Genomic hypomethylation in the human germline associates with selective structural mutability in the human genome," *PLoS Genetics*, vol. 8, no. 5, Article ID e1002692, 2012.

[166] R. C. Iskow, M. T. McCabe, R. E. Mills et al., "Natural mutagenesis of human genomes by endogenous retrotransposons," *Cell*, vol. 141, no. 7, pp. 1253–1261, 2010.

[167] R. M. LoPachin and D. S. Barber, "Synaptic cysteine sulfhydryl groups as targets of electrophilic neurotoxicants," *Toxicological Sciences*, vol. 94, no. 2, pp. 240–255, 2006.

[168] L. J. Chun, M. J. Tong, R. W. Busuttil, and J. R. Hiatt, "Acetaminophen hepatotoxicity and acute liver failure," *Journal of Clinical Gastroenterology*, vol. 43, no. 4, pp. 342–349, 2009.

[169] S. T. Schultz, "Does thimerosal or other mercury exposure increase the risk for autism? A review of current literature," *Acta Neurobiologiae Experimentalis*, vol. 70, no. 2, pp. 187–195, 2010.

[170] P. Good, "Did acetaminophen provoke the autism epidemic?" *Alternative Medicine Review*, vol. 14, no. 4, pp. 364–372, 2009.

[171] N. R. Pumford, B. M. Martin, and J. A. Hinson, "A metabolite of acetaminophen covalently binds to the 56 kDa selenium binding protein," *Biochemical and Biophysical Research Communications*, vol. 182, no. 3, pp. 1348–1355, 1992.

[172] D. J. Hoivik, J. E. Manautou, A. Tveit, D. C. Mankowski, E. A. Khairallah, and S. D. Cohen, "Evidence suggesting the 58-kDa acetaminophen binding protein is a preferential target for acetaminophen electrophile," *Fundamental and Applied Toxicology*, vol. 32, no. 1, pp. 79–86, 1996.

[173] T. Ishida, M. Abe, K. Oguri, and H. Yamada, "Enhancement of acetaminophen cytotoxicity in selenium-binding protein-overexpressed COS-1 cells," *Drug Metabolism and Pharmacokinetics*, vol. 19, no. 4, pp. 290–296, 2004.

[174] J. Mattow, I. Demuth, G. Haeselbarth, P. R. Jungblut, and J. Klose, "Selenium-binding protein 2, the major hepatic target for acetaminophen, shows sex differences in protein abundance," *Electrophoresis*, vol. 27, no. 8, pp. 1683–1691, 2006.

[175] Y. Masubuchi, J. Nakayama, and Y. Watanabe, "Sex difference in susceptibility to acetaminophen hepatotoxicity is reversed by buthionine sulfoximine," *Toxicology*, vol. 287, no. 1–3, pp. 54–60, 2011.

[176] K. J. Heard, "Acetylcysteine for acetaminophen poisoning," *The New England Journal of Medicine*, vol. 359, no. 3, pp. 285–292, 2008.

25

Autistic Traits Affect P300 Response to Unexpected Events, regardless of Mental State Inferences

Mitsuhiko Ishikawa,[1] Shoji Itakura,[1] and Hiroki C. Tanabe[2]

[1] *Graduate School of Letters, Kyoto University, Kyoto, Japan*
[2] *Graduate School of Environmental Studies, Nagoya University, Nagoya, Japan*

Correspondence should be addressed to Mitsuhiko Ishikawa; ishikawa.mitsuhiko.23r@st.kyoto-u.ac.jp

Academic Editor: Robert F. Berman

Limited use of contextual information has been suggested as a way of understanding cognition in people with autism spectrum disorder (ASD). However, it has also been argued that individuals with ASD may have difficulties inferring others' mental states. Here, we examined how individuals with different levels of autistic traits respond to contextual deviations by measuring event-related potentials that reflect context usage. The Autism Spectrum Quotient (AQ) was used to quantify autistic-like traits in 28 university students, and 19 participants were defined as Low or High AQ groups. To additionally examine inferences about mental state, two belief conditions (with or without false belief) were included. Participants read short stories in which the final sentence included either an expected or an unexpected word and rated the word's degree of deviation from expectation. P300 waveform analysis revealed that unexpected words were associated with larger P300 waveforms for the Low AQ group, but smaller P300 responses in the High AQ group. Additionally, AQ social skill subscores were positively correlated with evaluation times in the Unexpected condition, whether a character's belief was false or not. This suggests that autistic traits can affect responses to unexpected events, possibly because of decreased availability of context information.

1. Introduction

There is a general assumption that, in order to interact with and have smooth relationships with others in society, one must master certain social behaviors such as empathizing with others, understanding humour, seeing through lies, and comprehending ironies. A diagnosis of autism spectrum disorder (ASD) indicates difficulties with these social behaviors, which are required for understanding others' beliefs, desires, and intentions (termed "theory of mind" [1]).

It has been argued that the foundation of social difficulties may be the absence of a theory of mind [2]. However, Happé [3] revealed that children with ASD can obtain a theory of mind, albeit with some developmental delay. Subsequently, explanations for problems associated with ASD began to focus on the ways that theory of mind is used in social situations. One such explanation involves the idea of context blindness [4], which, for people with ASD, refers to difficulties with the spontaneous use of context in social situations. For instance, to accurately appraise emotions based on another person's facial expressions, we must think about contextual information, such as the events affecting or surrounding the person. Additionally, understanding irony and sarcasm depends heavily on context. There is an example in the Strange Stories test that assesses theory of mind [4]: Emma takes a banana, holds it against her ear, and then says "Look, this banana is a telephone!" In this story, what Emma said is not literally true, but we can understand through context that it is about pretending. Therefore, the use of theory of mind in social situations may be related to the spontaneous use of contextual information.

For the purposes of the context blindness hypothesis, context is defined as not only the flow of linguistic information, but also any type of global information, including that based on visual perceptual. The first global hypothesis states that weak central coherence (WCC [5, 6]) explains deficits in the use of global information in people with ASD. This theory asserts that people with ASD are not inclined to perceive stimuli as a coherent "big picture." WCC has been examined in some tasks measuring the use of visual and linguistic global information. One of the best known WCC tasks is called the Embedded Figures Test, which requires detection of target shapes within complex big pictures, so it can be expected that individuals with ASD perform better on such a task. Notably, it has been reported that linguistic central coherence was associated with performance in a theory of mind assessment that uses a second-order false-belief task. However, performance on a visual central coherence task was unaffected [7].

The use of linguistic context has also been examined in many studies. Pijnacker et al. [8] conducted an ERP study that examined contextual processing in people with ASD. They found that the N400 component, beginning at 400 ms after stimulus, was diminished in people with ASD compared with their typically developing peers. The N400 is the negative component that reflects semantic language processing, and many studies have reported that the typical N400 can be evoked when semantic deviation in a sentence is recognised [9–11]. Pijnacker et al. [8] argued that people with ASD may show a diminished response to deviation from context. One possible explanation of such a difference is that there is a deficit in the use of context.

The P300 component has also been examined in relation to the cognitive functioning reflected in the N400 [9, 10]. The P300 component had initially been assumed to be related to the recognition of unexpected stimuli [12]. In other words, the P300 can reflect recognition of a violation of expectancy, such that it has been observed in many cognitive tasks such as the oddball task, in which presentation of a so-called "target" or "rare" stimuli randomly mixed with nontarget (to be ignored) distractors. The P300 Speller is one of the most known paradigms used in the Brain Computer Interface [13]. The P300 Speller presents 6 rows and 6 columns containing the set of the characters including an item attended by the observer described as the rare set and the others described as the frequent set [14]. Participants need to focus on one of the items and the sequence of 12 flashes is used to detect the item attended by the observer. In this paradigm, flashing items from the rare set will elicit the P300 component because that is rare event in the context of other flashes. The P300 response is thought to be a positive component that reflects contextual and semantic processing. This component occurs approximately 300–500 ms after stimulus over parietal regions [15].

The oddball paradigm requires only a simple response and comprises relatively simple stimuli, but the P300 response has also been shown during more complex cognitive tasks. For instance, Meinhardt et al. [16] examined the ERP response upon seeing a character acting in either a belief-congruent or belief-incongruent way and found a stronger P300 response in the belief-incongruent condition. The authors suggested from this result that the P300 response could reflect the updating of "a mental model of the environment" and that the P300 amplitude reflects the unexpectedness of the eliciting event. Dunn et al. [17] used ERP to examine how autistic children were influenced by global semantic context. They found that reduced P300 responses were observed in autistic children compared to typically developing children when the target words expected from context were present. Therefore, this diminished P300 response in autistic children may reflect the contextual processing of linguistics.

Recently, the false-belief task was used in a violation-of-expectancy paradigm [18]. The false-belief task requires people to anticipate what a character will do next, which is possible if they have theory of mind and if they understand false belief. Senju et al. [18] reported that people with ASD showed reduced looking times when the character in the false-belief task acted unexpectedly, and they therefore suggested that people with ASD have difficulty using theory of mind spontaneously. However, as mentioned, people with ASD can show deficits in their use of contextual information. Recent theoretical works suggest that autistic behavioral traits can be explained by deficits in forming predictions and processing unexpected events [19–21]. Dungan et al. [22] also suggested the possibility that autistic traits influence how unexpected events are processed, primarily according to context. By measuring the P300, it is possible to know participants' degree of certainty in their predictions from context.

It has been asserted that people without a diagnosis of ASD but showing highly autistic traits may have a similar cognitive style to those with a formal diagnosis and may also experience similar difficulties in social relationships [23]. However, there are many confounding factors in people diagnosed with ASD, including language impairment and sensory hypersensitivity [24], factors that typically have less impact for typically developing people with autistic traits. We focused only on the relationship between individual social difficulties and the processing of contextual information, such that typical university students without a diagnosis were recruited.

Here, we examined whether individuals high in such traits have difficulty using context or thinking about others' mental states. If autistic people are deficient at using context, the P300 component should decrease when a character acts unexpectedly relative to contextual information, and this should occur with or without belief understanding (i.e., use of theory of mind). However, if autistic people show a specific difficulty in apprehending false beliefs and unmet expectations regarding others' mental states, the P300 should decrease only in the unexpected belief condition.

2. Materials and Methods

2.1. Participants. Twenty-eight university students (15 males and 13 females; age = 19.9±0.8 years) were randomly recruited for this study. All participants spoke Japanese as their first language. The mean Autism Spectrum Quotient (AQ) Japanese version [25] score was 21.89 (range: 10–39, SD = 6.61). This average score is similar to that obtained in other studies that examined the AQ in nonautistic Japanese populations [23]. There was no difference between males (range: 10–39; mean AQ = 21.92; SD = 8.37) and females (range: 11–28; mean AQ = 21.85; SD = 4.537) in AQ total scores. For the AQ, a score of 22 or above is indicative of the broader autism phenotype (subclinical expression of behaviors characteristic of ASD [26]).

Table 1: Examples of stimulus sentences (target words are italicized).

Condition	Context	Last sentence
Belief-Expected	Sally and Anne are in a room. Sally puts a marble inside the blue box While Sally is away Anne takes the marble from the box and puts inside the red box Then Sally comes back to the room	Sally looks for her marble in the *blue* box
Belief-Unexpected	Sally and Anne are in a room. Sally puts a marble inside the blue box While Sally is away Anne takes the marble from the box and puts inside the red box Then Sally comes back to the room	Sally looks for her marble in the *red* box
No-belief-Expected	Mark wakes up at six. Then he washes his face While Mark washes his face his mother put his breakfast on a table Mark comes to the dining room	After that Mark *pours* a cup of milk
No-belief-Unexpected	Mark wakes up at six. Then he washes his face While Mark washes his face his mother put his breakfast on a table Mark comes to the dining room	After that Mark *burns* a cup of milk

Prior to analysis, the experimental data were screened for univariate outliers (deviation scores that were more than two standard deviations from the mean) and as a result, one participant was excluded from analysis because this participant did not appear to understand the item content. In studies of autistic traits, it is common to use data only from participants who scored extremely high or extremely low on the AQ (e.g., [27]). To examine group differences, participants were divided into High AQ and Low AQ groups according to the frequency distribution of scores, and around 10 participants from the top and bottom of the AQ score distribution were extracted. The High and Low AQ groups comprised 10 and 9 participants, respectively (score range: 23–33, 4 males, mean AQ_{High} = 27.00, and SD = 3.46; score range: 10–19, 5 males, mean AQ_{Low} = 15.33, and SD = 3.57). As mentioned, there was no gender difference in AQ scores in this study, and we therefore did not further analyse this variable.

All participants were naïve to the purpose of this study, and all reported normal or corrected-to-normal vision. In this study, participants were told that the AQ questionnaire just measures personality traits, and AQ test was done only once. The protocol was approved by the ethical committee of the Psychology Department, Faculty of Letters, Nagoya University, Nagoya, Japan. All participants give their written informed consent to participate in the study.

2.2. Apparatus. Visual stimuli were presented through a RDT231WM-X monitor (Mitsubishi, Japan) and were controlled by PsychoPy version 1.83 [28]. EEG data were collected using BrainAmp-DC and ActiCap with 32 channels (Brain Products, Munich, Germany) at standard locations following the extended 10/20 international system referenced to the nose and grounded to the forehead. The sampling rate was 500 Hz, and the impedance was kept below 25 kΩ. The EEG filtering parameter was set to dc-to-70 Hz (12 dB/oct). All EEG data were recorded in a soundproof room using Brain Vision Recorder software from Brain Products.

2.3. Stimuli and Conditions. All our stimuli were presented visually. We set up four conditions for stories: No-belief-Expected; No-belief-Unexpected; Belief-Expected; and Belief-Unexpected. All stories comprised five 5-Japanese-word sentences (e.g., サリーと/アンの/2人が/部屋に/います), four sentences of which provided contextual information and the last sentence provided target words. The visual presentation of a "target word," centered on the monitor, was the ERP onset and determined whether the condition was expected or unexpected. In the Belief conditions (Table 1), two characters were first introduced, and one character placed an object in a given location. A second character was then described as moving the object to a new location. This action was missed by the first character, who initially placed the object. The first character then goes to retrieve the object. In the expected conditions, the first character looks for the object where he or she initially placed it. In the unexpected conditions, the first character looks where the second character placed the object. Additionally, in the No-belief conditions (Table 1), two characters are also introduced, but there is no mental state to infer; the characters are simply described as performing actions in daily situations. Each of the four conditions (Belief-Expected, Belief-Unexpected, No-belief-Expected, and No-belief-Unexpected) was composed of 40 trials, and different sentences were presented for each trial. All sentences were selected from the preliminary test. In the preliminary test, participants were required to evaluate how much the target words were predictable from the story's contextual flow, using a 5-point scale for which only the end anchor points (1 = unpredictable and 5 = predictable) were defined. Unexpected sentences were selected from sentences scored under 3 points; on the other hand, Expected sentences were selected from sentences scored over 3 points.

2.4. Assessment. The Japanese version of the AQ [25] was used to measure autistic traits. It comprises 50 items that assess five different areas, with 10 items each: social skills (e.g., finding social situations easy), attention switching (e.g., feeling anxious in new situations), attention to detail (e.g., noticing patterns in things all the time), communication (e.g., enjoying social chit-chat), and imagination (e.g., making up stories easily). Participants were required to choose one of four options (1 = "definitely agree," 2 = "slightly agree," 3 = "slightly disagree," and 4 = "definitely disagree"), and each of the item is scored 1 point if the respondent provides an abnormal response, whether mild or strong. The total score for a participant is hereafter known as the AQ score.

2.5. Procedure. After completing the questionnaire, participants performed 160 trials reading different stories, with 40 trials per condition, presented in a random order. Viewing distance was about 60 cm and each Japanese character was about 2° in width and height. All words were presented in a black on white format. The first four sentences of a story were presented initially to provide contextual information. Participants were required to read them once and push the "Enter" key after they understood what was happening in each situation. Next, after the blank (500 ms) and the fixation cross (500 ms) were presented, the last sentence was presented word by word (300 ms each with 200 ms blank), and target word was set to the third word, after 2000 ms from "Enter" key press, across all conditions. Because EEG recordings are affected by participants' fatigue (e.g., body movements), to shorten the experimental time, the remaining words appeared together after the target words were presented for 1500 ms. After the remaining words were presented, participants were required to evaluate how much the last sentence deviated from the story's contextual flow (i.e., they were instructed to rate how much the ending of the story deviated from the rest of the story) as soon as possible, using a 5-point scale for which only the end anchor points (1 = no deviation and 5 = high deviation) were defined. After all tasks were completed, participants were told the purpose of the study. The whole experiment took about 90 minutes.

3. Results

3.1. EEG Analysis. Raw EEG signals were first filtered between 0.01 Hz (high-pass) and 30-Hz (low-pass) digital filter. The time-locked epochs of 900 ms following the target event were extracted, with a 100-ms baseline. Next, to delete paroxysmal trials caused by large movements or eye blinks, trials showing potentials greater than ±75 μV were removed (5% of each condition). In many past studies, a single electrode has been used to index the P300 response (e.g., [29]). The location is typically *Pz*, which is on the midline and over the parietal region. Therefore, our ROI (region of interest) was only designated as *Pz*. The mean amplitude of P300 on the midline locations (*Pz*, *Cz*, and *Fz*) for each condition was shown in Table 2. Each ERP average contained a minimum of 36 artefact-free trials. Some previous studies have shown differences between ASD and typical development groups only in terms of ERP amplitudes, with no significant difference in ERP latencies [30], so we only analysed ERP amplitudes.

3.1.1. Amplitudes. We took the mean amplitude of the P300 component within the time window of 250–350 ms as the dependent variable. A 2 × 2 × 2 mixed analysis of variance (ANOVA) with two levels of AQ (High and Low), two levels of context condition (Expected and Unexpected), and two levels of belief (Belief and No-belief) was conducted (Table 2). The interaction effect between AQ and context was statistically significant (Figure 1), $F(1, 17) = 8.731$, $p = .009$, $\eta_p^2 = .339$. Post hoc t-tests corrected by the Bonferroni method indicated that the Low AQ group had larger P300 amplitudes in the Unexpected conditions (SD = 1.712) than in the Expected conditions (SD = 2.521; $p = .036$, $\eta_p^2 = .234$). In contrast, the High AQ group displayed marginally significantly smaller P300 responses in the Unexpected conditions (SD = 3.336) ($p = .076$, $\eta_p^2 = .174$).

We also examined the mean amplitude of the P100 component within the time window of 50–150 ms as a dependent variable. A mixed 2 × 2 × 2 analysis of variance (ANOVA) with two levels of AQ (High and Low), two levels of context condition (Expected and Unexpected), and two levels of belief (Belief and No-belief) was conducted. The interaction effect for AQ and context was statistically significant, $F(1, 17) = 4.659$, $p = .045$, $\eta_p^2 = .215$). Post hoc t-tests corrected by the Bonferroni method indicated that the Low AQ group had larger P100 amplitudes in the Expected conditions (SD = 2.094) than in the Unexpected conditions (SD = 1.575; $p = .052$, $\eta_p^2 = .205$). In contrast, the High AQ group displayed no significant difference between context conditions ($p = .366$, $\eta_p^2 = .048$).

Finally, we took the mean amplitude of the N200 component within the time window of 150–250 ms as a dependent variable. A 2 × 2 × 2 mixed analysis of variance (ANOVA) with two levels of AQ (High and Low), two levels of context condition (Expected and Unexpected), and two levels of belief (Belief and No-belief) was conducted. The interaction effect for context and belief was marginally significant, $F(1, 17) = 4.292$, $p = .071$, $\eta_p^2 = .179$. Post hoc t-tests corrected by the Bonferroni method indicated that the No-belief condition had larger N200 amplitudes in the Unexpected conditions (SD = 3.039) than in the Expected conditions (SD = 2.629; $p = .029$, $\eta_p^2 = .249$). In contrast, the Belief condition displayed no significant difference between the context conditions ($p = .809$, $\eta_p^2 = .004$).

3.1.2. Latencies. We took the peak latency of the P300, P100, and N200 component within the time window of 250–350, 50–150, and 150–250 ms, respectively, as the dependent variable. A 2 × 2 × 2 mixed analysis of variance (ANOVA) with two levels of AQ (High and Low), two levels of context condition (Expected and Unexpected), and two levels of belief (Belief and No-belief) was also conducted, respectively. As a result, only the N200 component showed the significant difference. The interaction effect for AQ, context, and belief was marginally significant, $F(1, 17) = 3.401$, $p = .083$, $\eta_p^2 = .167$. Post hoc t-tests corrected by the Bonferroni method

TABLE 2: Mean ERP amplitudes (μV) and latencies (ms) on Pz, Cz, and Fz (standard deviants in parentheses).

	Belief-Expected	Belief-Unexpected	No-belief-Expected	No-belief-Unexpected
		P100		
Amplitude (μV)				
Low AQ	2.84 (1.88), 0.27 (1.09), 0.27 (0.75)	3.52 (1.94), 0.26 (0.81), 0.26 (1.11)	3.01 (1.88), −0.02 (0.76), 0.33 (0.74)	2.90 (1.38), 0.61 (0.39), −0.05 (0.57)
High AQ	3.05 (1.68), 0.53 (0.73), 0.02 (0.92)	2.90 (1.43), 0.48 (0.91), −0.11 (0.62)	3.43 (1.50), 0.58 (0.79), −0.16 (0.74)	2.22 (1.18), 0.35 (0.49), −0.32 (0.76)
Latency (ms)				
Low AQ	113 (18.1), 107 (36.0), 92.9 (27.8)	107 (26.4), 113 (28.7), 112 (33.1)	114 (15.5), 107 (27.0), 106 (28.9)	110 (19.5), 110 (27.8), 101 (34.6)
High AQ	101 (32.1), 89.8 (34.1), 99.6 (38.5)	108 (25.1), 111 (34.9), 85 (22.5)	105 (25.3), 107 (27.4), 107 (32.3)	105 (23.5), 93.8 (27.4), 87.4 (38.7)
		N200		
Amplitude (μV)				
Low AQ	−0.62 (2.62), −0.2 (1.32), 0.22 (1.01)	0.04 (1.76), −0.15 (1.12), 0.36 (1.42)	−0.35 (1.55), −0.06 (0.87), 0.22 (0.77)	−0.35 (1.55), −0.06 (0.87), 0.35 (0.71)
High AQ	1.11 (2.50), 0.24 (0.96), −0.07 (1.03)	0.76 (1.66), 0.24 (0.80), −0.36 (0.57)	0.33 (2.67), −0.23 (0.87), −0.25 (−.80)	0.33 (2.69), −0.23 (0.87), −0.20 (0.60)
Latency (ms)				
Low AQ	186 (13.3), 186 (26.3), 194 (37.2)	181 (11.4), 181 (21.6), 208 (35.9)	185 (13.8), 179 (17.1), 190 (34.7)	188 (16.4), 296 (28.1), 186 (33.6)
High AQ	189 (23.9) 187 (28.9), 210 (29.5)	187 (25.5), 186 (29.3), 229 (46.0)	204 (27.1), 200 (31.1), 184 (29.7)	181 (14.5), 289 (26.6), 183 (26.7)
		P300		
Amplitude (μV)				
Low AQ	4.46 (2.80), 1.52 (0.95). 0.51 (0.68)	5.96 (1.64), 1.78 (0.89), 0.50 (1.36)	5.07 (3.29), 1.10 (0.78), 0.59 (0.68)	5.19 (2.05), 1.40 (0.97), 0.91 (0.63)
High AQ	5.76 (2.81), 2.15 (1.11), 0.03 (1.19)	5.52 (3.25), 2.19 (0.72), −0.13 (0.59)	5.52 (3.87), 1.56 (1.25), 0.36 (0.67)	4.48 (3.69), 1.27 (0.87), 0.65 (0.66)
Latency (ms)				
Low AQ	284 (27.6), 310 (33.8), 284 (44.6)	285 (22.2), 300 (16.8), 263 (34.2)	273 (20.2), 284 (34.1), 283 (36.0)	282 (26.2), 287.6 (40.1), 285 (40.0)
High AQ	288 (27.8), 306 (28.5), 285 (41.1)	287 (39), 301 (22.7), 264 (31.9)	288 (28.7), 303 (20.7), 308 (41.59)	287 (29.6), 298 (32.3), 295 (37.7)

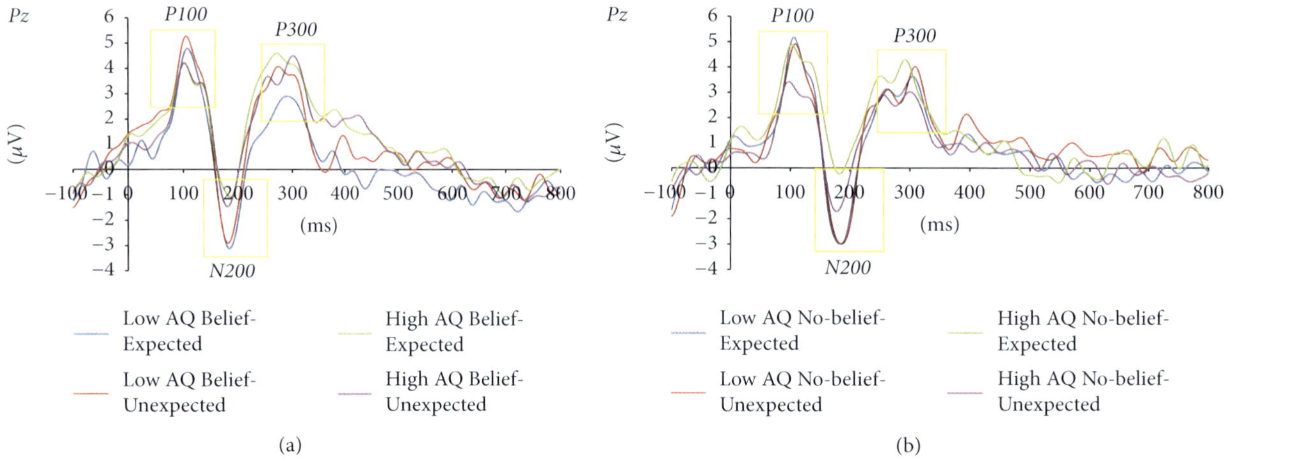

FIGURE 1: Grand mean ERPs on Pz elicited by target words for all conditions. (a) Four conditions in the Belief story condition and (b) four conditions in the No-belief condition.

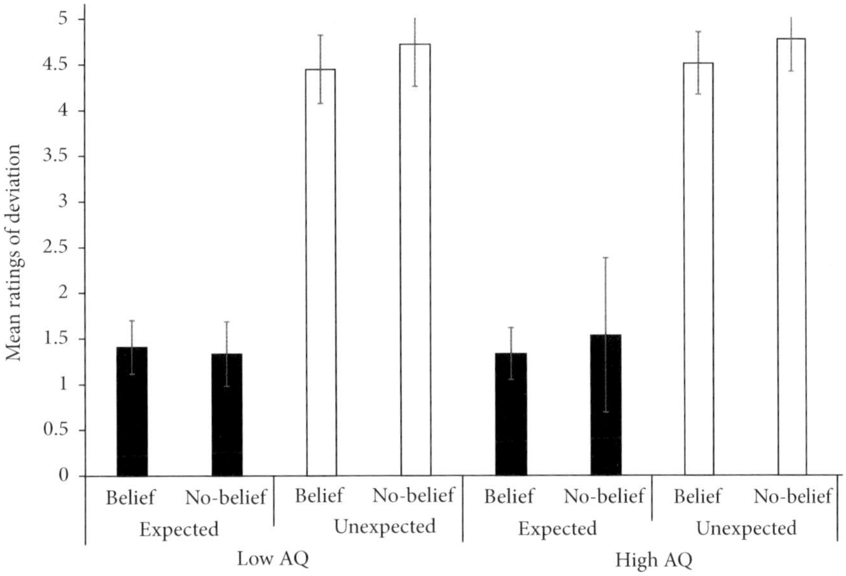

FIGURE 2: Mean ratings of deviation in all conditions.

indicated that, in the High AQ group, the Unexpected condition had shorter N200 latencies in the No-belief conditions (SD = 4.878) than in the Expected conditions (SD = 6.910; $p = .010$, $\eta_p^2 = .331$). In addition, the interaction effect between AQ and context was statistically significant, $F(1, 17) = 4.523$, $p = .048$, $\eta_p^2 = .210$. Post hoc t-tests corrected by the Bonferroni method indicated that the Unexpected conditions had shorter N200 latencies in the High AQ group (SD = 5.504) than in the Expected conditions (SD = 4.734; $p = .003$, $\eta_p^2 = .407$). Also, the main effect of context was significant, $F(1, 17) = 6.654$, $p = .019$, $\eta_p^2 = .281$, and the Unexpected conditions (SD = 3.439) had shorter N200 latencies than in the Expected conditions (SD = 3.999).

3.2. Behavioral Results. A separate ANOVA with participants' ratings of deviation as the dependent variable produced the anticipated significant main effect of context, with the Unexpected conditions evaluated as more deviant than the Expected conditions, $F(1, 17) = 725.719$, $p < .001$, $\eta_p^2 = .977$ (see Figure 2). Additionally, a main effect of belief was observed, wherein Belief was evaluated as less deviant than No-belief, $F(1, 17) = 3.213$, $p = .091$, $\eta_p^2 = .159$.

The response times for evaluating the level of deviation, measured from the evaluation options presented on the monitor, were also analysed via a 2 × 2 × 2 mixed ANOVA. The context × belief interaction was statistically significant, $F(1, 17) = 15.151$, $p = .001$, $\eta_p^2 = .471$. Post hoc t-tests revealed that the Belief condition (SD = 0.323) took less time than did No-belief in the Expected condition (SD = 0.474; $p = .007$, $\eta_p^2 = .356$). However, the reverse was true in the Unexpected condition: slower performance was seen in the Belief condition (SD = 0.492) than in the No-belief condition (SD = 0.482; $p = .060$, $\eta_p^2 = .193$). Additionally, in Belief trials, the Unexpected condition showed slower responses than did the Expected condition ($p = .002$, $\eta_p^2 = .447$). To consider the relationship between social difficulties and the use of context at the behavioral level, a correlation analysis was conducted that included both AQ total scores and subscale scores for 19 participants. Both of the Unexpected conditions (Belief and No-belief) were correlated positively only with the social skill subscale of the AQ ($r = .393$, $p = .096$; $r = .424$, $p = .070$; Figure 3). On the other hand, both of the Expected conditions (Belief and No-belief) did not show significant correlation with the social skill subscale of the AQ ($r = .143$, $p = .560$; $r = .134$, $p = .585$). The Expected conditions did not show significant correlations with AQ total score or any of the subscales.

3.3. Correlation Analysis between Behavioral and ERP Data. A correlation analysis was conducted between ERP components and behavioral data (ratings of deviation and response times) for 19 participants. Both of the ratings of deviation in Belief conditions (Expected and Unexpected) were correlated with P300 components, respectively ($r = .555$, $p = .014$; $r = -.549$, $p = .015$). No significant correlation was observed in both of the No-belief conditions (Expected and Unexpected) ($r = -.377$, $p = .111$; $r = .094$, $p = .703$). Also, there was no correlation between ERP components and response time.

4. Discussion

The purpose of this study was to examine how autistic traits influence responses when contextual deviation is recognised. We also examined whether a nonclinical population that scores high on autistic traits has difficulty using context or inferring mental states.

First, deviation was rated significantly higher in the Unexpected conditions than in the Expected conditions. This result served to confirm that our manipulation of expectations was effective. However, Belief conditions produced higher

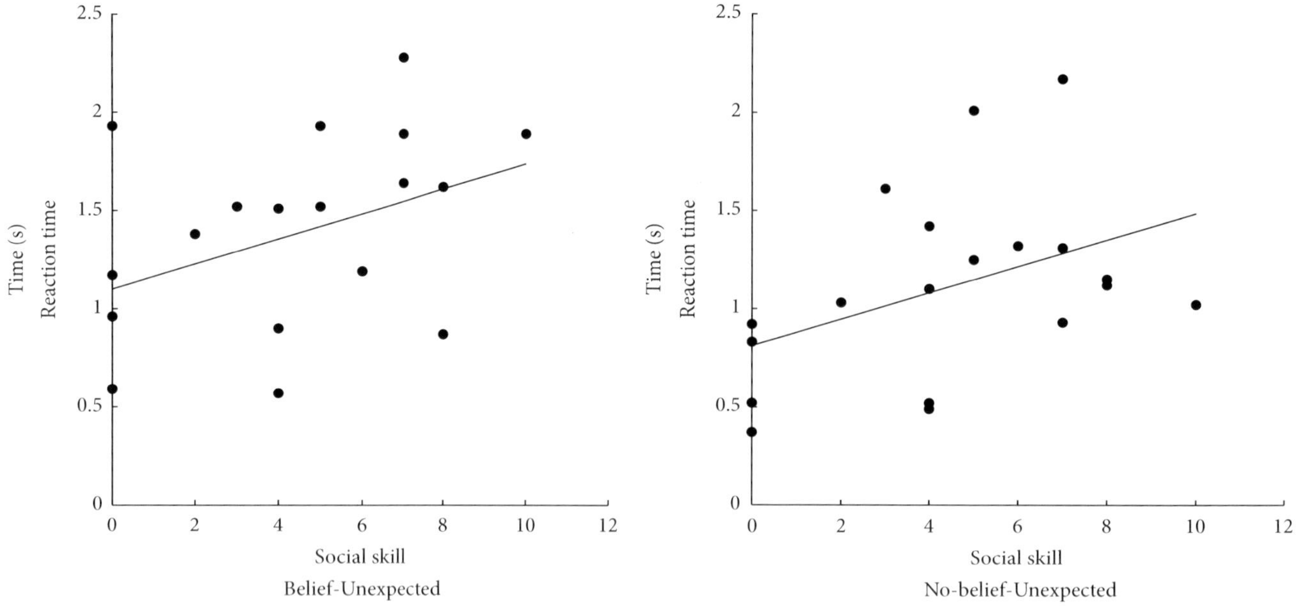

FIGURE 3: Correlation analysis of social skill and reaction time in the Belief Unexpected condition and in the No-belief Unexpected condition.

deviation ratings than did No-belief conditions. In addition, response times for evaluation in the Belief conditions were also slower compared with the No-belief conditions. It may be that the stories that entailed the mental states of others were more complex than stories without the attribution of mental states. The false-belief task has been used to measure linguistic Intelligence Quotient. Happé [3] argued that a certain level of linguistic Intelligence Quotient is required to succeed in the false-belief task, which implies that, all other things being equal, stories that imply another's beliefs should be linguistically more complex and difficult to understand than stories that do not.

In the analysis of evaluation times, regardless of Belief condition, social skill subscores of the AQ were positively correlated in both Unexpected conditions. In other words, people who find it difficult to deal with social situations took longer to evaluate the level of deviation that the stories presented. It may be that this delay is caused by lack of or less than optimal use of contextual information. With sufficient expectancy of contextual flow, the recognition and evaluation of deviation should proceed relatively quickly. Frith [5, 6] argued that, according to WCC theory, people with ASD can be assumed to have lower levels of integration of global contextual information than do non-ASD individuals. This lower level of contextual integration, in turn, produces difficulty that results in slower integration of the sentence flow and slower evaluation times. However, another possible explanation exists. Čeponienė et al. [31] examined the ERP response to deviant sounds in children with ASD. Their results suggested that the children could perceive deviation but that their attention toward it may be inhibited. Relatively low allocation of attention to deviant words could also cause slower evaluations of deviation. However, AQ score was not a significant factor in the ANOVA for evaluation scores. To summarise these results, people with autistic traits can evaluate contextual deviation properly but may require more time to do so. Also, the results of correlation analysis between the participant's ratings of deviant and P300 components showed the significant relationship between the subjective evaluation and ERP components only in Belief conditions. Independently of AQ scores, it has been suggested that P300 may be related with false-belief reasoning [32]. Therefore P300 components may have possibility of predicting the participant's ratings of deviant in Belief conditions.

ERP results indicated that the Low AQ group showed a greater P300 response; on the other hand the High AQ group showed a smaller response when deviation was present. This result revealed that the response to context deviation may be different depending on the level of autistic traits. Gomot and Wicker [33] suggested that the lower P300 response in people with ASD may reflect their weak use of contextual information and lesser inclination to use context for predictions. Bornkessel et al. [34] revealed that the P300 component can be observed when incorrect words in the context of sentences were recognised, and they concluded that P300 may be considered one index of linguistic contextual deviation. Therefore, the P300 response should also be involved in expectancy based on contextual flow in language. This hypothesis has been examined in relation to the linguistic ability of people with ASD. For example, particularly in English speaking countries, the homograph test has been widely used. In this test, where context in sentences has to be actively used to determine proper meanings of words, people with ASD perform more poorly than non-ASD controls (Lopez and Leekman, 2003). Happé [3] revealed that people with ASD have difficulties using contextual information during this test and suggested WCC theory as a framework for understanding such phenomena. WCC theory was first to focus on the reduced use of contextual information among people with ASD. The homograph test requires updating of contextual information as the words of the sentence are presented and prediction of the words that come next. Therefore, worse performance on this test may also suggest that people with ASD have difficulties using linguistic context more generally to build expectancy for what will happen next. This deficit in using context in ASD may also affect the ability to interpret ambiguous sentences, for example, "he bought some glasses" [35]. From our results, supporting context blindness or WCC theory, it can be considered that difficulties using contextual information are related to not only linguistic prediction but also linguistic interpretation. People with ASD has been reported to show language delay, although after their language skills develop they still continue to have communication difficulties in everyday life, such as understanding irony and metaphor [5, 6]. In addition, Happé [3] revealed a relationship between linguistic intelligence and theory of mind. Hence, it can be suggested that using linguistic context may be a cause of the social difficulties in ASD.

We did not have an a priori hypothesis but did analyse P100 and N200 components. Results indicated that the Low AQ group showed a reduced P100 response when deviation was present. In semantic priming tasks, it has been reported that a reduced P100 response is observed when untrained rare words were present [36]. P100 components may possibly reflect semantic processing of words. In the present study, this difference was only observed in the Low AQ group, such that the Low AQ group may predict the target words and realize deviation faster than the High AQ group. However, many studies report that the diminished P100 response in ASD is related to visual attention [37]. Therefore, our results may have been influenced by such a difference. In addition, in the No-belief condition, greater N200 amplitude was observed when deviation was present. We used words showing simple semantical deviation in the No-belief conditions. As a result, it can be considered that deviations in the No-belief conditions may be processed quickly and reflected in the N200 time window. N200, similar to P300, is elicited when participants attend to deviations in oddball paradigms [38]. It has been said that N200 also reflect the recognition of deviation from a mentally stored expectation of the standard stimulus [39]. Although the N400 response reflects semantic comprehension, we could not observe that component in this study. However, P300 response has been claimed to reflect similar cognitive processes to the N400 response [9, 10]. Hence, our P300 response results should be considered to be related to contextual interpretation of semantic processes in people with autistic traits.

Also, the analysis of latencies showed the significant effect of the context only in the N200 component. Shorter N200 latency was observed when deviation was present. Furthermore, the interaction effect for AQ, context and belief was marginally significant and the interaction effect between AQ and context was statistically significant. The post hoc t-tests indicated that the significant difference was only observed in the High AQ group No-belief conditions. This result may not be consistent with behavioral result which suggested that people in the High AQ group take longer time to judge context deviation. Frith and Snowling [40] indicated that autistic individuals fail to use semantic context. However, it can be a limitation that some of our sentences did not require using total semantic context. Also, some studies suggested that there may be differences in autistic traits between individuals with and without ASD [41]. Therefore, nonclinical people with autistic traits would have different cognitive styles from individuals with ASD. One possibility is that participants in the High AQ group used some strategies during the task. Recently, broader autism phenotype has been paid more attention [42]. It is necessary to examine the cognitive styles in the nonclinical populations having high autistic traits.

A functional magnetic resonance imaging study conducted by Dungan et al. [22] measured autistic traits and examined how individuals respond to expected or unexpected events. They found that, in the context of an agent's behavior, unexpected versus expected outcomes elicited an especially robust activation of the right temporoparietal junction, and the magnitude of this difference across participants was correlated negatively with autistic traits. Consistent with our study, this study showed that autistic traits can affect the processing of contextual expectations. While our correlational data were based on a small sample, our results are in line with those of previous studies and theoretical works related to autistic recognition.

Our results suggested some cognitive styles in the people having autistic traits; however, the small number of participants can be a limitation. Our results included marginally significant effects; also correlation analysis of AQ scores and behavioral data indicated only marginally significant relations. Although our sample sizes were small to mention firm conclusions, the effect size was seemed to be strong. Further research is required to examine the use of context in people with ASD or nonclinical participants with autistic traits.

Taken together, our findings suggest that the response to deviation is different for those with autistic traits, regardless of whether mental states must be inferred. Although our participants were a nonclinical sample of typical university students, we observed statistically significant differences in ERP responses as a function of relatively low or high levels of autistic traits. Therefore, autistic traits appear to influence recognition of contextual deviation. Furthermore, our results revealed that individuals with autistic traits may not have difficulties in inferring others' mental states, but rather in using contextual information. Level of social skill was correlated with evaluation times, such that the use of context and sociality may be related. Our results supported both WCC theory and the idea of context blindness, and it can be suggested that using contextual information is related to the deficits of sociality and language in ASD.

Recent neuroscientific studies suggest that people with ASD show functional underconnectivity between frontal and posterior brain regions [43]. This lower frontal-posterior synchronization was observed in the sentence comprehension task using linguistic context [44, 45]. Therefore, it is possible that this underconnectively is related to the deficit in using contextual information observed here. However, in this study, we only examined the response to contextual deviation.

Therefore, the differential use of contextual information as a function of autistic traits is somewhat speculative. Moreover, our sole focus was linguistic contextual information. Both WCC theory and the idea of context blindness focus not only on linguistic context, but also on more global context. Further research is necessary to clarify the relationship between autistic traits and the use of context.

References

[1] D. Premack and G. Woodruff, "Does the chimpanzee have a theory of mind?" *Behavioral and Brain Sciences*, vol. 1, no. 4, pp. 515–526, 1978.

[2] S. Baron-Cohen, *Mindblindness: An Essay on Autism and Theory of Mind*, MIT Press, Cambridge, MA, USA, 1997.

[3] F. G. Happé, "The role of age and verbal ability in the theory of mind task performance of subjects with autism," *Child Development*, vol. 66, no. 3, pp. 843–855, 1995.

[4] P. Vermeulen, *Autism as Context Blindness*, Autism Asperger Publishing, Kansas City, MO, USA, 2012.

[5] U. Frith, *Autism: Explaining the Enigma*, Basil Blackwell, Oxford, U.K, 1989.

[6] U. Frith, "A new look at language and communication in autism," *International Journal of Language & Communication Disorders*, vol. 24, no. 2, pp. 123–150.

[7] C. P. Burnette, P. C. Mundy, J. A. Meyer, S. K. Sutton, A. E. Vaughan, and D. Charak, "Weak central coherence and its relations to theory of mind and anxiety in autism," *Journal of Autism and Developmental Disorders*, vol. 35, no. 1, pp. 63–73, 2005.

[8] J. Pijnacker, B. Geurts, M. van Lambalgen, J. Buitelaar, and P. Hagoort, "Exceptions and anomalies: an ERP study on context sensitivity in autism," *Neuropsychologia*, vol. 48, no. 10, pp. 2940–2951, 2010.

[9] M. Kutas and S. A. Hillyard, "Event-related brain potentials to semantically inappropriate and surprisingly large words," *Biological Psychology*, vol. 11, no. 2, pp. 99–116, 1980.

[10] M. Kutas and S. A. Hillyard, "Reading senseless sentences: brain potentials reflect semantic incongruity," *Science*, vol. 207, no. 4427, pp. 203–205, 1980.

[11] M. Kutas and S. A. Hillyard, "Brain potentials during reading reflect word expectancy and semantic association," *Nature*, vol. 307, no. 5947, pp. 161–163, 1984.

[12] E. Donchin and M. G. H. Coles, "Is the P300 component a manifestation of cognitive updating?" *Behavioral and Brain Sciences*, vol. 11, no. 3, pp. 357–427, 1988.

[13] D. J. Krusienski, E. W. Sellers, F. Cabestaing et al., "A comparison of classification techniques for the P300 Speller," *Journal of Neural Engineering*, vol. 3, no. 4, article 007, pp. 299–305, 2006.

[14] L. A. Farwell and E. Donchin, "Talking off the top of your head: Toward a mental prosthesis utilizing event-related brain potentials," *Electroencephalography and Clinical Neurophysiology*, vol. 70, no. 6, pp. 510–523, 1988.

[15] J. Polich, "Updating P300: an integrative theory of P3a and P3b," *Clinical Neurophysiology*, vol. 118, no. 10, pp. 2128–2148, 2007.

[16] J. Meinhardt, B. Sodian, C. Thoermer, K. Döhnel, and M. Sommer, "True- and false-belief reasoning in children and adults: an event-related potential study of theory of mind," *Developmental Cognitive Neuroscience*, vol. 1, no. 1, pp. 67–76, 2011.

[17] M. Dunn, H. Vaughan Jr., J. Kreuzer, and D. Kurtzberg, "Electrophysiologic correlates of semantic classification in autistic and normal children," *Developmental Neuropsychology*, vol. 16, no. 1, pp. 79–99, 1999.

[18] A. Senju, V. Southgate, S. White, and U. Frith, "Mindblind eyes: an absence of spontaneous theory of mind in asperger syndrome," *Science*, vol. 325, no. 5942, pp. 883–885, 2009.

[19] R. P. Lawson, G. Rees, and K. J. Friston, "An aberrant precision account of autism," *Front Hum Neurosci*, vol. 8, p. 302, 2014.

[20] P. Sinha, M. M. Kjelgaard, T. K. Gandhi et al., "Autism as a disorder of prediction," *Proceedings of the National Academy of Sciences of the United States of America*, vol. 111, no. 42, pp. 15220–15225, 2014.

[21] S. van de Cruys, K. Evers, R. van der Hallen et al., "Precise minds in uncertain worlds: predictive coding in autism," *Psychological Review*, vol. 121, no. 4, pp. 649–675, 2014.

[22] J. A. Dungan, M. Stepanovic, and L. Young, "Theory of Mind for Processing Unexpected Events Across Contexts," *Social Cognitive and Affective Neuroscience*, nsw032, 2016.

[23] Y. Kunihira, A. Senju, H. Dairoku, A. Wakabayashi, and T. Hasegawa, "'Autistic' traits in non-autistic Japanese populations: relationships with personality traits and cognitive ability," *Journal of Autism and Developmental Disorders*, vol. 36, no. 4, pp. 553–566, 2006.

[24] B. Ingersoll and A. Wainer, "The broader autism phenotype," in *Handbook of Autism and Pervasive Developmental Disorders*, edition., F. R. Volkmar, S. J. Rogers, R. Paul, and K. A. Pelphrey, Eds., vol. 1, pp. 28–56, Wiley & Sons, New Jersey, NJ, USA, 4th edition, 2014.

[25] A. Wakabayashi, Y. Tojo, S. Baron-Cohen, and S. Wheelwright, "The Autism-Spectrum Quotient (AQ) Japanese version: evidence from high-functioning clinical group and normal adults," *Shinrigaku Kenkyu: The Japanese journal of psychology*, vol. 75, no. 1, pp. 78–84, 2004.

[26] S. Wheelwright, B. Auyeung, C. Allison, and S. Baron-Cohen, "Defining the broader, medium and narrow autism phenotype among parents using the autism spectrum quotient (AQ)," *Molecular Autism*, vol. 1, no. 1, 2010.

[27] E. J. Hermans, G. van Wingen, P. A. Bos, P. Putman, and J. van Honk, "Reduced spontaneous facial mimicry in women with autistic traits," *Biological Psychology*, vol. 80, no. 3, pp. 348–353, 2009.

[28] J. W. Peirce, "PsychoPy-Psychophysics software in Python," *Journal of Neuroscience Methods*, vol. 162, no. 1, pp. 8–13, 2007.

[29] S. J. Maclean, C. D. Hassall, Y. Ishigami, O. E. Krigolson, and G. A. Eskes, "Using brain potentials to understand prism adaptation: the error-related negativity and the P300," *Frontiers in Human Neuroscience*, vol. 9, 2015.

[30] A. Thillay, M. Lemaire, S. Roux et al., "Atypical brain mechanisms of prediction according to uncertainty in autism," *Frontiers in Neuroscience*, vol. 10, article 317, 2016.

[31] R. Ceponiene, T. Lepistö, A. Shestakova et al., "Speechsound-selective auditory impairment in children with autism: they can perceive but do not attend," *Proceedings of the National Academy of Sciences of the United States of America*, vol. 100, no. 9, pp. 5567–5572, 2003.

[32] M. A. Sabbagh and M. Taylor, "Neural correlates of theory-of-mind reasoning: An event-related potential study," *Psychological Science*, vol. 11, no. 1, pp. 46–50, 2000.

[33] M. Gomot and B. Wicker, "A challenging, unpredictable world

for people with autism spectrum disorder," *International Journal of Psychophysiology*, vol. 83, no. 2, pp. 240–247, 2012.

[34] I. Bornkessel, M. Schlesewsky, and A. D. Friederici, "Contextual information modulates initial processes of syntactic integration: the role of inter-versus intrasentential predictions," *Journal of Experimental Psychology: Learning Memory and Cognition*, vol. 29, no. 5, pp. 871–882, 2003.

[35] T. Jolliffe and S. Baron-Cohen, "The strange stories test: A replication with high-functioning adults with autism or Asperger syndrome," *Journal of Autism and Developmental Disorders*, vol. 29, no. 5, pp. 395–406, 1999.

[36] G. A. Frishkoff, C. A. Perfetti, and K. Collins-Thompson, "Lexical quality in the brain: ERP evidence for robust word learning from context," *Developmental Neuropsychology*, vol. 35, no. 4, pp. 376–403, 2010.

[37] C. Cantiani, N. A. Choudhury, H. Y. Yan, V. L. Shafer, R. G. Schwartz, and A. A. Benasich, "From sensory perception to lexical-semantic processing: an erp study in non-verbal children with autism," *PloS one*, vol. 11, no. 8, article e0161637, 2016.

[38] S. H. Patel and P. N. Azzam, "Characterization of N200 and P300: selected studies of the event-related potential," *International Journal of Medicine and Medical Sciences*, vol. 2, no. 4, pp. 147–154, 2005.

[39] M. Sams, K. Alho, and R. Näätänen, "Sequential effects on the ERP in discriminating two stimuli," *Biological Psychology*, vol. 17, no. 1, pp. 41–58, 1983.

[40] U. Frith and M. Snowling, "Reading for meaning and reading for sound in autistic and dyslexic children," *British Journal of Developmental Psychology*, vol. 1, no. 4, pp. 329–342, 1983.

[41] A. L. Murray, T. Booth, K. McKenzie, R. Kuenssberg, and M. O'Donnell, "Are autistic traits measured equivalently in individuals with and without an autism spectrum disorder? an invariance analysis of the autism spectrum quotient short form," *Journal of Autism and Developmental Disorders*, vol. 44, no. 1, pp. 55–64, 2014.

[42] E. Bora, A. Aydın, T. Saraç, M. T. Kadak, S. Köse, and A. Aydın, "Heterogeneity of subclinical autistic traits among parents of children with autism spectrum disorder: identifying the broader autism phenotype with a data-driven method," *Autism Research*, vol. 10, no. 2, pp. 321–326, 2016.

[43] M. A. Just, T. A. Keller, V. L. Malave, R. K. Kana, and S. Varma, "Autism as a neural systems disorder: a theory of frontal-posterior underconnectivity," *Neuroscience and Biobehavioral Reviews*, vol. 36, no. 4, pp. 1292–1313, 2012.

[44] M. A. Just, V. L. Cherkassky, T. A. Keller, and N. J. Minshew, "Cortical activation and synchronization during sentence comprehension in high-functioning autism: evidence of underconnectivity," *Brain*, vol. 127, no. 8, pp. 1811–1821, 2004.

[45] R. K. Kana, T. A. Keller, V. L. Cherkassky, N. J. Minshew, and M. A. Just, "Sentence comprehension in autism: thinking in pictures with decreased functional connectivity," *Brain*, vol. 129, no. 9, pp. 2484–2493, 2006.

26

Initial Development of the Early Intensive Behavioral Intervention Parental Self-Efficacy Scale

Aaron Blocher-Rubin[1] and Paige Krabill[2]

[1]*Arizona Autism United, 5025 E. Washington St. #212, Phoenix, AZ 85034, USA*
[2]*Capella University, Minneapolis, MN, USA*

Correspondence should be addressed to Aaron Blocher-Rubin; aaron@azaunited.org

Academic Editor: Herbert Roeyers

Early Intensive Behavioral Intervention (EIBI) is an effective treatment for children with autism. However, it is known that some parents struggle to fully implement the program, and providers are not always able to identify the specifics of each family's individualized challenges. The purpose of this pilot study was to begin the process of developing a new instrument, the EIBI Parental Self-Efficacy (EPSE) Scale, to help providers better assess and assist parents in regard to EIBI implementation. The methodology included four phases: scale construction, expert review, pretest administration, and a large sample pilot study ($N = 192$). The final 29-item EPSE Scale contained strong reliability properties (Cronbach's alpha = .900). Factor analysis established five subscales: *Family Well-Being, Preparing for Successful Sessions, Team Participation, Not Giving Up*, and *Working with your Child.* Following this pilot study, future research is recommended to refine and validate the EPSE Scale as a useful clinical tool for EIBI providers.

1. Introduction

This pilot study was conducted as a first step toward developing a new instrument, the EIBI Parental Self-Efficacy (EPSE) Scale. The purpose of the EPSE Scale is to assess parents of children with autism who are actively receiving Early Intensive Behavioral Intervention (EIBI), specifically in regard to any challenges they might be experiencing related to the demands of implementing an in-home EIBI program.

Research has repeatedly demonstrated that EIBI, a comprehensive treatment package based on the science of applied behavior analysis (ABA), is currently the most effective evidence-based treatment for young children with autism [1–5]. Although EIBI is known to be highly effective, it is also known that implementation can place heavy demands on parents [6–8]. EIBI is mostly home-based and requires thousands of one-to-one instructional hours with the child for several years, along with ongoing intensive parental involvement expectations. As such, EIBI implementation can also require major lifestyle adjustments for the whole family [8–10].

The ability of parents to be involved is key to the EIBI treatment approach [11, 12]. However, requiring too much from parents can actually be detrimental toward overall intervention effectiveness [13]. Providers need to be keenly aware of each parent's current capacity in order to determine an appropriate balance of expectations. Therefore, the potential value of the EPSE Scale is that it gives providers an objective method to identify any underlying problems experienced by parents, which may not be immediately obvious but could inhibit treatment effectiveness if not properly addressed.

1.1. Clinic-Directed versus Community-Based EIBI. As EIBI has evolved into a broad spectrum of intervention packages for children with autism over the past few decades, several publications have helped clarify its core elements [5, 8, 14, 15]. *Early* signifies that intervention should begin as soon as possible, typically following diagnosis and preferably by the age of 3. *Intensive* indicates that direct treatment hours should range from about 20 to 40 per week for at least two years, depending on the child's age and other factors. *Behavioral* means that all teaching methods are consistent with the science of ABA and guided by an individualized, developmental, and comprehensive curriculum that addresses a wide range of skills in all domains of functioning. *Intervention* refers to the entire treatment package, which involves creating a structured and predictable learning environment for the child to respond appropriately and be reinforced. Each child's treatment program must be designed and directed by a certified behavior analyst and delivered mostly in a one-to-one context by a team of trained paraprofessional behavioral therapists (i.e., technicians) in the child's natural environment.

Depending on available providers and funding sources, families may receive either a robust clinic-directed model with all services managed by an EIBI provider agency or a community-based model in which parents are responsible for significantly more program management duties [16, 17]. Although there are many variations of community-based models, the general distinctions are that far fewer resources are available and a significant portion of treatment management becomes the parents' responsibility [13, 15]. Staff typically receive less training and supervision, which requires parents to take a more active supervisory role. At times, parents must also recruit their own therapists from the community, as provider agencies may not always have enough capacity to meet demand. Funding is generally much lower than a clinic-directed model and supervisors have less time to spend on each case due to higher caseloads, which can result in diluted treatment with fewer research-based protocols. Parents may need to guide their teams between consultation visits from program supervisors, without necessarily knowing how to respond optimally to various challenges. It is important to note that studies do show that community-based EIBI is effective, but considerably less so than clinic-directed programs [2, 15, 18–20]. The benefit, however, is that community-based models can reach far more children and families in need. Therefore, as the need for EIBI grows, it is critical that providers have better tools to deliver more effective services in community-based models.

1.2. Demands on Parents. Implementing EIBI inevitably requires families to manage a wide range of tasks and challenges, especially within a community-based model. For example, parents must establish a robust in-home therapy environment in the context of their daily lives that involves frequent visits from therapists. They typically must be present for up to two sessions per day of about three hours each, in addition to weekly or monthly meetings and training with their therapy team [1, 15, 16, 21, 22]. Some programs require parents to act as cotherapists themselves, in varying capacities from highly structured to naturalistic, which can be stressful for some. Outside of direct therapy time, parents are usually tasked with implementing consistent behavioral strategies with their child, which at times may increase behavioral challenges and require extensive perseverance under pressure [8, 13, 23]. Sadly, these techniques are too often misunderstood by extended family or community members, leaving parents at risk for feeling stressed, socially unsupported, or judged as unable to control their child's behavior despite doing all they can to follow the EIBI program's recommendations [24–26].

Several studies have investigated how well families adapt to EIBI. One study interviewed parents that completed EIBI for at least two years, who believed it was beneficial but also had struggles [7]. The lack of in-home privacy was often difficult and not always respected by therapists. Administrative duties could also be stressful and take time away from the rest of the family. Additional frustration ensued when therapists had issues with reliability, punctuality, and maintaining confidentiality. The authors suggest that EIBI may at times exacerbate marital strain. Another study found that EIBI can be emotionally difficult for mothers, involving fatigue and a sense of sacrifice [6]. Some found it difficult to be both mother and therapist, feeling less effective than other therapists and struggling to transition back into the parent role, in addition to finding time for their other children. A separate study found that EIBI impacted the family's home environment, with requirements such as allocating space exclusively for therapists to work without distractions, and some families had little time for other social activities [10]. Each of these studies identifies different struggles that families have faced, yet the participants only represent parents who were able to complete the EIBI program. The impact of struggles faced by families who were unable to sustain the treatment is still unknown, which further emphasizes the need for a standardized assessment tool to identify risks before they significantly impede treatment implementation.

1.3. The Role of Self-Efficacy. Since it is known that EIBI implementation can pose significant challenges for parents, the logic follows that the odds of treatment success could be improved if providers have a way to predict which specific tasks and behaviors are most likely to be a struggle for any given family, so that they can give extra attention to those areas. In the psychological literature, a commonly measured predictor of behavior is self-efficacy, which is defined as the degree to which a person believes he or she is able to perform a particular skill or behavior [27, 28]. A person's level of self-efficacy for any given behavior serves as a predictor because it influences whether or not he or she will engage in that behavior, as well as persist, when confronted by challenges. For that reason, the EPSE Scale is constructed as a measure of self-efficacy for tasks and behaviors specifically related to EIBI implementation, to assess how likely parents are to continue completing those tasks over time as the treatment progresses.

According to Bandura [27], self-efficacy is most relevant when people have the skills, incentive, and opportunity to do the task, so that self-efficacy is the only remaining factor to alter their behavior. Parents implementing EIBI clearly have the incentive and opportunity, but some may not have adequate levels of self-efficacy for all necessary tasks to persist when circumstances are challenging. Utilizing self-efficacy as the guiding psychometric for the EPSE Scale is fitting because self-efficacy has been shown to predict positive parenting practices under stressful circumstances [29]. For the purposes of this study, EIBI implementation is conceptualized as a component of parenting because all parents are responsible for coordinating any treatment necessary for their child's well-being. It is also worthy to note that self-efficacy has been the construct of choice for domain measurement with many other conceptually similar scales, such as assessing one's ability to self-manage a treatment regimen for other health conditions [30, 31].

1.4. The Need for a New Instrument. As discussed, EIBI is a very unique and intensive treatment. The specific demands on parents are not easily comparable to other early intervention services that consist of far fewer hours and in general a much less comprehensive approach. No other measurement tool has been published that specifically targets a parent's ability to carry out the tasks and behaviors uniquely related to EIBI implementation, even though it is the most evidence-based treatment available for young children with autism. One other publication, the Early Intervention Parenting Self-Efficacy Scale [32], appears similar on the surface but is not specific to autism or EIBI. Instead, it measures self-efficacy related to feeling competent as a parent and helping the child make progress, while receiving early intervention services such as speech and occupational therapy. This scale may have value for the same target population for which the EPSE Scale is intended, but it measures an entirely different construct and would not be appropriate to specifically identify EIBI treatment implementation challenges.

Bandura [28] emphasizes that self-efficacy measurement tools must be designed to examine specific domains of functioning. It is not useful (or accurate) to simply say that someone has a high level of self-efficacy, for example, because it is not a global construct that applies equally to everything a person does. Instead, the recommended approach to developing self-efficacy based scales is to measure a defined class of performances under various classes of relevant conditions. The EPSE Scale achieves this goal by assessing common tasks specifically associated with implementing EIBI in a variety of circumstances that parents are known to experience. Additionally, because self-efficacy beliefs can vary over time [28], the EPSE Scale is designed to be administered at multiple times throughout the EIBI treatment process as needed so that new concerns can be identified and addressed anytime. The intended outcome is for providers to use the resulting information to facilitate discussion with parents to find solutions and improve their self-efficacy in those areas. In theory, this process should ultimately help families overcome EIBI challenges because improving self-efficacy can change the perception of treatment barriers [33].

For decades, researchers have focused on demonstrating EIBI as an effective treatment, but only recently are researchers noting a need for parental assessment to understand their readiness for such a taxing treatment regimen [12, 34–36]. Currently, EIBI providers do not typically assess barriers experienced by families that affect implementation and adherence [37]. Instead, it is often just assumed that parents can fulfill their requirements [35]. Since not all families complete the recommended treatment time to maximize EIBI outcomes [38], researchers must identify more effective methods to support parents with successful ongoing implementation, especially in community-based models.

Challenges faced by families are an individualized combination of circumstances. Schreibman [39] has noted that practitioners need to be more responsive to feedback from families, as EIBI requires the involvement of the child's total environment. The overall rationale for this study was to develop a tool to identify what each individual family is facing on a case-by-case basis as they attempt to implement EIBI in their home, so that solutions can be equally individualized. The goal of the EPSE Scale is to provide a practical tool to assess parental capabilities related to completing tasks and behaviors necessary for EIBI implementation, which in turn gives providers a clearer insight into what they need to focus on to help each family succeed, thereby adding to the overall social validity of EIBI.

2. Methods

This study was completed in four phases: (a) scale construction, (b) expert review field test, (c) pretest administration, and (d) large sample pilot study. The first step involved creating and revising items using best practice guidelines [40]. This draft was shared with subject matter experts for suggestions on individual items and the scale as a whole. The second draft was used for pretest administration with a small sample of the target population, followed by additional feedback to assist with making further improvements. The final phase involved 192 participants completing the scale and providing demographic information. Statistical analyses were conducted to establish key scale properties including reliability, validity, and factor structure. In summary, this pilot study completed a rigorous development and initial testing process for the EPSE Scale, as a first step toward preparing it for future use in research and practice.

2.1. Scale Construction. Two primary sources were used to guide the development of the scale's first draft. DeVellis [40] provides a comprehensive overview of best practices for scale development in the social and behavioral sciences, while Bandura [41] offers specific guidelines for developing self-efficacy based scales. As per DeVellis, initial scale construction is done in three steps: (a) determining item format, (b) brainstorming a large pool of possible items, and (c) refining the initial item list.

As recommended by Bandura [41], the items on the EPSE Scale ask participants to rate how certain they are that they can do a given task or behavior under various challenging conditions, consistent with the construct of self-efficacy. The phrasing of items follows a consistent format to avoid confusion. Participants respond using a Likert scale to indicate level of belief in their capabilities, consistent with Bandura's approach and other widely used scales [40]. Each item describes a specific task or behavior associated with implementing EIBI. Although Bandura recommends a scoring range of 0–100, DeVellis cautions against false estimates of precision. Therefore, a 7-point scale is used instead, which DeVellis identifies as a standard approach for measuring attitudes and beliefs. This range also provides enough response variation to conduct robust reliability testing and factor analysis.

A series of best practice guidelines [40] were followed to optimize the initial list of possible items, including testing the reading level to ensure it was not above seventh grade, avoiding any ambiguous words or phrases, and limiting each item to a single task or behavior. Since parental responsibilities associated with EIBI are broad, categories were established based on the literature review to ensure that items were brainstormed within all facets of the domain for a wide range of possible situations.

The literature review followed a comprehensive process involving a wide variety of search terms related to autism, EIBI, treatment efficacy in real world settings, parental adherence and experiences, barriers to treatment, community-based and clinic-directed models, and the role of self-efficacy. Robust online databases were utilized, and references within retrieved articles were analyzed for additional leads as part of a snowball approach. Over 200 peer-reviewed journal articles and several dozen textbook chapters were examined in all. Content was categorized and coded to identify the most common and relevant themes for scale construction.

Using this information, an initial list of 343 items was developed and then refined by identifying items that most clearly represented a range of tasks related to EIBI implementation. The primary considerations were avoiding redundancy, picking items most relevant to the construct, and eliminating wording confusion or vagueness. When finished, the first draft of the scale contained 100 items and a set of instructions that were created in accordance with Bandura's [41] guidelines of clarifying that participants are to rate their perceived capabilities now, rather than what they expect to be able to do in the future.

2.2. Expert Review Field Test. The field test followed best practices [40] and included 14 subject matter experts from the following categories: (a) behavior analysts with extensive EIBI experience; (b) parents who had completed EIBI and helped other families; and (c) published researchers in the fields of autism, EIBI, and self-efficacy. Experts were asked to rate each item on the scale as excellent, average, or poor based on the following considerations: (a) readability, (b) relevance, (c) likelihood that people would understand the question, (d) specificity of task or behavior, and (e) representativeness of EIBI parental responsibilities. Comment fields were also available to give feedback on each item, as well as the scale instructions. Experts were also asked for general feedback on (a) how well the tasks and behaviors listed relate to successful EIBI, (b) changes to how the scale should be organized, (c) potential problems, (d) other examples or themes that should be included, (e) concerns for items that might upset or embarrass participants, and (f) other suggestions.

Expert feedback was analyzed to identify common themes and specific suggestions to improve the scale. Ten experts agreed that all of the items represented tasks and behaviors associated with parents successfully implementing EIBI, while four noted that some items did and some did not. Several experts noted that care should be taken to avoid describing any tasks as too difficult, to minimize the risk of parents feeling discouraged.

DeVellis [40] stresses that expert feedback should be strongly considered, but final decisions belong to the researcher as experts may not fully understand the process of scale development. All suggestions were considered in a systematic way by calculating the expert rating scores and categorizing common feedback themes. This input was used to make decisions around revising some items and deleting others. The process concluded with 49 items for the second draft of the EPSE Scale.

2.3. Pretest Administration. The pretest administration tested the draft scale with a small sample ($n = 10$) of the target population, to identify any problems before recruiting a large sample and obtain final feedback for revisions. Inclusion criteria were parents or guardians currently implementing EIBI for a child with autism under the age of six. Participants also had to be at least 18 years old, fluent in English, living with the child, and responsible for coordinating services. All recruitment materials directed participants to a website that contained all information, consent forms, and questions for the study. Participation was anonymous. An option was given to provide contact information to participate in a voluntary phone call to provide additional feedback. General questions were asked about the participation experience, including whether the length was reasonable, instructions were clear, the layout was easy, and if they experienced any distress. All items were then displayed again with an optional comment box for participants to share suggestions to improve any particular item.

A simplified item analysis was conducted to observe response patterns, including highest, lowest, and average scores for each item. The range and mean scores were analyzed to determine whether any items were not achieving variation. All items had some variation in scores. After additional revisions based on participant feedback, observations, and reconsideration of scale development guidelines, 29 items were kept as is and five revised, for a total of 34 items.

Participants reported that it took five to 20 minutes to complete the scale, but all felt it was a reasonable amount of time. All stated that the layout was easy to read, they understood what each item was asking, and the rating scale gave them the right amount of response choices. Six participants participated in an optional phone interview and said they felt the scale was easy to complete with straightforward questions. No problems with the scale or experiences of distress or embarrassment were reported. Participants felt they could express their real beliefs and answer all questions accurately. They had no opposition to any of the topics or questions and did not think any items needed to be worded differently to suit the target population.

2.4. Large Sample Pilot Study. In the final phase, the EPSE Scale was tested with 192 participants, followed by statistical analyses of psychometric properties to complete final decisions for item elimination. Participants were recruited across the country through many autism organizations and EIBI providers. All materials were available online and participation was anonymous. The website included participant eligibility screening, consent forms, and a demographic survey. For ethical considerations, it was stated clearly that the purpose of the study was to better understand what factors help families succeed with EIBI. It was explicitly noted that the purpose was not to determine whether someone is able to implement EIBI and that it is not yet known whether these items are necessary to be successful. It was also clarified that this scale would not be used in any way to determine eligibility for treatment, in case any participants were concerned that their answers or future use of the scale could have a negative effect on families seeking services.

Following data collection, four major analyses were conducted: (a) initial item analysis, (b) item correlation analysis, (c) reliability analysis, and (d) factor analysis. When all analyses were complete, final decisions were made regarding items to eliminate and factor interpretation, guided by recommendations from several scale development publications [40, 42–44].

3. Results

Data analysis involved identifying factor structure, determining items to eliminate, and establishing psychometric properties for the EPSE Scale. The final scale consisted of 29 items and five factors, with exceptionally strong reliability scores. Basic construct and content validity were also established, and an item analysis revealed additional key properties of the scale.

3.1. Sample Characteristics. The initial eligibility criteria required that the participant's child be less than six years old and receiving at least 20 hours per week of home-based EIBI, and 41 participants completed the study under these criteria. Unfortunately, the researcher experienced significant recruitment challenges and had to modify the eligibility criteria beyond the intended target population in order to secure enough participants for statistically significant data analysis. A decision was made to expand the parameters to include parents who had limited experience implementing EIBI but could likely relate to the items asked in a meaningful way. Following IRB approval, the age limit was increased to less than nine years old, and hours per week were decreased to five or more. Additionally, parents whose child had received EIBI in the past before the age of nine were accepted, with instructions to respond to the best of their memory regarding how they felt on average while their child was receiving EIBI. The modified sample criteria are clearly the biggest limitation to this pilot study, and all findings should be interpreted accordingly. However, the changes did facilitate more successful recruitment as an additional 151 participants then completed the study for a total of 192, achieving the scale development sample size standards put forth by DeVellis [40].

Participant demographics revealed a broad distribution of household income and employment status, as well as geographical locations from 26 states. The most common categories for respondents were biological parent (97%), over the age of 30 (91%), female (89%), married (78%), and Caucasian (77%). In total, 75% had a child currently receiving EIBI, with 57% meeting the initial eligibility criteria and target population definition of under age six.

3.2. Reliability. Reliability was assessed using Cronbach's alpha [45], which is generally recommended for scale development. Cronbach's alpha for the final 29-item EPSE Scale was .900, which is essentially an ideal score according to DeVellis [40]. A split-half analysis was also conducted. Cronbach's alpha for the first half was .852, compared to .865 for the second half. The correlation between forms was .622, and the Spearman-Brown coefficient was .767. Clark and Watson [42] also recommend examining the interitem correlation. The mean interitem correlation for this scale was .245, with a minimum of −.098 and a maximum of .652.

Table 1: Means and ranges for scale item scores.

Statistic	*M*	Lowest	Highest
Mean item scores	5.88	3.98	6.68
Standard deviations	1.17	0.63	1.75
Variances	1.44	0.39	3.06
Ranges	5.41	3	6
Minimum scores	1.59	1	4
Maximum scores	7.00	7	7

Note. M: mean score.

3.3. Validity. The process used to develop the EPSE Scale allowed for two forms of basic validity to be established, using standards defined by DeVellis [40]. Construct validity was established by strictly adhering to the guidelines of self-efficacy theory and the boundaries of the scale's primary construct of parental ability to continue implementing EIBI. Content validity was established by conducting the field test, wherein subject matter experts helped determine whether the EPSE Scale was easy to understand, representative of the construct, and appropriate for the target population.

3.4. Item Analysis. The item analysis analyzed the mean, standard deviation, variance, range, minimum, and maximum scores. As per DeVellis [40], items with the following characteristics are candidates for elimination: (a) mean near the extremes, (b) low standard deviation, (c) low variance, (d) low range, or (e) minimum or maximum not approaching the extremes. Table 1 summarizes the mean, lowest, and highest numbers for item scores within each of the identified categories.

Most items had means closer to the maximum than midpoint. Standard deviation and variance averaged above 1.0, and range averaged at least 5. As such, the following criteria were established to mark items for possible deletion: (a) mean above 6.5, (b) standard deviation below 1.0, (c) variance below 1.0, (d) range below 4, (e) minimum above 3, and (f) maximum below 5.

In general, all items had high mean scores. However, since the purpose of the EPSE Scale is to identify struggles, it may not be appropriate to assume that a midpoint score should be the average. One ethical theme from the expert review was that items should not portray EIBI as too difficult, which could discourage families. Therefore, a higher average may be appropriate.

Descriptive statistics were obtained for total scale scores across participants. The range between minimum and maximum scores was 130. The mean scale score was 199.96, with a standard deviation of 20.32, which equals three standard deviations above the midpoint of 136.

The total number of responses for each possible item score was analyzed, and the results revealed a negative skew of −1.288. This result was not surprising since, as previously noted, mean item scores were high, but in general participant data did not display a normal distribution.

For an item correlation analysis, the Pearson product-moment correlation coefficient (r) was obtained for all items. Floyd and Widaman [44] state that the minimum score should be 0.20, and Field [43] cautions that items with very high correlations of 0.90 or above may be problematic due to multicollinearity. The matrix revealed no correlations above 0.90, but nearly half were below 0.20. The risk of low correlations is that they may perform poorly in factor analysis. However, as explained in the next section, no such issues arose.

3.5. Factor Analysis. Factor analysis identified how many factors were causing item response variation. Items that did not fit into a factor were eliminated. The four major steps conducted were (a) factor extraction, (b) factor rotation, (c) factor loadings, and (d) interpretation of factors.

Factor extraction involves determining how many factors to analyze, using either exploratory or confirmatory methods [40]. Exploratory methods are recommended when there are no firm expectations regarding the number of factors based on theory or prior research [44]. Since the goal of this study was to measure something not previously researched, exploratory factor analysis was utilized. This process was conducted in two ways, using both a principal components analysis (PCA) and a common factor analysis (CFA).

The extraction procedure was conducted with the eigenvalue level set at over one. A scree plot was generated, and the extraction sums of squared loadings for all eigenvalues over 1.0 were examined, separated by PCA versus CFA. The eigenvalue rule [46] states that factors with eigenvalues of less than 1.0 should not be retained. However, DeVellis [40] explains that 1.0 is equivalent to the effect of a single item, so a value just above 1.0 may not be worth retaining either. For this test, eigenvalues showed six factors clearly above 1.0 with the lowest at 1.273, followed by 1.098. Therefore, only the top six factors were retained.

Field [43] also recommends checking the value for the Kaiser-Meyer-Olkin (KMO) measure of sampling adequacy. A value greater than 0.5 signifies that the sample size is adequate for factor analysis, and the KMO value for this sample was .863.

The next step was to conduct factor rotation so that meaningful groupings of items could emerge. Both orthogonal and oblique rotations were conducted with PCA and CFA analyses. Floyd and Widaman [44] state that a high cumulative percentage such as 80% is ideal, so that these factors are accounting for most of the variance. These analyses did not quite achieve that goal, as PCA rotation represented 55.5% of the variance and CFA represented 46.4 percent.

In total, factor extraction and rotation were conducted in four ways: (a) PCA orthogonal, (b) CFA orthogonal, (c) PCA oblique, and (d) CFA oblique. The factor loading results for each combination were analyzed, and CFA orthogonal provided the clearest factor structure.

Several considerations were important to arrive at this conclusion. First, the oblique rotations did not provide enough clarity. Both PCA and CFA factor loading results showed at least seven items that did not meet the minimum strength requirements of .400 for PCA or .350 for CFA. Deleting these items solely on this basis would have put the scale at risk as more items may have been deleted later for other reasons, resulting in potentially too few items overall to accomplish the scale's goals. Additionally, both oblique analyses contained one factor with no items even achieving a minimal loading requirement of .300. Floyd and Widaman [44] state that factor loadings are most meaningful when they exceed .300 or .400 and that at least three items should have significant loadings to retain a factor. Clark and Watson [42] state that factors should load at least .350 in CFA or .400 in PCA and that items loading strongly on only one factor are the best candidates to keep.

By contrast, both orthogonal extractions had strong results with almost all items clustering clearly around all six factors with good distribution. PCA, however, did not clearly reveal which items should be deleted, as too many items loaded strongly on more than one factor. The only area in which PCA outperformed CFA was total variance explained (55.5% versus 46.4%, resp.). However, the initial eigenvalues showed that 14 factors would be required to reach the desired goal of 80 percent, which would be too many for the practical purposes of this scale and would contain six eigenvalues below 1.0.

The process of interpreting factors involves qualitatively examining items loading on each factor. If similarities can be explained as indicators of a theoretical construct, the factor can be interpreted [40]. Loading values were considered as well, with scores below .350 eliminated. Upon examining the items, five factors were interpreted as follows: (a) *Family Well-Being*, (b) *Preparing for Successful Sessions*, (c) *Team Participation*, (d) *Not Giving Up*, and (e) *Working with Your Child*. A sixth factor, *Motivating Others*, was also identified but later eliminated as it only contained two items.

All items for *Family Well-Being* allude to promoting healthy relationships and a balanced life for family members. The *Preparing for Successful Sessions* items focus on daily procedures to facilitate operational aspects of EIBI. The elements of *Team Participation* reflect parent involvement in the design and implementation of the child's program and working with team members. *Not Giving Up* includes items presenting challenges that require perseverance in the face of obstacles. The items in *Working with Your Child* discuss parents doing activities directly with their child that support the behavior change procedures established in the EIBI program.

After rerunning CFA orthogonal analysis with these five factors, cumulative amount of variance was 46.2 percent, just below the score obtained in the original analysis with six factors, thus maintaining the amount of total variance explained despite eliminating one factor. The final rotated factor loadings are provided in Table 2, along with all items and their interpreted factor themes. Reliability scores for all factors are also shown, ranging from .695 to .835, which rates as acceptable to very good [40]. All items loaded above the CFA

Table 2: Factor loadings with orthogonal rotation for the final five factors.

Factors and items	1	2	3	4	5
Factor 1: Family Well-Being (α = *.812*)					
Spend enough time with each of your other family members	.721				
Support each other if EIBI is causing any stress for people in your home	.693				
Make time to celebrate small steps of progress with your family	.659				
Find time to take breaks and take care of yourself	.616				
Find a way to have bonding time with your child, which might be separate from therapy time	.533				
Help your extended family understand why EIBI is so important for your child	.479				
Get your family members to join in on some of the home program activities	.417				
Factor 2: Preparing for Successful Sessions (α = *.835*)					
Have your home ready when therapists come over to work with your child		.705			
Get your child ready for each session before the therapist arrives		.670			
Set up your home in a way that works for the program and also works for your family		.570			
Set up areas in your home where therapists can work with your child without interruptions		.548			
Keep all program materials organized so therapists can find what they need		.524			
Make sure therapists feel welcome in your home at all times		.471			
Help everyone who lives with you get used to having the therapists in the home		.461			
Factor 3: Team Participation (α = *.792*)					
Take good notes during team meetings and discussions with your program supervisor			.728		
Make sure you have a say in choosing your child's goals and designing the program			.657		
Talk to the supervisor if you have concerns about one of the therapists			.537		
Participate in training with your team so you know how to use all the strategies			.520		
Host meetings in your home with your child's therapy team, at least once a month			.506		
Help therapists plan their daily activities with your child			.445		
Observe what the therapists are doing each day			.415		
Factor 4: Not Giving Up (α = *.695*)					
Make EIBI one of your top priorities				.709	
Be willing to change parts of your family's lifestyle so that your child can continue EIBI				.691	
Allow therapy sessions to continue when your child is upset				.373	
Continue EIBI even if your child's school is not supportive of it				.356	
Factor 5: Working with Your Child (α = *.738*)					
When working with your child, be consistent with what you have been trained to do, even if your child gets upset					.636
Be one of your child's therapists, and balance this role with also being a parent					.578
Be persistent and try different things to get your child to engage in activities with you					.578
Be enthusiastic when you work with your child, even if you feel sad about other things	.550				.473

Note. Varimax rotation procedure used in SPSS. Numbers across header row represent extracted factors. Item loadings lower than the assigned factor are not shown. Cronbach's alpha scores for each factor are provided.

significance cutoff of .350 on their identified factor group. Some items loaded above .350 for more than one factor, but all except one loaded highest on the correct factor. This item was included in factor five even though its primary loading was on factor one. As shown in Table 2, both scores were above the defined significance level of .400, but factor five was a better conceptual fit with the interpreted themes. Factor one also had the most items while factor five had the fewest. Thus, the move was made to achieve better overall scale composition. This approach is supported by Field [43], as factor analysis is an exploratory tool to use only as a guide for making decisions.

DeVellis [40] states that item elimination decisions should never be made solely on a statistical basis. Original intent of the scale needs to be considered along with statistical evidence. Following researcher review of all data analysis, five items were eliminated that had undesirable qualities from the item analysis and did not fit into one of the established factors.

The final version of the EPSE Scale contains 29 items within five subscales. The instructions state that the scale is intended for parents/guardians of a child diagnosed with autism (or at-risk), who lives at home with this parent/guardian and is currently receiving home-based EIBI. Participants are asked to read each item and rate how certain they are that they can do the stated task regularly on a scale of 1 to 7, with 1 representing that they can never do it and 7 signifying they can always do it. Tasks that they do now should be scored based on their certainty of being able to continue doing it, whereas items they have not done yet should be scored based on their belief that they could do it regularly if they had to start now.

3.6. Limitations. The first major limitation was that the methodology did not allow for robust validity. Two basic forms of validity were demonstrated—content and construct validity. The most powerful form, especially for self-efficacy scales, is predictive validity [40, 41], which involves first administering the scale and then observing future behavior to see if there is a clear correlation. For the EPSE Scale, that would require a longitudinal study to see if scale scores accurately predict ongoing parent struggles. Presumably, families with low scores would be at higher risk for discontinuing or reducing the intensity of EIBI treatment. This limitation was known before the study began, as the scope of this pilot study did not allow for a comprehensive long-term evaluation of participants.

The next major limitation, as discussed previously, was not expected and arose due to recruiting challenges. The initial goal was 150 participants, but the planned strategy yielded only 41. Since the target sample size needed to be met for factor analysis, the criteria were modified so that more people would qualify. Of the final sample, more than half did meet the initial eligibility criteria and defined target population for whom the scale is intended. However, a good portion of the participants did not. The participants who only met the revised criteria were likely to have had a good understanding of the items as they did have related experience with implementing EIBI, but all findings should be considered in light of this significant limitation.

The demographics also revealed some limitations. Nearly 90% of respondents were female, and almost all were biological parents. More than 70% were over the age of 35, more than 75% were Caucasian, and nearly 80% were married to the other biological parent. Less than 10% had household income under $30,000, and all had at least a high school diploma or GED. These proportions suggest a potentially more stable subpopulation with fewer barriers than some parents of children with autism. There was low representation from minorities, single parents, younger parents, and low income families who may be at higher risk for implementation difficulties. The sample was built on participants independently responding to announcements from support groups, providers, or autism organizations. It is possible that these parents were more likely to be actively involved in their child's treatment and thus scored higher on their capability confidence levels. Overall, however, nearly every demographic category did have some participant representation.

4. Discussion

The results of this pilot study provide an initial framework for researchers to further develop this new instrument that focuses on understanding parental roles within EIBI treatment. As such, the EPSE Scale is the first of its kind, in that it measures self-efficacy specifically related to the tasks and behaviors that facilitate successful implementation of a very unique and comprehensive autism treatment program. Now that initial development of the scale has been completed, future research is warranted to refine and validate the measure.

The area in which this pilot study offers the most promise is in potential implications for practice. The EPSE Scale was designed with a vision of improving outcomes and family experiences through its use in real world settings, most notably in community-based EIBI models. If additional research successfully validates the scale, it can then be made available to EIBI providers around the world as a tool to help objectively identify any challenges parents are experiencing related to implementation. In practice, use of the EPSE Scale could serve to improve overall communication between parents and providers as part of a commitment to finding family-centered solutions.

The purpose of this scale is not to determine whether a family will succeed with EIBI, but rather to identify any critical areas that are presenting a challenge, so that practitioners have the opportunity to provide assistance proactively and increase the odds of success. This study adds to a growing body of research on how to make EIBI consistently successful in real world and community-based settings.

Once a family has begun implementing EIBI, there are as of yet no defined time intervals regarding when to administer the EPSE Scale. It is clearly not appropriate to administer before treatment begins, as parents will not have any implementation experience to relate to when answering the questions. It does appear to be appropriate early on in the treatment process, such as within the first three months of implementation, and again at various points thereafter (e.g., every six to 12 months). Until further research providers clear recommendations, practitioners should use clinical judgment regarding overall frequency, and it may vary based on the client. However, overuse of the instrument through frequent administrations could be detrimental, as participants could become overly familiar with the questions and exhibit response bias. It is also possible that, in some cases, simply administering the tool once and engaging in follow-up conversation to discuss identified challenges might be enough to establish a relationship of open dialogue and proactive support, which could last throughout the remainder of treatment and not require additional formal administrations of the scale. As stated, further research is necessary to determine the optimal schedule for recurring administrations.

Another limitation of this pilot study is that it does not specify exactly how to interpret any given participant's scale and subscale scores. There is, for example, no identified cutoff point that signifies a problem for either an individual item or a group of items making up a themed subscale. Additionally, this pilot study does not provide evidence-based direction as to what the resulting actions should be if a practitioner assesses a family and finds low scores in certain areas that suggest help is needed. The intended concept is that practitioners would use the scale as a way to objectively collect information from families, followed by a supportive conversation to collaboratively discuss identified challenges. Perhaps modifications can then be made to the treatment protocols as needed with the goal of integrating the program as smoothly as possible into the family's life, thereby maximizing a family-centered approach to EIBI. Additional studies will be necessary to determine how to best interpret variability in scores.

As intended, this pilot study provides multiple opportunities for additional research. The first and most important step is to test the current version of the EPSE Scale with participants that strictly align with the intended target population of children less than six years old who are actively receiving at least 20 hours per week of EIBI. To maximize confidence in the findings, such a study should include a very large sample size, and each demographic characteristic should have significant representation to establish strong evidence for the validity of the tool with all members of the target population. As with any scale, overall validation is only achieved over time by repeated use in research with a variety of populations and circumstances [40].

Another critical recommendation is to conduct a longitudinal study that tracks participants for up to several years, to see how scale scores correlate with EIBI treatment outcomes and ongoing challenges. Doing so would assess the highly desired predictive validity of the EPSE Scale, which Bandura [41] cites as the most important property to validate any self-efficacy based scale. If it is found that the scale does have clear predictive power, another question arises as to how far into the future the prediction goes. For example, if the scale identifies a challenge that the family is currently experiencing, does that predict struggles for the next two months, six months, or duration of treatment? How many challenges constitute a risk of early treatment termination? Are there particular combinations of challenges that lead to higher risk? The more that such issues are investigated, the more valuable the EPSE Scale will become in real world settings.

Researchers should also examine what types of practitioner response procedures are most effective. The assumption made here is that practitioners could use scale response data to initiate constructive dialogue with parents about possible solutions. For example, perhaps the EIBI program could be modified to better fit the family's needs, or other community resources could be secured to help struggling families. The general principle is that knowing is better than not knowing, and addressing a problem together will ultimately improve the likelihood of positive treatment outcomes and experiences. That being said, however, it would be ideal to know how to best alleviate a problem once it has been discovered. For that reason, it is recommended that future researchers investigate optimal responses for each EPSE Scale item or domain.

If other studies pursue the recommendations noted thus far of diverse sampling, predictive power, and how to best help after assessment, researchers could then closely investigate the specifics of scale scores. Individual items and subscales all have a wide range of possible scores, and with enough data it could be possible to identify what to expect for specific scoring ranges. The more clearly this relationship is understood, the easier it will be to establish consistent follow-up procedures that are based on an exact score. From the current study alone, it is not yet possible to determine what constitutes a score within a normal range.

4.1. Conclusion. This pilot study completed an initial development and evaluation process for a new instrument, the EIBI Parental Self-Efficacy (EPSE) Scale. This 29-item, five-factor tool measures the perceived self-efficacy for parents implementing home-based Early Intensive Behavioral Intervention (EIBI) for their child with autism. The scale demonstrated a series of sound psychometric properties, including a Cronbach's alpha reliability score of .900.

The four phases of this pilot study followed best practice guidelines for scale development in the social and behavioral sciences, thereby contributing to construct validity. These phases involved item generation and scale construction, a field test with expert reviewers, a pretest administration with the target population, and a large sample pilot study with 192 participants. Factor analysis revealed a clear structure of five factors with at least three items each, which were interpreted as follows: (a) *Family Well-Being*, (b) *Preparing for Successful Sessions*, (c) *Team Participation*, (d) *Not Giving Up*, and (e) *Working with Your Child*. The EPSE Scale is now ready for researchers to conduct additional studies toward validation.

This study also contributed to the literature surrounding challenges that parents face when implementing EIBI. Through the processes of a comprehensive literature review, item development, expert review, and participant data analysis, a significant amount of evidence was obtained that suggests these items and factor themes represent real issues that parents face when trying to implement EIBI for their child. It is clear that providers should never take it for granted that parents are adequately equipped to tackle the varying amount of responsibilities they must embrace in order to sustain a successful treatment experience for their child. Providers need to be sensitive to the obstacles parents may face, and work in partnership with them to ensure a successful treatment experience. Hopefully, tools such as the EPSE Scale will facilitate that process and ultimately improve access to effective treatment for all children and families living with autism.

Ethical Approval

The university's IRB approved all components of the study. All procedures performed in studies involving human participants were in accordance with the ethical standards of the institutional and/or national research committee and with the 1964 Helsinki Declaration and its later amendments or comparable ethical standards.

Disclosure

This article does not contain any studies with animals performed by any of the authors. Aaron Blocher-Rubin, Ph.D., BCBA, was a doctoral student at Capella University in Minnesota while completing this study. Dr. Paige Krabill, PsyD, served as dissertation mentor for this study and is currently a faculty member for Multidisciplinary Human Services graduate programs through the School of Public Service Leadership at Capella University in Minnesota. Dr. Blocher-Rubin is now at Arizona Autism United, a nonprofit organization in Phoenix. This study was completed as part of Dr. Blocher-Rubin's doctoral dissertation. A copy of the EPSE Scale form with instructions is available for practitioners and researchers to download for free at www.EPSEscale.com.

References

[1] S. Eldevik, R. P. Hastings, J. C. Hughes, E. Jahr, S. Eikeseth, and S. Cross, "Meta-analysis of early intensive behavioral intervention for children with autism," *Journal of Clinical Child & Adolescent Psychology*, vol. 38, no. 3, pp. 439–450, 2009.

[2] H. E. Flanagan, A. Perry, and N. L. Freeman, "Effectiveness of large-scale community-based intensive behavioral intervention: a waitlist comparison study exploring outcomes and predictors," *Research in Autism Spectrum Disorders*, vol. 6, no. 2, pp. 673–682, 2012.

[3] N. Peters-Scheffer, R. Didden, H. Korzilius, and P. Sturmey, "A meta-analytic study on the effectiveness of comprehensive ABA-based early intervention programs for children with Autism Spectrum Disorders," *Research in Autism Spectrum Disorders*, vol. 5, no. 1, pp. 60–69, 2011.

[4] B. Reichow, "Overview of meta-analyses on early intensive behavioral intervention for young children with autism spectrum disorders," *Journal of Autism and Developmental Disorders*, vol. 42, no. 4, pp. 512–520, 2012.

[5] J. Virués-Ortega, "Applied behavior analytic intervention for autism in early childhood: meta-analysis, meta-regression and dose-response meta-analysis of multiple outcomes," *Clinical Psychology Review*, vol. 30, no. 4, pp. 387–399, 2010.

[6] S. Granger, C. Des Rivières-Pigeon, G. Sabourin, and J. Forget, "Mothers' reports of their involvement in early intensive behavioral intervention," *Topics in Early Childhood Special Education*, vol. 32, no. 2, pp. 68–77, 2012.

[7] C. Grindle, H. Kovshoff, R. Hastings, and B. Remington, "Parents' experiences of home-based applied behavior analysis programs for young children with autism," *Journal of Autism & Developmental Disorders*, vol. 39, no. 1, pp. 42–56, 2009.

[8] J. R. Love, J. E. Carr, S. M. Almason, and A. I. Petursdottir, "Early and intensive behavioral intervention for autism: a survey of clinical practices," *Research in Autism Spectrum Disorders*, vol. 3, no. 2, pp. 421–428, 2009.

[9] K. R. Cebula, "Applied behavior analysis programs for autism: Sibling psychosocial adjustment during and following intervention use," *Journal of Autism and Developmental Disorders*, vol. 42, no. 5, pp. 847–862, 2012.

[10] C. Trudgeon and D. Carr, "The impacts of home-based early behavioural intervention programmes on families of children with autism," *Journal of Applied Research in Intellectual Disabilities*, vol. 20, no. 4, pp. 285–296, 2007.

[11] S. J. Sheinkopf and B. Siegel, "Home-based behavioral treatment of young children with autism," *Journal of Autism & Developmental Disorders*, vol. 28, no. 1, pp. 15–23, 1998.

[12] A. Solish and A. Perry, "Parents' involvement in their children's behavioral intervention programs: parent and therapist perspectives," *Research in Autism Spectrum Disorders*, vol. 2, no. 4, pp. 728–738, 2008.

[13] T. Smith, G. A. Buch, and T. E. Gamby, "Parent-directed, intensive early intervention for children with pervasive developmental disorder," *Research in Developmental Disabilities*, vol. 21, no. 4, pp. 297–309, 2000.

[14] Behavior Analyst Certification Board, *Guidelines, Health Plan Coverage of Applied Behavior Analysis Treatment for Autism Spectrum Disorder*, Behavior Analyst Certification Board, 2012, http://www.bacb.com/Downloadfiles/ABA_Guidelines_for_ASD.pdf.

[15] A. Perry, A. Cummings, J. Dunn Geier et al., "Effectiveness of intensive behavioral intervention in a large, community-based program," *Research in Autism Spectrum Disorders*, vol. 2, no. 4, pp. 621–642, 2008.

[16] E. M. Butter, J. Wynn, and J. A. Mulick, "Early intervention critical to autism treatment," *Pediatric Annals*, vol. 32, no. 10, pp. 677–684, 2003.

[17] B. Reichow and M. J. Wolery, "Comprehensive synthesis of early intensive behavioral interventions for young children with autism based on the UCLA young autism project model," *Journal of Autism and Developmental Disorders*, vol. 39, no. 1, pp. 23–41, 2009.

[18] R. D. Boyd and M. J. Corley, "Outcome survey of early intensive behavioral intervention for young children with autism in a community setting," *Autism*, vol. 5, no. 4, pp. 430–441, 2001.

[19] H. Cohen, M. Amerine-Dickens, and T. Smith, "Early intensive behavioral treatment: Replication of the UCLA model in a community setting," *Journal of Developmental and Behavioral Pediatrics*, vol. 27, no. 2, pp. 145–155, 2006.

[20] I. Magiati, T. Charman, and P. Howlin, "A two-year prospective follow-up study of community-based early intensive behavioural intervention and specialist nursery provision for children with autism spectrum disorders," *Journal of Child Psychology Psychiatry*, vol. 48, no. 8, pp. 803–812, 2007.

[21] G. Green, L. C. Brennan, and D. Fein, "Intensive behavioral treatment for a toddler at high risk for autism," *Behavior Modification*, vol. 26, no. 1, pp. 69–102, 2002.

[22] P. Tzanakaki, C. Grindle, R. P. Hastings, J. C. Hughes, H. Kovshoff, and B. Remington, "How and why do parents choose early intensive behavioral intervention for their young child with autism?" *Education and Training in Autism and Developmental Disabilities*, vol. 47, no. 1, pp. 58–71, 2012.

[23] J. S. Howard, C. R. Sparkman, H. G. Cohen, G. Green, and H. Stanislaw, "A comparison of intensive behavior analytic and eclectic treatments for young children with autism," *Research in Developmental Disabilities*, vol. 26, no. 4, pp. 359–383, 2005.

[24] V. K. Jensen and L. V. Sinclair, "Treatment of autism in young children: behavioral intervention and applied behavior analysis," *Infants Young Children: An Interdisciplinary Journal of Special Care Practices*, vol. 14, no. 4, pp. 42–52, 2002.

[25] T. R. Moore and F. J. Symons, "Adherence to treatment in a behavioral intervention curriculum for parents of children with autism spectrum disorder," *Behavior Modification*, vol. 35, no. 6, pp. 570–594, 2011.

[26] S. Phetrasuwan and M. Shandor Miles, "Parenting stress in mothers of children with autism spectrum disorders," *Journal for Specialists in Pediatric Nursing*, vol. 14, no. 3, pp. 157–165, 2009.

[27] A. Bandura, "Self-efficacy: toward a unifying theory of behavioral change," *Psychological Review*, vol. 84, no. 2, pp. 191–215, 1977.

[28] A. Bandura, "The nature and structure of self-efficacy," in *Self-Efficacy: The Exercise of Control*, S. F. Brennan and C. Hastings, Eds., pp. 36–78, W. H. Freeman, New York, NY, USA, 1997.
[29] P. K. Coleman and K. H. Karraker, "Self-efficacy and parenting quality: findings and future applications," *Developmental Review*, vol. 18, no. 1, pp. 47–85, 1998.
[30] J. V. D. Bijl, A. V. Poelgeest-Eeltink, and L. Shortridge-Baggett, "The psychometric properties of the diabetes management self-efficacy scale for patients with type 2 diabetes mellitus," *Journal of Advanced Nursing*, vol. 30, no. 2, pp. 352–359, 1999.
[31] M. L. Horan, K. K. Kim, P. Gendler, R. D. Froman, and M. D. Patel, "Development and evaluation of the osteoporosis self-efficacy scale," *Research in Nursing and Health*, vol. 21, no. 5, pp. 395–403, 1998.
[32] A. B. Guimond, M. J. Wilcox, and S. G. Lamorey, "The early intervention parenting self-efficacy scale (EIPSES): scale construction and initial psychometric evidence," *Journal of Early Intervention*, vol. 30, no. 4, pp. 295–320, 2008.
[33] K. E. Hoagwood, "Family-based services in children's mental health: a research review and synthesis," *Journal of Child Psychology and Psychiatry*, vol. 46, no. 7, pp. 690–713, 2005.
[34] L. A. Osborne, L. McHugh, J. Saunders, and P. Reed, "Parenting stress reduces the effectiveness of early teaching interventions for autistic spectrum disorders," *Journal of Autism and Developmental Disorders*, vol. 38, no. 6, pp. 1092–1103, 2008.
[35] B. Remington, "Early intensive behavioral intervention and family psychological adjustment," *Inside Behavior Analysis*, vol. 2, no. 3, 2010.
[36] L. M. T. Silva and M. Schalock, "Autism Parenting Stress Index: Initial psychometric evidence," *Journal of Autism & Developmental Disorders*, vol. 42, pp. 566–574, 2012.
[37] C. Springer and L. Reddy, "Measuring adherence in behavior therapy: opportunities for practice and research," *The Behavior Therapist*, vol. 27, no. 5, pp. 99–101, 2004.
[38] C. Lord, A. Wagner, S. Rogers et al., "Challenges in evaluating psychosocial interventions for autistic spectrum disorders," *Journal of Autism and Developmental Disorders*, vol. 35, no. 6, pp. 695–708, 2005.
[39] L. Schreibman, "Intensive behavioral/psychoeducational treatments for autism: research needs and future directions," *Journal of Autism and Developmental Disorders*, vol. 30, no. 5, pp. 373–378, 2000.
[40] R. F. DeVellis, *Scale Development—Theory and Applications*, Sage Publications, Thousand Oaks, Calif, USA, 3rd edition, 2012.
[41] A. Bandura, "Guide to constructing self-efficacy scales," in *Self-Efficacy Beliefs of Adolescents*, T. Urdan and F. Pajares, Eds., pp. 307–337, Information Age Publishing, Charlotte, NC, USA, 2006.
[42] L. A. Clark and D. Watson, "Constructing validity: basic issues in objective scale development," *Psychological Assessment*, vol. 7, no. 3, pp. 309–319, 1995.
[43] A. Field, *Discovering Statistics Using SPSS*, Sage Publications, Thousand Oaks, Calif, USA, 2nd edition, 2005.
[44] F. J. Floyd and K. F. Widaman, "Factor analysis in the development and refinement of clinical assessment instruments," *Psychological Assessment*, vol. 7, no. 3, pp. 286–299, 1995.
[45] L. J. Cronbach, "Coefficient alpha and the internal structure of tests," *Psychometrika*, vol. 16, no. 3, pp. 297–334, 1951.
[46] H. F. Kaiser, "The application of electronic computers to factor analysis," *Educational and Psychological Measurement*, vol. 20, pp. 141–151, 1960.

27

Physical Activity and Physical Fitness of School-Aged Children and Youth with Autism Spectrum Disorders

Kiley Tyler,[1] Megan MacDonald,[1] and Kristi Menear[2]

[1] *College of Public Health and Human Sciences, Oregon State University, Corvallis, OR 97331, USA*
[2] *School of Education, University of Alabama at Birmingham, Birmingham, AL 35294, USA*

Correspondence should be addressed to Megan MacDonald; megan.macdonald@oregonstate.edu

Academic Editor: Geraldine Dawson

Autism spectrum disorder (ASD) is characterized by impairments in social communication deficits and the presence of restricted and repetitive behaviors, interests, or activities. Literature comparing the physical activity and fitness of children with ASD to typically developing peers is in need of attention. The purpose of this investigation was to examine the physical activity and fitness of school-aged children with ASD ($N = 17$) in comparison to typically developing peers ($N = 12$). Participants with ASD completed diagnostic and developmental assessments and a series of physical fitness assessments: 20-meter multistage shuttle, sit-and-reach test, handgrip strength, and body mass index. Physical activity was measured using accelerometry and preestablished cut-points of physical activity (Freedson et al., 2005). MANCOVA revealed significant between-group effects in strength ($P = .03$), while ANCOVA revealed significant between-group effects in sedentary ($P = .00$), light ($P = .00$), moderate ($P = .00$), and total moderate-to-vigorous ($P = .01$) physical activity. Children with ASD are less physically active and fit than typically developing peers. Adapted physical activity programs are one avenue with intervention potential to combat these lower levels of physical activity and fitness found in children with ASD.

1. Introduction

As the incidence rate of autism spectrum disorder (ASD) increases, so does the interest in the health and wellness of these individuals. Similar to their typically developing peers, youth with ASD face increased rates of obesity [1, 2] and decreased engagement in physical activities [3]. Reviews of physical activity patterns indicated that older adolescents with ASD are less physically active than their younger peers with ASD [4–6]. The contributing factors to the obesity and physical inactivity epidemic in this population may be both diagnosis-specific and environmental [7].

Profiles of motor skills and physical fitness in children and youth with ASD have documented delayed performance levels. Pan [8] assessed 62 adolescent males with ($n = 31$) and without ($n = 31$) ASD aged 10–17 years using the Bruininks-Oseretsky Test of Motor Proficiency (2nd edition), the BROCKPORT Physical Fitness Test, and the bioelectrical impedance analysis. Results indicated that adolescents with ASD had significantly lower scores on all motor proficiency and fitness measures, except body composition, than adolescents without ASD and that the types of associations between the two measures differed significantly across the groups. Staples and Reid [9] compared the fundamental movement skills of 25 children and youth with ASD (ages 9–12 years) to three typically developing groups of children using the Test of Gross Motor Development (TGMD-2). Their results suggested that children and youth with ASD experience more than just delays in movement abilities but that movement deficits in motor skill performance existed.

Literature that compares the physical activity and fitness of children and youth with ASD to their typically developing peers is scarce, but what does exist uses common fitness measures such as the shuttle run, sit-and-reach, and handgrip dynamometer [8] and activity measures such as accelerometry [3]. Health-related physical fitness, which is embedded in physical activity through physical exercise, consists of body composition, aerobic fitness (aerobic capacity, power, and endurance), flexibility, and muscular fitness (muscular strength and muscular endurance) [10–12]. Our study includes these physical fitness measures, in addition to a physical activity measure. The indicated measures are used to describe the physical activity and physical fitness of school-aged children with ASD in comparison to typically developing peers. By using a similar age range to the studies cited above, including both male and female participants with a range of severity (as indicated through calibrated autism severity scores), and adding additional measures of physical fitness compared to other studies, our study provides further evidence of the profiles of this population compared to their typically developed peers as it relates to physical activity and physical fitness. Thus, the purpose of this study is to determine the physical fitness and physical activity of children with ASD, compared to their typically developed peers.

2. Method

2.1. Participants. Children and youth with ASD ($N = 17$, $M = 9$, $F = 8$) and without ASD ($N = 12$, $M = 6$, $F = 6$) between the ages of 9 and 18 years were recruited for this study. Recruitment occurred through the dissemination of study flyers, autism-based programs, local schools, local rehabilitation facilities, and word of mouth. Participants were not excluded based on race/ethnicity or gender.

2.2. Procedure. Each parent/caregiver of each participant completed a supplemental questionnaire, which included demographic information such as age of participant, maternal education, income, ethnicity, and diagnosis of an ASD. Data collection took place in a lab-based setting, where participants completed the majority of assessments over the course of two days. Each assessment session took into consideration the comfort and scheduling needs of each participant and family. The order of assessments typically consisted of the diagnostic assessment and developmental assessment, followed by a series of physical fitness assessments in aerobic fitness, muscular strength, flexibility, and anthropometric measures (height and weight). Physical activity was measured through accelerometry. The assessments are described below.

2.2.1. Diagnostic Assessment. Participants with ASD, per parental report, were administered the autism diagnostic observation schedule (ADOS) [13–15] by a trained research administrator. The senior investigator on this project was research trained and reliable on ADOS administration. Each member of the research team attained interrater reliability of ADOS administration exceeding 80% exact agreement over the course of three consecutive administrations before the study began with the senior investigator on this project. Thus, within site reliability was obtained. The ADOS is a semistructured standardized assessment of communication, social interaction, and play for individuals with autism spectrum disorder or suspected of having autism. This diagnostic tool is commonly used in practice and research and is considered the "gold standard" in terms of standardized diagnostic assessments [16]. Calibrated severity scores [13] were used in this study to confirm diagnosis; these scores are consistent with ADOS-2 criteria [13].

2.2.2. Developmental Assessment. The Stanford-Binet Intelligence Scale Fifth Edition (SB5) was administered to assess cognitive abilities of each participant [17]. The SB5 is an individually administered assessment of cognitive abilities for individual of 2–85 years. If the participant was unable to progress through the SB5, typically based on limited language, the Differential Ability Scale Second Edition (DAS-II) was administered. The DAS-II is a standardized comprehensive assessment of cognitive abilities [18]. The DAS-II consists of a variety of subtests including verbal and visual working memory, immediate and delayed recall, visual recognition and matching, process and naming speed, phonological processing, and understanding of basic number concepts [18]. Ratio verbal and nonverbal IQ scores were calculated from the SB-5 and the DAS-II, allowing for comparison of verbal and nonverbal abilities across tests. Ratio nonverbal IQ was calculated by dividing the average age equivalent across nonverbal subtest scales, by chronological age in months, and then multiplying by 100. Ratio verbal IQ was calculated in the same manner using the verbal subtest.

2.2.3. Aerobic Fitness Assessment. Aerobic fitness was assessed using the 20-meter multistage shuttle run [19]. The 20-meter multistage shuttle run is a valid and reliable assessment of aerobic power in children [19], with good test-retest reliability for children ($r = .89$, $P = .05$). Each participant was provided with a shuttle run demonstration by the examiner as well as a practice trial before the trials began. During each measured trial, an undergraduate student served as the participant's running partner in an effort to help with the pacing of each shuttle run. The procedures for the 20-meter multistage shuttle run include the participant running back and forth between two sets of cones (shuttles) spaced 20 meters apart. The rate at which the participant runs is controlled by an audio recording that "beeps" when the participant should reach the opposing set of cones. The beeps are equally spaced within one-minute "stages," starting slowly and accelerating incrementally every minute thereafter. If the participant was unable to complete two consecutive stages in accordance with the prompted "beeps," the test was terminated and the final distance was recorded. The velocity of the final shuttle completed by the individual was used to determine the estimated maximal aerobic power ($VO_{2\,max}$) for that individual [19]. The 20-meter multistage shuttle was converted into $VO_{2\,max}$ (Y, $mL\,kg^{-1}\,min^{-1}$) values. These values were obtained from the maximal shuttle run speed (Xlt $km\,h^{-1}$) and age ($X2$, year rounded to the lower integer) for children between the ages of 6 and 18 years ($y = 31.025 + 3.238X1 - 3.248X'2 + 0.1536X^{r}1X'2$) [19].

2.2.4. Flexibility Assessment. Flexibility was assessed using the sit-and-reach test [20]. The sit-and-reach test is a valid and reliable measure used to determine trunk and lower

TABLE 1: Participant demographic information.

	Children with autism (N = 17)		Children without autism (N = 12)		F value	P
	M ± SD/frequency	Min–max	M ± SD/frequency	Min–max		
Age	12.6 ± 2.3	9–17	9.0 ± 1.8	9–14	1.49	0.23
Ratio verbal IQ	60.1 ± 25.2	16–110	112.3 ± 99.0	45–385	2.20	0.14
Ratio nonverbal IQ	65.7 ± 40.0	16–172	73.1 ± 19.3	49–105	1.42	0.24
CSS	8.6 ± 1.54	4–10				
Weight (kg)	52.0 ± 27.1	24–128	46.2 ± 14.1	31–81	3.81	0.06
Height (cm)	154.4 ± 15.38	128–184	153.9 ± 14.1	134–176	0.35	0.85
Gender	M = 9/F = 7		M = 6/F = 6			
Maternal education ethnicity	4 no college/12 college 12 Caucasian/4 other		2 no college/11 college 10 Caucasian/3 other			

Note: M: mean; SD: standard deviation. $^*P \leq 0.05$.

TABLE 2: Physical fitness by group.

	Children with autism (N = 17)		Children without autism (N = 12)		F value	P
	M ± SD	Min–max	M ± SD	Min–max		
VO_{2max}	39.9 ± 5.8	31–57	42.0 ± 5.3	32–53	0.07	0.93
Strength	17.5 ± 8.7	6–38	21.1 ± 11.1	10–40	4.7	0.03*
Flexibility	23.7 ± 8.3	12–41	31.5 ± 10.0	15–44	3.5	0.06
BMI (kg/m^2)	20.4 ± 6.6	11–34	19.1 ± 4.3	14–30	0.30	0.58

$^*P \geq 0.05$.

body flexibility in children [21]. Standardized protocols were followed [20] in addition to several bouts of verbal and nonverbal direction (i.e., reminders to keep the legs straight during the stretch forward). Each participant was initially shown how to perform the sit-and-reach test by the examiner and was provided a practice trial before the trials began.

2.2.5. Strength Assessment. Strength was measured using a handgrip strength assessment. In this test, the participant was asked to stand and grip a Jamar Hydraulic Hand Dynamometer [22] with the dominant hand. The participant forcefully squeezed the dynamometer while holding the arm at 90 degrees of flexion and continued squeezing the instrument while straightening the arm to full flexion. The entire action was performed over the course of three separate trials. Each participant was provided with an initial practice trial and task demonstration. During the three trials, each participant was encouraged to squeeze the instrument to full potential while simultaneously straightening their arm to full flexion. The maximal force production, derived from the average of all three trials, was recorded by the examiner. Handgrip strength is a valid and reliable measure of upper-body muscular strength (r = .90) in typically developing children ages of 6–12 years [23].

2.2.6. Physical Activity Assessment. Physical activity was measured using an accelerometer, the ActiGraph GTX3+ (Pensacola, FL), over a seven-day period. This is a valid and reliable measure of physical activity for children with disabilities [24]. All participants were asked to wear the monitor for all waking hours of the day on the right hip using an elastic belt. The monitor was worn for all activities except swimming, showering/bathing, and sleeping and was indicated through self-report logs. The parents/caregivers of the participants were provided with a self-report log to record any times when the monitor was not worn (i.e., forgetting to put it on in the morning, taking it off for comfort, or any other reasons for which it may have been removed). Accelerometry data was compared to parent logs and reduced to physical activity categories of sedentary, light, moderate, and moderate-to-vigorous these were derived from established cut-points [25]. Data were reduced into average time spent in the physical activity categories described. Zero activity counts lasting for a period longer than 5 minutes were considered a nonwear period and therefore excluded from data analysis [26].

2.2.7. Anthropometric Measures. Height and weight of each participant was measured without shoes. Each participant was provided with an initial task demonstration and practice trial if needed. Height was measured in centimeters to the nearest tenth of a millimeter with the portable stadiometer, model: SECA S-214. Weight was measured in kilograms to the nearest gram with the Health O Meter H-349KL digital scale. Each participant's body mass index (BMI) was calculated using the standard formula: body mass (in kilograms) divided by height squared (in meters) [12, 27]. BMI is a valid and reliable (r = .90) means of assessing body composition (height in relation to weight) in children [12]. Measurements were taken twice at each site and rounded to the nearest tenth of a millimeter.

2.3. Data Analysis. Multivariate analysis of covariance (MANCOVA) was used to determine each physical fitness variable of aerobic fitness, flexibility, strength, and BMI of school-aged participants with an ASD compared to typically developing peers. Analysis of covariance (ANCOVA) was used to determine the physical activity of school-aged participants with an ASD compared to participants without an ASD. Covariates for all analyses included age. IQ was highly correlated with age; thus only age was used in these analyses.

3. Results

A total of 17 participants with an ASD ($n = 9$ males and $n = 8$ females) and 12 participants without an ASD ($n = 6$ males and $n = 6$ females) between the ages of 9 and 17 years (mean = 12.6 years) were included in this study. Demographic information is presented in Table 1. There were no relationships between physical fitness and income, maternal education, or ethnicity. Missing values were resolved through single mean substitution [28] by group for the variable of interest. Missing variables of physical fitness accounted for less than 10% of missing data. The most common missing variable was physical activity; less than 20% of data were missing in this variable.

3.1. Physical Fitness. MANCOVA was used to determine the physical fitness of school-aged participants with ASD and typically developing peers. Age was used as a covariate in this model because the distribution of age was different across groups. Participants with an ASD had more 15-year-olds than any other age, whereas participants without an ASD had a higher distribution of 9-year-olds. The MANCOVA revealed nonsignificant effects ($F = 1.59; P = .21$) between groups, indicating that no significant differences existed in physical fitness between participants with an ASD and participants without an ASD. Between-group effects reached significance in strength ($P = .03; F = 3.5$), suggesting that participants with ASD have lower strength compared to participants without an ASD. Flexibility, BMI, and $VO_{2\,max}$ (calculated from the 20-meter multistage shuttle run) did not have a significant result. Physical fitness by group is presented in Table 2.

3.2. Physical Activity. ANCOVA resulted in between-group effects in sedentary ($P = .00$), light ($P = .00$), moderate ($P = .00$), and moderate-to-vigorous (MVPA) ($P = .01$) physical activity. Children with ASD spent less time in light, moderate, and moderate-to-vigorous physical activity and spent more time in sedentary behavior when compared to typically developing peers. Physical activity results by group are presented in Table 3.

4. Discussion and Future Directions

Children with an ASD are less physically fit in the strength domain and less physically active than their peers without disabilities. Yet physical fitness in flexibility, aerobic fitness ($VO_{2\,max}$), and BMI demonstrates similar results compared to peers without disabilities. Although these results provide further evidence that children with an ASD face known health disparities, they also indicate that aspects of physical fitness are attainable and comparable to peers without ASD.

Our data indicated that children and youth with an ASD performed the shuttle run at only slightly lower levels than their peers without an ASD. This finding, although discrepant, is encouraging given the potentially negative overall health impact of low cardiovascular endurance. This finding further suggests that children with an ASD are more similar to their peers in this area; thus physical education, community-based programs, and other physical activity opportunities may provide an opportunity to further bridge the gap and health disparity between children with an ASD and their peers without an ASD. Supporting the use of peer mentoring in data collection efforts was an encouraging tool for success (i.e., children with ASD completing the task). Knowledge of how shuttle-run performance, ultimately peak oxygen uptake, associates with gender, BMI, age, height, and weight in children and youth with ASD may further aid in better understanding, where to intervene, and how to improve the fitness of school-aged children with ASD [29].

The finding of lower levels of strength (strength with ASD $M = 20.3$, $F = 14.3$, without ASD $M = 26.4$, $F = 15.9$) indicated a weak area of physical fitness for children with an ASD. Based on the results of this study, strength is in need of improvement, suggesting a clear starting point for physical fitness-based interventions.

It is important to note the practical implications of this research methodology as it relates to physical education. The physical fitness and physical activity assessments we employed are common approaches used by physical educators. Too often, students with disabilities, and particularly students with an ASD, are left out of physical fitness assessment data collection. Our participants with an ASD were able to complete all assessments as were their peers. Not only does federal special education law (i.e., Individuals with Disabilities Education Act and 20 U.S.C. § 1400) addresses the right of students with disabilities to participate in physical education, but also research indicates that children and youth with an ASD have a higher prevalence of obesity compared to children without an ASD [2, 30]. Additionally, Memari et al. [5] found a substantial reduction in physical activity across the adolescent years in youth with an ASD. Therefore, we encourage parents, teachers, and administrators to include students with an ASD in physical fitness and physical activity assessments and provide them with individualized information about associated behaviors that can impact their health into adulthood.

Our ability to complete physical fitness and physical activity assessments of children and youth with an ASD has additional educational implications. The relationship between academics and physical activity is a current topic of discussion in the United States [31–33] and federal initiatives aimed at improving the fitness of our youth have been implemented nationwide, with health and education in mind (e.g., Let's Move, Healthy People 2020). Eveland-Sayers et al. [34] investigated physical fitness and

Table 3: Daily average time spent in physical activity by group.

	Children with autism (N = 17)		Children without autism (N = 12)		F value	P
	M ± SD	Min–max	M ± SD	Min–max		
Sedentary	$452.1 \pm 100.5^{***}$	218–572	369.14 ± 105.7	143–518	13.9	0.00^{*}
Light	$104.6 \pm 36.1^{***}$	54–195	122.7 ± 22.2	66–159	33.4	0.00^{*}
Moderate	$154.9 \pm 50.1^{***}$	85–263	210.8 ± 51.1	139–304	16.4	0.00^{*}
Total MVPA	$165.9 \pm 58.7^{**}$	86–286	218.3 ± 65.6	143–358	13.7	0.01^{*}

Note: M: mean; SD: standard deviation. $^{*}P \leq 0.05$.
$^{**}P \geq 0.01$.
$^{***}P \geq 0.001$.

academic achievement in elementary school children and found a link between specific components of physical fitness and academic achievement. Future research might consider applying a similar approach for students with an ASD.

In this study, participants with ASD were less physically fit, in the strength domain, and less physically active than their peers without disabilities. Similarly, previous research confirms these findings [8, 35]. Our participants met the 2008 Physical Activity Guidelines, set by the U.S. Department of Health and Human Services, of 60 minutes/day of moderate-to-vigorous physical activity but had significantly lower activity time than their peers without disabilities. These results are not tremendously different from those of Bandini et al. [3] who found that children with an ASD and those without an ASD spent a similar amount of time in moderate and vigorous physical activity. Contributing factors to the physical activity health disparity present in children with ASD may be the result of diagnostic and environmental determinants [7]. Yet there are many known determinants of physical inactivity in children; more research is needed on the physical activity determinants specific to children with ASD. In conclusion, our results are encouraging as they indicate that children and youth with an ASD show capacity to meet daily guidelines for physical fitness and activity.

4.1. Limitations. Limitations to this study include unequal sample sizes and unmatched controls; however, these limitations were accounted for in analyses. This sample of children with ASD consisted of more females (N = 17, males = 9, females = 8) than would be expected given the current ratio 5 males : 1 female [36]. Participants completed all assessment, yet individual accommodations were implemented when needed (i.e., all assessments were performed in a single day or assessments were split over two days based on participant/familial needs). Finally, this study consisted of a small sample size; thus additional studies with larger sample sizes are needed.

5. Conclusion

These results provide further evidence that children with an ASD face known health disparities, and efforts to promote physical activity in school and through public health initiatives need to include children and youth with an ASD.

Ethical Approval

Consent/assent process: parental/caregiver consent and participant assent were obtained from all participants. All methods and procedures were approved by the Institutional Review Board at Oregon State University.

Acknowledgments

The contents of this presentation were developed under a grant from the US Department of Education, no. H325D100061. However, the contents do not necessarily represent the policy of the US Department of Education, and you should not assume endorsement by the Federal Government. Project Officer Louise Tripoli. Funding for this project was also awarded to Dr. MacDonald from the Oregon State University General Research Fund.

References

[1] C. Curtin, M. Jojic, and L. G. Bandini, "Obesity in children with autism spectrum disorder," *Harvard Review of Psychiatry*, vol. 22, no. 2, pp. 93–103, 2014.

[2] A. M. Egan, M. L. Dreyer, C. C. Odar, M. Beckwith, and C. B. Garrison, "Obesity in young children with autism spectrum disorders: Prevalence and associated factors," *Childhood Obesity*, vol. 9, no. 2, pp. 125–131, 2013.

[3] L. G. Bandini, J. Gleason, C. Curtin et al., "Comparison of physical activity between children with autism spectrum disorders and typically developing children," *Autism*, vol. 17, no. 1, pp. 44–54, 2013.

[4] M. MacDonald, P. Esposito, and D. Ulrich, "The physical activity patterns of children with autism," *BMC Research Notes*, vol. 4, article 422, 2011.

[5] A. H. Memari, B. Ghaheri, V. Ziaee, R. Kordi, S. Hafizi, and P. Moshayedi, "Physical activity in children and adolescents with

autism assessed by triaxial accelerometry," *Pediatric Obesity*, vol. 8, no. 2, pp. 150–158, 2013.

[6] C.-Y. Pan and G. C. Frey, "Physical activity patterns in youth with autism spectrum disorders," *Journal of Autism and Developmental Disorders*, vol. 36, no. 5, pp. 597–606, 2006.

[7] S. M. Srinivasan, L. S. Pescatello, and A. N. Bhat, "Current perspectives on physical activity and exercise recommendations for children and adolescents with autism spectrum disorders," *Physical Therapy*, vol. 94, no. 6, pp. 875–889, 2014.

[8] C.-Y. Pan, "Motor proficiency and physical fitness in adolescent males with and without autism spectrum disorders," *Autism*, vol. 18, no. 2, pp. 156–165, 2014.

[9] K. L. Staples and G. Reid, "Fundamental movement skills and autism spectrum disorders," *Journal of Autism and Developmental Disorders*, vol. 40, no. 2, pp. 209–217, 2010.

[10] J. R. Morrow Jr., J. S. Tucker, A. W. Jackson, S. B. Martin, C. A. Greenleaf, and T. A. Petrie, "Meeting physical activity guidelines and health-related fitness in youth," *The American Journal of Preventive Medicine*, vol. 44, no. 5, pp. 439–444, 2013.

[11] F. B. Ortega, J. R. Ruiz, M. J. Castillo, and M. Sjöström, "Physical fitness in childhood and adolescence: a powerful marker of health," *International Journal of Obesity*, vol. 32, no. 1, pp. 1–11, 2008.

[12] J. P. Winnick and F. X. Short, "Conceptual framework for the brockport physical fitness test," *Adapted Physical Activity Quarterly*, vol. 22, no. 4, pp. 323–332, 2005.

[13] K. Gotham, A. Pickles, and C. Lord, "Standardizing ADOS scores for a measure of severity in autism spectrum disorders," *Journal of Autism and Developmental Disorders*, vol. 39, no. 5, pp. 693–705, 2009.

[14] C. Lord, M. Rutter, P. DiLavore, and S. Risi, *Autism Diagnostic Observation Schedule: Manual*, Western Psychological Services, Los Angeles, LA, USA, 1999.

[15] C. Lord, S. Risi, L. Lambrecht et al., "The Autism Diagnostic Observation Schedule—generic: a standard measure of social and communication deficits associated with the spectrum of autism," *Journal of Autism and Developmental Disorders*, vol. 30, no. 3, pp. 205–223, 2000.

[16] J. L. Matson and M. Sipes, "Methods of early diagnosis and tracking for autism and pervasive developmental disorder not otherwise specified (PDDNOS)," *Journal of Developmental and Physical Disabilities*, vol. 22, no. 4, pp. 343–358, 2010.

[17] G. H. Roid, *Stanford-Binet Intelligence Scales: Technical Manual*, Riverside Publishing, Rolling Meadows, Ill, USA, 5th edition, 2003.

[18] C. D. Elliot, *Differential Ability Scales-Second Edition, Technical Manual*, Pearson, Minneapolis, Minn, USA, 2007.

[19] L. A. Léger, D. Mercier, C. Gadoury, and J. Lambert, "The multistage 20 metre shuttle run test for aerobic fitness.," *Journal of Sports Sciences*, vol. 6, no. 2, pp. 93–101, 1988.

[20] W. Liemohn, G. Sharpe, and J. Wasserman, "Criterion related validity of sit-and-reach test," *The Journal of Strength & Conditioning Research*, vol. 8, no. 2, pp. 65–124, 1994.

[21] F. Ayala, P. S. de Baranda, M. de Ste Croix, and F. Santonja, "Comparison of active stretching technique in males with normal and limited hamstring flexibility," *Physical Therapy in Sport*, vol. 14, no. 2, pp. 98–104, 2013.

[22] V. Mathiowetz, D. M. Wiemer, and S. M. Federman, "Grip and pinch strength: norms for 6- to 19-year-olds," *The American Journal of Occumpational Therapy*, vol. 40, no. 10, pp. 705–711, 1986.

[23] L. A. Milliken, A. D. Faigenbaum, R. L. Loud, and W. L. Westcott, "Correlates of upper and lower body muscular strength in children," *Journal of Strength and Conditioning Research*, vol. 22, no. 4, pp. 1339–1346, 2008.

[24] S.-Y. Kim and J. Yun, "Determining daily physical activity levels of youth with developmental disabilities: days of monitoring required?" *Adapted Physical Activity Quarterly*, vol. 26, no. 3, pp. 220–235, 2009.

[25] P. Freedson, D. Pober, and K. F. Janz, "Calibration of accelerometer output for children," *Medicine and Science in Sports and Exercise*, vol. 37, no. 11, pp. S523–S530, 2005.

[26] I. Jeong, *Measuring physical activity in youth with Down syndrome and autism spectrum disorder: Identifying data-based measurement conditions [Ph.D. thesis]*, 2012.

[27] L. D. Hammer, H. C. Kraemer, D. M. Wilson, P. L. Ritter, and S. M. Dornbusch, "Standardized percentile curves of body-mass index for children and adolescents," *The American Journal of Diseases of Children*, vol. 145, no. 3, pp. 259–263, 1991.

[28] D. Howell, *Statistical Methods for Psychology*, Wadsworth, 7th edition, 2010.

[29] S. Agiovlasitis, K. H. Pitetti, M. Guerra, and B. Fernhall, "Prediction of vo_{2peak} from the 20-m shuttle-run test in youth with down syndrome," *Adapted Physical Activity Quarterly*, vol. 28, no. 2, pp. 146–156, 2011.

[30] C. Curtin, S. E. Anderson, A. Must, and L. Bandini, "The prevalence of obesity in children with autism: a secondary data analysis using nationally representative data from the National Survey of Children's Health," *BMC Pediatrics*, vol. 10, article 11, 2010.

[31] D. N. Ardoy, J. M. Fernández-Rodríguez, D. Jiménez-Pavón, R. Castillo, J. R. Ruiz, and F. B. Ortega, "A physical education trial improves adolescents' cognitive performance and academic achievement: The EDUFIT study," *Scandinavian Journal of Medicine and Science in Sports*, vol. 24, no. 1, pp. e52–e61, 2014.

[32] J. N. Booth, S. D. Leary, C. Joinson et al., "Associations between objectively measured physical activity and academic attainment in adolescents from a UK cohort," *British Journal of Sports Medicine*, vol. 48, no. 3, pp. 265–270, 2014.

[33] P. Correa-Burrows, R. Burrows, C. Ibaceta, Y. Orellana, and D. Ivanovic, "Physically active Chilean school kids perform better in language and mathematics," *Health Promotion International*, 2014.

[34] B. M. Eveland-Sayers, R. S. Farley, D. K. Fuller, D. W. Morgan, and J. L. Caputo, "Physical fitness and academic achievement in elementary school children," *Journal of Physical Activity and Health*, vol. 6, no. 1, pp. 99–104, 2009.

[35] E. Borremans, P. Rintala, and J. A. McCubbin, "Physical fitness and physical activity in adolescents with asperger syndrome: a comparative study," *Adapted Physical Activity Quarterly*, vol. 27, no. 4, pp. 308–320, 2010.

[36] J. Baio, "Prevalence of autism spectrum disorder among children aged 8 years—autism and developmental disabilities monitoring network, 11 sites, United States, 2010," *MMWR Surveillance Summaries*, vol. 63, no. 1, pp. 1–21, 2014.

28

Measuring Outcome in an Early Intervention Program for Toddlers with Autism Spectrum Disorder: Use of a Curriculum-Based Assessment

Elizabeth C. Bacon,[1] Sarah Dufek,[1,2] Laura Schreibman,[1] Aubyn C. Stahmer,[3,4] Karen Pierce,[5] and Eric Courchesne[5]

[1] *Department of Psychology, University of California, San Diego, 9500 Gilman Drive, La Jolla, CA 92093-0109, USA*
[2] *Department of Psychiatry, Weill Cornell Medical College, 21 Bloomingdale Road, Rogers Building, White Plains, NY 10605, USA*
[3] *Department of Psychiatry, University of California, San Diego, 9500 Gilman Drive, La Jolla, CA 92093, USA*
[4] *Child and Adolescent Services Research Center and Autism Discovery Institute, Rady Children's Hospital San Diego, 3020 Children's Way, San Diego, CA 92123, USA*
[5] *Department of Neurosciences, University of California, San Diego, 9500 Gilman Drive, La Jolla, CA 92093, USA*

Correspondence should be addressed to Elizabeth C. Bacon; ebacon@ucsd.edu

Academic Editor: Herbert Roeyers

Measuring progress of children with autism spectrum disorder (ASD) during intervention programs is a challenge faced by researchers and clinicians. Typically, standardized assessments of child development are used within research settings to measure the effects of early intervention programs. However, the use of standardized assessments is not without limitations, including lack of sensitivity of some assessments to measure small or slow progress, testing constraints that may affect the child's performance, and the lack of information provided by the assessments that can be used to guide treatment planning. The utility of a curriculum-based assessment is discussed in comparison to the use of standardized assessments to measure child functioning and progress throughout an early intervention program for toddlers with risk for ASD. Scores derived from the curriculum-based assessment were positively correlated with standardized assessments, captured progress masked by standardized assessments, and early scores were predictive of later outcomes. These results support the use of a curriculum-based assessment as an additional and appropriate method for measuring child progress in an early intervention program. Further benefits of the use of curriculum-based measures for use within community settings are discussed.

1. Introduction

Advancements in the identification, diagnosis, and treatment of very young children with autism spectrum disorder (ASD) have challenged researchers and clinicians to examine alternative assessments of child progress and outcome in early intervention programs. The most common assessments evaluating change across developmental domains (i.e., cognition, communication, social skills, adaptive behavior, and behavior challenges) are standardized assessments [1–5]. However, several limitations to this type of measurement approach have been noted in the literature, including lack of sensitivity, testing constraints, and contextual issues [6, 7]. Furthermore, standardized assessments, in particular assessments of intelligence, are not as stable in toddlers and young children as they are at older ages [8]. Given the surge of early identification and early treatment programs, novel methods for tracking treatment progress are essential.

A recurrent theme throughout the intervention literature is the lack of sensitivity of standardized measures for children with ASD. For example, a child may show maintenance or decrease in standardized scores over time while simultaneously increasing in raw scores [9–13]. Discrepancy between standard scores and raw scores may occur because over time a child is expected to gain skills due to maturation. Therefore, when a child is not maintaining an expected rate of development, standardized scores can be affected negatively over time as the gap between chronological age and expected skills becomes larger as the child ages [14]. In the case of a developmentally delayed child (as is common in ASD), these children often are not progressing at the same pace as their typically developing peers. This may result in a decline in standardized scores, despite the absence of any actual regression and the presence of some progress. Thus, many children with ASD will still show measured impairment after, or experience slow progress during, intervention because standardized tests may not measure change in such small increments, masking progress made by the child [6]. While standardized assessments are useful for comparing groups of children receiving intervention and comparing progress of children with ASD in relation to typical development, they are not designed to measure the progress of an individual child in an intervention program. In addition, because standardized assessments measure broad ability level, they are not designed to be used for treatment planning and individualization. Often, more detailed information about progress toward specific goals is needed. As such, standardized assessments in isolation may not be the most informative tool to measure child progress during intervention.

Another concern related to use of standardized measures with children with ASD is the influence of constraints during test administration. Administration of standardized assessments is usually highly structured, with the intention of keeping the administration consistent across many participants and true to established norms. Due to these restrictions, it is likely that a child's behavior may be very different when assessed by an unfamiliar clinician in an unfamiliar clinic than during normal routines [9, 11]. Additionally, the lack of administration flexibility may be especially detrimental to the measurement of populations such as children with ASD, where lack of social motivation, attention deficits, and disruptive behaviors are frequently present. Koegel et al. [15] found improved scores on several assessments implemented with children with ASD when the clinician incorporated motivational and attentional strategies such as giving breaks to do preferred activities contingent upon compliance during testing. Koegel and colleagues [15] concluded that standardized assessments may be erroneously measuring test taking skills rather than actual abilities for the children in their study.

Ideally, child testing would provide valuable information that may be incorporated into an individual child's ongoing intervention program. However, standardized assessments were not designed to provide detailed information relating to treatment goal development. In fact, developing intervention goals based on a child's performance on standardized assessments is discouraged in order to avoid "teaching to the test." Clinicians are advised to let at least six months pass before readministering the same standardized assessment to the same child as practice effects often are seen with multiple presentations of the same material within a recent time frame, making the results an invalid representation of the individual's abilities [16, 17]. The limitations of goal-specific information gathered from standardized testing combined with the restrictions regarding how often a test can be administered pose a problem for timely tracking of child progress and goal planning.

In order to address the issues discussed above, we propose that standardized testing be supplemented with the use of curriculum-based assessments to provide finer detail on child progress and to assist with treatment individualization and planning. This paper presents the results of an evaluation of the utility of the adapted student learning profile (aSLP) to measure progress of children in an early intervention program specific to the aSLP curriculum. The aSLP is a curriculum-based measure that assesses mastery of targeted skills to measure a child's progress during, and outcome after, an intervention program. The aSLP has the potential to measure child progress throughout ongoing intervention in a systematic way that better allows comparison of child progress and rate of learning in intervention within and across programs. We posit that using a combination of curriculum-based and standardized assessments to measure child functioning will provide a greater understanding of child progress and outcomes in early intervention.

2. Method

2.1. Participants. The toddlers and families in this investigation were participants in a larger multidisciplinary research project examining early neurobiological features and development of ASD at the University of California, San Diego. Toddlers at risk for an ASD were obtained from one of two sources: general community referral (e.g., website or outside agency) and a population-based screening method called the 1-Year Well-Baby Check-Up Approach [18]. Using this method, toddlers at risk for an ASD as young as 12 months were identified in pediatric offices with a broadband screening instrument, the Communication and Symbolic Behavior Scales-Developmental Profile Infant Toddler Checklist [19]. Toddlers were evaluated and tracked every six months until their third birthday when a final diagnosis was given. Experienced clinicians with expertise in the evaluation and diagnosis of ASD identified children at risk for an ASD by incorporating criteria for ASD on the Autism Diagnostic Observation Schedule [20] along with the clinician's clinical judgment. Child participants who were determined to be at risk for ASD were offered intervention at a university-affiliated clinical research program. Seventy-two families were referred for intervention, and 49 families chose to receive treatment at our program. Of the 49 children who received treatment from our program, 45 of the children (mean age = 22.67 months, r = 13–27 months) were included in the analyses. Inclusion criteria included completion of six months or more of early intervention treatment as well as completion of diagnostic and cognitive assessments prior to and at the end of the intervention program. Three children were excluded because they received less than six months of treatment; one child was excluded because of parental failure to complete assessments after intervention. Additional participant demographic information can be found in Table 1.

Table 1: Participant demographics.

Gender	
Male	36
Female	9
Age (months)	
Intake	22.67 (4.13)
Exit	34.06 (3.25)
Length of treatment program	
Months in intervention	11.53 (4.04)
Ethnicity	
Hispanic or Latino	12
Not-Hispanic or Latino	21
Not reported	12
Race	
American Indian or Alaska Native	0
Asian	3
Black or African American	4
Native Hawaiian or other Pacific Islander	1
White	25
Not reported	12

Note: averages listed with standard deviations within parentheses.

Forty-two of the 45 children continued to meet criteria for an ASD upon exit of the intervention program while three children did not.

2.2. Early Intervention Program

2.2.1. Curriculum. The Strategies for Teaching Based on Autism Research (STAR) curriculum [21] was used as the basis for the early intervention in-home programming. The STAR program is a comprehensive behavioral intervention program with a curriculum designed specifically for children with ASD and includes instructional strategies of Discrete Trial Training [22–24], Pivotal Response Training [25, 26], and teaching in Functional Routines [27, 28]. In an effort to improve the developmental appropriateness of the curriculum for these very young children, the STAR curriculum was augmented with developmental approaches applied through Teaching Social Communication (TSC) to Children with Autism. TSC is a manualized curriculum developed by Ingersoll and Dvortcsak [29] used to target social-communication goals in young children with ASD. TSC focuses on the relationship between adult responsivity and children's social-communicative development. In the TSC curriculum, an early childhood interventionist (ECI) combines naturalistic behavioral strategies and developmental strategies. For example, the interventionist would respond to all communicative attempts by the child as if they were purposeful and recast expanded communication to facilitate communicative growth.

2.2.2. Treatment Delivery. Each child received approximately 6–12 hours per week of direct one-on-one intervention with a trained ECI at home until 36 months of age ($M = 9.044$; $r = 4.5–12$). ECIs were bachelor's degree or undergraduate-level research assistants with previous experience with young children with ASD. Each ECI received extensive didactic and hands-on training in behavioral principles and the STAR and TSC programs discussed above. Fidelity of implementation was reached for each intervention strategy as determined by using all components of the intervention correctly at least 80% of the time across two different children. Programs were developed and supervised by master's degree-level clinicians (i.e., in-home coordinator) experienced in ASD, with oversight from two doctorate-level clinical psychologists with extensive experience in early behavioral intervention for this population. In addition, parent training was provided throughout the course of participation. As the focus of this paper is on the evaluation of a curriculum-based measure to assess children during intervention, details regarding the assessments rather than the intervention are emphasized. However, additional details regarding the intervention provided can be obtained from the authors.

2.3. Measures

2.3.1. The Adapted Student Learning Profile. The aSLP is a curriculum-based assessment for determining student learning goals and was adapted from the STAR curriculum to include additional goals from the TSC curriculum (see [21, 29]; e.g., Table 2). The aSLP provides an extensive list of skills targeted in the STAR and TSC curricula and allows for the assessor to indicate the child's performance level on each skill across six domains, receptive language, expressive language, spontaneous language, functional routines, preacademic concepts, and play and social interaction concepts. Data were analyzed using overall scores only for ease of analysis. The aSLP is administered by presenting each item up to five times to the child and observing the child's response. This is conducted in a structured format, and no teaching was done during the assessment. The assessor then rates the child's response, indicating if the child did not demonstrate the skill or showed partial demonstration of the skill or mastery of the skill (e.g., see Table 2). The entire aSLP takes about 30–45 minutes to complete. Each child's in-home coordinator completed an aSLP at intake and every three months thereafter to determine performance and progress. This method of measurement resulted in a variable number of aSLP assessments across children depending on how long they participated in the early intervention program ($M = 4.53$, $r = 2–8$ aSLPs). All available scores were used to examine learning trajectories. All toddlers had aSLP scores at intake into the program and at age three when they exited the program. Scores on the aSLP reflected child performance on items related to the six domains. The amount of progress made during intervention was quantified by taking the aSLP score at exit and subtracting the aSLP score at intake, yielding a change score for each child (aSLP exit score minus aSLP intake score).

2.3.2. Mullen Scales of Early Learning (MSEL). The MSEL assesses developmental functioning of children between birth and 68 months [30]. An examiner measures child functioning

Table 2: aSLP assessment example.

Lesson	Concept	Example instruction cue	Target skill	Student response		
Preverbal communication	Goal directed reach to request	Teacher holds up object	Child reaches toward desired object	Rarely	Sometimes	Usually
	Eye contact to request	Teacher blocks access/withholds desired object	Child makes eye contact to obtain desired object	Rarely	Sometimes	Usually
	Proximal point to request	Teacher holds up object	Child points to desired object	Rarely	Sometimes	Usually
		Teacher holds up two objects	Child points to indicate a choice between two objects	Rarely	Sometimes	Usually
Expanded learning to play	Multiple-step imitation	Verbal cue: "Do this." Nonverbal play model: teacher puts man in toy car and then pushes the car	Student models teacher's action (e.g., student puts man in a toy car and then student pushes car)	Never	If prompted	Independently
Expanded playing with toys	Following two- or three-step play commands	Teacher gives verbal cue (e.g., "Put man in car and push car")	Student responds to teacher cue without need for initiation (e.g., student puts man in the toy car and pushes it)	Never	If prompted	Independently
	Independent construction or functional play	No specific cue is needed	Child plays appropriately with toy during reinforcement phase of PRT lessons	Never	If prompted	Independently

level through a series of play-like tasks over five domains, gross motor, fine motor, receptive language, expressive language, and visual reception skills. Children were assessed on the MSEL at intake and exit from the program. For each scale, the assessment derives a T-score with a mean of 50 and standard deviation of 10, a percentile score, and an age equivalent indicating at what developmental age the child is performing. An early learning composite (ELC) score is calculated from the total of scores on all scales (excepting the gross motor scale) with a mean of 100 and standard deviation of 15. Change on the MSEL while in intervention was calculated using changes on the ELC from intake to exit from the program (MSEL ELC Exit Score minus MSEL ELC Intake Score).

2.3.3. Wechsler Preschool and Primary Scale of Intelligence, 3rd Edition (WPPSI). Three children were administered the WPPSI rather than the MSEL at exit as these children were performing at ceiling levels on the MSEL at the close of their early intervention program. The WPPSI assesses cognitive development in children between two years, six months and seven years, three months [31]. It provides composite scores that represent intellectual functioning in verbal and performance domains as well as a full scale intelligence quotient (FSIQ) that represents a child's general intellectual ability. Each composite score has an average of 100 with a standard deviation of 15. For the three children who received the WPPSI, the FSIQ was used in lieu of the MSEL ELC score at exit.

2.3.4. Vineland Adaptive Behavior Scales, 2nd Edition (VABS). The VABS provides a measure of adaptive skills used to cope with challenges of daily living [32]. A caregiver completes a questionnaire regarding the individual's current level of functioning across five domains: communication, daily living skills, socialization, motor skills, and maladaptive behavior. The Vineland Scales are applicable to children with and without delays from birth to 18 years, 11 months. Standardization of the instrument included national samples of both "handicapped" and "nonhandicapped" children. All scales use standard scores with a mean of 100 and a standard deviation of 15, a percentile score, and an age equivalent indicating at what developmental age the individual is performing. Scores on all scales are combined to obtain an overall adaptive behavior composite (ABC) with a mean of 100 and a standard deviation of 15. Change on the VABS while in intervention program was quantified by calculating the changes on the ABC from intake to exit from the program (VABS ABC exit score minus VABS ABC intake score).

2.4. Statistical Analyses. Means with standard deviations were calculated for all assessments at intake into the program, exit, and change scores from intake to exit. In order to analyze whether the aSLP measured progress in intervention similarly to the MSEL and VABS, partial correlations were conducted controlling for the amount of time the child was in treatment. Lastly, a linear regression was conducted to analyze if aSLP scores at three months into intervention were predictive of aSLP scores at exit. This analysis was included to examine if early treatment progress on the aSLP is

Table 3: Summary of assessment scores.

MSEL ELC	
Intake	75.44 (14.87)
Exit	83.51 (21.76)*
Change scores	8.07 (16.46)
VABS ABC	
Intake	84.38 (11.46)
Exit	83.13 (10.85)
Change scores	−1.24 (11.58)
aSLP score	
Intake	23.56 (24.27)
Exit	120.58 (61.87)*
Change scores	97 (50.96)

Note: average scores listed with standard deviations within parentheses.
*Indicates statistically significant change from intake to exit.

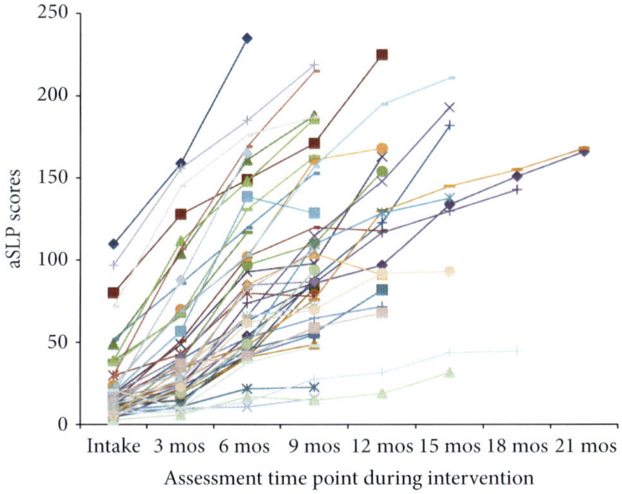

Figure 1: aSLP scores for each participant over time. Each participant is depicted by one line. The aSLP was administered to each child at intake into the early intervention program and every 3 months thereafter. The aSLP score depicts the number of skills mastered at each assessment. Significant changes were seen in aSLP scores from intake to exit from the early intervention program.

indicative of later outcomes, which would give practitioners information about the importance of early performance, and insight into the type of outcome that could be expected. Analyses were conducted using the IBM SPSS Statistics 22 statistical analysis package.

3. Results

Results for all assessments are summarized in Table 3. Children showed variable rates and amount of progress as measured by the aSLP (see Figure 1). On average, participants entered the intervention program with 23.56 (r = 3–110) skills that were part of the curriculum and exited the program on average with a mastery of 120.58 skills (r = 16–235). A repeated measures t-test revealed significant differences in the number of skills measured on the aSLP between intake and exit from the program ($t(44) = 12.778$; $P < 0.001$). Children mastered an average of 97 (r = 8–187) skills while being in treatment. There was a very large range in scores with some children learning very few skills and others mastering many. Similar heterogeneity in scores was seen on the MSEL ELC (intake: $M = 75.44$, r = 44–115, exit: $M = 83.51$, r = 49–128; change scores: $M = 8.07$, r = −20–56) and VABS ABC (intake: $M = 84.38$, r = 65–130, exit: $M = 83.13$, r = 59–111; change scores: $M = -1.24$, r = −42–21). A repeated measures t-test revealed significant differences in MSEL scores at intake and exit ($t(44) = 3.287$, $P = 0.002$). There were no significant differences between intake and exit scores on the VABS.

3.1. Relationship between aSLP and Standardized Test Measures. Partial correlations between the MSEL, VABS, and aSLP scores, controlling for the number of months the children were in the treatment program, were conducted. Since child age or time passing is not controlled for on the aSLP as it is not a standardized measure, the effect of the amount of time the child spent in treatment on aSLP scores was investigated. The amount of time the child was in treatment had a small negative correlation with the aSLP scores at intake ($r = -0.332$, $P = 0.026$) and a significant correlation with aSLP change scores ($r = 0.422$, $P < 0.005$). Time in treatment was not correlated with aSLP scores at exit, or scores on the MSEL or VABS at any time point. It appears that the amount of time the child was in treatment may influence aSLP scores and therefore may impact the relationship observed between the aSLP and the MSEL and VABS. Thus, partial correlations were conducted holding the amount of time in treatment constant to adjust for the effect time in treatment may have on the aSLP, MSEL, and VABS. aSLP scores at intake were positively correlated with the MSEL ELC at intake ($r = 0.580$, $P < 0.001$) and the VABS ABC at intake ($r = 0.654$, $P < 0.001$; see Figure 2). aSLP scores at exit were positively correlated with the MSEL ELC ($r = 0.713$, $P < 0.001$) and VABS ABC ($r = 0.643$, $P < 0.001$) at exit (see Figure 2). aSLP change scores were also positively correlated with MSEL ELC change scores ($r = 0.548$, $P < 0.001$) and VABS ABC change scores ($r = 0.354$, $P = 0.019$; see Figures 3 and 4). Notably, 33% of the sample (i.e., 15 toddlers) showed a decrease or no gain in their MSEL ELC and 36% of the sample showed a decrease or no gain in their VABS ABC scores, while the aSLP captured a skill gain for these children that averaged a change of 97 (r = 8–187) newly learned skills (see Figures 3 and 4). A linear regression was conducted to evaluate whether aSLP scores at three months into the intervention program predicted aSLP scores when the participants exited the program. The results of the regression indicated aSLP scores at three months into intervention explained 54.8% of the variance ($R^2 = 0.547$, $F(1, 43) = 51.907$, $P < 0.001$; see Figure 5). aSLP scores at three months into intervention significantly predicted aSLP scores at exit ($\beta = 0.72$, $P < 0.001$).

Two of the children displayed very high scores across all three assessments at intake. These children were the only participants to score two standard deviations above the mean

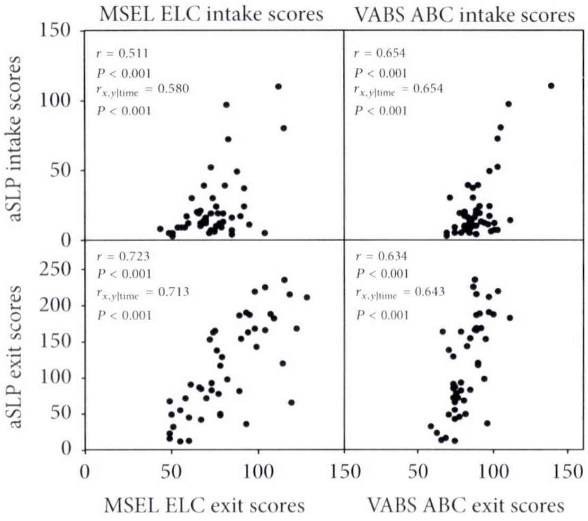

FIGURE 2: Correlations between the aSLP scores and MSEL ELC and VABS ABC at intake and exit of the early intervention program. Correlation coefficients are reported for Pearson correlations and partial correlations controlling for the amount of time in intervention. Significant positive correlations were found between all measures.

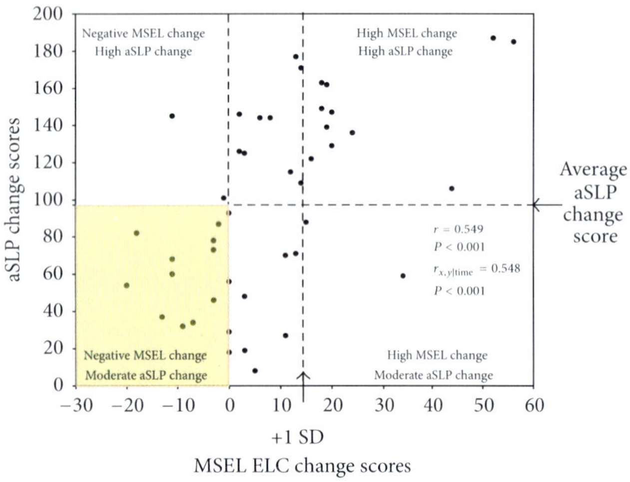

FIGURE 3: Correlation between MSEL ELC change scores and aSLP change scores (i.e., change in scores from intake to exit). Correlation coefficients are reported for the Pearson correlation and partial correlation controlling for the amount of time each child was in treatment. A significant positive correlation was found. Children exhibited an average of 97 aSLP skills learned on average and an average change score of 8 on the MSEL ELC.

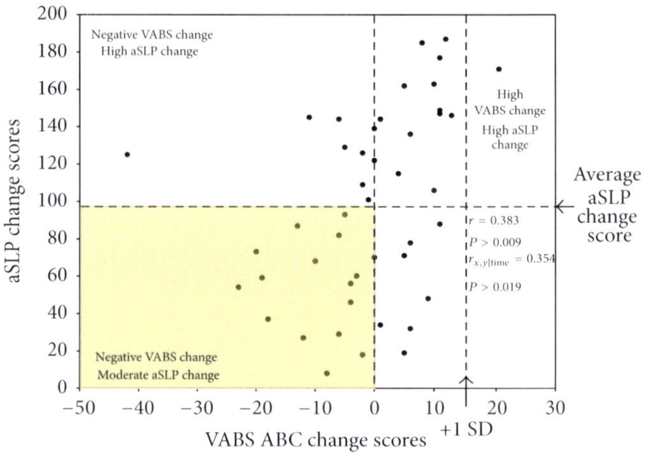

FIGURE 4: Correlation (controlling for the amount of time each child was in treatment) between VABS ABC change scores and aSLP change scores (i.e., change in scores from intake to exit). Correlation coefficients are reported for the Pearson correlation and partial correlation controlling for the amount of time each child was in treatment. A significant positive correlation was found. Children exhibited an average of 97 aSLP skills learned on average and an average change score of −1 on the VABS ABC.

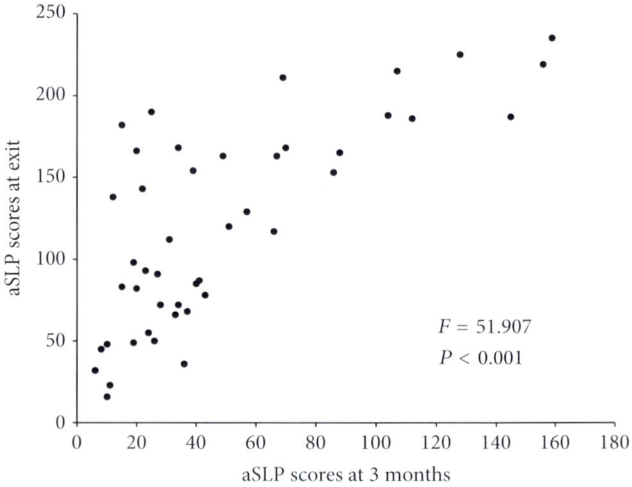

FIGURE 5: A linear regression between aSLP scores at 3 months and exit. aSLP scores at 3 months into treatment significantly predicted aSLP scores when participants exited the program.

score on at least two of the three assessments. Therefore, the following analyses also were conducted excluding these two participants. Partial correlations controlling for the number of months the children were in treatment were conducted. aSLP scores at intake were positively correlated with the MSEL ELC at intake ($r = 0.336$, $P = 0.030$) and VABS ABC at intake ($r = 0.440$, $P = 0.004$). aSLP scores at exit were positively correlated with the MSEL ELC ($r = 0.738$, $P < 0.001$) and VABS ABC ($r = 0.684$, $P < 0.001$) at exit. aSLP change scores were also positively correlated with MSEL ELC change scores ($r = 0.648$, $P < 0.001$) and VABS ABC change scores ($r = 0.585$, $P < 0.001$). A linear regression was conducted to evaluate whether aSLP scores at three months into the intervention program predicted aSLP scores when the participants exited the program. aSLP scores at three months into intervention explained 47% of the variance ($R^2 = 0.470$, $F(1, 41) = 36.360$, $P < 0.001$). aSLP scores at three months into intervention significantly predicted aSLP scores at exit ($\beta = 0.686$, $P < 0.001$).

4. Discussion

The results of this study provide support for the supplemental use of a curriculum-based assessment, the aSLP, for determining the benefits of an early intervention program for children with ASD. While standardized assessments such as the MSEL and the VABS are valuable tools in evaluating child outcome, they have some limitations that suggest the need for the addition of a curriculum-based measure such as the aSLP. High variability in scores among participants was seen across all assessments. Assessments were highly correlated, likely indicating that children who had higher overall cognitive and adaptive functioning were more likely to have mastered more skills, which is not surprising but may support the validity of a curriculum-based assessment. The VABS standard scores were not sensitive to change in the children's skills during intervention as evidenced by nonsignificant changes in VABS standard scores over time. The MSEL and aSLP showed significant changes in scores over time. This may indicate that the aSLP and MSEL are sensitive to change in skill acquisition and development but do not capture change in adaptive functioning. One explanation may be that the STAR program is more heavily focused on behaviors related to cognitive gains for these very young children. Alternatively, the children may be showing specific changes in skill acquisition during treatment and testing sessions, but these skills may not generalize to daily functioning and use across multiple environments. The assessments may simply be measuring very different skills, or the age of the children may be a factor given the limited change in adaptive behavior expected on the VABS at this young age.

Given that the children's scores on the aSLP were positively correlated with the MSEL and VABS at all time points and over time, it is likely that the aSLP is a comparable measure of child progress despite its lack of standardized norms. Two participants displayed high scores across all three assessments at intake. Correlations between the aSLP and MSEL and VABS were stronger with these participants included; however, intake, exit, and change scores were still moderately correlated when these participants were removed from the analyses. The evidence of significant positive correlations with or without these two participants suggests that the extreme scores of these two participants were not driving the correlations between the assessments and rather supports the use of the aSLP across a wide range of children with varying levels of functioning.

The addition of the aSLP in this study was very informative, in terms of ongoing child response to treatment, treatment trajectory, and overall outcome at the conclusion of the study. For example, over 1/3 of the children showed a decrease or no gain in MSEL or VABS standardized scores. However, all children showed an increase in skills mastered as measured by the aSLP. Tracking progress of children can become complicated when utilizing standardized measures as standardized scores are determined by comparing raw scores on the assessment to norms of children of the same chronological age. Thus, when evaluating children who may be progressing slower than typically expected, those children may actually exhibit no gain or a decrease in standardized scores since the children are not keeping up with the expected progress. Thus, interpreting the treatment success for this particular group of children based on the MSEL or VABS alone makes it difficult to determine rate of progress. It is important to have a measure of treatment progress in children who are developing more slowly to make appropriate changes to intervention strategies, determine rate of learning, and make predictions regarding service needs.

Additionally, the aSLP allowed the children's in-home treatment coordinators to quickly and easily determine the children's intervention progress throughout the intervention period. The results of the aSLP provided detailed information about specific behaviors, rather than general information about the child's ability level, which is provided by standardized assessments. This allowed for easy analysis of child functioning at the skill by skill level, which is particularly beneficial for treatment planning. Very young children, like those in the current study, have very little experience with testing and may not do well on standardized tests, which makes using them to guide early treatment even more problematic. In contrast, the aSLP may be useful for early goal development and allow for a systematic yet individualized process for the child's treatment program to follow. Additionally, the aSLP provided some information to hypothesize child's trajectory of treatment. aSLP scores after 3 months of treatment predicted aSLP scores at exit. The aSLP scores provide information early on regarding the child's predicted treatment trajectory. Early information on responsivity to treatment may provide valuable information for individualization of treatment. The utility of the aSLP for assessing and detecting treatment trajectory information so early on gives it a unique advantage for practical use within community settings, beyond what a standardized assessment might provide. Information about child progression through a curriculum such as the aSLP can be a very useful complement to standardized assessments as it gives a researcher or practitioner the opportunity to observe the real-world effects of treatment.

4.1. Limitations. The main limitation of the current study is that the in-home coordinator for each child administered the aSLP, rather than employing a blind rater to assess the children. It is possible that the in-home coordinators had an expectancy bias when assessing the children, which may have influenced the scores derived from the aSLP. However, the in-home coordinators were not providing direct service to the children. Children were familiar with them but did not receive intervention directly from the person doing the testing. Blind raters were not employed due to the amount of additional resources that would be needed to carry out a blind rating system and because the purpose of the aSLP was to provide clinical data. Another limitation was the lack of formalized procedures to ensure interrater reliability of the aSLP ratings between in-home coordinators. Although the scoring procedure is straightforward and in-home coordinators were trained in the same manner, there is a potential for differences to occur between aSLP raters. Another concern with the use of the aSLP over time is the possibility of practice effects.

Specific steps were taken to try to limit practice effects. The aSLP was given only every three months and tested items not specifically targeted during treatment. Feedback was not provided to the children regarding appropriate or correct responses. The task format was similar to that of intervention and familiar procedures tend to lead to fewer practice effects. However, it remains possible that practice effects may account for some of the increase in skills measures on the aSLP.

Additional limitations include the use of a small, young sample. Forty-five children under the age of three were evaluated throughout participation in an early intervention program. Future research should evaluate the usefulness of a curriculum-based measure such as the aSLP in a larger and older population. Likely, the benefits of a curriculum-based measure would generalize across populations, as the same benefits of ease of implementation, frequency of use, and direct translation to informing programming would be applicable. Additionally, as the aSLP is not a normed, standardized measure, we do not have a good understanding of the validity and reliability of the measure beyond what was explored in the current study. As such, the aSLP provides limited information in regard to the functioning level of the child with respect to same-aged peers and rather focuses on the skills learned in the treatment program. Therefore we are suggesting the use of a curriculum based assessment in conjunction with, not as a replacement for, standardized assessments. Also, although the items on the aSLP were not directly taught, the aSLP was used to develop treatment goals which may have inflated progress. However, skill gain was the important variable for these analyses. Additionally, these limitations are generalizable to how the assessment would be used in community practice; therefore this study represents an examination of the utility of the measure in community care.

4.2. Future Research. The aSLP shows promise as a useful tool for measuring intervention progress and assisting with intervention development; however future research is needed to fully determine accuracy and limitations of the measure. Future studies should compare progress across groups of children in various intervention programs, including those not using the aSLP to develop curriculum items, to examine sensitivity to specific treatment changes. This will also help reduce issues of children learning items that are directly related to the assessment. Studies of the psychometric properties of the aSLP are imperative. Future research should establish interrater reliability with blind raters to further evaluate the rigor of this type of measure. Examination of the generalization of skills assessed by the aSLP is needed, including the relationship between the specific items on the aSLP and those on standardized measures of adaptive and cognitive functioning.

4.3. Summary. One of the greatest challenges facing early intervention researchers and community providers today is finding accurate and useful methods for assessing child response to treatment and overall outcome during and after a course of early intervention [33]. There is a large amount of money spent on early intervention and this spending is likely to increase over time. As such, it is important to have a recommended set of assessments that effectively measure child functioning and progress during early intervention [34]. In addition, with the increased responsibility of insurance companies over the coming years, use of the aSLP may offer assistance to ASD service providers who are challenged with providing information on child response to treatment. ASD service providers will most likely need information about child progress, treatment planning, and whether an intervention program is beneficial to the child overall. Standardized cognitive and adaptive behavior assessments are invaluable but the addition of a detailed curriculum-based measure that can be repeated often throughout intervention is critical to both obtaining an accurate measure of a child's abilities and being able to quickly and effectively keep up with the child's progress in a way that maximizes treatment benefit for the child. Curriculum-based measures such as the aSLP may allow providers to gather all these pieces of information on a regular basis. Thus while standardized assessments such as the MSEL and the VABS are valuable tools in evaluating child outcome, the results of this study provide support for the additional use of a curriculum-based measure, the aSLP, for determining the benefits of an early intervention program for children with ASD.

Disclosure

See http://www.autism-center.ucsd.edu/ for more information regarding the larger multidisciplinary research project referenced within the paper.

Acknowledgments

This research was supported by the National Institutes of Health P50-MH081755 awarded to Eric Courchesne and R01-MH080134 awarded to Karen Pierce. The authors would like to thank Kevin Smith and Cory Rieth for assistance with statistical analyses as well as the families and children who participated in the study.

References

[1] C. Aldred, J. Green, and C. Adams, "A new social communication intervention for children with autism: pilot randomised controlled treatment study suggesting effectiveness," *Journal of Child Psychology and Psychiatry and Allied Disciplines*, vol. 45, no. 8, pp. 1420–1430, 2004.

[2] E. Ben-Itzchak and D. A. Zachor, "The effects of intellectual functioning and autism severity on outcome of early behavioral intervention for children with autism," *Research in Developmental Disabilities*, vol. 28, no. 3, pp. 287–303, 2007.

[3] T. Charman, E. Taylor, A. Drew, H. Cockerill, J.-A. Brown, and G. Baird, "Outcome at 7 years of children diagnosed with autism at age 2: predictive validity of assessments conducted at 2 and 3

years of age and pattern of symptom change over time," *Journal of Child Psychology and Psychiatry and Allied Disciplines*, vol. 46, no. 5, pp. 500–513, 2005.

[4] R. Luyster, S. Qiu, K. Lopez, and C. Lord, "Predicting outcomes of children referred for autism using the MacArthur-Bates Communicative Development Inventory," *Journal of Speech, Language, and Hearing Research*, vol. 50, no. 3, pp. 667–681, 2007.

[5] A. L. Rickards, J. E. Walstab, R. A. Wright-Rossi, J. Simpson, and D. S. Reddihough, "One-year follow-up of the outcome of a randomized controlled trial of a home-based intervention programme for children with autism and developmental delay and their families," *Child*, vol. 35, no. 5, pp. 593–602, 2009.

[6] J. L. Matson, "Determining treatment outcome in early intervention programs for autism spectrum disorders: a critical analysis of measurement issues in learning based interventions," *Research in Developmental Disabilities*, vol. 28, no. 2, pp. 207–218, 2007.

[7] P. Yoder and D. Compton, "Identifying predictors of treatment response," *Mental Retardation and Developmental Disabilities Research Reviews*, vol. 10, no. 3, pp. 162–168, 2004.

[8] I. Rapin, "Value and limitations of preschool cognitive tests, with an emphasis on longitudinal study of children on the autistic spectrum," *Brain and Development*, vol. 25, no. 8, pp. 546–548, 2003.

[9] N. Akshoomoff, "Use of the Mullen Scales of Early Learning for the assessment of young children with Autism Spectrum Disorders," *Child Neuropsychology*, vol. 12, no. 4-5, pp. 269–277, 2006.

[10] N. Akshoomoff, A. C. Stahmer, C. Corsello, and N. E. Mahrer, "What happens next? Follow-up from the children's toddler school program," *Journal of Positive Behavior Interventions*, vol. 12, no. 4, pp. 245–253, 2010.

[11] P. Rosenbaum, "Screening tests and standardized assessments used to identify and characterize developmental delays," *Seminars in Pediatric Neurology*, vol. 5, no. 1, pp. 27–32, 1998.

[12] A. C. Stahmer and C. Carter, "An empirical examination of toddler development in inclusive childcare," *Early Child Development and Care*, vol. 175, no. 4, pp. 321–333, 2005.

[13] A. C. Stahmer and B. Ingersoll, "Inclusive programming for toddlers with autism spectrum disorders: outcomes from the children's toddler school," *Journal of Positive Behavior Interventions*, vol. 6, no. 2, pp. 67–82, 2004.

[14] S. M. Kanne, A. J. Gerber, L. M. Quirmbach, S. S. Sparrow, D. V. Cicchetti, and C. A. Saulnier, "The role of adaptive behavior in autism spectrum disorders: implications for functional outcome," *Journal of Autism and Developmental Disorders*, vol. 41, no. 8, pp. 1007–1018, 2011.

[15] L. K. Koegel, R. L. Koegel, and A. Smith, "Variables related to differences in standardized test outcomes for children with autism," *Journal of Autism and Developmental Disorders*, vol. 27, no. 3, pp. 233–243, 1997.

[16] A. S. Kaufman, "Practice effects," in *Encyclopedia of Human Intelligence*, R. Sternberg, Ed., pp. 828–833, Macmillan Publishing Company, New York, NY, USA, 1994.

[17] J. M. Sattler, *Assessment of Children, Jerome*, M. Sattler Publisher, San Diego, Calif, USA, 3rd edition, 1986.

[18] K. Pierce, C. Carter, M. Weinfeld et al., "Detecting, studying, and treating autism early: the one-year well-baby check-up approach," *Journal of Pediatrics*, vol. 159, no. 3, pp. 458–465, 2011.

[19] A. Wetherby and B. Prizant, *Communication and Symbolic Behavior Scales Developmental Profile*, Paul H. Brookes, Baltimore, Md, USA, 1st edition, 2002.

[20] C. Lord, M. Rutter, P. C. DiLavore, and S. Risi, *Autism Diagnostic Observation Schedule*, Western Psychological Services, Los Angeles, Calif, USA, 1999.

[21] J. Arick, L. Loos, R. Falco, and D. Krug, *The Star Program: Strategies for Teaching Based on Autism Research*, Pro-Ed, Austin, Tex, USA, 2004.

[22] O. I. Lovaas, "Behavioral treatment and normal educational and intellectual functioning in young autistic children," *Journal of Consulting and Clinical Psychology*, vol. 55, no. 1, pp. 3–9, 1987.

[23] C. Maurice, G. Green, and S. Luce, *Behavioral Intervention For Young Children With Autism: A Manual For Parents and Professionals*, Pro-Ed, Austin, Tex, USA, 1996.

[24] T. Smith, "Discrete trial training in the treatment of autism," *Focus on Autism and Other Developmental Disabilities*, vol. 16, no. 2, pp. 86–92, 2001.

[25] R. L. Koegel, M. C. O'Dell, and L. K. Koegel, "A natural language teaching paradigm for nonverbal autistic children," *Journal of Autism and Developmental Disorders*, vol. 17, no. 2, pp. 187–200, 1987.

[26] R. L. Koegel, L. Schreibman, A. Good, L. Cerniglia, C. Murphy, and L. Koegel, *How to Teach Pivotal Behaviors to Children with Autism: A Training Manual*, University of California, Santa Barbara, Calif, USA, 1989.

[27] F. Brown, I. M. Evans, K. A. Weed, and V. Owen, "Delineating functional competencies: component model," *The Association for Persons with Severe Handicaps*, vol. 12, no. 2, pp. 117–124, 1987.

[28] L. E. McClannahan and P. J. Krantz, *Activity Schedules for Children With Autism: Teaching Independent Behavior*, Woodbine House, Bethesda, Md, USA, 1999.

[29] B. Ingersoll and A. Dvortcsak, *Teaching Social Communication to Children with Autism*, The Guildford Press, New York, NY, USA, 2010.

[30] E. M. Mullen, *Mullen Scales of Early Learning*, American Guidance Service, Circle Pines, Minn, USA, 1995.

[31] D. Wechsler, *Wechsler Preschool and Primary Scale of Intelligence*, Psychological Corporation, San Antonio, Tex, USA, 3rd edition, 2002.

[32] S. S. Sparrow, D. V. Cicchetti, and D. A. Balla, *Vineland Adaptive Behavior Scales*, American Guidance Service, Circle Pines, Minn, USA, 1984.

[33] J. L. Matson and M. J. Konst, "What is the evidence for long term effects of early autism interventions?" *Research in Autism Spectrum Disorders*, vol. 7, no. 3, pp. 475–479, 2013.

[34] E. E. Bolte and J. J. Diehl, "Measurement tools and target symptoms/skills used to assess treatment response for individuals with autism spectrum disorder," *Journal of Autism and Developmental Disorders*, vol. 43, no. 11, pp. 2491–2501, 2013.

29

An Analysis of Canadian Institute for Health Research Funding for Research on Autism Spectrum Disorder

R. Deonandan,[1] E. Y. Liu,[2] B. Kolisnyk,[3] and A. T. M. Konkle[1,4]

[1] *Interdisciplinary School of Health Sciences, Faculty of Health Sciences, University of Ottawa, 25 University Private, THN 208, Ottawa, ON, Canada K1N 6N5*
[2] *Department of Public Health Sciences, Queen's University, Kingston, ON, Canada K7L 3N6*
[3] *Neuroscience, Schulich School of Medicine and Dentistry, University of Western Ontario, London, ON, Canada N6A 5B7*
[4] *School of Psychology, Faculty of Social Sciences, University of Ottawa, Ottawa, ON, Canada K1N 6N5*

Correspondence should be addressed to R. Deonandan; rdeonand@uottawa.ca

Academic Editor: Geraldine Dawson

We examined patterns of Canadian Institute for Health Research (CIHR) funding on autism spectrum disorder (ASD) research. From 1999 to 2013, CIHR funded 190 ASD grants worth $48 million. Biomedical research received 43% of grants (46% of dollars), clinical research 27% (41%), health services 10% (7%), and population health research 8% (3%). The greatest number of grants was given in 2009, but 2003 saw the greatest amount. Funding is clustered in a handful of provinces and institutions, favouring biomedical research and disfavouring behavioural interventions, adaptation, and institutional response. Preference for biomedical research may be due to the detriment of clinical research.

1. Introduction

Government-sponsored medical research funding is always scarce, but recent policy decisions at the federal level have further constrained academic research budgets [1] such that funding priority setting has become a prime task for policy makers and institution administrators alike.

At the same time, more important challenges to population health are entering the public consciousness, and with them calls for deeper and broader investigations. One such challenge is autism spectrum disorder (ASD), whose prevalence in the Canadian population is largely unknown, but whose prominence in the national media and discourse is high, as is its perceived social burden. No other neurodevelopmental disorder has seen such a recent explosion in fundraising and lobbying activities [2]. In the USA, from 1995 to 2001, research funding for ASD quintupled from $US 11 million to $US 56 million [3]. The public demand, as least as seen through the eyes of parents with ASD children, appears to be for immediate breakthroughs in treatment and in utero detection [4, 5].

While it is important to understand the underlying biological basis of ASD, it is equally as important to understand the nonbiological risk factors for the disease, as well as opportunities for social or behavioural interventions, and economic factors useful for modelling the burden of disease. In other words, in an era of compressed research funding, attention must be paid to the domains of research within a given subject area that funding decisions tend not to reward. This is particularly relevant for funding decisions made by the Canadian Institutes of Health Research (CIHR), which is Canada's principle funding body for human health-related research.

Thus, with this study we examined the distribution and temporal trends in CIHR's funding grants for topics in ASD, for the purpose of refocusing the public debate on research priorities. We feel that this approach can be applied to other areas of health research that rely upon a small number of principle funding sources and is useful for achieving high

TABLE 1: Variables extracted from CIHR funded grants.

Variable name	Description
Amount	Total amount of funds released by CIHR
Year	Fiscal year in which grant was awarded
Grant type	(i) Capacity building; (ii) knowledge creation; (iii) knowledge translation
Theme of research	(i) Biomedical; (ii) clinical; (iii) health systems/services; (iv) social/cultural/environmental/population health
Province	Province in which administering institution is located
CIHR Institute	CIHR institute from which funds originated: (i) Neurosciences, Mental Health and Addiction; (ii) Human Development, Child and Youth Health; (iii) Genetics; (iv) Health Services and Policy Research; (v) Aging; (vi) Population and Public Health

TABLE 2: Distribution by research theme of all grants and all ASD-related grants awarded by CIHR from 1991 to 2013.

Research theme	Percentage of number of ASD-related grants funded	Percentage of dollar value of ASD-related grants given	Percentage of dollar value of all CIHR grants given
Biomedical	43%	46%	53%
Clinical	27%	41%	13%
Not applicable or not specified	12%	3%	21%
Health systems/services	10%	7%	5%
Social/cultural/environmental/population health	8%	3%	8%

level perspective on the extent to which funding decisions reflect national research values.

2. Methods

We conducted a search of CIHR's public funding database, which includes bilingual (English and French) information on successful grant applications, using the following keywords and their French equivalents: autism, autistic, ASD, Asperger syndrome, pervasive developmental disorder, PDD-NOS, Rett's syndrome, and Childhood Disintegrative Disorder. The initial search was conducted on Nov 28th, 2012, and then updated on June 2nd, 2013.

First, titles and abstracts were reviewed by a single investigator for probable relevance to ASD. In the event of uncertainty, the abstract was reviewed by a second investigator who then decided whether the project should be included in our set of studies to be analyzed. Grants that focused on multiple neurological disorders were disqualified. Grants were included if their abstracts indicated a dedicated focus on ASD or its effects and implications.

Demographic, geographical, thematic, and financial information were then extracted from the resulting grants. The collected variables are summarized in Table 1. Note that responses to "Theme of research" are coded in the funding database, having been preselected by each grant writer at the time of their project's submission to CIHR.

The distributive and temporal trends in funding were explored using descriptive statistics.

A sensitivity analysis was also conducted to determine if inclusion or exclusion of the grants reviewed by a second investigator would alter the results appreciably.

3. Results

Of 329 projects resulting from our keyword search, 252 were deemed relevant based upon their titles and abstract content, with 62 rejected due to lack of relevance and 15 rejected since there was no abstract to review. Of the 252 relevant grants, further 62 were excluded by the second reviewer due to lack of perceived relevance or due to lack of sufficient specific focus on ASD. In our sensitivity analysis, reinclusion of the latter 62 grants rejected by the second reviewer resulted in no appreciable change to our results, based upon a <5% change in total grant dollars.

Of all the years analyzed, the highest number of ASD-related grants (28) was funded in 2009, while 2003 saw the peak in the total dollar investment in ASD funding ($6.9 million).

A plurality of funding was allocated to biomedical research (see Table 2). Also, Ontario, Quebec, and British Columbia received 77% of all ASD-related grants (see Table 3). The lion's share of dollars, unsurprisingly, was granted by two CIHR Institutes: Neurosciences, Mental Health and Addiction (52%) and Human Development, Child and Youth Health (30%). The majority of grants were given for capacity building and knowledge creation purposes (see Table 4).

The top 3 institutions receiving the most money for ASD research were all in Ontario. Together, they received just over $19 million in ASD-related funding, which is almost 40% of the total dollars allocated nationally. Three institutions also received the most number of grants, accounting for 46% of all ASD-related grants. A few non-Canadian institutions, located in the USA and UK, were recipients of 6.9% of the grants.

TABLE 3: Distribution by region of all grants and all ASD-related grants awarded by CIHR from 1991 to 2013.

Province	Percentage of number of ASD grants funded	Percentage of dollar value of ASD grants given	Percentage of dollar value of all CIHR grants given
Ontario	48%	60%	41%
Quebec	18%	18%	29%
British Columbia	11%	3%	12%
Alberta	7%	12%	10%
Nova Scotia	4%	2%	3%
The rest of the country and out of country	12% (no single province was >2%)	5% (no single province was >1%)	5%

TABLE 4: Distribution by type of CIHR ASD grants from 1991 to 2013.

Type of grant	Percentage of number of grants funded	Percentage of dollar value of grants given
Capacity building	44%	14%
Knowledge creation	31%	53%
Not classified	19%	31%
Knowledge translation	6%	2%

In terms of temporal trends, both the number of grants and total funding dollars saw no obvious trend over the time period considered; however, both saw a steady yearly decrease from 2010 (27 grants totalling over $4 million) to 2013 (5 grants totalling under $1 million).

4. Discussion

According to our results, the lion's share of CIHR ASD funding is granted to researchers in Ontario and Quebec and to a handful of key institutions in those provinces. This is in line with the overall CIHR funding pattern, which dramatically benefits institutions in Ontario. A plurality of the ASD-related funding, in terms of both dollars (46%) and number of grants (43%), is earmarked for biomedical research, which is characterized by basic, "wet laboratory" studies, often dependent upon expensive equipment. And while overall ASD research funding has decreased over the past 3 years, most divestment has come from the areas of clinical, health systems, and social/cultural/population health research.

These results are somewhat aligned to similar findings in the USA [2], where funding data from the National Institutes of Health revealed that American ASD funding also favours basic medical research (65% of funded projects), though their system shows a steady growth in overall ASD funding, increasing at about 15% per year, while Canadian funding is in decline.

Our methodology suffers from a reliance on titles, abstracts, and researcher-chosen keywords to determine projects' applicability to ASD research. As well, we have no information on the number or nature of submitted or unfunded grant applications, raising the possibility that funding trends might actually correlate well with trends in actual researcher interest, but not in funder interest.

Most problematic is our reliance on a single source of research funding, specifically CIHR. However, in Canada the only major funders of ASD research outside of CIHR are a collection of autism-specific foundations, such as Autism Speaks Canada, the Spectrum Intervention Group, L'Amitient, the Canadian National Autism Foundation, and some international foundations with interest in Canada, such as the Geneva Centre for Autism. In 2012, these groups provided a combined total of just over $500,000 in research funding [6], which is significantly smaller than that provided by CIHR. The Ontario Brain Institute, as well, embraces a multidisciplinary funding approach to autism, though we could not identify the dollar amount offered by that funder.

In addition, for the last few years, CIHR has been responsible for disbursing all federal health-related research funds, whereas historically the Social Sciences and Humanities Research Council (SSHRC) might have funded some social/cultural projects related to ASD. A quick search of 1998–2013 SSHRC competition results, using the keyword "autism" without a deeper search for relevance, reveals about 100 funded grants totalling approximately $2 million, which is very small compared to CIHR funding over the same time period [7]. A similar search of the NSERC grants database found just over $3 million in monies associated ASD, which includes funds earmarked for both research and student support [8], though earlier records may not be accessible through NSERC's online portal.

While it would have been ideal to have included NSERC and SSHRC funding data in our general analyses, our initial intent was to specifically examine the extent to which CIHR ASD funding was aligned with societal priorities, with an understanding that CIHR's granting activities would be most reflective of the Canadian government's policies on this manner. Our cursory search of NSERC and SSHRC ASD-related activities indicated that those agencies' contributions were of insufficient size and scope to have altered our findings or conclusions.

It is worth pointing out that while our results suggest an overall national trend in focusing on the strict biomedical dimensions of ASD, there exist pockets of researchers who strive to more comprehensively approach disorders of national interest. A notable example is the Ontario Brain Institute, which embraces a multidisciplinary approach to disorders of the nervous system with an explicit focus on prevention, detection, and treatment, an approach that necessarily includes nonbench related science as well as basic biomedical research. Thus, our findings should not suggest that researchers in Canada are unaware of the need for a diverse and multidisciplinary approach to addressing a given health issue, but rather that funding priorities may be constraining the extent to which a diverse set of research tools is indeed being permitted to enter the fray.

Moreover, the importance of our results lies not in their description of funding patterns relating specifically to ASD, but rather in the implications for the extent to which these patterns reflect values underlying research priorities. Our finding that an increase in funding of what we call biomedical research, which seeks to explore the biological causes and treatments of the disease, coincides with a decrease in funding of projects seeking to address clinical (i.e., treatment oriented) or social/cultural/population aspects of the disease, which include studies on comorbidities, environmental associations, economic impacts, and social adaptation approaches. This is despite both literatures' stressing of the value of interventions to relive the stress of caregivers to ASD children [9] and the announcement of CIHR's doubling of its clinical research budget in 2012 [10]. While researchers and clinicians dealing with ASD typically do not view the disease through the dualistic lens that we have proposed, that of biomedical versus nonbiomedical approaches, it is our contention that the funding administrative dynamic artificially imposes such a false choice, necessitating the preference of one approach over the others. The underlying question is whether this funding preference is expressive of society's true priorities or is either an unintended consequence of the funding decision-making process or indeed a reflection of an unstated policy. This study, then, represents but one approach to explore this necessary alignment of research expenditure with societal priorities.

A similar approach was undertaken by Leroy et al. [11], who examined National Institutes of Health (NIH) and Gates Foundation granting data to determine the extent to which research funding aimed at reducing global child mortality was earmarked for technological improvement. They found that 97% of grants were for developing new technologies and expressed concern that insufficient research attention was thus being directed toward increased efficacy of treatment and delivery and use of technology. This discrepancy can be interpreted as a misalignment of funding priorities with both researcher values and the actual needs of the sector.

Scholarly research into the so-called "research values" is relatively scarce in the peer-reviewed biomedical literature. However, management and communication sciences have long acknowledged the extent to which social, political, and cultural agendas are necessarily reflected in money management strategies, including national research priorities. Despite this, there is conspicuous lack of agreement on what values actually are and the degree to which social values can affect individual decision making within the research milieu [12].

Accepting that Canadian values, expressed through research funding, are in some ways decided upon by Parliamentarians, researchers in 2007 measured Members of Parliament attitudes toward health research funding [13]. They found that while 84% of 308 federal Members of Parliament knew of CIHR, 32% knew nothing about its role; 66% believed that the business sector should be the primary source of health research funding; and 57% most frequently defined health research as study into cures or treatments of disease, rather than a disease's determinants, accommodations, role in societal interplay, sociolegal interactions, and so forth. Our results reflect a preference for a biological, cure-based research agenda and are thus seemingly in line with politicians' expectations, but there appears to be little opportunity or incentive for the private sector to fund the remaining types of research, as seemingly would be preferred by Parliamentarians. Seeking a cure is understandably society's priority for most illnesses. But diseases with strong lifestyle, psychological, social, and accommodative considerations, like ASD and other neurological disorders, distinct from dissimilar diseases, may have funding priorities beyond finding a cure or a preventative measure.

Perhaps an approach, like that pioneered by Sivananthan and Chambers [14], in which health research priority setting was systematically measured amongst researchers, caregivers, and policymakers, is warranted for a larger Canadian health research agenda. Similarly, Fleurence and Torgerson [15] point out that setting priorities for research should be conducted to make the most efficient use of scarce resources and that the uptake by policymakers of methods for identifying such priorities has been slow. In 2010, the World Health Organization had similarly conducted a process for identifying research priorities best aligned with its membership's values [16]. In the Canadian case, our national dialogue must go beyond prioritizing topics and delve into the intent of the research at hand, to determine the relative valuation of biomedical, clinical, health systems, and social/cultural/population health approaches for the long term wherewithal of our population.

To better address the issue, further investigations are warranted, preferably including funding sources beyond CIHR, embracing topics beyond ASD, and, critically, considering the nature of unfunded projects, as well, in order to determine whether patterns of funded research only reflect decision-makers' priorities, or whether the topics sought by the researchers themselves are also in line with these patterns. As health research funding dwindles, each nation is well-advised to consider the values that must determine the facets of individual health problems that are most important to its citizenry, and therefore most deserving of taxpayer money.

References

[1] Canadian Institutes of Health Research (CIHR), "Message from the President of CIHR: Budget 2012," 2012, http://www.cihr-irsc.gc.ca/e/45207.html.

[2] J. Singh, J. Illes, L. Lazzeroni, and J. Hallmayer, "Trends in US autism research funding," *Journal of Autism and Developmental Disorders*, vol. 39, no. 5, pp. 788–795, 2009.

[3] C. J. Newschaffer and L. K. Curran, "Autism: an emerging public health problem," *Public Health Reports*, vol. 118, no. 5, pp. 393–399, 2003.

[4] M. Aarons and T. Gittens, *The Handbook of Autism. A Guide for Parents and Professionals*, Routledge, New York, NY, USA, 2nd edition, 1999.

[5] R. Bazell, "Parents push for autism cure," 2005, http://www.msnbc.msn.com/id/7012176.

[6] Unity for Autism Website, 2014, http://www.unityforautism.ca/grants/recipients/.

[7] Social Sciences and Humanities Research Council Awards Search Engine (SSHRC), 2014, http://www.sshrc-crsh.gc.ca/results-resultats/award_search-recherche_attributions/index-eng.aspx.

[8] Natural Sciences and Engineering Research Council Awards Search Engine (NSERC), 2014, http://www.nserc-crsng.gc.ca/onlineservices-servicesenligne/index_eng.asp.

[9] T. Lerthattasilp, T. Charernboon, I. Chunsuwan, and P. Siriumpunkul, "Depression and burden among caregivers of children with autistic spectrum disorder," *Journal of the Medical Association of Thailand*, vol. 98, supplement 2, pp. S45–S52, 2015.

[10] L. Vogel, "CIHR doubles support for clinical research," *Canadian Medical Association Journal*, vol. 184, no. 7, pp. E343–E344, 2012.

[11] J. L. Leroy, J.-P. Habicht, G. Pelto, and S. M. Bertozzi, "Current priorities in health research funding and lack of impact on the number of child deaths per year," *American Journal of Public Health*, vol. 97, no. 2, pp. 219–223, 2007.

[12] B. M. Meglino and E. C. Ravlin, "Individual values in organizations: concepts, controversies, and research," *Journal of Management*, vol. 24, no. 3, pp. 351–389, 1998.

[13] D. R. Clark, P. J. McGrath, and N. MacDonald, "Members' of Parliament knowledge of and attitudes toward health research and funding," *CMAJ*, vol. 177, no. 9, pp. 1045–1051, 2007.

[14] S. N. Sivananthan and L. W. Chambers, "A method for identifying research priorities for health systems research on health and aging," *Healthcare Management Forum*, vol. 26, no. 1, pp. 33–36, 2013.

[15] R. L. Fleurence and D. J. Torgerson, "Setting priorities for research," *Health Policy*, vol. 69, no. 1, pp. 1–10, 2004.

[16] R. F. Viergever, *Health Research Prioritization at WHO: An Overview of Methodology and High Level Analysis of WHO Led Health Research Priority Setting Exercises*, World Health Organization, Geneva, Switzerland, 2010, http://www.who.int/rpc/publications/Health_research_prioritization_at_WHO.pdf.

Conceptualisation and Development of a Quality of Life Measure for Parents of Children with Autism Spectrum Disorder

Valsamma Eapen,[1,2] Rudi Črnčec,[1,2] Amelia Walter,[1,2] and Kwok Ping Tay[2]

[1] *Academic Unit of Child Psychiatry, South Western Sydney Local Health District (AUCS), Liverpool Hospital, Mental Health Centre (Level 1: ICAMHS), Locked Bag 7103, Liverpool BC, NSW 1871, Australia*
[2] *University of New South Wales, Sydney, NSW 2052, Australia*

Correspondence should be addressed to Valsamma Eapen; v.eapen@unsw.edu.au

Academic Editor: Herbert Roeyers

Parents of children with autism spectrum disorder (ASD) tend to experience greater psychological distress than parents of typically developing children or children with other disabilities. Quality of Life (QoL) is increasingly recognised as a critical outcome measure for planning and treatment purposes in ASD. There is a need for ASD-specific QoL measures as generic measures may not capture all relevant aspects of living with ASD. This paper describes the conceptualisation and development of an autism-specific measure of QoL, the Quality of Life in Autism Questionnaire (QoLA) for parents and caregivers of children with ASD, that is suitable to clinical and research settings. Preliminary psychometric properties (reliability and validity) of the measure are also presented. The QoLA has 48 items in two subscales: one comprising QoL items and the second a parent report of how problematic their child's ASD symptoms are. A study involving 39 families suggested the QoLA has excellent internal consistency as well as good known-groups validity between parents of children with ASD and those who were typically developing. The QoLA also showed good convergent validity with other measures of QoL and ASD symptom severity, respectively. The QoLA may be a valuable assessment tool and merits further psychometric evaluation.

1. Introduction

Autism spectrum disorder (ASD) is a lifelong neurodevelopmental disorder characterised by impairments in social interaction, verbal and nonverbal communication, and a restricted repertoire of activities and interests [1]. The prevalence of ASD appears to be rising worldwide [2] with ASD estimated to affect around 1 in every 88 persons [3]. Building on genetic vulnerability [4], it has been hypothesised that ASD emerges from a developmental cascade in which a deficit in attention to social stimuli leads to impaired interactions with primary caregivers. This results in abnormal development of the neurocircuitry responsible for social cognition, which in turn adversely affects later behavioural and functional domains dependent on these early processes [5, 6].

Parenting children with ASD can be emotionally, socially, financially, and physically challenging. Studies have consistently found higher levels of psychological distress in parents of children with ASD when compared to parents of typically developing children or children with other disabilities [7–10]. For example, mothers of individuals with ASD have been shown to display lower levels of wellbeing and higher levels of stress than mothers of individuals with Down syndrome, fragile X syndrome, and cerebral palsy [7, 8]. Similarly, families of children with ASD are reported to experience higher levels of family stress and more family problems than families of children with Down syndrome [11, 12], attention deficit hyperactivity disorder [13], and medical conditions such as cystic fibrosis [14].

In addition to measuring mental health related factors such as stress and psychological wellbeing, a broader and encompassing construct that is important to assess in families of children with ASD is Quality of Life (QoL). In 1995 the World Health Organisation defined QoL as an individual's "perception of their position in life in the context of the culture and value systems in which they live and in relation to their goals, expectations, standards and concerns" [15]. The term "Quality of Life" first appeared in the literature in around 1920, but it was not until the middle of the century that the concept became a part of public discourse. This increased awareness of QoL followed the duel effects of the World Health Organisation broadening the definition of "health" within its 1948 constitution to include physical, emotional, and social wellbeing [16], and of a generally increased cognisance of social inequity in Western societies [17]. Wood-Dauphine notes that between 1966 and 1974 there were 40 references related to QoL identified within a MEDLINE database search, whereas between 1986 and 1994 there were over 10,000—highlighting the proliferation of research, including in the development of generic QoL measures, that began during the 1970s [17, 18]. A wide range of disorder-specific QoL measures have been developed in recent years given the general acknowledgement of the importance of tailoring QoL measures to specific populations [19].

QoL is a multidimensional construct and includes health- and non-health-related domains of functioning. Various models of QoL are available with differing foci, including some that concentrate on health-related aspects of QoL; however, a widely accepted model for assessing QoL in the context of disabilities has been put forward by Schalock et al. [20]. This model proposes eight core QoL domains: personal development, self-determination, interpersonal relations, social inclusion, rights, emotional wellbeing, physical wellbeing, and material wellbeing.

QoL thus offers the potential to be a useful index of parents' adjustment to their child's ASD and is an important component in obtaining a full understanding of the experiences of, and difficulties faced by, individuals with ASD and their families [21–23]. Research in this area is also important as QoL has been identified as a potential mediator of psychological adjustment and treatment outcome for people with ASD and is also pertinent to service planning and evaluation [21].

While advances in the accurate diagnosis of ASD at increasingly earlier ages have been made, as well as the development of evidence-based early interventions [24, 25], QoL research in ASD is in its infancy. In this regard, a recent review of the literature on QoL measures for use in ASD identified a lack of focus on QoL in ASD research and suggested that a new condition-specific measure of QoL was needed [26].

Recent studies have used generic QoL measures to assess QoL among parents whose children have ASD, including the World Health Organisation QoL measures [27]; Short-Form Health Surveys [28, 29]; and EuroQol Five Dimensional Questionnaire (EQ-5D-3L, [30]). Khanna et al. found that the EQ-5D-3L showed good convergent, discriminant, and known-groups validity, and satisfactory internal consistency, when used among caregivers of children with ASD [30]. Similarly, when parents are asked to make QoL ratings on behalf of a young person, generic measures tend to be used [31]. Several instruments, such as the Beach Centre Family Quality of Life Scale [32], have been developed for families of children with intellectual and developmental disabilities and may have some relevance and utility to the ASD population. One ASD-specific QoL measure that has been developed for parents of children with ASD is the 102-item Quality of Life Scale [33], although this measure is presently only available in French.

While generic QoL measures often have large normative data sets and well-articulated psychometric properties underpinning their use, such measures may not prove sufficiently sensitive to the unique challenges faced by individuals with ASD or parents of children with ASD, particularly with respect to social and emotional aspects [34]. Therefore, the power of studies investigating treatment effects may be affected, and the ability to enhance knowledge where QoL is a dependent variable may be compromised. Similarly, within clinical contexts the ability to use a QoL measure to help target and assess treatment outcomes is reduced when a generic measure is utilised. For example, in the context of ASD, generic QoL measures or measures developed for use in intellectual disability do not typically ask specific questions regarding the impact of, say, restricted/repetitive behaviours; sensory difficulties; or difficulties with social understanding.

The present study aimed to develop an autism-specific measure of QoL, the Quality of Life in Autism Questionnaire (QoLA) for parents of children with ASD that is suitable to clinical and research settings. The clinical utility of such a measure would be improved by having a relatively small number of items, as well as subscales that are relevant to service and treatment planning: these were goals of the proposed measure. Furthermore, the present study aimed to investigate the preliminary psychometric properties of the QoLA. The internal reliability of the measure (the consistency of scores across items) was assessed, in addition to its known-groups validity (an index of construct validity measuring a questionnaire's ability to discriminate between groups); concurrent validity (the correlation of the QoLA with an existing validated measure of QoL); and convergent validity (the extent to which scores on the QoLA were associated with scores on theoretically-related measures).

2. Materials and Methods

2.1. Ethical Approval. The study had the approval of the Human Research Ethics Committees of the Local Health Service as well as the University where the research was conducted. All families recruited to the study provided informed consent to participate, and the research was conducted in accordance with the ethical standards outlined in the Helsinki Declaration.

2.2. Development of the Quality of Life in Autism Questionnaire (QoLA). The QoLA was designed to provide a measure of QoL in parents of children with ASD. The scale was developed for parents of children aged 2–18 years; however specific experimental work in this study was conducted with parents of preschool aged children. This was undertaken for several reasons. First, given increased efforts at early ASD identification in recent years, this group is of particular clinical interest. Second, as this is the first study using the

QoLA, the provision of some homogeneity of sample age was considered to be important.

The QoLA was developed following initial consultation and semistructured interviews regarding the impact of caring for a child with ASD upon QoL. These interviews were conducted with consumers and clinicians experienced in working with young people who have ASD and their families. Interviews were transcribed, and a thematic cluster analysis of transcripts was conducted to identify key themes. Item selection and refinement was guided by an expert panel that included several academic clinicians experienced in working with children with ASD from disciplines including psychiatry, psychology, and occupational and speech therapy. Early drafts of the measure were also provided to ASD service provider managers and consumer group representatives for feedback regarding relevance of items and readability. Item selection was ultimately guided by these qualitative data, together with (1) extant models of QoL (e.g., [20]) and (2) review of several widely-used generic QoL measures, as well as (3) consideration of the diagnostic criteria for ASD. An expanded version of the QoL was then piloted with 20 families attending local ASD support services. During the pilot phase, participants were specifically asked whether they felt each item should be included in the measure and were also asked to provide their general thoughts about any areas for improvement. Items rated as not important for inclusion in the scale by >60% of participants during the piloting phase were discussed within the expert panel and all were ultimately omitted in the final QoLA version that was used in the study. Several minor amendments to the wording of questions were also made at that stage based upon the comments of pilot participants so as to improve the readability of the QoLA.

To aid in the clinical utility of the tool and to provide ASD specificity, the QoLA was designed with two subscales (Parts A and B) that are described below. Part A contains some items that are reverse scored. Parents are asked to rate each item based on their experiences over the preceding four weeks.

Part A (QoL subscale) includes 28 items designed to measure parents' overall perception of their quality of life. Items include "I feel happy and content," "I am satisfied with my social life," and "I am satisfied with my close relationships". Each item is measured on a five-point Likert scale ranging from one (not very much) to five (very much). Thus, scores on Part A can range from 28 to 140, with higher scores indicating greater perceived QoL. Items in Part A reflect each of Schalock et al.'s eight domains [20], with a particular weighting on emotional wellbeing, social inclusion, and interpersonal relationships.

Part B (impact of ASD symptoms subscale) was designed to assess parents' perception of how problematic their child's autism-specific difficulties are for them. A list of 20 difficulties that children with ASD can experience was provided (e.g., "socialising with people," "needing to stick to a routine," "destructive behaviours including anger and aggression"). Parents are asked to rate how problematic these difficulties have been for them, on a five-point Likert scale from five (not much of a problem for me) to one (very much of a problem for me). Thus, scores on part B can range from 20 to 100, with higher scores denoting fewer problems for parents regarding their child's ASD-related behaviours.

The potential range for the QoLA total score is therefore 48–240. A total score can be computed for overall comparisons; however, Parts A and B were intended to be scored separately and reflect separate subscales within the instrument.

The final version of the QoLA is available free of charge from the study authors and items are outlined in Table 1.

2.3. Participants. Two participant groups were recruited: a clinical group comprising parents of children with ASD (ASD group) and a control group comprising parents of children without ASD (control group). Participants were recruited in metropolitan Sydney, Australia, and demographic information for both groups is presented in Table 2. No statistical differences emerged between groups with respect to child age, child sex, parent age, parent sex, or family cultural background. A greater proportion of parents in the control group had a tertiary education.

The ASD group consisted of 23 mothers of children on the waitlist for, or having recently (within the previous month) commenced at, an Autism Specific Early Learning and Care Centre. These children had a mean age of 46.8 months (SD = 9.8, range = 30–71 months), and all had a DSM-IV-TR diagnosis of Autistic Disorder, made by a community-based physician, with the exception of one child who had a diagnosis of Pervasive Developmental Disorder - Not Otherwise Specified. These children would have met DSM-5 criteria for autism spectrum disorder.

A control group was recruited to assist in ascertaining the known-groups validity of the QoLA. This group comprised 16 parents (13 mothers and three fathers) of children attending a childcare centre. None of the children had been diagnosed with ASD or any other developmental problems. The mean age of these children was 43.2 months (SD = 12.1, range = 22–59 months). The absence of an ASD diagnosis among children in the control sample was supported by screening with the Modified Checklist for Autism in Toddlers (M-CHAT, [35]). While several cut-offs are available for the M-CHAT, amongst the most conservative is that advocated by Wong et al, who reported a failing score of six or more of the 23 items using a modified graded scoring system [36]. No children in the control sample failed six or more items on the M-CHAT.

2.4. Measures of Quality of Life. In addition to the QoLA, participants in the ASD group also completed the World Health Organisation Quality of Life Questionnaire: WHOQoL-BREF [37]. The WHOQoL-BREF is a 26-item brief version of the original WHOQOL-100 that is designed to assess perceptions of overall quality of life. It generates scores with a range of 0 to 100 on four domains: Physical Health, Psychological Health, Social Relations, and Environment, with higher scores indicating greater perceived quality of life. The WHOQoL-BREF has strong psychometric properties [37] and was the key measure used in the determination of the concurrent validity of QoLA Part A. The WHOQoL-BREF was not completed by the control group due to constraints in

Table 1: QoLA items.

	QoLA—Part A (QoL subscale)	QoLA—Part B (impact of ASD symptoms subscale)
(1)	I am satisfied with my life	Socialising with people
(2)	I feel stressed*	Having friends
(3)	I feel happy and content	Understanding others' feelings
(4)	I feel depressed or anxious*	Holding a conversation
(5)	I feel good about myself as a person	Communicating needs
(6)	I am satisfied with my close relationships	Taking a literal meaning of comments
(7)	People are there for me when I need them	Saying things that are socially embarrassing
(8)	I am satisfied with my social life	Needing to stick to a routine
(9)	I am satisfied with my family life	Being overly interested in a particular topic
(10)	I am satisfied with my financial situation	Getting anxious in a specific situation or during changes
(11)	I am satisfied with where I live	Sensitivity to certain sensations
(12)	I have enough money to meet my needs	Understanding the rules of social interaction
(13)	I am satisfied with my achievements	Managing emotional responses
(14)	I am satisfied with my general health	Needing to do things a certain way
(15)	I have a healthy lifestyle	Destructive behaviours including anger and aggression
(16)	I am satisfied with my leisure activities	Showing inappropriate emotional reactions
(17)	Health problems stop me doing things that I want to*	Unusual repetitive behaviours or body movements
(18)	I feel in control of my life	Engaging in reckless or tactless behaviours
(19)	I set and achieve goals in my life	Doing daily living tasks independently
(20)	I can make a plan of action and follow it	Responding when approached socially
(21)	I make my own decisions	
(22)	I feel guilty*	
(23)	I am part of a community	
(24)	I can get the support that I need from the community	
(25)	I am able to get to where I need to	
(26)	I feel safe in my everyday life	
(27)	I feel respected in my everyday life	
(28)	I am satisfied with the availability of health services	

*Item is reverse scored.

Table 2: Demographic information for the ASD and control groups.

	ASD group	Control (non-ASD) group
n	23	16
Mean child age in months (SD)	49.39 (16.75)	43.19 (12.13)
Number with ASD	23	0
Child gender Male : Female	17 : 6	10 : 6
Mean parent age in years (SD)	35.10 (4.50)	37.88 (3.40)
Parent gender Male : Female	0 : 23	3 : 13
Parent's education background	47% tertiary 48% secondary 5% no formal education	100% tertiary
Parent's ethnic background	47% Australian or New Zealander 32% South-East Asian 16% European 5% Middle Eastern	63% Australian or New Zealander 25% South-East Asian 6% European 6% Southern Asian

Table 3: Descriptive statistics and internal consistency coefficients for all measures used.

Variable	Mean	Range	SD	Cronbach's α
QoLA Part A: ASD group	86.96	46–138	21.53	0.94
QoLA Part A: control group	110.00	65–138	17.58	0.96
QoLA Part B: ASD group	68.52	30–99	17.56	0.92
QoLA Part B: control group	94.31	78–100	6.14	0.86
WHOQOL-BREF: Physical[a]	59.32	28.57–89.29	17.45	0.85
WHOQOL-BREF: Psychological[a]	55.98	33.33–91.67	15.38	0.75
WHOQOL-BREF: Social relations[a]	55.07	16.67–100	22.15	0.72
WHOQOL-BREF: Environmental[a]	58.70	28–97	17.12	0.84
DASS-21: Depression[a]	4.91	0–13	3.57	0.86
DASS-21: Anxiety[a]	3.30	0–10	3.01	0.75
DASS-21: Stress[a]	6.74	0–14	3.70	0.81
PSOC: Satisfaction[a]	3.16	1–5.4	1.02	0.81
PSOC: Efficacy[a]	4.35	2.14–6	0.95	0.89
PSOC: Interest[a]	4.59	2–6	1.35	0.78

[a]Measure administered to ASD group only.

the number of measures that could be administered within that setting.

2.5. Measures of Severity of Child's Autism Symptoms and Adaptive Functioning. Parents in the ASD group completed two measures to assess the severity of their child's autism symptoms and adaptive functioning. The Social Communication Questionnaire (SCQ: [38]) is a 40-item measure of autism-specific symptoms where scores of 15 or more indicate probable ASD. The SCQ has robust psychometric properties [39, 40]. The Vineland Adaptive Behaviour Scales Second Edition (Parent Form) (VABS-II: [41]) assesses parents' perceptions of their child's everyday adaptive functioning in the domains of Communication (including expressive and receptive language), Daily Living Skills, Socialisation, and Motor Skills. For each domain, including an overall Adaptive Behaviour Composite, a norm-referenced standardised score with a mean of 100 and SD of 15 is calculated. For the maladaptive behaviour index, a *v*-scale score with a mean of 15 and a SD of three is calculated. The VABS-II has well established strong psychometric properties [41]. The SCQ and VABS-II maladaptive behaviour index were used to assist with determining the convergent validity of QoLA Part B. That is, it is reasonable to hypothesise that parent-rated child autism severity (SCQ) and child adaptive functioning (VABS-II) would be related to parents' ratings of how problematic their child's ASD symptoms were for them (QoLA Part B).

2.6. Measures of Parental Wellbeing. Participants in the ASD group also completed two additional measures of parental wellbeing. The Depression Anxiety Stress Scales (DASS-21: [42]) is a 21-item self-report measure that assesses negative affect. The measure generates separate scores for the subscales of Depression, Anxiety, and Stress, with higher scores on each subscale indicating greater symptomatology. The DASS-21 has been shown to have excellent psychometric properties [42–44]. The Parenting Sense of Competence Scale (PSOC: [45]) includes 17 items designed to measure parental self-efficacy. Based on the factor structure found in Australian populations [46], the scale generates scores on three subscales: Satisfaction, Efficacy, and Interest, with higher scores indicative of higher levels of parental satisfaction and self-efficacy. The PSOC has been found to have strong psychometric properties [46]. Given the body of research suggesting an association between low QoL and poorer mental health (e.g., [47]), these measures were included to help in the assessment of the convergent validity of the QoLA. The measures were also included to provide additional data regarding the wellbeing of parents whose children have ASD.

2.7. Statistical Analysis. Analyses were conducted using SPSS statistical software. Cronbach's alpha values were computed to assess the internal consistency of both Parts A and B of the QoLA. Known-groups validity was evaluated by comparing group QoLA scores in the ASD and control groups. In cases where Levene's test was significant, equal variances were not assumed. Pearson's product-moment correlations were computed to examine the concurrent and convergent validity of the QoLA with the WHOQoL-BREF, parental wellbeing measures, and child functioning measures. Alpha was set at 0.05 for all comparisons, following recommendations by Saville [48] who argues for this per-comparison level rather than a family-wise approach when conducting research in novel areas.

3. Results

3.1. Descriptive Statistics and Internal Consistency. Descriptive statistics and internal consistency for all measures are summarised in Table 3.

Internal consistency coefficients for the QoLA were $\alpha = 0.94$ for Part A and $\alpha = 0.92$ for Part B in the ASD group, and $\alpha = 0.96$ for Part A and $\alpha = 0.86$ for Part B in the control group. A Cronbach's alpha value of 0.7 to 0.9 is considered to be adequate and greater than 0.9 as excellent [49].

There was some evidence of positive skew in QoLA Part B responses, with parents in the ASD group endorsing the highest response category (very much of a problem for me) 31% of the time on average. This ranged from 65% of parents endorsing the highest response on the item relating to destructive behaviours and aggression to 9% endorsing the highest response for their child needing to stick to a routine.

3.2. Construct (Known-Groups) Validity. Independent samples t-tests were performed to compare total scores between the clinical and control groups on the QoLA Part A and QoLA Part B. Parents in the ASD group reported significantly lower total scores on the QoLA Part A (mean = 86.96, SD = 21.53) than parents in the control group (mean = 110.00; SD = 17.58), $t(37) = -3.54$, $P < 0.01$). This equates to a Cohen's d effect size of 1.17, which is large. Parents in the ASD group also reported significantly lower total scores on the QoLA Part B (mean = 68.52, SD = 17.56) than parents in the control group (mean = 94.31, SD = 6.14), $t(29.09) = -6.50$, $P < 0.001$, equivalent to Cohen's d of 1.96, which is again large.

In terms of the QoLA total score, the ASD group reported significantly lower scores (mean = 155.48, SD = 26.86) than parents in the control group (mean = 204.31, SD = 19.64), $t(36.87) = -6.59$, $P < 0.001$, equivalent to Cohen's d of 2.08.

3.3. Concurrent and Convergent Validity. Scores on the QoLA Part A were positively correlated with scores on all four subscales of the WHOQOL-BREF ($r = 0.74$ to 0.91, all $Ps < 0.01$) suggesting strong concurrent validity. Furthermore, QoLA Part A was associated negatively with maternal depression ($r = -0.49$, $P < 0.05$) and stress ($r = -0.57$, $P < 0.01$) and positively with maternal satisfaction ($r = 0.74$, $P < 0.01$). Moderate sized correlations (>0.30) in the expected direction were also observed with maternal anxiety and maternal efficacy.

Scores on the QoLA Part B approached significance in correlation with the SCQ ($r = -0.37$, $P = 0.086$) and a moderate and identical sized correlation of $r = -0.37$ was also observed with the VABS-II maladaptive behaviour index. This provides some support for the convergent validity of the QoLA Part B. QoLA Part B scores were not significantly correlated with scores on the QoLA Part A, nor any of the subscales of the WHOQOL-BREF, DASS-21, or PSOC. See Table 4.

3.4. Comparison with Normative Data. To further explore the psychosocial functioning of parents in the ASD group, mean scores for the WHOQOL-BREF, DASS-21, and PSOC in the clinical group sample were compared to Australian population norms [37, 43, 46] using Welch t tests. Mothers in the ASD group had significantly lower scores on the Physical ($t(24) = 4.43$, $P < 0.0001$), Psychological ($t(24) = 5.06$, $P < 0.0001$), Social Relations ($t(23) = 3.64$, $P < 0.01$), and Environmental ($t(23) = 4.43$, $P < 0.001$) domains of the WHOQOL-BREF than the Australian population norms [37]. Mothers in the current sample also reported significantly higher levels of Depression ($t(43) = 3.07$, $P < 0.01$), Anxiety ($t(29) = 3.08$, $P < 0.01$), and Stress ($t(44) = 3.43$, $P < 0.01$) on the DASS-21 than nonclinical volunteers in the study by Antony et al. [43]. There were no significant differences between mothers' scores on Satisfaction ($t(23) = 1.31$, $P = 0.20$) or Interest ($t(22) = 1.85$, $P = 0.08$) in the ASD group and those reported by Rogers and Matthews [46], but mothers in the current sample were found to have significantly higher scores on Efficacy ($t(23) = 5.69$, $P < 0.0001$).

3.5. Association between ASD Symptoms and Parental Wellbeing. There were no significant correlations between scores on the QoLA Part B or SCQ and scores on any measures of parental wellbeing (QoLA, WHOQoL-BREF, DASS-21, or PSOC). See Table 4.

4. Discussion

To date the assessment of QoL in parents of children with ASD and the broader incorporation of this construct into clinical settings have been complicated by the lack of an English speaking ASD-specific measure. The results of the present study suggest that the QoLA may provide an initial step toward remedying this situation.

The primary aim of this paper was to describe the conceptualisation and development of the QoLA. Given the relatively small sample size involved in the study, the psychometric properties reported should be considered preliminary. Nonetheless, QoLA Part A shows excellent internal consistency as well as strong concurrent validity with the WHOQOL-BREF and good convergent validity with measures of maternal depression, stress, and parenting satisfaction. QoLA Part B also showed excellent internal consistency, approached significance in its convergent association with a measure of ASD symptomatology, the Social Communication Questionnaire, and showed a moderate correlation with the VABS-II maladaptive behaviour index. Both QoLA Part A and B and the QoLA total score showed strong known-groups validity between an ASD and nonclinical cohort. Together, these results provide promising initial data on the reliability and validity of the QoLA.

Given the QoLA Part B is relatively unique in asking parents of children with ASD how much of a problem a range of ASD-specific behaviours are for the parent, locating a measure that was directly comparable for the establishment of validity was problematic. More specifically, while the SCQ enquires about ASD symptoms and the VABS-II maladaptive behaviour scale about challenging behaviours, neither specifically enquires after the parent's perceptions of how much of an issue these behaviours are to the parent. In this regard, the medium sized associations observed ($r = 0.37$) between QoLA Part B and both the SCQ and VABS-II maladaptive behaviour index do not necessarily challenge the validity of this part of the scale. Moreover, given QoLA Part B was constructed in part with reference to DSM criteria, the face validity of items and relevance to clinical practice is high. The authors would contend that QoLA Part B also offers clinical utility in identifying those families for targeted additional support where the child's ASD symptoms are perceived as highly problematic to the parent.

Table 4: Correlations between all measures in the ASD sample.

	Measure	2	3	4	5	6	7	8	9	10	11	12	13	14	15	16	17	18	19
(1)	QoLA Part A	−.07	.74**	.82**	.78**	.91**	−.49*	−.40	−.57**	.74**	.38	.26	−.12	.12	.09	.08	.10	−.02	.15
(2)	QoLA Part B	—	−.03	−.16	−.18	−.22	.19	.17	.14	.26	−.05	.22	−.37	.29	.25	−.18	.05	−.37	.23
(3)	WHO Physical		—	.63**	.69**	.75**	−.26	−.26	−.46*	.62**	.16	−.00	−.25	−.13	−.22	.23	.06	−.25	.08
(4)	WHO Psychological			—	.64**	.87**	−.45*	−.28	−.38	.52*	.26	.23	−.15	.31	.18	.33	.18	.20	.34
(5)	WHO Social				—	.72**	−.36	−.33	−.50*	.67**	.32	.21	.21	.02	−.11	−.04	.17	.07	−.02
(6)	WHO Environment					—	−.56**	−.44*	−.59**	.69**	.29	.23	−.22	.00	.14	.08	−.03	.06	.05
(7)	DASS-21: Depression						—	.66**	.81**	−.43*	−.45*	−.18	−.18	−.10	−.20	−.24	−.03	−.17	−.16
(8)	DASS-21: Anxiety							—	.73**	−.47*	−.27	−.17	−.00	.14	−.10	−.01	.15	.22	.09
(9)	DASS-21: Stress								—	−.58**	−.56**	.04	.09	.17	−.02	−.06	.13	.13	.10
(10)	PSOC: Satisfaction									—	.23	.30	−.24	.05	.12	−.07	.16	−.18	.13
(11)	PSOC: Efficacy										—	.31	.04	.25	.06	−.01	.28	.01	.19
(12)	PSOC: Interest											—	.10	.49*	.05	−.26	.26	.25	.22
(13)	SCQ Total												—	−.00	−.55**	−.44*	−.04	.29	−.33
(14)	VABS Communication													—	.39	.18	.50*	.45*	.74**
(15)	VABS Socialisation														—	.45*	.48*	−.05	.75**
(16)	VABS Daily Living															—	.42	.28	.63**
(17)	VABS Motor Skills																—	.30	.82**
(18)	VABS Maladaptive																	—	.35
(19)	VABS Adaptive Behaviour Composite																		—

Note: ** $P < .01$; * $P < .05$. QoLA: Quality of Life in Autism Questionnaire; WHO: World Health Organisation Quality of Life Questionnaire: brief version; DASS-21: Depression, Anxiety, Stress Scale 21; PSOC: Parent Sense of Competence Questionnaire; SCQ: Social Communication Questionnaire; VABS: Vineland Adaptive Behaviour Scales 2nd Edition.

Results of this study provided support to the extensive existing literature highlighting the psychosocial difficulties faced by parents of children with ASD [50] and help to extend these findings to parents of preschool aged children. Specifically, when compared to available nonclinical normative data, participants in this study showed lower QoL scores across the WHOQoL-BREF domains of Physical, Psychological, Social Relations, and Environmental QoL. In addition, mothers of children with ASD in the present sample were found to have higher depression, anxiety, and stress scores than those reported in nonclinical normative data. Interestingly, mothers of children with ASD in the current sample were found to have higher efficacy scores than those reported in Australian nonclinical normative data. The Efficacy subscale of the PSOC includes items assessing parents' perceptions of their parenting capability. It is conceivable that, due to the unique challenges associated with parenting a child with ASD and the availability of specialist assistance to parents in our cohort, some parents may develop greater confidence in their ability as parents to manage difficult situations. Replication of this finding would be necessary before firm conclusions could be drawn, however.

While the primary aim of the present study was to develop the QoLA, one unexpected set of findings generated in the conduct of the study related to the apparent lack of relationship between ASD symptomatology and measures of parental QoL and parental wellbeing. That is, there were no significant correlations between either the QoLA Part B or SCQ (i.e., measures, broadly speaking, of ASD symptomatology) and the QoLA Part A, WHOQOL-BREF, or DASS-21 subscales (i.e., measures of QoL and parental wellbeing). This may suggest that the children's ASD symptoms themselves may not necessarily be the primary factor affecting QoL and other indices of wellbeing among parents and caregivers. This finding is consistent with studies that have reported that factors outside of ASD symptom severity per se may contribute to increased psychological distress among parents of children. These factors include low levels of perceived social support [51–53] and psychological characteristics of the parent such as low perceived self-efficacy [54], external locus of control, and emotion-focused coping styles [23, 53]. This finding is also consistent with literature demonstrating that QoL among adults with ASD is not predicted by the severity of their disability but rather by the availability of social support [55].

Scores on the Environmental subscale of the WHOQOL-BREF in the present study were found to be negatively correlated with maternal depression, anxiety, and stress and positively correlated with all other domains on the WHOQOL-BREF and the QoLA Part A. This observation is consistent with research demonstrating that parents with greater perceived access to social support have lower levels of psychological distress [51–53]. Bromley et al. [51] observed that mothers were more likely to report lower levels of support if they were a lone parent, were living in poor housing, or were the mother of a boy with ASD.

It also appears that the age of the child may be an important mediator in determining parental wellbeing, with one study observing that there was greater family stress when the child with autism was an older adolescent or adult (aged 15–21.9 years) as compared to a younger adolescent (aged 10–14.9 years) [11]. In this regard, by four years of age—the approximate average age of ASD probands in the present study—a cumulative psychosocial burden may not yet have developed for some parents.

Nonetheless, numerous studies have shown that parents' level of psychological distress is associated with the severity of their child's ASD symptoms and challenging behaviours [51, 52, 56–59]. In particular, it has been shown that disruptive behaviours, fixed schedules, and difficulties for families participating in activities outside home are the main reasons for family burden [60]. Parents of children with ASD have also been found to be at increased risk of experiencing both physical and psychological distress [14, 61, 62] with the demands of caring for a child with special needs such as ASD resulting in parents having less time to meet their own needs as well as limited opportunities for participation in employment and leisure activities.

Given children in the present sample had a relatively high level of ASD symptomatology and were from a group that warranted receipt of early intensive behavioural intervention, it is also possible that a modest ceiling effect was in operation in the data for ASD symptomatology, potentially limiting variability, and experimental power for detecting effects of ASD symptoms upon wellbeing.

Limitations of the current study need to be taken into account when interpreting findings. The preliminary nature of the psychometric data given the small sample size has been noted above. Further, while the QoLA is thought to be useful for parents of children aged up to 18 years, given the present study focused upon preschool aged children, it is not yet clear whether results will generalise to cohorts with older children. Similarly, while the authors would contend that the QoLA is applicable to fathers, further research with fathers is required before this can be substantiated as the present clinical sample involved only mothers. In addition, only parent self-report measures were utilised to ascertain the child's level of autism severity and adaptive functioning, rather than a standardised observational measure of ASD diagnosis and severity. Finally, we did not directly ascertain challenging behaviours in the child or the availability of psychosocial support for the parents, factors known to impact on parental wellbeing. Future research will need to address these issues, in addition to examining the QoLA in older children as well as determining the utility of a parallel self-report version of the measure that has been designed for use amongst adolescents and adults with ASD. Further work examining the psychometric properties of the scale will also be crucial, particularly its test retest reliability and factor structure, as will additional experimental work examining the levels of agreement between parents with respect to their perceptions of their quality of life.

5. Conclusions

The present study reports on the conceptualisation and development of the QoLA. To the authors' knowledge, this is the first English-speaking measure of autism-specific QoL for parents of children with ASD that has been developed. The preliminary psychometric properties of the scale are encouraging with each of the two subscales of the QoLA showing strong internal consistency and good convergent validity. Moreover, the QoLA subscales and total score showed excellent discrimination between an ASD and control sample. Future work expanding on the psychometric properties of the QoLA would appear to be indicated, as is research more generally that examines QoL in families of young people affected by ASD.

Acknowledgments

The authors would like to acknowledge the research funding from the Australian Government (FaHCSIA) for the establishment of KU Marcia Burgess Autism Specific Early Learning and Care Centre in Liverpool, Australia, by KU Children's Services with University of New South Wales (UNSW) as research partner. The authors would like to thank the staff and families who participated in the project and in particular Kate Piromalli and Jack Lynch who assisted in setting up and collecting the data in the initial phase of the study. The authors also appreciate the helpful comments of the anonymous paper reviewers.

References

[1] American Psychiatric Association, *Diagnostic and Statistical Manual of Mental Disorders*, American Psychiatric, Arlington, Va, USA, 5th edition, 2013.

[2] M. Elsabbagh, G. Divan, Y. L. Koh et al., "Global prevalence of autism and other pervasive developmental disorders," *Autism Research*, vol. 5, no. 3, pp. 160–179, 2012.

[3] Centers for Disease Control and Prevention, "Prevalence of autism spectrum disorders—autism and developmental disabilities monitoring Network, 14 sites, United States, 2008," *MMWR Surveillance Summaries*, vol. 61, no. 3, pp. 1–19, 2012.

[4] V. Eapen, "Genetic basis of autism: is there a way forward?" *Current Opinion in Psychiatry*, vol. 24, no. 3, pp. 226–236, 2011.

[5] G. Dawson, "Early behavioral intervention, brain plasticity, and the prevention of autism spectrum disorder," *Development and Psychopathology*, vol. 20, no. 3, pp. 775–803, 2008.

[6] V. Eapen, R. Črnčec, and A. Walter, "Exploring links between genotypes, phenotypes, and clinical predictors of response to early intensive behavioral intervention in autism spectrum disorder," *Frontiers in Human Neuroscience*, vol. 7, article 567, 2013.

[7] L. Abbeduto, M. M. Seltzer, P. Shattuck et al., "Psychological well-being and coping in mothers of youths with autism, down syndrome, orfragile X syndrome," *American Journal of Mental Retardation*, vol. 109, no. 3, pp. 237–254, 2004.

[8] A. Eisenhower, B. L. Baker, and J. Blacher, "Preschool children with intellectual disability: syndrome specificity, behaviour problems, and maternal well-being," *Journal of Intellectual Disability Research*, vol. 49, no. 9, pp. 657–671, 2005.

[9] A. Estes, J. Munson, G. Dawson, E. Koehler, X.-H. Zhou, and R. Abbott, "Parenting stress and psychological functioning among mothers of preschool children with autism and developmental delay," *Autism*, vol. 13, no. 4, pp. 375–387, 2009.

[10] D. Mugno, L. Ruta, V. G. D'Arrigo, and L. Mazzone, "Impairment of quality of life in parents of children and adolescents with pervasive developmental disorder," *Health and Quality of Life Outcomes*, vol. 5, article 22, 2007.

[11] A. M. Donovan, "Family stress and ways of coping with adolescents who have handicaps: maternal perceptions," *American Journal on Mental Retardation*, vol. 92, no. 6, pp. 502–509, 1988.

[12] J. Holroyd and D. Mcarthur, "Mental retardation and stress on the parents: a contrast between down's syndrome and childhood autism," *American Journal of Mental Deficiency*, vol. 80, no. 4, pp. 431–436, 1976.

[13] L.-C. Lee, R. A. Harrington, B. B. Louie, and C. J. Newschaffer, "Children with autism: quality of life and parental concerns," *Journal of Autism and Developmental Disorders*, vol. 38, no. 6, pp. 1147–1160, 2008.

[14] R. Bouma and R. Schweitzer, "The impact of chronic childhood illness on family stress: a comparison between autism and cystic fibrosis," *Journal of Clinical Psychology*, vol. 46, no. 6, pp. 722–730, 1990.

[15] The World Health Organization Quality of Life Group, "The World Health Organization quality of life assessment (WHOQOL): position paper from the World Health Organization," *Social Science and Medicine*, vol. 41, no. 10, pp. 1403–1409, 1995.

[16] World Health Organization, WHO Constitution, Geneva, Switzerland, 1948.

[17] S. Wood-Dauphinee, "Assessing quality of life in clinical research: from where have we come and where are we going?" *Journal of Clinical Epidemiology*, vol. 52, no. 4, pp. 355–363, 1999.

[18] G. Albrecht, "Subjective health assessment," in *Measuring Health and Medical Outcomes*, C. Jenkinson, Ed., pp. 7–26, University College London, London, UK, 1994.

[19] S. King, H. Schwellnus, D. Russell, L. Shapiro, and O. Aboelele, "Assessing Quality of Life of Children and Youth with Disabilities: A Review of Available Measures," Keeping Current, 2005.

[20] R. L. Schalock, G. S. Bonham, and M. A. Verdugo, "The conceptualization and measurement of quality of life: implications for program planning and evaluation in the field of intellectual disabilities," *Evaluation and Program Planning*, vol. 31, no. 2, pp. 181–190, 2008.

[21] A. F. Burgess and S. E. Gutstein, "Quality of life for people with autism: raising the standard for evaluating successful outcomes," *Child and Adolescent Mental Health*, vol. 12, no. 2, pp. 80–86, 2007.

[22] F. Gerber, M. A. Baud, M. Giroud, and G. Galli Carminati, "Quality of life of adults with pervasive developmental disorders and intellectual disabilities," *Journal of Autism and Developmental Disorders*, vol. 38, no. 9, pp. 1654–1665, 2008.

[23] E. Cappe, M. Wolff, R. Bobet, and J.-L. Adrien, "Quality of life: a key variable to consider in the evaluation of adjustment in parents of children with autism spectrum disorders and in the development of relevant support and assistance programmes," *Quality of Life Research*, vol. 20, no. 8, pp. 1279–1294, 2011.

[24] G. Dawson, S. Rogers, J. Munson et al., "Randomized, controlled trial of an intervention for toddlers with autism: the Early Start Denver Model," *Pediatrics*, vol. 125, no. 1, pp. e17–e23, 2010.

[25] V. Eapen, R. Črnčec, and A. Walter, "Clinical outcomes of an early intervention program for preschool children with autism spectrum disorder in a community group setting," *BMC Pediatrics*, vol. 13, article 3, 2013.

[26] L. Tavernor, E. Barron, J. Rodgers, and H. Mcconachie, "Finding out what matters: validity of quality of life measurement in young people with ASD," *Child*, vol. 39, no. 4, pp. 592–601, 2013.

[27] B.-C. Shu, "Quality of life of family caregivers of children with autism: the mother's perspective," *Autism*, vol. 13, no. 1, pp. 81–91, 2009.

[28] N. Kheir, O. Ghoneim, A. L. Sandridge, M. Al-Ismail, S. Hayder, and F. Al-Rawi, "Quality of life of caregivers of children with autism in Qatar," *Autism*, vol. 16, no. 3, pp. 293–298, 2012.

[29] S. Rizk, K. Pizur-Barnekow, and A. R. Darragh, "Leisure and social participation and health-related quality of life in caregivers of children with autism," *OTJR Occupation, Participation and Health*, vol. 31, no. 4, pp. 164–171, 2011.

[30] R. Khanna, K. Jariwala, and J. P. Bentley, "Psychometric properties of the EuroQol Five Dimensional Questionnaire (EQ-5D-3L) in caregivers of autistic children," *Quality of Life Research*, vol. 22, pp. 2909–2920, 2013.

[31] S. Kose, S. Erermis, O. Ozturk et al., "Health related quality of life in children with autism spectrum disorders: the clinical and demographic related factors in Turkey," *Research in Autism Spectrum Disorders*, vol. 7, no. 2, pp. 213–220, 2013.

[32] J. Park, L. Hoffman, J. Marquis et al., "Toward assessing family outcomes of service delivery: validation of a family quality of life survey," *Journal of Intellectual Disability Research*, vol. 47, no. 4-5, pp. 367–384, 2003.

[33] E. Cappe, R. Bobet, M. P. Gattegno, A. Fernier, and J.-L. Adrien, "Effet d'un programme spécialisé pour enfants avec autisme sur la qualité de vie des parents," *Revue Québécoise de Psychologie*, vol. 30, no. 2, pp. 137–159, 2009.

[34] N. Payakachat, J. M. Tilford, E. Kovacs, and K. Kuhlthau, "Autism spectrum disorders: a review of measures for clinical, health services and cost-effectiveness applications," *Expert Review of Pharmacoeconomics & Outcomes Research*, vol. 12, no. 4, pp. 485–503, 2012.

[35] D. L. Robins, D. Fein, M. L. Barton, and J. A. Green, "The modified checklist for autism in toddlers: an initial study investigating the early detection of autism and pervasive developmental disorders," *Journal of Autism and Developmental Disorders*, vol. 31, no. 2, pp. 131–144, 2001.

[36] V. Wong, L.-H. S. Hui, W.-C. Lee et al., "A modified screening tool for autism (Checklist for Autism in Toddlers [CHAT-23]) for Chinese children," *Pediatrics*, vol. 114, no. 2, pp. e166–e176, 2004.

[37] B. Murphy, B. Murphy, H. Herrman, G. Hawthorne, T. Pinzone, and H. Evert, "The World Health Organization Quality of Life (WHOQOL) Study: Australian WHOQOL-100, WHOQOL-BREF and CA-WHOQOL instruments user's manual and interpretation guide," Melbourne: WHOQOL Field Study Centre, Department of Psychiatry, University of Melbourne and St Vincent's Mental Health Service, 2000.

[38] M. Rutter, A. Bailey, and C. Lord, *The Social Communication Questionnaire: Manual*, Western Psychological Services, 2003.

[39] S. Chandler, T. Charman, G. Baird et al., "Validation of the social communication questionnaire in a population cohort of children with autism spectrum disorders," *Journal of the American Academy of Child & Adolescent Psychiatry*, vol. 46, no. 10, pp. 1324–1332, 2007.

[40] A. V. Snow and L. Lecavalier, "Sensitivity and specificity of the modified checklist for autism in toddlers and the social communication questionnaire in preschoolers suspected of having pervasive developmental disorders," *Autism*, vol. 12, no. 6, pp. 627–644, 2008.

[41] S. Sparrow, D. Cicchetti, and D. Balla, *Vineland Adaptive Behavior Scales*, Vineland, Pearson Assessments, Livonia, Minn, USA, 2nd edition, 2005.

[42] S. Lovibond and P. F. Lovibond, *Manual For the Depression Anxiety Stress Scales*, 1995.

[43] M. M. Antony, B. J. Cox, M. W. Enns, P. J. Bieling, and R. P. Swinson, "Psychometric properties of the 42-item and 21-item versions of the depression anxiety stress scales in clinical groups and a community sample," *Psychological Assessment*, vol. 10, no. 2, pp. 176–181, 1998.

[44] J. D. Henry and J. R. Crawford, "The short-form version of the Depression Anxiety Stress Scales (DASS-21): construct validity and normative data in a large non-clinical sample," *British Journal of Clinical Psychology*, vol. 44, no. 2, pp. 227–239, 2005.

[45] C. Johnston and E. J. Mash, "A measure of parenting satisfaction and efficacy," *Journal of Clinical Child Psychology*, vol. 18, no. 2, pp. 167–175, 1989.

[46] H. Rogers and J. Matthews, "The parenting sense of competence scale: investigation of the factor structure, reliability, and validity for an Australian sample," *Australian Psychologist*, vol. 39, no. 1, pp. 88–96, 2004.

[47] B. Zablotsky, C. Anderson, and P. Law, "The association between child autism symptomatology, maternal quality of life, and risk for depression," *Journal of Autism and Developmental Disorders*, pp. 1–10, 2012.

[48] D. J. Saville, "Multiple comparison procedures: the practical solution," *The American Statistician*, vol. 44, no. 2, pp. 174–180, 1990.

[49] J. C. Nunnally and I. H. Bernstein, *Psychometric Theory*, McGraw-Hill, New York, NY, USA, 1978.

[50] B. Zablotsky, C. P. Bradshaw, and E. A. Stuart, "The association between mental health, stress, and coping supports in mothers of children with autism spectrum disorders," *Journal of Autism and Developmental Disorders*, pp. 1–14, 2012.

[51] J. Bromley, D. J. Hare, K. Davison, and E. Emerson, "Mothers supporting children with autistic spectrum disorders: social support, mental health status and satisfaction with services," *Autism*, vol. 8, no. 4, pp. 409–423, 2004.

[52] M. Stuart and J. H. McGrew, "Caregiver burden after receiving a diagnosis of an autism spectrum disorder," *Research in Autism Spectrum Disorders*, vol. 3, no. 1, pp. 86–97, 2009.

[53] M. E. Dunn, T. Burbine, C. A. Bowers, and S. Tantleff-Dunn, "Moderators of stress in parents of children with autism," *Community Mental Health Journal*, vol. 37, no. 1, pp. 39–52, 2001.

[54] R. P. Hastings and T. Brown, "Behavior problems of children with autism, parental self-efficacy, and mental health," *Journal Information*, vol. 107, no. 3, 2002.

[55] J. Renty and H. Roeyers, "Quality of life in high-functioning adults with autism spectrum disorder: the predictive value of disability and support characteristics," *Autism*, vol. 10, no. 5, pp. 511–524, 2006.

[56] H. Allik, J.-O. Larsson, and H. Smedje, "Health-related quality of life in parents of school-age children with Asperger syndrome or high-functioning autism," *Health and Quality of Life Outcomes*, vol. 4, article 1, 2006.

[57] N. O. Davis and A. S. Carter, "Parenting stress in mothers and fathers of toddlers with autism spectrum disorders: associations with child characteristics," *Journal of Autism and Developmental Disorders*, vol. 38, no. 7, pp. 1278–1291, 2008.

[58] M. M. Konstantareas and V. Papageorgiou, "Effects of temperament, symptom severity and level of functioning on maternal stress in Greek children and youth with ASD," *Autism*, vol. 10, no. 6, pp. 593–607, 2006.

[59] S. Tomanik, G. E. Harris, and J. Hawkins, "The relationship between behaviours exhibited by children with autism and maternal stress," *Journal of Intellectual and Developmental Disability*, vol. 29, no. 1, pp. 16–26, 2004.

[60] L. Fox, B. J. Vaughn, M. L. Wyatte, and G. Dunlap, "'We can't expect other people to understand': family perspectives on problem behavior," *Exceptional Children*, vol. 68, no. 4, pp. 437–450, 2002.

[61] E. Fombonne, H. Simmons, T. Ford, H. Meltzer, and R. Goodman, "Prevalence of pervasive developmental disorders in the British nationwide survey of child mental health," *Journal of the American Academy of Child & Adolescent Psychiatry*, vol. 40, no. 7, pp. 820–827, 2001.

[62] M. M. Seltzer, L. Abbeduto, M. W. Krauss, J. Greenberg, and A. Swe, "Comparison groups in autism family research: down syndrome, fragile X syndrome, and schizophrenia," *Journal of Autism and Developmental Disorders*, vol. 34, no. 1, pp. 41–48, 2004.

Permissions

All chapters in this book were first published in AR&T, by Hindawi Publishing Corporation; hereby published with permission under the Creative Commons Attribution License or equivalent. Every chapter published in this book has been scrutinized by our experts. Their significance has been extensively debated. The topics covered herein carry significant findings which will fuel the growth of the discipline. They may even be implemented as practical applications or may be referred to as a beginning point for another development.

The contributors of this book come from diverse backgrounds, making this book a truly international effort. This book will bring forth new frontiers with its revolutionizing research information and detailed analysis of the nascent developments around the world.

We would like to thank all the contributing authors for lending their expertise to make the book truly unique. They have played a crucial role in the development of this book. Without their invaluable contributions this book wouldn't have been possible. They have made vital efforts to compile up to date information on the varied aspects of this subject to make this book a valuable addition to the collection of many professionals and students.

This book was conceptualized with the vision of imparting up-to-date information and advanced data in this field. To ensure the same, a matchless editorial board was set up. Every individual on the board went through rigorous rounds of assessment to prove their worth. After which they invested a large part of their time researching and compiling the most relevant data for our readers.

The editorial board has been involved in producing this book since its inception. They have spent rigorous hours researching and exploring the diverse topics which have resulted in the successful publishing of this book. They have passed on their knowledge of decades through this book. To expedite this challenging task, the publisher supported the team at every step. A small team of assistant editors was also appointed to further simplify the editing procedure and attain best results for the readers.

Apart from the editorial board, the designing team has also invested a significant amount of their time in understanding the subject and creating the most relevant covers. They scrutinized every image to scout for the most suitable representation of the subject and create an appropriate cover for the book.

The publishing team has been an ardent support to the editorial, designing and production team. Their endless efforts to recruit the best for this project, has resulted in the accomplishment of this book. They are a veteran in the field of academics and their pool of knowledge is as vast as their experience in printing. Their expertise and guidance has proved useful at every step. Their uncompromising quality standards have made this book an exceptional effort. Their encouragement from time to time has been an inspiration for everyone.

The publisher and the editorial board hope that this book will prove to be a valuable piece of knowledge for researchers, students, practitioners and scholars across the globe.

List of Contributors

Miguel Ángel Romero-Munguía
Outpatient Service, "Dr. Samuel Ram´ırez Moreno" Psychiatric Hospital, Health Secretariat, Autopista M´exico-Puebla Km 5.5 Santa Catarina, Tl´ahuac, 13100 Mexico, DF, Mexico

Jay R. Lucker
Howard University, Washington, DC, USA

Alex Doman
Advanced Brain Technologies, Ogden, UT, USA

Kris Evers and Johan Wagemans
Laboratory of Experimental Psychology, KU Leuven, Tiensestraat 102, 3000 Leuven, Bel-gium

Kris Evers and Jean Steyaert
Department of Child Psychiatry, UPC-KU Leuven, 3000 Leuven, Belgium

Kris Evers, Jean Steyaert, Ilse Noens and Johan Wagemans
Leuven Autism Research (LAuRes), KU Leuven, 3000 Leuven, Belgium

Inneke Kerkhof
Quantitative Psychology and Individual Differences, KU Leuven, 3000 Leuven, Belgium

Jean Steyaert
Department of Clinical Genetics, University Hospital Maastricht, 6200 Maastricht,The Netherlands

Ilse Noens
Parenting and Special Education Research Unit, KU Leuven, 3000 Leuven, Belgium
Psychiatric and Neurodevelopmental Genetics Unit, Massachusetts General Hospital, MA, Boston, USA

Grace T. Baranek, Linda R. Watson, Lauren Turner-Brown, Samuel H. Field, Elizabeth R. Crais, Linn Wakeford, Lauren M. Little and J. Steven Reznick
University of North Carolina at Chapel Hill, Chapel Hill, NC 27599-7122, USA

T. May
Deakin Child Study Centre, Deakin University, Melbourne Burwood Campus, 221 Burwood Highway, Burwood, VIC 3125, Australia

K. Cornish
School of Psychological Sciences and Monash Institute for Brain Development and Repair, Monash University, Clayton Campus, Building 17,Wellington Road, Clayton, VIC 3800, Australia

N. J. Rinehart
Deakin Child Study Centre, School of Psychology, Deakin University, Melbourne Burwood Campus, 221 Burwood Highway, Burwood, VIC 3125, Australia

Greet Lambrechts, Jarymke Maljaars, Hannah Boonen, Lotte van Esch, Karla Van Leeuwen and Ilse Noens
Parenting and Special Education Research Unit, University of Leuven (KU Leuven), Leopold Vanderkelenstraat 32, 3000 Leuven, Belgium

Greet Lambrechts, Jarymke Maljaars, Hannah Boonen, Lotte van Esch and Ilse Noens
Leuven Autism Research (LAuRes), University of Leuven (KU Leuven), 3000 Leuven, Belgium

Louisa M. T. Silva and Kristen R. Gabrielsen
Teaching Research Institute, Western Oregon University, McMinnville, OR 97128, USA

Mark Schalock
Teaching Research Institute, Western Oregon University, 345 N. Monmouth Avenue, Monmouth, OR 97361, USA

Manabu Oi and Sanae Tanaka
Research Center for Child Mental Development, United Graduate School of Child Development, Kanazawa University, B-b43, 13-1 Takaramachi, Kanazawa 920-8640, Japan

Harue Ohoka
Nihon Fukushi University Chuo College of Social Services, 3-27-11 Chiyoda, Naka-ku, Nagoya 460-0012, Japan

Elena Patten
Department of Communication Sciences and Disorders,The University of North Carolina, Greensboro, 300 Ferguson Building, Greensboro, NC 27412, USA

Karla K. Ausderau
The University ofWisconsin-Madison, 3195 Medical Sciences Center, 1300 University Avenue, Madison, WI 53706, USA

Linda R. Watson
Division of Speech and Hearing Sciences, The University of North Carolina at Chapel Hill, CB No. 7190 Chapel Hill, NC 27599, USA

Grace T. Baranek
Division of Occupational Science and Occupational Therapy,The University of North Carolina at Chapel Hill, CB No. 7122 Chapel Hill, NC 27599, USA

Deirdre Kindregan and John Gormley
Discipline of Physiotherapy, School of Medicine, Trinity College Dublin, Dublin, Ireland

Louise Gallagher
Discipline of Psychiatry, School of Medicine, Trinity College Dublin, Dublin, Ireland

Irina Manouilenko, Jonna M. Eriksson and Susanne Bejerot
Department of Clinical Neuroscience, Karolinska Institutet, Stockholm, Sweden

Irina Manouilenko
Järva Psychiatric Outpatient Clinic, Rinkebysvängen 70A, 4tr, 163 74 Spånga, Sweden

Mats B. Humble
School of Health and Medical Sciences, Psychiatric Research Center, Örebro University, Örebro, Sweden

Dina Tell
Department of Health Promotion, Loyola University Chicago, Marcella Niehoff School of Nursing, 2160 S. First Avenue, Maywood, IL 60153, USA

Denise Davidson
Department of Psychology, Loyola University Chicago, 1032W. Sheridan Road, Chicago, IL 60660,USA

Linda A. Camras
Department of Psychology, DePaul University, 2219 N. Kenmore Avenue, Chicago, IL 60614, USA

Stephen J. Sheinkopf, Todd P. Levine, Cynthia Miller-Loncar and Barry Lester
Department of Psychiatry and Human Behavior,Warren Alpert Medical School of Brown University, Providence, RI 02912, USA
Brown Center for the Study of Children at Risk,Women and Infants Hospital, 101 Dudley Street, Providence, RI 02905, USA

Stephen J. Sheinkopf, Cynthia Miller-Loncar and Barry Lester
Department of Pediatrics,Warren Alpert Medical School of Brown University, Providence, RI 02912, USA

A. Rebecca Neal-Beevers
Department of Psychology, University of Texas at Austin, 108 E. Dean Keeton Street, Austin, TX 78712, USA

Muhammad Mustafa Arif, Ayesha Niazy, Bilal Hassan and Farah Ahmed
Department of Community Health Sciences, Ziauddin University, 4/B, Shahrah-e-Ghalib, Block 6, Clifton, Karachi 75600, Pakistan

Paul T. Shattuck and Anne M. Roux
A. J. Drexel Autism Institute, Drexel University, 3020 Market Street, Suite 560, Philadelphia, PA 19104, USA

Benjamin P. Cooper
Washington University, One Brookings Drive, St. Louis, MO 63130, USA

Jennifer Yu, Xin Wei and Lynn Newman
SRI International, 333 Ravenswood Avenue, BS169, Menlo Park, CA 94025-3493, USA

Elena Patten
Department of Audiology and Speech Pathology, University of Tennessee Health Science Center, 434 South Stadium Hall, Knoxville, TN 37996, USA

Linda R. Watson
Division of Speech and Hearing Sciences, CB No. 7190, University of North Carolina at Chapel Hill, Chapel Hill, NC 27599, USA

Grace T. Baranek
Division of Occupational Sciences, CB No. 7122, University of North Carolina at Chapel Hill, Chapel Hill, NC 27599, USA

M. Mackus, D. de Kruijff, L. S. Otten, A. D. Kraneveld, J. Garssen and J. C. Verster
Division of Pharmacology, Utrecht University, Utrecht, Netherlands

A. D. Kraneveld and J. C. Verster
Institute for Risk Assessment Sciences (IRAS), Utrecht University, Utrecht, Netherlands

J. Garssen
Nutricia Research, Utrecht, Netherlands

J. C. Verster
Centre for Human Psychopharmacology, Swinburne University, Melbourne, VIC, Australia

Jenna Mendelson
Department of Psychology,The University of North Carolina at Greensboro, Greensboro, NC, USA

Yasmine White and Geraldine Dawson
Department of Psychiatry and Behavioral Sciences, Duke University, Durham, NC, USA

Laura Hans, Richard Adebari, Lorrie Schmid, Ali Goldsmith, Burcu Ozler, Kristen Buehne, Sarah Jones and Jennifer Shapleton
Education and Human Development Incubator and Social Science Research Institute, Duke University, Durham, NC, USA

Jan Riggsbee
Program in Education, Duke University, Durham, NC, USA

Giorgio Pini, Laura Congiu, Alberto Benincasa, Pietro DiMarco, Stefania Bigoni and Daniela Tropea
Tuscany Rett Center, Ospedale Versilia, 55043 Lido di Camaiore, Italy

Adam H. Dyer, Sean O'Leary and Rachel McNamara
School of Medicine, Trinity College Dublin, College Green, Dublin 2, Ireland

Niall Mortimer and Kevin J.Mitchell
Department of Genetics, Trinity College Dublin, College Green, Dublin 2, Ireland

Andrea Della-Chiesa
Trinity College Institute of Neuroscience, College Green, Dublin 2, Ireland

Michael Gill and Daniela Tropea
Department of Psychiatry, Trinity College Dublin, College Green, Dublin 2, Ireland

Daniela Tropea
Neuropsychiatric Genetics, Trinity Centre for Health Sciences, St. James Hospital, Dublin 8, Ireland

Ann M. Sam, Yi Pan, Kara Hume and Samuel L. Odom
Frank Porter Graham Child Development Institute, University of North Carolina, Chapel Hill, 517 S. Greensboro Road, Carrboro, NC 27510, USA

Stephanie S. Reszka and Brian A. Boyd,
Department of Allied Health, University of North Carolina, Chapel Hill, NC 27599, USA

Tawny Tsang
Department of Psychology, University of California, Los Angeles, CA 90024, USA

Kristen Gillespie-Lynch
Department of Psychology, College of Staten Island andThe Graduate Center, CUNY, New York, NY 10314, USA

Ted Hutman
Department of Psychiatry and Bio-Behavioral Sciences, David Geffen School of Medicine at UCLA, University of California, Los Angeles, CA 90024, USA

Kavita Ruparelia
Open University, Milton Keynes, UK

Kavita Ruparelia and Karim Manji
Department of Pediatrics and Child Health, Muhimbili University of Health and Allied Sciences, Dar es Salaam, Tanzania

Amina Abubakar
KEMRI-Wellcome Trust Research Programme, Centre for Geographic Medicine Research (Coast), Kilifi, Kenya

Charles R. Newton
Department of Psychiatry, University of Oxford, Oxford, UK

Shylaja Srinivasan and Madhusmita Misra
Pediatric Endocrinology, Massachusetts General Hospital and Harvard Medical School, Boston, MA, USA

Julia O'Rourke, Sara Bersche Golas and Ann Neumeyer
Lurie Center for Autism, Massachusetts General Hospital for Children, Boston, MA, USA

Sara Bersche Golas and Ann Neumeyer
Pediatric Neurology, Massachusetts General Hospital and Harvard Medical School, Boston, MA, USA

Laura J. Raymond and V. C. Ralston
Energy and Environmental Research Center, University of North Dakota, 15 North 23rd Street, Stop 9018, Grand Forks, ND 58202, USA

Richard C. Deth
Department of Pharmaceutical Sciences, Northeastern University, Boston, MA 02115, USA

Mitsuhiko Ishikawa and Shoji Itakura
Graduate School of Letters, Kyoto University, Kyoto, Japan

Hiroki C. Tanabe
Graduate School of Environmental Studies, Nagoya University, Nagoya, Japan

Aaron Blocher-Rubin
Arizona Autism United, 5025 E.Washington St. #212, Phoenix, AZ 85034, USA

Paige Krabill
Capella University, Minneapolis, MN, USA

Kiley Tyler and Megan MacDonald
College of Public Health andHuman Sciences,Oregon State University, Corvallis,OR 97331,USA

Kristi Menea
School of Education, University of Alabama at Birmingham, Birmingham, AL 35294, USA

Elizabeth C. Bacon, Sarah Dufek and Laura Schreibman
Department of Psychology, University of California, San Diego, 9500 Gilman Drive, La Jolla, CA 92093-0109, USA

Sarah Dufek
Department of Psychiatry,Weill Cornell Medical College, 21 Bloomingdale Road, Rogers Building, White Plains, NY 10605, USA

Aubyn C. Stahmer
Department of Psychiatry, University of California, San Diego, 9500 Gilman Drive, La Jolla, CA 92093, USA
Child and Adolescent Services Research Center and Autism Discovery Institute, Rady Children's Hospital San Diego, 3020 Children'sWay, San Diego, CA 92123, USA

Karen Pierce and and Eric Courchesne
Department of Neurosciences, University of California, San Diego, 9500 Gilman Drive, La Jolla, CA 92093, USA

R. Deonandan and A. T. M. Konkle
Interdisciplinary School of Health Sciences, Faculty of Health Sciences, University of Ottawa, 25 University Private, THN 208, Ottawa,ON, Canada K1N6N5

E. Y. Liu
Department of Public Health Sciences, Queen's University, Kingston, ON, Canada K7L 3N6

B. Kolisnyk
Neuroscience, Schulich School of Medicine and Dentistry, University ofWestern Ontario, London, ON, Canada N6A 5B7

A. T. M. Konkle
School of Psychology, Faculty of Social Sciences, University of Ottawa, Ottawa, ON, Canada K1N 6N5

Valsamma Eapen, Rudi Hrnlec and Amelia Walter
Academic Unit of Child Psychiatry, SouthWestern Sydney Local Health District (AUCS), Liverpool Hospital, Mental Health Centre (Level 1: ICAMHS), Locked Bag 7103, Liverpool BC, NSW1871, Australia

Valsamma Eapen, Rudi Črnčec, Amelia Walter and and Kwok Ping Tay
University of New SouthWales, Sydney, NSW2052, Australia

Index